ADA®/PDR®

MEDICATIONS FOR THE TREATMENT OF DIABETES

John R. White, Jr., PharmD, PA
Professor of Pharmacotherapy
College of Pharmacy
Washington State University
Spokane, WA

R. Keith Campbell, PharmB, MBA, CDE
Distinguished Pr...
College of Phar...
Washington Sta...
Pullman, WA

D1212195

ADA®/PDR® Medications for the Treatment of Diabetes

Senior Director, Editorial & Publishing: Bette LaGow
Manager, Clinical Services: Nermin Shenouda, PharmD
Drug Information Specialists: Anila Patel, PharmD; Christine Sunwoo, PharmD;
  Greg Tallis, RPh
Contributing Clinical Editors: Michael DeLuca, PharmD, MBA; Majid Kerolous, PharmD
Manager, Editorial Services: Lori Murray
Project Editors: Sabina Borza, Kathleen Engel
Associate Editor: Jennifer Reed
Senior Director, Client Services: Stephanie Struble
Project Manager: Christina Klinger
Manager, Production Purchasing: Thomas Westburgh
Manager, Art Department: Livio Udina
Electronic Publishing Designers: Deana DiVizio, Carrie Faeth

Senior Director, Copy Sales: Bill Gaffney
Senior Product Manager: Richard Buchwald

PHYSICIANS' DESK REFERENCE
Executive Vice President, PDR: Thomas F. Rice
Vice President, Product Management: Cy Caine
Vice President, Publishing & Operations: Valerie Berger
Vice President, Pharmaceutical Sales: Anthony Sorce
Vice President, Clinical Relations: Mukesh Mehta, RPh
Vice President, Strategy & Business Development: Ray Zoeller
Vice President, Manufacturing & Vendor Management: Brian Holland

Copyright © 2008 and published by the Healthcare business of Thomson Reuters at Montvale, NJ 07645-1725. All rights reserved. None of the content of this publication may be reproduced, stored in a retrieval system, resold, redistributed, or transmitted in any form or by any means (electronic, mechanical, photocopying, recording, or otherwise) without the prior written permission of the publisher. Physicians' Desk Reference® and PDR® are registered trademarks of Thomson Reuters.

ADA® and the American Diabetes Association® are registered trademarks of the American Diabetes Association, Inc.

American Diabetes Association
1701 North Beauregard Street
Alexandria, VA 22311
1-800-DIABETES
www.diabetes.org

Thomson Reuters, Healthcare
Physicians' Desk Reference
5 Paragon Drive
Montvale, NJ 07645
800-232-7379
www.thomsonreuters.com

Officers of the Healthcare business of Thomson Reuters: *President & Chief Executive Officer,* Mike Boswood; *Senior Vice President & Chief Technology Officer,* Frank Licata; *Chief Strategy Officer,* Courtney Morris; *Executive Vice President, Payer Decision Support,* Jon Newpol; *Executive Vice President, Provider Management Decision Support,* Terry Cameron; *Executive Vice President, Provider Clinical Decision Support,* Thomas Hegelund; *Executive Vice President, PDR,* Tom Rice; *Executive Vice President, Marketing & Innovation,* Doug Schneider; *Senior Vice President, Finance,* Phil Buckingham; *General Counsel,* Darren Pocsik

ISBN: 978-1-56363-734-6   Printed in the United States

Table of Contents

Introduction

Diabetes is a fascinating, yet devastating disorder that is exploding in incidence and continues to be a major cause of morbidity and mortality throughout the world. In the past 15 years, our understanding of hyperglycemia and its causes and consequences has grown dramatically but with the realization that there is still much to learn. The management of diabetes has been vigorously expanded from trying to just lower blood glucose to also normalizing blood lipids, blood pressure, coagulation and inflammatory factors. We know that diabetes equals cardiovascular disease, and all aspects of cardiovascular disease prevention need attention. New treatments for diabetes complications have been approved, and new devices and treatments are being announced on a weekly basis to help health care providers (HCPs) and patients more easily achieve target levels.

Our appreciation of the complexity of diabetes and the efforts that people with diabetes need to undertake each day to try to reach near-normal blood glucose levels is at an all-time high. The basic formula to achieve treatment objectives has been known for a long time, however. Patients need to be empowered through education and motivation to follow a daily treatment program that includes nutrition, exercise, drug therapy, education, and self-monitoring. It is essential that the patient and the HCP understand and use each step in the treatment program to manage blood glucose, blood lipids, blood pressure and other factors to slow the development of diabetes complications. Fortunately we now have a sophisticated group of new and old medications that can be used alone or in combination that impact various organ systems to near normalize blood glucose levels. It is known that the most clinically and cost-effective way to manage diabetes is through the use of medication intervention by well-informed patients and HCPs.

In the past 13 years, the tool chest of medications has grown significantly to treat elevated blood glucose, lipids, and pressure. For blood glucose, we have progressed from just insulin and sulfonylureas to new and more sophisticated medications that reduce the liver's release of glucose; slow the absorption of carbohydrates; improve insulin sensitivity and decrease insulin resistance; diminish the effect of glucagon; and promote the timely release of insulin from the pancreas. We also have better choices of medications and studies that have proved that certain new classes of medications to treat high cholesterol and triglycerides work and lower cardiovascular risk. The same is true of medications to lower blood pressure and protect the kidneys. New medications have also been approved to treat diabetes complications. It is critical to remember that these medications are always most successful when used in combination with nutrition, exercise, and self-monitoring in an empowered patient who takes charge of his/her diabetes management.

The *ADA/PDR Medications for the Treatment of Diabetes* was specifically written to provide physicians, nurses, nurse practitioners, pharmacists, physician assistants, dietitians, other HCPs and motivated patients with an in-depth but easy-to-use summary of the medications used to treat both type 1 and type 2 diabetes patients as well as patients with complications of diabetes. The book is written in a manner that allows you to read background information that explains how and why a medication can assist in caring for your patient. Easy-to-use tables provide you with the ability to look up information in a quick manner. Each class of drugs presently used to manage blood glucose is covered, as well as medications for dyslipidemias, hypertension, and other commonly encountered problems. Information is also covered concerning the treatment of specific diabetes complications. A chapter that provides a glimpse into the future types of medications in development is also presented.

The editors and authors plus the American Diabetes Association and Thomson Reuters believe that you will find this book of great value in understanding and using medications to improve the care of your patients with diabetes.

How to Use This Book

This new edition of the *ADA®/PDR® Medications for the Treatment of Diabetes* marks the collaboration of the American Diabetes Association® and *Physicians' Desk Reference®*, making it one of the most comprehensive drug references of its kind—the only one authoritative enough to bear the ADA name.

The chapters are organized into four sections according to therapeutic area: drugs used to manage hyperglycemia; management of macrovascular disease; management of microvascular disease and other comorbidities; and future medications. Within each chapter, the information is arranged to allow easy reference to the specific area of interest:

An overview appears first, with each topic researched and written by clinicians affiliated with the American Diabetes Association. Chapters are organized by drug or therapeutic class and include:

- Pharmacology, including mechanism of action and pharmacokinetics
- Treatment advantages and disadvantages
- Therapeutic considerations, such as contraindications and precautions, adverse effects and monitoring, and special populations (eg, hepatic or renal impairment, pregnancy, and pediatrics)
- Drug interactions
- Dosage and administration
- Suggested references and further reading

Drug tables containing prescribing and interactions information are found at the end of the overview section, as applicable. The tables were created by a staff of experienced pharmacists at *PDR* and contain concise drug entries, organized alphabetically by therapeutic class and generic drug name. **A key to the abbreviations used in these tables appears on page xv.** Prescribing tables are shown first and give pertinent details on the following:

- *Generic name:* Listed in bold, with brand names appearing in parentheses, when available.
- *Drug forms and strengths:* Indicates whether the drug comes as a tablet, capsule, injection, etc. Scored tablets are noted with an asterisk.
- *Dosage:* Highlights adult and pediatric dosages in bold italics. Dosages are arranged according to each drug's indication, shown in bold type. When available, special dosing considerations—maximum dose, titration, dosage reductions for special patient groups—are also provided.
- *Warnings/precautions and contraindications:* Lists any black box warnings and other crucial warnings and precautions first (denoted with **BB** or **W/P**), followed by contraindications (denoted with **Contra**) and pregnancy/nursing information (denoted with **P/N**). Pregnancy categories are defined at the end of this section.

- *Adverse effects:* Lists serious and most common side effects occurring in ≥3% of patients as noted in the manufacturer's product labeling.

Tables with drug interactions appear after the prescribing information. These are also organized alphabetically by therapeutic class and generic name. Please keep in mind that only common and dangerous adverse reactions and interactions are included here, and that numerous less-prevalent adverse effects may be reported in the complete labeling. In addition, the chance of an interaction varies among patients, and previously undocumented drug interactions are always a possibility.

The drug information in both types of tables contains FDA-approved product labeling as published in the *Physicians' Desk Reference* or supplied by the manufacturer. This information is drawn from the *PDR* database, which is compiled and updated on a regular basis by a staff of experienced pharmacists. While diligent efforts have been made to ensure the accuracy of each drug entry, it is essential to bear in mind that the information presented here is merely a synopsis of key points in the official labeling, and that the complete labeling contains additional precautionary information that may be of significance in specific cases. If an entry leaves any question unanswered, be sure to consult *Physicians' Desk Reference* or the manufacturer for additional information.

ADA Guidelines—including position statements and clinical practice recommendations—appear after the drug tables, when available. These cover not only the treatment of type 2 diabetes but also the management of comorbidities associated with this disease.

Definitions for the ADA evidence-grading system used in these guidelines are shown at the end of this section.

Important note about the information in this book

The American Diabetes Association (ADA), *Physicians' Desk Reference* (PDR), Thomson Reuters, and the authors and contributors of the *ADA/PDR Medications for the Treatment of Diabetes* have used care to confirm that the drugs and treatment schedules set forth in this book are in accordance with current recommendations and practice at the time of publication. The suggestions and information contained herein are generally consistent with the Clinical Practice Recommendations and other policies of the ADA, but they do not represent the policy or position of the Association or any of its boards or committees. Reasonable steps have been taken to ensure the accuracy of the information presented. However, the ADA and Thomson Reuters cannot ensure the safety or efficacy of any product or service described in this publication. Individuals are advised to consult a physician or other appropriate healthcare professional before undertaking any diet or exercise program or taking any medication referred to in this publication. Professionals must use and apply their own professional judgment, experience, and training and should not rely solely on the information contained in this publication before prescribing any diet, exercise program, or medication. The ADA—its officers, directors, employees, volunteers, and members—and Thomson Reuters assume no responsibility or liability for personal or other injury, loss, or damage that may result from the suggestions or information in this publication.

Chapter 1

Management Strategies for Patients with Type 1 Diabetes

R. Keith Campbell, PharmB, MBA, CDE
Joshua J. Neumiller, PharmD, CGP, FASCP

INTRODUCTION

Insulin therapy is a medical necessity for all patients with type 1 diabetes. Because of this fact, type 1 diabetes was historically termed insulin-dependent diabetes mellitus. Type 1 diabetes results from the inability of the β-cell of the pancreas to secrete insulin when blood glucose levels are increasing. The onset of the condition is usually rapid and occurs primarily in children, adolescents, and young adults; but can occur in patients at any age. Because of the high incidence in children it was formerly called juvenile-onset diabetes.

Since insulin is a protein and would be digested if administered orally, insulin has traditionally been administered via subcutaneous injections. Understanding proper use and administration of insulin is vital to patients, their families, and health care practitioners. It is important to note that insulin is also often used in type 2 diabetes to achieve treatment objectives.

Insulin has essentially unlimited power to reduce plasma glucose levels. Insulin both increases glucose uptake by adipose and muscle tissues, and suppresses hepatic glucose release. The primary limitation to its usefulness as a diabetes drug is hypoglycemia. In addition, insulin use often leads to weight gain, a negative effect for the commonly overweight or obese type 2 diabetes patient. Insulin has proven to be the most clinically and cost-effective treatment to normalize blood glucose levels. There are many common challenges involved in prescribing insulin—from choosing insulin regimens, to dealing with patient reluctance to start insulin therapy, to minimizing the hypoglycemia and weight gain that often accompanies improved glycemic control.

Until the late 1970s, most patients requiring insulin were prescribed one or two injections of insulin each day. This lowered the number of injections the patient had to administer but did not provide a normal physiological replacement of insulin. Without good management of blood glucose levels, the development of diabetes microvascular complications was rampant. In an attempt to simulate how insulin is released in people without diabetes, the concept of basal/bolus insulin administration emerged. In the basal/bolus concept, a long-acting insulin is administered that mimics the basal insulin release of nondiabetic individuals where approximately one unit of insulin is secreted every hour to handle the non-fed insulin needs of the liver and muscle cells. Short- or rapid-acting insulin is also administered in conjunction with the ingestion of carbohydrates (approximately 1 unit for every 10 g of carbohydrate) that simulates the rapid release of insulin (bolus) that typically occurs in the fed state. Thus by giving patients a long-acting insulin once or twice a day and then an injection of rapid-acting insulin with meals, a much better and more physiologically normal management of blood glucose occurs. Both long- and rapid-acting insulins were developed in unlimited supplies via recombinant technology that allowed a more efficient ability to copy the basal/bolus concept of insulin replacement in diabetes patients requiring insulin (all type 1 and many type 2). Rapid-acting and longer-acting insulin analogs were also developed that made the use of the basal/bolus insulin regimen easier and more effective.

Please be aware that there are no standards for how to best use insulin therapy. Every patient is unique, and the insulin regimen must be individualized. Self-monitoring of blood glucose (SMBG) and the utilization of proven titration strategies will allow for optimal insulin therapies and outcomes. Choosing an initial insulin dose and making adjustments dependent upon blood glucose measurements allows the patient to achieve excellent blood glucose management and minimize problems.

It is also known that diabetes patients who do not secrete and receive insulin from an injection do not secrete a hormone called amylin. A molecule of amylin is secreted with each secreted molecule of insulin. It turns out that amylin has a significant impact on the body and when an agonist of amylin called pramlintide was developed and injected with meals, blood glucose levels improved, people were able to decrease their insulin doses, and weight gain was avoided or minimized. Thus the two general classes of drugs used to treat type 1 diabetes are insulins and amylin agonists. As of mid 2008, the medical community has not yet embraced the wide spread use of pramlintide, possibly due to the fact that most people require three injections of pramlintide daily, and it can cause noticeable nausea.

Pramlintide use has been shown to result in significant weight loss in patients with type 1 diabetes who have gained considerable weight and is now available in an easy-to-use pen device. See Chapter 12 for more detailed information on this drug.

It should be noted that one barrier to insulin use in type 2 diabetes patients is physician and patient reluctance to injections. This is due in large part to concerns about a prospective patient's unwillingness to self-administer injections and/or the fear of low blood glucose levels. It must be emphasized that insulin can be effectively and safely used, and the HCP who gives positive support to the patient using insulin can help ensure optimal management of blood glucose. It is important to consider the needs of the individual when deciding the best mode of administration to minimize concerns regarding self-administration. Options of administering insulin include insulin pens, insulin pumps, and the old standby of using insulin from a vial with an insulin syringe and needle. Insulin pens and pumps can often help people overcome the fear and anxiety associated with self-injection.

PATIENT SELECTION

Insulin therapy is required for **all patients with type 1 diabetes** and is appropriate for many type 2 diabetes patients.

The absolute insulin deficiency of established type 1 diabetes can most effectively be treated with multiple daily insulin injections (basal/bolus concept), continuous subcutaneous insulin infusion (the insulin pump). An inhaled, dry-powdered insulin formulation was approved by the FDA but was not well accepted by physicians or patients and has been voluntarily removed from the market by the manufacturer due to disappointing sales. The Mannkind Corporation has a pulmonary insulin in development and insulin that is sprayed into the mouth called OraLyn is being evaluated and will be discussed in Chapter 21 on future medications to treat diabetes.

It is important to stress that the insulin requirements of each patient may differ significantly. Basic guidelines based on the weight of the patient, the patient's age, and the patient's blood glucose readings can be used to try to determine the amount of insulin that should be injected for a total daily insulin dose. Tremendous variability in the recommended amount of insulin can range from 0.2 unit/kg/day in a child to up to several units/kg/day depending on the patient's degree of insulin resistance and other factors. Many diabetes centers begin adult patients on 0.5 unit/kg/day. This rough estimate calculation can then be divided into what amount is given as a long-acting (basal) dose and what should be given as a bolus before or with each meal. The process is almost always a trial and error approach that has been greatly enhanced by the ability of the patient to utilize SMBG. By testing, keeping track of blood glucose levels throughout the various times of the day, and knowing the impact of a unit of insulin for both basal and bolus needs, a determination can be made as to the patient's degree of insulin resistance. The basal insulin dose can be fine-tuned as well as the amount of insulin required with each meal to cover carbohydrates consumed. This process is often called "pattern management" of insulin since the SMBG records are evaluated and insulin doses fine-tuned based on consistently high or low readings at various times of the day. In recent years, a strong emphasis on measuring and managing after meal (postprandial) blood glucose levels has occurred. Near normalizing blood glucose requires a well educated and motivated patient who takes charge of his/her condition. **Therefore, it is critical that patients are empowered to manage their own insulin needs and perform injections related to blood glucose levels,** **consumption of carbohydrates, and type and duration of exercise.** Time spent with a registered dietitian is time well spent in assisting the patient to count carbohydrates. Record keeping allows an analysis of how well blood glucose levels are being managed before and after meals and at other times during the day. Dose adjustments based on blood glucose records make it easier to fine tune the insulin doses and achieve target blood glucose levels. Patients are also taught to take correction doses of insulin to bring blood glucose levels to near normal if they are too high.

TREATMENT GUIDELINES FOR TYPE 1 DIABETES

Health care practitioners who follow the ADA's Standards of Diabetes Care for their patients ensure improved outcomes of care. Patients who fine-tune their insulin regimens and, if necessary, add pramlintide not only can achieve target blood glucose levels but also live healthy, relatively normal lives. These patients also lessen the chance of developing both microvascular and macrovascular blood vessel disease. It is important to have an awareness of the Standards of Diabetes Care and to make sure that patients meet with their practitioner several times a year to:
- have their eyes, ears, feet, teeth, and gums checked
- receive flu and pneumovax vaccinations on schedule
- practice SMBG and keep records
- normalize blood pressure and blood lipids
- take an aspirin daily, if indicated
- receive HbA_{1c} testing several times per year

SUGGESTED READING

Bangstad HJ, Danne T, Deeb LC, et al. ISPAD clinical practice consensus guidelines 2006-2007. *Pediatric Diabetes*. 2007;8:88-102.

Bode B. *Medical Management of Type 1 Diabetes, 4th Edition*. American Diabetes Association. Alexandria, VA; 2003.

Oiknine R, Bernbaum M, Mooradian AD. A critical appraisal of the role of insulin analogues in the management of diabetes mellitus. *Drugs*. 2005;65(3):325-340.

Campbell RK. *Practical Insulin, 2nd Edition*. American Diabetes Association. Alexandria, VA; 2007.

Ryan GJ, Jobe LJ, Martin R. Pramlintide in the treatment of type 1 and type 2 diabetes mellitus. *Clin Ther*. 2005;27(10):1500-1512.

Walsh J, Roberts R, Varma C, et al. *Using Insulin*. San Diego: Torrey Pines Press; 2003.

Wolpert H. *Smart Pumping: A Practical Approach to Mastering the Insulin Pump*. American Diabetes Association. Alexandria, VA; 2002.

Chapter 2

Overview of Medications Used to Treat Type 2 Diabetes

John R. White, Jr., PharmD, PA
R. Keith Campbell, PharmB, MBA, CDE

INTRODUCTION

The options available to clinicians in the U.S. for the management of hyperglycemia secondary to type 2 diabetes have changed dramatically in the past two decades. Currently there are nine categories of medications that may be used in the management of diabetes, including insulins, sulfonylureas, thiazolidinediones, glinides, biguanides, amylin derivatives, gliptins (DPP-4 inhibitors), α-glucosidase inhibitors, bile-acid sequestrants, and GLP analogues. The efficacy associated with various permutations of multiple drug combinations continues to be evaluated as newer agents are released. The selection of the best medication or combinations of medications for the management of hyperglycemia in patients with type 2 diabetes, while based in science, remains to a large degree in the realm of "art." Although in some situations the choice of medication is relatively simple, in the majority of situations the decision-making process is complex and does not necessarily lead to a clear-cut choice. While algorithms can sometimes provide an overall framework through which decisions can be made, they often ignore pertinent patient specific characteristics, and are not powerful enough to provide specific recommendations for the best medications the multitude of complex situations often encountered in clinical practice.

Hopefully, as more is learned about the natural history of diabetes and the pharmacology of the medications used to manage it, the rationale behind medication choice will become more straightforward.

Several factors should be considered when choosing a medication, including degree of glycemic lowering needed to get the patient into target goal ranges, ease of compliance, effect of the medication on lipid profiles, contraindications, side effects, cost and patient insurance coverage, and potential level of adherence of the patient to the regimen. This chapter will briefly review the use of the above-mentioned categories of medications and will include brief discussions of mechanisms of action, efficacy, effects of the medications on lipid profiles, common side effects, contraindications for use of the medications, and patient adherence to the regimens. **Tables 2.1** and **2.2** provide an overview of usual costs, pro/cons, and a suggested overall ranking of each category of medication. **Table 2.3** provides a more detailed list of potential considerations to consider when prescribing a particular antihyperglycemic medication. All tables appear at the end of this chapter.

This chapter also suggests a ranking of medications based on where they might best be positioned in order of use. This type of ranking is fraught with problems, since it can not be designed with all patients in mind. The suggested ranking in this chapter is based on a "typical patient with type 2." Clearly, these rankings are not appropriate in all cases but will hopefully provide a starting point for consideration and discussion. **More detailed information regarding specific medications is provided in chapters 3 through 12.**

SULFONYLUREAS

Sulfonylureas (SUs) have been widely used in the management of type 2 diabetes since their introduction in the late 1950s. In the past it was estimated that 40% of all type 2 diabetes patients were treated with sulfonylureas. However, since the introduction of newer oral agents, this number has probably been reduced. The sulfonylureas exhibit both pancreatic and extrapancreatic effects and are useful only in patients with viable β-cells. The primary effect of the sulfonylureas is due to direct stimulation of insulin release. In vivo studies of sulfonylureas show that they sensitize β-cells to glucose, increasing insulin secretion indirectly. Therefore, under the influence of sulfonylureas, more insulin is secreted at all glucose levels than would be expected in the absence of sulfonylureas. Sulfonylureas may also affect glucose metabolism via several extrapancreatic mechanisms, such as increasing insulin's effect by a postreceptor action, decreasing hepatic insulin extraction, and increasing insulin receptor number and receptor binding affinity; however, the relative clinical relevance of each of these mechanisms of action is still subject to research and debate.

In terms of glycemic lowering, sulfonylureas can be expected to reduce HbA$_{1c}$ values between 1% and 2%. The SUs have also been associated with weight gain. Lastly, the SUs are true hypoglycemic agents and can cause significant hypoglycemia. However, their long track record of relative safety, their efficacy in reducing hypoglycemia, and very low cost, probably makes them a reasonable choice early on in the treatment of type 2 diabetes.

GLINIDES

Repaglinide and nateglinide are nonsulfonylurea insulinotropic agents whose biochemical mechanism of action—closure of ATP-sensitive potassium channels in β-cells—is similar to that of sulfonylureas. Closure of ATP-sensitive potassium channels causes an influx of calcium by way of voltage-dependent calcium channels. Insulin release is stimulated after intercellular calcium concentrations reach a threshold. Therefore, similar to sulfonylureas, the glinides reduce blood glucose levels by stimulating insulin release from the pancreas.

The glycemic lowering afforded by the glinides is generally less than that of the SUs. Typically, HbA$_{1c}$ lowering of about 1%-1.5% can be expected in a secretagogue naïve patient. These agents do not work in patients who do not respond to SUs. The glinides are associated with a lower incidence of hypoglycemia than the SUs. The major disadvantages of the glinides are the need for multiple daily doses, less HbA$_{1c}$ lowering capacity than the SUs, and cost. These compounds are probably most appropriately positioned as fourth- or fifth-step agents in most cases.

INSULIN

Insulin has been used widely for monotherapy since its introduction in 1922 and has been used in combination with oral agents since the late 1950s. Today, about 40% of patients with type 2 diabetes use insulin as part of their effort to control hyperglycemia. **Overall, insulin is probably underutilized in this population.** It is the one type of therapy that, with appropriate titration, can consistently bring a patient's blood sugar levels into the target range.

Insulin binds to the α-subunit of the insulin receptor, activating tyrosine kinase activity of the β-subunit. Activation of tyrosine kinase initiates a cascade of reactions resulting in several physiological events, including inhibition of hepatic glucose production, stimulation of hepatic glucose uptake, stimulation of glucose uptake by muscle, and mild stimulation of glucose uptake by adipose tissue. Insulin therapy has been associated with as much as a 44% reduction in hepatic glucose production and between a 17% and 80% increase in peripheral glucose uptake.

The most significant side effects of insulin in patients with type 2 diabetes include hypoglycemia and weight gain. Severe hypoglycemia, while a major concern in patients with type 2 diabetes, probably occurs much less frequently than in patients with type 1 diabetes. In clinical trials where patients were treated towards an A1C of <7% rates of severe hypoglycemia occurred at about 1/50th (1-3 episodes per 100 patient-years) of the rate encountered in type 1 patients during the DCCT trial.

Insulin has also been associated with significant weight gain. Studies in patients treated with insulin for between 6 and 12 months have reported weight gains of up to 6 kg, but are more commonly on the order of 2-4 kg.

The hypoglycemic lowering capacity of insulin therapy in patients with type 2 diabetes is limited only by dose and eventual development of hypoglycemia if too much insulin is used. It is very effective in combination with other pharmacologic modalities. Its titration can be simplified, in many instances, to a point that allows the patient to continue to titrate doses between visits to the provider. One of the most successful studies in the management of type 2 diabetes (The Treat to Target Trial) demonstrated that the

majority of patients evaluated could achieve HbA_{1c} values of <7% with the addition of a simple insulin regimen to their management plan. Generally speaking, insulin is relatively inexpensive, very effective, and relatively safe in this population. It may be considered as a first-line agent in some cases and probably should be considered as a second or third step in almost all other cases.

The use of insulin is reviewed in detail in the next chapter.

BIGUANIDES

The biguanide metformin (Glucophage) was first introduced in 1959 as an antihyperglycemic agent for use in patients with type 2 diabetes, but was not approved for use in the U.S. until the 1990s. Metformin causes several metabolic effects, including changes in lipoprotein and carbohydrate metabolism. The effects of this compound on carbohydrate metabolism occur primarily at the level of the liver, inhibiting hepatic glucose production. Metformin has no direct effect on β-cell function.

Patients treated with metformin may experience a 30% higher incidence of abdominal bloating, nausea, cramping, feeling of fullness, and diarrhea. These side effects can be a particular problem during the initiation phases of therapy. However, these side effects are usually self-limiting and transient and can be mitigated by starting with a low dose, titrating up slowly, and taking the medication with food.

Less common side effects include a reduction in cyanocobalamin levels (vitamin B_{12}) and a metallic taste in the mouth. Lactic acidosis can occur with the administration of metformin, but it is extremely rare (0.03 cases per 1,000 patient-years) and has occurred primarily in patients with significant renal dysfunction. Currently, there is question as to whether or not metformin use is truly associated with lactic acidosis. Metformin is contraindicated in patients with renal dysfunction (serum creatinine >1.5 mg/dL in men, >1.4 mg/dL in women). This is due to the fact that metformin is excreted entirely unchanged via the kidneys and can accumulate in patients with significant renal dysfunction.

Metformin should be avoided in patients with congestive heart failure (CHF), unstable heart disease, hypoxic lung disease, or advanced age (>80 years). Because lactic acidosis is sometimes associated with hepatic dysfunction, metformin is contraindicated in patients with clinical or laboratory evidence of hepatic dysfunction. Metformin is also contraindicated in patients with a history of alcoholism or binge drinking and in patients with acute or chronic acidosis. Metformin should also be withheld temporarily in patients with acute conditions predisposing them to acute renal failure or acidosis, such as exacerbation of CHF, major surgical procedure, cardiovascular collapse, or acute myocardial infarction. Lastly, metformin should be discontinued just before the administration of intravenous iodinated contrast media and reinstituted 48 hours or so after the procedure, after the patient's renal function has been verified.

Metformin could arguably be the drug of first choice in the management of hyperglycemia in obese patients with type 2 diabetes. Metformin therapy, unlike sulfonlyureas or thiazolidinediones, is not related to an increase in weight. In fact, many patients experience a mild degree of weight loss when treated with metformin. Additionally, metformin therapy may also result in a modest reduction in plasma triglyceride and low-density lipoprotein concentrations. Metformin may also be used effectively with other oral agents and insulin. Also, metformin is available generically and is inexpensive. Metformin therapy can be expected to cause about a 1.5% reduction in HbA$_{1c}$ levels. Metformin's positive effect on weight, lipids, and glycemic control along with its low cost make it a very attractive first-line agent in many cases, particularly in overweight individuals, who account for ~85% of all newly diagnosed type 2 patients.

α-GLUCOSIDASE INHIBITORS

Two drugs in the α-glucosidase inhibitor (AGI) category have been approved for use in the U.S.: acarbose and miglitol. These drugs exhibit mild antihyperglycemic activity. They may be used as monotherapy in new onset or mild type 2 diabetes and are also useful in combination with insulin or other oral agents in more severe type 2 diabetes.

The primary mechanism of action of α-glucosidase inhibitors is competitive inhibition of the α-glucosidase enzymes in the brush border of the small intestine. Additionally, they may inhibit pancreatic α-amylase, the enzyme responsible for the hydrolysis of complex starches to oligosaccharides in the lumen of the small intestine. α-glucosidase enzymes are responsible for the breakdown of oligosaccharides, trisaccharides, and disaccharides in the brush border of the small intestine. These enzymes include maltase, isomaltase, glucoamylase, and sucrase. Inhibition of these enzyme systems effectively reduces the rate of absorption of carbohydrates without altering the absolute absorption. The result is reduced postprandial glucose levels. There is a modest effect on fasting glucose.

The most common side effects of the AGIs are dose-related gastrointestinal complaints, abdominal pain, flatulence, and diarrhea. In many cases these side effects may be mitigated with continued administration of the drug and with slow stepwise titration.

Elevated hepatic enzymes have been reported at higher doses of acarbose (200 and 300 mg tid); however, the occurrence of hepatic dysfunction with doses of ≤100 mg tid is rare. In fact, elevated serum transaminase levels are no more frequent than those observed with placebo when doses of ≤100 mg tid were used.

One problem that may be encountered in patients treated with acarbose and hypoglycemic agents (eg, insulin or sulfonylureas) is difficulty in treating hypoglycemic episodes with oral complex carbohydrates. The absorption rates of complex carbohydrates are drastically reduced with the administration of acarbose, so their use will not resolve hypoglycemia. Therefore, patients treated with AGIs and oral hypoglycemic agents should be advised to have a source of glucose such as glucose tablets or gel on hand in the event of a hypoglycemic episode.

Contraindications for the use of AGIs primarily revolve around gastrointestinal side effects. Acarbose should be avoided in patients with inflammatory bowel disease, colonic ulceration, or obstructive bowel disorders. Relative contraindications include medical conditions that might deteriorate with increased intestinal gas formation and chronic intestinal disorders of digestion or absorption.

Acarbose should be avoided in patients with serum creatinine levels >2.0 mg/dL.

Typically an HbA_{1c} reduction of about 0.5%-1% can be expected with AGIs. However, they must be dosed three times daily and are sometimes avoided secondary to their gastrointestinal side effects. AGIs should probably be viewed as third- or fourth-line agents in most cases.

THIAZOLIDINEDIONES

Currently, two thiazolidinediones (TZDs) are available for use in the U.S.: pioglitazone and rosiglitazone. These medications appear to work by affecting insulin action without affecting insulin secretion. They are sometimes referred to as insulin sensitizers. Although several mechanisms of action may contribute to their antihyperglycemic properties, it is known that these compounds stimulate receptors on the nuclear surface, PPARγ (peroxisome-proliferator-activated receptor gamma). Therefore, the thiazolidinediones are also referred to as PPAR activators. Stimulation of PPARγ leads to increased glucose uptake by mechanisms that are still unclear. Additionally, these compounds have mild to moderate effects on lipid metabolism.

Several studies have suggested a link between the use of TZDs and reduced bone density and fractures. While it has been demonstrated that patients with type 2 diabetes are at increased risk of fracture compared to their euglycemic peers, recent evidence has been suggested that use of TZDs in patients at risk for osteoporosis may result in a higher fracture rate. Providers should be mindful of this possibility when prescribing oral antihyperglycemic agents. The most salient suggested mechanism for TZD-induced osteoporosis is via inhibition of bone formation by PPAR-mediated diversion of mesenchymal progenitor cells into the adipocytes rather than osteoblasts.

TZDs have also been associated with mild to moderate weight gain (1-5 kg) in some patients. Initially, this weight gain was thought to be due primarily to edema but has since been shown to be nonedema weight gain.

Rosiglitazone and pioglitazone have different effects on lipid profiles. This difference may be related to relative effect of these agents on the nuclear receptor. Pioglitazone has a higher affinity for PPARα and is associated with mild improvements in lipid profiles (reduction of TG and increases in HDL). Both agents may cause an increase in LDL. Indirect comparisons of pioglitazone and rosiglitazone suggest that rosiglitazone probably causes more LDL elevation than pioglitazone.

Both agents can cause edema. This may in turn increase the incidence of exacerbations of CHF in patients who have underlying disease. This effect seems to be more pronounced in patients who are also treated with insulin. Edema, if it occurs, can sometimes be mitigated via the use of diuretics. However, TZDs are contraindicated in patients with NYHA class III or IV failure.

The published conclusions regarding the impact of TZDs on overall cardiovascular mortality are conflicting. A handful of contradictory manuscripts and a plethora of opposing opinions and editorials on this subject have been published. While it is clear that untreated hyperglycemia is a major risk factor for cardiovascular mortality, it is not clear that treating hyperglycemia in patients with TZDs results in significantly more cardiovascular mortality than is encountered in patients treated with other modalities.

HbA$_{1c}$ lowering can be expected somewhere between 0.5%-1.5% in most patients. Significant differences between the two available agents, in terms of glycemic lowering, are not obvious. However, the TZDs are less effective than insulin and slightly less effective than metformin or sulfonlyureas. In most cases, the later agents should probably be used initially.

sion of exendin-4, was approved for use in the U.S. in 2005 and is administered twice per day by subcutaneous injection.

The mechanism of action of exenatide is complex and multifaceted. It stimulates insulin secretion from functional β-cells. Secondly, it suppresses glucagon secretion and slows gastric motility. It probably also has a central effect on satiety and is associated with reduced food intake. While exenatide is not associated with hypoglycemia, it has been associated with a relatively high frequency of gastrointestinal side effects. As many as 45% of treated patients reported experiencing one or more episodes of nausea, vomiting, or diarrhea. Also, several cases of acute pancreatitis have been reported in patients treated with exenatide. Exenatide labeling now carries a warning to this effect.

Exenatide has been associated with weight loss of 2 to 3 kg over 6 months in some studies. Part of this (as with metformin) may be a result of its gastrointestinal side effects. Exenatide should be injected twice daily, but is available as a convenient pen. HbA$_{1c}$ lowering of 0.5%-1% can be expected with the use of exenatide. While patients treated with exenatide can expect some weight loss, exenatide's cost, its need for multiple daily injections, and its relatively mild glycemic lowering ability probably position it as a third- or fourth-line agent in most cases.

GLP-1 AGONISTS

Glucagon-like peptide 1 (GLP-1) 7-37 is a naturally occurring peptide that stimulates insulin secretion. It is secreted by the influence of glucose by the L-cells of the small intestine. A compound isolated from the gila monster, exendin-4, has homology with the human GLP-1 sequence but has a longer circulating half-life. Exenatide, a synthetic ver-

GLIPTINS (DPP-4 INHIBITORS)

GLP-1, the hormone mentioned in the section above, under normal conditions has a very short half-life and short duration of action. This short half-life is due to degradation of GLP by an enzyme system known as dipeptidyl peptidase-4 (DPP-4). Pharmacologic inhibition of this system results in prolonged activity of the incretin hormones, which in turn are associated with enhanced insulin secretion and a reduction in glucagon secretion. Currently, one DPP-4 inhibitor is available in the U.S., sitagliptin.

Sitagliptin is associated with a number of desirable characteristics. It is dosed orally, once daily. There is minimal risk of hypoglycemia when sitagliptin is used as monotherapy. Overall, sitagliptin has a relatively mild side effect profile when compared to other agents used in the treatment of type 2 diabetes. While sitagliptin was not associated with weight loss, it was found to be weight neutral in clinical trials.

Unfortunately, sitagliptin therapy generally results in a modest HbA_{1c} reduction. A reduction in HbA_{1c} of about 0.5%-1% can be expected in most cases with sitagliptin monotherapy. Sitagliptin's modest glycemic lowering and high cost probably position it as a third- or fourth-line agent in most cases.

AMYLIN AGONIST

Pramlintide is a synthetic form of the β-cell hormone amylin. Pramlintide is only approved for use in the U.S. in patients with type 1 or type 2 diabetes as adjunctive therapy with insulin.

Endogenous amylin is cosecreted with insulin from normal β-cells. Amylin's primary effects are to reduce glucagon secretion and delay gastric emptying. It may also reduce food intake via a central effect on satiety. Amylin concentrations are reduced in patients with diabetes. Pramlintide's effects mimic those of endogenous amylin. Pramlintide, when administered subcutaneously before meals, slows gastric emptying, inhibits glucagon production in a glucose-dependent fashion. Its primary affect on glucose control is via reduction in postprandial glucose excursions.

The major clinical side effects of this drug are gastrointestinal in nature. Approximately 30% of treated participants in the clinical trials evaluating pramlintide reported nausea. Pramlintide has been associated with weight loss of around 1-1.5 kg. The etiology of this weight loss is not clear. It may be due to reduced food intake mediated through a central effect or may be the result of gastrointestinal side effects. In clinical studies, HbA_{1c} has been decreased in type 2 patients by about 0.7% with the administration of pramlintide. At this time, pramlintide is probably most appropriately positioned as a fourth- or fifth-line agent in the management of the type 2 patient.

BILE ACID SEQUESTRANT

The bile acid sequestrant (BAS) colesevelam is the most recent medication approved for glycemic reduction in patients with diabetes. It was specifically developed for its ability to bind with bile acids, removing them from circulation, ultimately lowering LDL concentration. Studies in diabetes patients with high cholesterol and elevated LDL-C showed that glucose levels decreased by 13% after 24 weeks of treatment. Subsequent studies evaluated colesevelam as adjunctive therapy for improving glycemic control. In patients with inadequate glycemic control on sulfonylureas and/or metformin therapy, 12 weeks of colesevelam HCl treatment significantly improved HbA_{1c} and levels of fructosamine and postprandial glucose as well as reduced levels of LDL-C, total cholesterol, and apolipoprotein B. Thus, colesevelam has an antihyperglycemic effect. However, the mechanism by which colesevelam improves glycemic control is unknown. For information about potential MOAs, please refer to the BAS chapter.

Recently, the American Association of Clinical Endocrinologists (AACE) placed colesevelam in their Road Map to Achieve Glycemic Goals in patients naïve to therapy (type 2) at level 2 for patients with an initial HbA_{1c} between 7% and 8% and who should be using combination therapy, especially metformin. It would also seem appropriate to target type 2 patients who have not quite been able to achieve an HbA_{1c} of 7% or less who have elevated LDL-C. Lowering the HbA_{1c} of the many type 2 patients who cannot quite achieve a target HbA_{1c} of 7% or less with an oral medication with relatively few side effects and little weight gain that drops HbA_{1c} by 0.5% seems a reasonable alternative.

This drug is not absorbed systemically and is not associated with systemic side effects. Additionally, its use is not associated with significant weight gain.

One of the barriers to the use of this compound is that patients need to take 6 tablets a day or 3 tablets twice daily with food and plenty of fluid; and, many patients develop constipation. The tablet size of colesevelam can cause dysphagia or esophageal obstruction and should be used with caution in patients with dysphagia or swallowing disorders. In general, colesevelam is a useful addition to options available to treat type 2 diabetes. As an oral antihyperglycemic agent alone it probably ranks as a fourth- or fifth-line agent. However, because it may be primarily used as an antilipid drug it may be viewed as much more attractive agent in many cases.

CONCLUSIONS

At present, the development of a meaningful, clinically effective, and relevant medication treatment regimen for type 2 diabetes is complex and providers do not find it easy to decide which medication to prescribe. The prescriber must consider the patient's weight, diabetes duration, lipid and blood pressure status, dexterity, and liver and kidney function, as well as the medications that have been tried previously. Fasting plasma glucose, HbA_{1c} levels, postprandial glucose levels, allergies, insurance coverage, cost of therapy, dosing complexity and the time it takes to titrate to effective doses, degree of insulin resistance, and whether or not the β-cell is still capable of producing and releasing insulin are all additional considerations. For these reasons, an exact step-by-step treatment algorithm is difficult to develop and various clinics follow different guidelines.

As mentioned above, the hyperglycemia encountered in patients with type 2 diabetes is often accompanied by other metabolic abnormalities, such as hyperlipidemia, hyperinsulinemia, hypertension, and weight gain. In the past several years many new medications have been introduced that address not only glycemic abnormalities but also other metabolic abnormalities in patients with type 2 diabetes. While the cost of medication should be considered, the most effective method of achieving cost savings in the management of type 2 diabetes is via strict glycemic control with medications that do not adversely affect the patient's metabolic profile and do not carry contraindications to the patient's specific situation. When designing a therapeutic regimen for a given patient, the practitioner should consider the amount of glycemic lowering needed to bring that patient into glycemic control (achieving American Diabetes Association goals for treatment), the contraindications of the medication, the side effects of the medication, the effect of the medication on insulin resistance, the expected degree of patient adherence, and lastly, medication costs. Clinicians presently have an expanded medication tool chest from which to select drug therapy that will allow achievement of metabolic objectives and still allow patients a flexible and near-normal lifestyle.

Table 2.1. Summary of Antidiabetic Medication Attributes in a Typical Patient

Interventions	Expected decrease in HbA$_{1c}$ (%)	Advantages	Disadvantages
Metformin	1.5	Weight neutral, inexpensive	GI side effects, rare to questionable lactic acidosis
Insulin	Dose dependent	No dose limit, inexpensive, improved lipid profile	Injections, monitoring, hypoglycemia, weight gain
Sulfonylureas	1-2	Inexpensive	Weight gain, hypoglycemia
TZDs	0.5-1.5	Low rates of hypoglycemia	Fluid retention, weight gain, expensive
Glinides	1-1.5	Short duration	Three times/day dosing, expensive
Exenatide	0.5-1.0	Weight loss, available in a pen	Injections, frequent GI side effects, expensive
Gliptins	0.5-1.0	Once-daily oral dosing	Moderate glycemic lowering, expensive
Pramlintide	0.7	Weight loss, available in a pen	Injections, three times/day dosing, frequent GI side effects, expensive
BAS	0.5	Positive impact on lipids, nonsystemic	Moderate glycemic lowering, large tablets

Table 2.2. Medication Costs*

Interventions	Expected decrease in HbA$_{1c}$ (%)	Cost per Month ($)	HbA$_{1c}$ lowering cost ($ monthly cost/mean lowering)
Sulfonylureas (glimepiride 4 mg/day)	1-2	14.00	9.33
Metformin (1000 mg bid)	1.5	32.00	21.33
Insulin (Lantus 50 units per day)	Dose dependent (2% used for example)	138.00	69.00**
Glinides (nateglinide 120 mg tid)	1-1.5	132.00	105.60
TZDs (pioglitazone 45 mg/day)	0.5-1.5	196.00	196.00
Gliptins (sitagliptin 100 mg/day)	0.5-1.0	181.00	241.33
Exenatide (10 mcg bid)	0.5-1.0	152.00	202.66
BAS (colesevelam 625 mg, 6/day)	0.5	196.00	392.00
Pramlintide (120 mcg bid)	0.7	290.00	414.30

*Prices accessed from Drugstore.com, June 5, 2008.   **Cost of supplies not included.

Table 2.3. Patient Has Type 2 Diabetes According to American Diabetes Association Criteria

At BASELINE, determine or implement the following:

HbA_{1c} level

Serum creatinine, microalbuminuria

Kidney function status ok?

Blood pressure, body mass index, waist-to-hip ratio

Liver function tests normal or not?

Lipid profile: HDL, LDL, total cholesterol, triglycerides

Cardiovascular risk?

Candidate for statin therapy?

History of pancreatitis?

Has patient had a flu shot and Pneumovax?

Have eyes been examined for retinopathy?

Determine if any neuropathies, gastroparesis

Has patient been referred for nutrition and exercise training?

Is patient using an ACE-I or ARB for kidney protection?

Has patient recieved foot examination and training in preventative foot care?

Has patient been trained to self-monitor blood glucose daily and know what to do with results?

Refer for in-depth diabetes education?

Has daily aspirin therapy been prescribed?

Recommend daily micronutrient supplements?

CONSIDER the following:

Duration of diabetes

Degree of insulin resistance

Degree of obesity

Postprandial blood glucose

Is FPG >140 mg/dL?

Is HbA_{1c} >7%?

Can β-cell be preserved?

Determine comorbidities and other patient-care needs.

Candidate for pump therapy?

Restrictions of insurance carrier?

Willingness to self-inject?

SUGGESTED READING

Bolen S, Feldman L, Vassy J, et al. Systematic review: comparative effectiveness and safety of oral medications for type 2 diabetes mellitus. *Ann Int Med*. 2007;147:386-389.

DeWitt DE, Hirsch IB. Outpatient insulin therapy in type 1 and type 2 diabetes mellitus. *JAMA*. 2003;289:2254-2264.

Fowler M. Diabetes treatment, part 2: oral agents for glycemic management. *Clinical Diabetes.* 2007;25;4:131-139.

Fowler M. Diabetes treatment, part 3: insulin and incretins. *Clinical Diabetes.* 2008;26;1:35-39.

Inzucchi SE. Oral antihyperglycemic therapy for type 2 diabetes: scientific review. *JAMA.* 2002;287:360-372.

Kahn SE, Haffner SM, Heise MA, et al; ADOPT Study Group. Glycemic durability of rosiglitazone, metformin, or glyburide monotherapy. *N Engl J Med.* 2006;355:2427-2443.

Kosi RR. Practical review of oral antihyperglycemic agents for type 2 diabetes mellitus. *Diabetes Educator.* 2006;32:869-876.

Nathan DM, Buse JB, Davidson MJ, Holmon RR, Sherwin R, Zinman B. Management of hyperglycemia in type 2 diabetes: a consensus algorithm for initiation and adjustment of therapy. *Diabetes Care.* 2006;29:1963-1972.

Management of Hyperglycemia in Type 2 Diabetes:

A Consensus Algorithm for the Initiation and Adjustment of Therapy

David M. Nathan, MD[1], John B. Buse, MD, PHD[2], Mayer B. Davidson, MD[3],
Robert J. Heine, MD[4], Rury R. Holman, FRCP[5], Robert Sherwin, MD[6],
Bernard Zinman, MD[7]B. Ellen Byrne, R.Ph., D.D.S., Ph.D.;
Leonard S. Tibbetts, D.D.S., M.S.D.

INTRODUCTION

The epidemic of type 2 diabetes in the latter part of the 20th and in the early 21st century, and the recognition that achieving specific glycemic goals can substantially reduce morbidity, have made the effective treatment of hyperglycemia a top priority (1–3). While the management of hyperglycemia, the hallmark metabolic abnormality associated with

From the [1]Diabetes Center, Massachusetts General Hospital and Harvard Medical School, Boston, Massachusetts; the [2]University of North Carolina School of Medicine, Chapel Hill, North Carolina; the [3]Clinical Trials Unit, Charles R. Drew University, Los Angeles, California; the [4]Diabetes Center, VU University Medical Center, Amsterdam, the Netherlands; the [5]Diabetes Trials Unit, Oxford Centre for Diabetes, Endocrinology and Metabolism, Oxford University, Oxford, U.K.; the [6]Department of Internal Medicine and Endocrinology, Yale University School of Medicine, New Haven, Connecticut; and the [7]Departments of Endocrinology and Metabolism, Mount Sinai Hospital, University of Toronto, Toronto, Canada.

type 2 diabetes, has historically had center stage in the treatment of diabetes, therapies directed at other coincident features, such as dyslipidemia, hypertension, hypercoagulability, obesity, and insulin resistance, have also been a major focus of research and therapy. Maintaining glycemic levels as close to the nondiabetic range as possible has been demonstrated to have a powerful beneficial impact on diabetes-specific complications, including retinopathy, nephropathy, and neuropathy in the setting of type 1 diabetes (4,5); in type 2 diabetes, more intensive treatment strategies have likewise been demonstrated to reduce complications (6–8). Intensive glycemic management resulting in lower HbA$_{1c}$ (A1C) levels has also been shown to have a beneficial effect on cardiovascular disease (CVD) complications in type 1 diabetes (9,10); however, the role of intensive diabetes therapy on CVD in type 2 diabetes remains under active investigation (11,12). Some therapies directed at lowering

Abbreviations: CVD, cardiovascular disease; DCCT, Diabetes Control and Complications Trial; GLP-1, glucagon-like peptide 1; SMBG, self-monitoring of blood glucose; TZD, thiazolidinedione; UKPDS, U.K. Prospective Diabetes Study.

glucose levels have additional benefits with regard to CVD risk factors, while others lower glucose without additional benefits.

The development of new classes of blood glucose–lowering medications to supplement the older therapies, such as lifestyle-directed interventions, insulin, sulfonylureas, and metformin, has increased the treatment options for type 2 diabetes. Whether used alone or in combination with other blood glucose–lowering interventions, the availability of the newer agents has provided an increased number of choices for practitioners and patients and heightened uncertainty regarding the most appropriate means of treating this widespread disease. Although numerous reviews on the management of type 2 diabetes have been published in recent years (13–16), practitioners are often left without a clear pathway of therapy to follow. We developed the following consensus approach to the management of hyperglycemia in the nonpregnant adult to help guide health care providers in choosing the most appropriate interventions for their patients with type 2 diabetes.

PROCESS

The guidelines and algorithm that follow are based on clinical trials that have examined different modalities of therapy of type 2 diabetes and on the authors' clinical experience and judgment, keeping in mind the primary goal of achieving and maintaining glucose levels as close to the nondiabetic range as possible. The paucity of high-quality evidence in the form of clinical trials that directly compare different diabetes treatment regimens remains a major impediment to recommending one class of drugs, or a particular combination of therapies, over another. While the algorithm that we propose is likely to engender debate, we hope that the recommendations will help guide the therapy of type 2 diabetes and result in improved glycemic control and health status over time.

GLYCEMIC GOALS OF THERAPY

Controlled clinical trials, such as the Diabetes Control and Complications Trial (DCCT) (4) and the Stockholm Diabetes Intervention Study (5) in type 1 diabetes and the U.K. Prospective Diabetes Study (UKPDS) (6,7) and Kumamoto Study (8) in type 2 diabetes, have helped to establish the glycemic goals of therapy that result in improved long-term outcomes. Although the various clinical trials have had different designs, interventions, and measured outcomes, the trials, in concert with epidemiologic data (17,18), support decreasing glycemia as an effective means of reducing long-term microvascular and neuropathic complications. The most appropriate target levels for blood glucose, on a day-to-day basis, and A1C, as an index of chronic glycemia, have not been systematically studied. However, both the DCCT (4) and the UKPDS (6,7) had as their goals the achievement of glycemic levels in the nondiabetic range. Neither study was able to sustain A1C levels in the nondiabetic range in their intensive treatment groups, achieving mean levels over time of ~7%, 4 SDs above the nondiabetic mean.

The most recent glycemic goal recommended by the American Diabetes Association, selected on the basis of practicality and the projected reduction in complications over time, is "in general" an A1C level <7% (19). For "the individual patient," the A1C should be "as close to normal (<6%) as possible without significant hypoglycemia." The most recent glycemic goal set by the European Union–International Diabetes Federation is an A1C level <6.5%.

The upper limit of the nondiabetic range is 6.1% (mean A1C of 5% + 2 SD) with the DCCT-standardized assay, which has been promulgated through the National Glycohemoglobin Standardization Program (NGSP) and adopted by the vast majority of commercially available assays (20). Our consensus is that an A1C of ≥7% should serve as a call to action to initiate or change therapy with the goal of achieving an A1C level as close to the nondiabetic range as possible or, at a minimum, decreasing the A1C to <7%. We are mindful that this goal is not appropriate or practical for some patients, and clinical judgment, based on the potential benefits and risks of a more intensified regimen, needs to be applied for every patient. Factors such as life expectancy and risk for hypoglycemia need to be considered for every patient before intensifying therapeutic regimens.

Assiduous attention to abnormalities other than hyperglycemia that accompany type 2 diabetes, such as hypertension and dyslipidemia, has been shown to improve microvascular and cardiovascular complications. Readers are referred to published guidelines for a discussion of the rationale and goals of therapy for the nonglycemic risk factors, as well as recommendations as to how to achieve them (1,21,22).

PRINCIPLES IN SELECTING ANTIHYPERGLYCEMIC INTERVENTIONS

Choosing specific antihyperglycemic agents is predicated on their effectiveness in lowering glucose, extraglycemic effects that may reduce long-term complications, safety profiles, tolerability, and expense.

Effectiveness in Lowering Glycemia

Apart from their differential effects on glycemia, there are insufficient data at this time to support a recommendation of one class of glucose-lowering agents, or one combination of medications, over others with regard to effects on complications. In other words, the salutary effects of therapy on long-term complications appear to be predicated predominantly on the level of glycemic control achieved rather than on any other specific attributes of the intervention(s) used to achieve glycemic goals. The UKPDS compared three classes of glucose-lowering medications (sulfonylurea, metformin, or insulin) but was unable to demonstrate clear superiority of any one drug over the others with regard to complications (6,7). However, the different classes do have variable effectiveness in decreasing glycemic levels (**Table 1**), and the overarching principle in selecting a particular intervention will be its ability to achieve and maintain glycemic goals. In addition to the intention-to-treat analyses demonstrating the superiority of intensive versus conventional interventions, the DCCT and UKPDS demonstrated a strong correlation between mean A1C levels over time and the development and progression of retinopathy and nephropathy (23,24). Therefore, we think it is reasonable to judge and compare blood glucose–lowering medications, and the combinations of such agents, primarily on the basis of the A1C levels that are achieved and on their specific side effects, tolerability, and expense.

Nonglycemic Effects of Medications

In addition to variable effects on glycemia, specific effects of individual therapies on CVD risk factors, such as hypertension or dyslipidemia, were also considered important. We also included the effects of interventions that may benefit or worsen the prospects for long-term glycemic control in our recommendations. Examples of these would be changes in body mass, insulin resistance, or insulin secretory capacity in type 2 diabetic patients.

CHOOSING SPECIFIC DIABETES INTERVENTIONS AND THEIR ROLES IN TREATING TYPE 2 DIABETES

Numerous reviews have focused on the characteristics of the specific diabetes interventions listed below (25–33). The aim here is to provide enough information to justify the choices of medications, the order in which they are recommended, and the utility of combinations of therapies. Unfortunately, there is a dearth of high-quality studies that provide head-to-head comparisons of the ability of the medications to achieve the currently recommended glycemic levels. The authors highly recommend that such studies be conducted. However, even in the absence of rigorous, comprehensive studies that directly compare the efficacy of all available glucose-lowering treatments, and their combinations, we feel that there are enough data regarding the characteristics of the individual interventions to provide the guidelines below.

An important intervention that is likely to improve the probability that a patient will have better long-term control of diabetes is to make the diagnosis early, when the metabolic abnormalities of diabetes are usually less severe. Lower levels of glycemia at time of initial therapy are associated with lower A1C over time and decreased long-term complications (34).

Lifestyle Interventions

The major environmental factors that increase the risk of type 2 diabetes, presumably in the setting of genetic risk, are overnutrition and a sedentary lifestyle, with consequent overweight and obesity (35). Not surprisingly, interventions that reverse or improve these factors have been demonstrated to have a beneficial effect on control of glycemia in established type 2 diabetes (36). While there is still active debate regarding the most beneficial types of diet and exercise, weight loss almost always improves glycemic levels. Unfortunately, the high rate of weight regain has limited the role of lifestyle interventions as an effective means of controlling glycemia long term. The most convincing long-term data that weight loss effectively lowers glycemia have been generated in the follow-up of type 2 diabetic patients who have had bariatric surgery (37,38). In this setting, diabetes is virtually erased, with a mean sustained weight loss of >20 kg (37,38). Studies of the pharmacologic treatment of obesity have been characterized by high drop-out rates, low sustainability, and side effects; weight loss medications cannot be recommended as a primary therapy for diabetes at this time. In addition to the beneficial effects of weight loss on glycemia, weight loss and exercise improve coincident CVD risk factors, such as blood pressure and atherogenic lipid profiles, and ameliorate other consequences of obesity (37–40). There are few adverse consequences of such lifestyle interventions other than the difficulty in incorporating them into usual lifestyle and sustaining them and the usually minor musculoskeletal injuries and potential problems associated with neuropathy, such as foot trauma and ulcers, that may occur with increased activity. Theoretically, effective weight loss, with its pleiotropic benefits, safety profile, and low cost, should be the most cost-effective means of controlling diabetes, if it could be achieved and maintained long term.

Given these beneficial effects, a lifestyle intervention program to promote weight loss and increase activity levels should, with rare exceptions, be included as part of diabetes management. The beneficial effects of such programs are usually seen rapidly, within weeks to months, and often before there has been substantial weight loss (41). Weight loss of as little as 4 kg will often ameliorate hyperglycemia. However, the limited

Table 1. Summary of Antidiabetic Interventions as Monotherapy

Interventions	Expected decrease in A1C (%)	Advantages	Disadvantages
Step 1: initial			
Lifestyle to decrease weight and increase activity	1–2	Low cost, many benefits	Fails for most in 1st year
Metformin	1.5	Weight neutral, inexpensive	GI side effects, rare lactic acidosis
Step 2: additional therapy			
Insulin	1.5–2.5	No dose limit, inexpensive, improved lipid profile	Injections, monitoring, hypoglycemia, weight gain
Sulfonylureas	1.5	Inexpensive	Weight gain, hypoglycemia*
TZDs	0.5–1.4	Improved lipid profile	Fluid retention, weight gain, expensive
Other drugs			
α-Glucosidase inhibitors	0.5–0.8	Weight neutral	Frequent GI side effects, three times/day dosing, expensive
Exenatide	0.5–1.0	Weight loss	Injections, frequent GI side effects, expensive, little experience
Glinides	1–1.5†	Short duration	Three times/day dosing, expensive
Pramlintide	0.5–1.0	Weight loss	Injections, three times/day dosing, frequent GI side effects, expensive, little experience

*Severe hypoglycemia is relatively infrequent with sulfonylurea therapy. The longer-acting agents (e.g., chlorpropamide, glyburide [glibenclamide], and sustained-release glipizide) are more likely to cause hypoglycemia than glipizide, glimepiride, and gliclazide.

†Repaglinide is more effective at lowering A1C than nateglinide.

GI, gastrointestinal.

long-term success of lifestyle programs to maintain glycemic goals in patients with type 2 diabetes suggests that a large majority of patients will require the addition of medications over the course of their diabetes.

Medications

The characteristics of currently available antidiabetic interventions, when used as monotherapy, are summarized in **Table 1**. The glucose-lowering effectiveness of individual therapies and combinations demonstrated in clinical trials is predicated not only on the intrinsic characteristics of the intervention, but also on the baseline glycemia, duration of diabetes, previous therapy, and other factors. A major factor in selecting a class of drugs, or a specific medication within a class, to initiate therapy or when changing therapy, is the ambient level of glycemic control. When levels of glycemia are high (e.g., A1C >8.5%), classes with greater and more rapid glucose-lowering effectiveness, or potentially earlier initiation of combination therapy, are recommended; conversely, when glycemic levels are closer to the target levels (e.g., A1C <7.5%), medications with lesser potential to lower glycemia and/or a slower onset of action may be considered. Obviously, the choice of glycemic goals and the medications used to achieve them must be individualized for each patient, balancing the potential for lowering A1C and anticipated long-term benefit with specific safety issues, as well as other characteristics of regimens, including side effects, tolerability, patient burden and long-term adherence, expense, and the non-glycemic effects of the medications. Finally, type 2 diabetes is a progressive disease with worsening glycemia over time. Therefore, addition of medications is the rule, not the exception, if treatment goals are to be met over time.

Metformin

Metformin is the only biguanide available in most of the world. Its major effect is to decrease hepatic glucose output and lower fasting glycemia. Typically, metformin monotherapy will lower A1C by ~1.5 percentage points (27,42). It is generally well tolerated, with the most common adverse effects being gastrointestinal. Although always a matter of concern because of its potentially fatal outcome, lactic acidosis is quite rare (<1 case per 100,000 treated patients) (43). Metformin monotherapy is usually not accompanied by hypoglycemia and has been used safely, without causing hypoglycemia, in patients with pre-diabetic hyperglycemia (44). The major nonglycemic effect of metformin is either weight stability or modest weight loss, in contrast to many of the other blood glucose-lowering medications. The UKPDS demonstrated a beneficial effect of metformin therapy on CVD outcomes that needs to be confirmed (7).

Sulfonylureas

Sulfonylureas lower glycemia by enhancing insulin secretion. They appear to have an effect similar to metformin, and they lower A1C by ~1.5 percentage points (26). The major adverse side effect is hypoglycemia, but severe episodes, characterized by need for assistance, coma, or seizure, are infrequent. However, such episodes are more frequent in the elderly. Episodes can be both prolonged and life threatening, although

these are very rare. Several of the newer sulfonylureas have a relatively lower risk for hypoglycemia (**Table 1**) (45,46). In addition, weight gain of ~2 kg is common with the initiation of sulfonylurea therapy. This may have an adverse impact on CVD risk, although it has not been established. Finally, sulfonylurea therapy was implicated as a potential cause of increased CVD mortality in the University Group Diabetes Program (47). Concerns raised by the University Group Diabetes Program study that sulfonylurea therapy may increase CVD mortality in type 2 diabetes were not substantiated by the UKPDS (6).

Glinides

Like the sulfonylureas, the glinides stimulate insulin secretion, although they bind to a different site within the sulfonylurea receptor (28). They have a shorter circulating half-life than the sulfonylureas and must be administered more frequently. Of the two glinides currently available in the U.S., repaglinide is almost as effective as metformin or the sulfonylureas, decreasing A1C by ~1.5 percentage points. Nateglinide is somewhat less effective in lowering A1C than repaglinide when used as monotherapy or in combination therapy (48,49). The glinides have a similar risk for weight gain as the sulfonylureas, but hypoglycemia may be less frequent, at least with nateglinide, than with some sulfonylureas (49,50).

α-Glucosidase Inhibitors

α-Glucosidase inhibitors reduce the rate of digestion of polysaccharides in the proximal small intestine, primarily lowering postprandial glucose levels without causing hypoglycemia. They are less effective in lowering glycemia than metformin or the sulfonylureas, reducing A1C by 0.5–0.8 percentage points (29). Since carbohydrate is absorbed more distally, malabsorption and weight loss do not occur; however, increased delivery of carbohydrate to the colon commonly results in increased gas production and gastrointestinal symptoms. This side effect has led to discontinuation of the α-glucosidase inhibitors by 25–45% of participants in clinical trials (29,51). One clinical trial examining acarbose as a means of preventing the development of diabetes in high-risk subjects with impaired glucose tolerance showed an unexpected reduction in severe CVD outcomes (51). This potential benefit of α-glucosidase inhibitors needs to be confirmed.

Thiazolidinediones

Thiazolidinediones (TZDs or glitazones) are peroxisome proliferator–activated receptor γ modulators; they increase the sensitivity of muscle, fat, and liver to endogenous and exogenous insulin ("insulin sensitizers") (31). The limited data regarding the blood glucose–lowering effectiveness of TZDs when used as monotherapy have demonstrated a 0.5–1.4% decrease in A1C. The most common adverse effects with TZDs are weight gain and fluid retention. There is an increase in adiposity, largely subcutaneous, with redistribution of fat from visceral deposits shown in some studies. The fluid retention usually manifests as peripheral edema, though new or worsened heart failure can occur. The TZDs either have a beneficial or neutral effect on atherogenic lipid profiles, with pioglitazone having a more beneficial effect than rosiglitazone (52,53). The PROactive (PROspective pioglitAzone Clinical Trial In macroVascular Events) study demonstrated no significant effects of pioglitazone compared with placebo on the primary CVD outcome (composite of all-cause mortality, nonfatal and silent myocardial infarction, stroke, major leg amputation, acute coronary syndrome, coronary artery bypass graft or percutaneous coronary intervention, and leg revascularization) after 3 years of follow-up, but a 16% reduction in death, myocardial infarction, and stroke, a secondary end point, was reported with marginal statistical significance (54).

Insulin

Insulin is the oldest of the currently available medications and has the most clinical experience. Although initially developed to treat the insulin-deficient type 1 diabetic patient, in whom it is life saving, insulin was used early on to treat the insulin-resistant form of diabetes recognized by Himsworth and Kerr (55). Insulin is the most effective of diabetes medications in lowering glycemia. It can, when used in adequate doses, decrease any level of elevated A1C to, or close to, the therapeutic goal. Unlike the other blood glucose–lowering medications, there is no maximum dose of insulin beyond which a therapeutic effect will not occur. Relatively large doses of insulin (≥1 unit/kg), compared with those required to treat type 1 diabetes, may be necessary to overcome the insulin resistance of type 2 diabetes and lower A1C to goal. Although initial therapy is aimed at increasing basal insulin supply, usually with intermediate- or long-acting insulins, patients may also require prandial therapy with short- or rapid-acting insulins as well (Fig. 1). Insulin therapy has beneficial effects on triglyceride and HDL cholesterol levels (56) but is associated with weight gain of ~2–4 kg, probably proportional to the correction of glycemia and owing predominantly to the reduction of glycosuria. As with sulfonylurea therapy, the weight gain may have an adverse effect on cardiovascular risk. Insulin therapy is also associated with hypoglycemia, albeit much less frequently than in type 1 diabetes. In clinical trials aimed at normoglycemia and achieving a mean A1C of ~7%, severe hypoglycemic episodes (defined as requiring help from another person to treat) occurred at a rate of between 1 and 3 per 100 patient-years (8,56–59) compared with 61 per 100 patient-years in the DCCT intensive-therapy group

(4). Insulin analogs with longer, nonpeaking profiles may decrease the risk of hypoglycemia compared with NPH, and analogs with very short durations of action may reduce the risk of hypoglycemia compared with regular insulin (60,61). Inhaled insulin was approved in the U.S. in 2006 for the treatment of type 2 diabetes. Published clinical studies to date have not demonstrated whether inhaled insulin, given as monotherapy (62,63) or in combination with an injection of long-acting insulin (64), can lower A1C to ≤7%.

Glucagon-like Peptide 1 Agonists (Exenatide)

Glucagon-like peptide 1 (GLP-1) 7-37, a naturally occurring peptide produced by the L-cells of the small intestine, stimulates insulin secretion. Exendin-4 has homology with the human GLP-1 sequence but has a longer circulating half-life. It binds avidly to the GLP-1 receptor on the pancreatic β-cell and potentiates glucose-mediated insulin secretion (32). Synthetic exendin-4 (exenatide) was approved for use in the U.S. in 2005 and is administered twice per day by subcutaneous injection. Although there are far less published data on this new compound than the other blood glucose–lowering medications, exendin-4 appears to lower A1C by 0.5–1 percentage points, mainly by lowering postprandial blood glucose levels (65–68). Exenatide also suppresses glucagon secretion and slows gastric motility. It is not associated with hypoglycemia but has a relatively high frequency of gastrointestinal side effects, with 30–45% of treated patients experiencing one or more episodes of nausea, vomiting, or diarrhea (65–68). In published trials, exenatide is associated with an ~2- to 3-kg weight loss over 6 months, some of which may be a result of its gastrointestinal side effects. Currently, exenatide is approved for use in the U.S. with sulfonylurea and/or metformin.

Amylin Agonists (Pramlintide)

Pramlintide is a synthetic analog of the β-cell hormone amylin. Currently, pramlintide is approved for use in the U.S. only as adjunctive therapy with insulin.

Pramlintide is administered subcutaneously before meals and slows gastric emptying, inhibits glucagon production in a glucose-dependent fashion, and predominantly decreases postprandial glucose excursions (33). In clinical studies, A1C has been decreased by 0.5–0.7 percentage points (69). The major clinical side effects of this drug, which is injected before meals, are gastrointestinal in nature. Approximately 30% of treated participants in the clinical trials have developed nausea. Weight loss associated with this medication is ~1–1.5 kg over 6 months; as with exenatide, some of the weight loss may be the result of gastrointestinal side effects.

HOW TO INITIATE DIABETES THERAPY AND ADVANCE INTERVENTIONS

Except in rare circumstances, such as patients who are extremely catabolic or hyperosmolar, who are unable to hydrate themselves adequately, or with diabetic ketoacidosis (see SPECIAL CONSIDERATIONS/ PATIENTS later in this article), hospitalization is not required to initiate or adjust therapy. The patient is the key player in the diabetes care team and should be trained and empowered to prevent and treat hypoglycemia, as well as to adjust medications with the guidance of health care providers to achieve glycemic goals. Many patients may be managed effectively with monotherapy; however, the progressive nature of the disease will require the use of combination therapy in many, if not most, patients over time to achieve and maintain glycemia in the target range.

The measures of glycemia that are initially targeted on a day-to-day basis are the fasting and preprandial glucose levels. Self-monitoring of blood glucose (SMBG) is an important element in adjusting or adding new interventions and, in particular, in titrating insulin doses. The need for and number of required SMBG measurements are not clear (70) but are dependent on the medications used. Oral hypoglycemic regimens that do not include sulfonylureas, and are therefore not likely to cause hypoglycemia, usually do not require SMBG. However, SMBG may be used to determine whether therapeutic blood glucose targets are being achieved and to adjust treatment regimens without requiring the patient to have laboratory-based blood glucose testing. A fasting glucose level measured several times per week generally correlates well with the A1C level. Insulin therapy requires more frequent monitoring.

The levels of plasma or capillary glucose (most meters that measure fingerstick capillary samples are adjusted to provide values equivalent to plasma glucose) that should result in long-term glycemia in the nondiabetic target range, as measured by A1C, are fasting and preprandial levels between 70 and 130 mg/dL (3.89 and 7.22 mmol/L). If these levels are not consistently achieved, or A1C remains above the desired target, postprandial levels, usually measured 90–120 min after a meal, may be checked. They should be less than 180 mg/dL (10 mmol/L) to achieve A1C levels in the target range.

Attempts to achieve target glycemic levels with regimens including sulfonylureas or insulin may be associated with modest hypoglycemia, with glucose levels in the 55- to 70-mg/dL (3.06- to 3.89-mmol) range. These episodes are generally well tolerated, easily treated with oral carbohydrate, such as glucose tablets or 4–6 oz (120–180 mL) juice or non-diet soda, and rarely progress to more severe hypoglycemia, including loss of consciousness or seizures.

ALGORITHM

The algorithm (**Fig. 2**) takes into account the characteristics of the individual interventions, their synergies, and expense. The goal is to achieve and maintain glycemic levels as close to the nondiabetic range as possible and to change interventions at as rapid a pace as titration of medications allows. Pramlintide, exenatide, α-glucosidase inhibitors, and the glinides are not included in this algorithm, owing to their generally lower overall glucoselowering effectiveness, limited clinical data, and/or relative expense (**Table 1**). However, they may be appropriate choices in selected patients.

Step 1:
Lifestyle Intervention and Metformin

Based on the numerous demonstrated short- and long-term benefits that accrue when weight loss and increased levels of activity are achieved and maintained, and the cost-effectiveness of lifestyle interventions when they succeed, the consensus is that lifestyle interventions should be initiated as the first step in treating new-onset type 2 diabetes (**Fig. 2**). These interventions should be implemented by health care professionals with appropriate training, usually registered dietitians with training in behavioral modification, and be sensitive to ethnic and cultural differences among populations. Moreover, lifestyle interventions to improve glucose, blood pressure, and lipids levels and to promote weight loss or at least avoid weight gain should remain an underlying theme throughout the management of type 2 diabetes, even after medications are used. For the 10–20% of patients with type 2 diabetes who are not obese or overweight, modification of dietary composition and activity levels may play a supporting role, but medications are generally required earlier (see SPECIAL CONSIDERATIONS/PATIENTS later in this article).

Table 2. Titration of Metformin

1) Begin with low-dose metformin (500 mg) taken once or twice per day with meals (breakfast and/or dinner).

2) After 5–7 days, if GI side effects have not occurred, advance dose to 850 or 1,000 mg before breakfast and dinner.

3) If GI side effects appear as doses advanced, can decrease to previous lower dose and try to advance dose at a later time.

4) The maximum effective dose is usually 850 mg twice per day, with modestly greater effectiveness with doses up to 3 g per day. GI side effects may limit the dose that can be used.

5) Based on cost considerations, generic metformin is the first choice of therapy. A longer-acting formulation is available in some countries and can be given once per day.

GI, gastrointestinal.

The authors recognize that for most individuals with type 2 diabetes, lifestyle interventions fail to achieve or maintain metabolic goals, either because of failure to lose weight, weight regain, progressive disease or a combination of factors. Therefore, our consensus is that metformin therapy should be initiated concurrent with lifestyle intervention at diagnosis. Metformin is recommended as the initial pharmacologic therapy, in the absence of specific contraindications, for its effect on glycemia, absence of weight gain or hypoglycemia, generally low level of side effects, high level of acceptance, and relatively low cost. Metformin treatment should be titrated to its maximally effective dose over 1–2 months, as tolerated (**Table 2**). Rapid addition of other glucose-lowering medications should be considered in the setting of persistent symptomatic hyperglycemia.

Step 2: Additional Medications

If lifestyle intervention and maximal tolerated dose of metformin fail to achieve or sustain glycemic goals, another medication should be added within 2–3 months of the initiation of therapy or at any time when A1C goal is not achieved. There was no strong consensus regarding the second medication added after metformin other than to choose among insulin, a sulfonylurea, or a TZD (**Fig. 2**). As discussed above, the A1C level will determine in part which agent is selected next, with consideration given to the more effective glycemia-lowering agent, insulin, for patients with A1C >8.5% or with symptoms secondary to hyperglycemia. Insulin can be initiated with a basal (intermediate- or long-acting) insulin (**see Fig. 1 for suggested initial insulin regimens**) (71). The relative increased cost of the newer agents that are only available as brand medications must be balanced against their relative benefits.

Step 3: Further Adjustments

If lifestyle, metformin, and a second medication do not result in goal glycemia, the next step should be to start, or intensify, insulin therapy (**Fig. 1**). When A1C is close to goal (<8.0%), addition of a third oral agent could be considered; however, this approach is relatively more costly and potentially not as effective in lowering glycemia compared with adding or intensifying insulin (72). Intensification of insulin therapy usually consists of additional injections that might include a short- or rapid-acting insulin given before selected meals to reduce postprandial glucose excursions (**Fig. 1**). When prandial rapid- or very-rapid-acting insulin injections are started, insulin secretagogues (sulfonylurea or glinides) should be discontinued, or tapered and then discontinued, since they are not considered synergistic with administered insulin.

RATIONALE IN SELECTING SPECIFIC COMBINATIONS

More than one medication will be necessary for the majority of patients over time.

Figure 1. Initiation and Adjustment of Insulin Regimens.

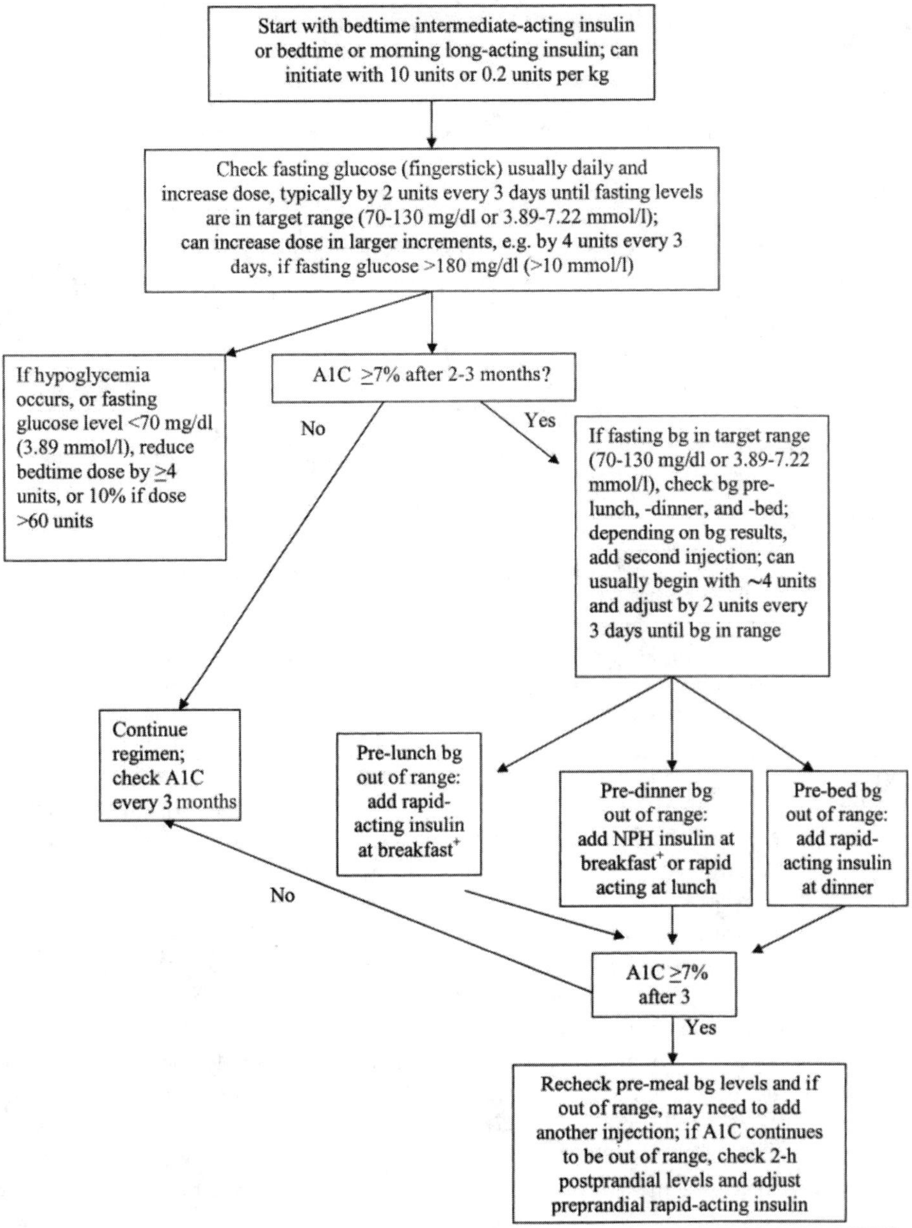

Start with bedtime intermediate-acting insulin or bedtime or morning long-acting insulin; can initiate with 10 units or 0.2 units per kg

Check fasting glucose (fingerstick) usually daily and increase dose, typically by 2 units every 3 days until fasting levels are in target range (70-130 mg/dl or 3.89-7.22 mmol/l); can increase dose in larger increments, e.g. by 4 units every 3 days, if fasting glucose >180 mg/dl (>10 mmol/l)

If hypoglycemia occurs, or fasting glucose level <70 mg/dl (3.89 mmol/l), reduce bedtime dose by ≥4 units, or 10% if dose >60 units

A1C ≥7% after 2-3 months?

No   Yes

If fasting bg in target range (70-130 mg/dl or 3.89-7.22 mmol/l), check bg pre-lunch, -dinner, and -bed; depending on bg results, add second injection; can usually begin with ~4 units and adjust by 2 units every 3 days until bg in range

Continue regimen; check A1C every 3 months

Pre-lunch bg out of range: add rapid-acting insulin at breakfast+

Pre-dinner bg out of range: add NPH insulin at breakfast+ or rapid acting at lunch

Pre-bed bg out of range: add rapid-acting insulin at dinner

No

A1C ≥7% after 3

Yes

Recheck pre-meal bg levels and if out of range, may need to add another injection; if A1C continues to be out of range, check 2-h postprandial levels and adjust preprandial rapid-acting insulin

Insulin regimens should be designed taking lifestyle and meal schedule into account. The algorithm can only provide basic guidelines for initiation and adjustment of insulin. See ref. 71 for more detailed instructions. +Premixed insulins are not recommended during adjustment of doses; however, they can be used conveniently, usually before breakfast and/or dinner if proportion of rapid- and intermediate-acting insulins is similar to the fixed proportions available.
bg, blood glucose.

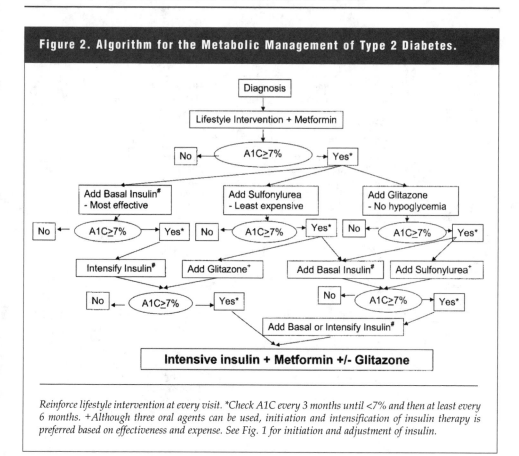

Figure 2. Algorithm for the Metabolic Management of Type 2 Diabetes.

*Reinforce lifestyle intervention at every visit. *Check A1C every 3 months until <7% and then at least every 6 months. +Although three oral agents can be used, initiation and intensification of insulin therapy is preferred based on effectiveness and expense. See Fig. 1 for initiation and adjustment of insulin.*

Selection of the individual agents should be made on the basis of their glucose-lowering effectiveness and other characteristics listed in **Table 1**. However, when adding second and potentially third antihyperglycemic medications, the synergy of particular combinations and other interactions should be considered. In general, antihyperglycemic drugs with different mechanisms of action will have the greatest synergy. Insulin plus metformin (73) and insulin plus a TZD (74) are particularly effective means of lowering glycemia. The increased risk of fluid retention with the latter combination must be considered. (TZD in combination with insulin is not currently approved in the European Union.) Although both TZDs and metformin effectively increase sensitivity to insulin, they have different target organs and have

been shown to have modest additive effects, with addition of TZD to metformin lowering A1C by 0.3–0.8% (75,76).

SPECIAL CONSIDERATIONS/ PATIENTS

In the setting of severely uncontrolled diabetes with catabolism, defined as fasting plasma glucose levels >250 mg/dL (13.9 mmol/L), random glucose levels consistently >300 mg/dL (16.7 mmol/L), A1C >10%, or the presence of ketonuria, or as symptomatic diabetes with polyuria, polydipsia, and weight loss, insulin therapy in combination with lifestyle intervention is the treatment of choice. Some patients with these characteristics will have unrecognized type 1 diabetes; others will have type 2 diabetes but with severe insulin deficiency. Insulin can be titrated rapidly and is associated with the greatest likelihood of returning glucose levels rapidly to target levels. After symptoms are relieved, oral agents can often be added and it may be possible to withdraw insulin, if preferred.

CONCLUSIONS/SUMMARY

Type 2 diabetes is epidemic. Its long-term consequences translate into enormous human suffering and economic costs. We now understand that much of the morbidity associated with long-term complications can be substantially reduced with interventions that achieve glucose levels close to the non-diabetic range. Although new classes of medications, and numerous combinations, have been demonstrated to lower glycemia, current-day management has failed to achieve and maintain the glycemic levels most likely to provide optimal health care status for people with diabetes.

The guidelines and treatment algorithm presented here emphasize
- achievement and maintenance of normal glycemic goals;
- initial therapy with lifestyle intervention and metformin;
- rapid addition of medications, and transition to new regimens, when target glycemic goals are not achieved or sustained; and
- early addition of insulin therapy in patients who do not meet target goals.

REFERENCES

1. American Diabetes Association. Standards of medical care of diabetes. *Diabetes Care* 28 (Suppl. 1):S15–S35, 2005
2. European Diabetes Policy Group: A desktop guide to type 2 diabetes mellitus. *Diabet Med* 16:716–730, 1999
3. The Royal College of General Practitioners Effective Clinical Practice Unit: Clinical guidelines for type 2 diabetes mellitus: management of blood glucose [article online], 2002. Available from http://www.nice.org.uk/pdf/ NICE_full_blood_glucose.pdf
4. Diabetes Control and Complications Trial Research Group: The effect of intensive diabetes treatment on the development and progression of long-term complications in insulin-dependent diabetes mellitus: the Diabetes Control and Complications Trial. *N Engl J Med* 329:978–986, 1993
5. Reichard P, Nilsson B-Y, Rosenqvist U: The effect of long-term intensified insulin treatment on the development of microvascular complications of diabetes mellitus. *N Engl J Med* 329:304–309, 1993

Address correspondence and reprint requests to David M. Nathan, MD, Diabetes Center, Massachusetts General Hospital, Boston, MA 02114. E-mail: dnathan@partners.org.

This document was reviewed and approved by the Professional Practice Committee of the American Diabetes Association and by an ad hoc committee of the European Association for the Study of Diabetes (Ulf Smith, Gothenburg, Sweden; Stefano Del Prato, Pisa, Italy; Clifford Bailey, Birmingham U.K.; and Bernard Charbonnel, Nantes, France).

D.M.N. has received research grants for investigator-initiated research from Aventis and Novo Nordisk. J.B.B. has conducted research and/or served on advisory boards under contract between the University of North Carolina and Amylin, Becton Dickinson, Bristol-Myers Squibb, Hoffman-LaRoche, Lilly, Novo Nordisk, Merck, Novartis, Pfizer, and Sanofi-Aventis. M.B.D. has received research support from Eli Lilly, Merck, and Pfizer; has served on advisory boards for GlaxoSmithKline, Merck, Sanofi-Aventis; and has been on speakers bureaus for Amylin, Eli Lilly, GlaxoSmithKline, and Pfizer. R.J.H. has received research support from GlaxoSmithKline, Minimed-Medtronic, Novartis, and Novo Nordisk and has served on advisory boards for Amylin, Bristol-Myers Squibb, Merck, Novartis, Novo Nordisk, Pfizer, and Sanofi-Aventis. R.R.H. has received research support from Bristol-Myers Squibb, GlaxoSmithKline, Merck Sante´, Novo Nordisk, Pfizer, and Pronova and has served on advisory boards and/or received honoraria for speaking engagements from Amylin, GlaxoSmithKline, Lilly, Merck Sharp & Dome, Novartis, and Sanofi-Aventis. R.S. has served on advisory boards for Amylin, Bristol-Myers Squibb, Eli Lilly, Merck, and Takeda. B.Z. has received research support from Eli Lilly, GlaxoSmithKline, Novartis, and Novo Nordisk and has been a member of scientific advisory boards and/or received honoraria for speaking engagements from Amylin, Eli Lilly, GlaxoSmith-Kline, Johnson & Johnson, Merck, Novartis, Pfizer, Sanofi-Aventis, and Smiths Medical.

Simultaneous publication: This article was simultaneously published in 2006 in *Diabetes Care* and *Diabetologia* by the American Diabetes Association and the European Association for the Study of Diabetes.

6. UK Prospective Diabetes Study (UKPDS) Group: Intensive blood glucose control with sulphonylureas or insulin compared with conventional treatment and risk of complication in patients with type 2 diabetes (UKPDS 33). *Lancet* 352: 837–853, 1998

7. UK Prospective Diabetes Study (UKPDS) Group: Effect of intensive blood glucose control with metformin on complication in overweight patients with type 2 diabetes (UKPDS 34). *Lancet* 352:854–865, 1998

8. Ohkubo Y, Kishikawa H, Araki E, Takao M, Isami S, Motoyoshi S, Kojima Y, Furuyoshi N, Shichiri M: Intensive insulin therapy prevents the progression of diabetic microvascular complications in Japanese patients with NIDDM: a randomized prospective 6-year study. *Diabetes Res Clin Pract* 28:103–117, 1995

9. Diabetes Control and Complications Trial /Epidemiology of Diabetes Interventions and Complications Research Group: Intensive diabetes therapy and carotid intimamedia thickness in type 1 diabetes. *N Engl J Med* 348:2294–2303, 2003

10. Diabetes Control and Complications Trial/ Epidemiology of Diabetes Interventions and Complications Research Group: Intensive diabetes treatment and cardiovascular disease in patients with type 1 diabetes. *N Engl J Med* 353: 2643–2653, 2005

11. Advance Collaborative Group: ADVANCE: Action in Diabetes and Vascular Disease: patient recruitment and characteristics of the study population at baseline. *Diabet Med* 22:882–888, 2005

12. Bastien A: The ACCORD trial: a multidisciplinary approach to control cardiovascular risk in type 2 diabetes mellitus. *Pract Diabetol* 23:6–11, 2004

13. Nathan DM: Initial management of glycemia in type 2 diabetes mellitus. *N Engl J Med* 347:1342–1349, 2002

14. Deeg MA: Basic approach to managing hyperglycemia for the nonendocrinologist. *Am J Cardiol* 96 (Suppl. 1):37E–40E, 2005

15. Sheehan MT: Current therapeutic options in type 2 diabetes mellitus: a practical approach. *Clin Med Res* 1:189–200, 2003

16. Inzucchi SE: Oral antihyperglycemic therapy for type 2 diabetes. *JAMA* 287: 360–372, 2002

17. Klein R, Klein BEK, Moss SE, Davis MD, DeMets DL: Glycosylated hemoglobin predicts the incidence and progression of diabetic retinopathy. *JAMA* 260:2864–2871, 1988

18. Chase HP, Jackson WE, Hoops, SL, Cockerham RS, Archer PG, O'Brien D: Glucose control and the renal and retinal complications of insulin-dependent diabetes. *JAMA* 261: 1155–1160, 1989

19. American Diabetes Association: Standards of medical care in diabetes–2006. *Diabetes Care* 29 (Suppl. 1):S4–42, 2006

20. Little RR, Rohlfing CL, Wiedmeyer H-M, Myers GL, Sacks DB, Goldstein DE: The National Glycohemoglobin Standardization Program (NGSP): a five year progress report. *Clin Chem* 47:1985–1992, 2001

21. Expert Panel on Detection, Evaluation, and Treatment of High Blood Cholesterol in Adults: Executive summary of the Third Report of the National Cholesterol Education Program (NCEP) Expert Panel on Detection, Evaluation, and Treatment of High Blood Cholesterol in Adults (Adult Treatment Panel III). *JAMA* 285: 2486–2497, 2001

22. Chobanian AV, Bakris GL, Black HR, Cushman WC, Green LA, Izzo JL, Jones DW, Materson BJ, Oparil S, Wright JT, Rocella EJ, the National Heart, Lung, and Blood Institute Joint National Committee on Prevention, Detection, Evaluation and Treatment of High Blood Pressure, the National High Blood Pressure Education Program Coordinating Committee: The seventh report of the Joint National Committee on Prevention, Detection, Evaluation and Treatment of High Blood Pressure: the JNC 7 report. *JAMA* 289: 2560–2571, 2003

23. DCCT Research Group: The association between glycemic exposure and longterm diabetic complications in the Diabetes Control and Complications Trial. *Diabetes* 44:968– 983, 1995

24. Stratton IM, Adler AI, Neil HA, Matthews DR, Manley SE, Cull CA, Hadden D, Turner RC, Holman RR: Association of glycaemia with macrovascular and microvascular complications of type 2 diabetes (UKPDS 35): prospective observational study. *BMJ* 321:405–412, 2000

25. National Institutes of Health: *Clinical Guidelines on the Identification, Evaluation, and Treatment of Overweight and Obesity in Adults: The Evidence Report.* Bethesda, MD, National Institutes of Health, 1999 (NIH publ. no. 98-4083)

26. Groop L: Sulfonylureas in NIDDM. *Diabetes Care* 15: 737–747, 1992

27. Bailey CJ, Turner RC: Metformin. *N Engl J Med* 334: 574–583, 1996

28. Malaisse WJ: Pharmacology of the meglitinide analogs: new treatment options for type 2 diabetes mellitus. *Treat Endocrinol* 2:401– 414, 2003

29. Van de Laar FA, Lucassen PL, Akkermans RP, Van de Lisdonk EH, Rutten GE, Van Weel C: Alpha-glucosidase inhibitors for type 2 diabetes mellitus. *Cochrane Database Syst Rev* CD003639, 2005

30. Genuth S: Insulin use in NIDDM. *Diabetes Care* 13: 1240–1264, 1990

31. Yki-Jarvinen H: Drug therapy: thiazolidinediones. *N Engl J Med* 351:1106, 2004

32. Drucker DJ: Biologic actions and therapeutic potential of the proglucagon-derived peptides. *Nature Endocrinol Metab* 1: 22–31, 2005

33. Schmitz O, Brock B, Rungby J: Amylin agonists: a novel approach in the treatment of diabetes. *Diabetes* 53 (Suppl. 3): S233–S238, 2004

34. Colagiuri S, Cull CA, Holman RR, UKPDS Group: Are lower fasting plasma glucose levels at diagnosis of type 2 diabetes associated with improved outcomes? *Diabetes Care* 25:1410–1417, 2002

35. Harris MI: Epidemiologic correlates of NIDDM in Hispanics, whites and blacks in the U.S. population. *Diabetes Care* 14 (Suppl. 3):639–648, 1991

36. Rewers M, Hamman RF: Risk factors for non-insulin dependent diabetes. In Dia- betes in America. 2nd ed. Harris M, Ed. Bethesda, MD, *National Institutes of Health*, 1995, p. 179–220 (NIH publ. no. 95-1468)

37. Pories WJ, Swanson MS, MacDonald KG, Long SB, Morris PG, Brown BM, Barakat HA, daRamon RA, Israel G, Dolezal JM: Whowould have thought it? An operation proves to be the most effective therapy for adult-onset diabetes mellitus. *Ann Surg* 222:339–350, 1995

38. Sjostrom L, Lindroos AK, Peltonen M, Torgerson J, Bouchard C, Carlsson B, Dahlgren S, Larrson B, Narbro K, Sjostrom CD, Sullivan M, Wedel H, Swedish Obese Subjects Study Scientific Group: Lifestyle, diabetes, and cardiovascular risk factors 10 years after bariatric surgery. *N Engl J Med* 351:2683–2693, 2004

39. Pontiroli AE, Folli F, Paganelli M, Micheletto G, Pizzocri P, Vedani P, Luisi F, Perego L, Morabito A, Doldi SB: Laparoscopic gastric banding prevents type 2 diabetes and arterial hypertension and induces their remission in morbid obesity. *Diabetes Care* 28:2703–2709, 2005

40. Diabetes Prevention Program Research Group: Impact of intensive lifestyle and metformin therapy on cardiovascular disease risk factors in the Diabetes Prevention Program. *Diabetes Care* 28:888–894, 2005

41. Hadden DR, Montgomery DAD, Skelly RJ, Trimble ER, Weaver JA, Wilson EA, Buchanan KD: Maturity onset diabetes mellitus: response to intensive dietary management. *BMJ* 3:276–278, 1975

42. DeFronzo R, Goodman A, Multicenter Metformin Study Group: Efficacy of metformin in patients with non-insulin-dependent diabetes mellitus. *N Engl J Med* 333:541, 1995

43. Salpeter S, Greyber E, Pasternak G, Salpeter E: Risk of fatal and nonfatal lactic acidosis with metfromin use in type 2 diabetes mellitus. *Cochrane Database Syst Rev* CD002967, 2006

44. Diabetes Prevention Program Research Group: Reduction in incidence of type 2 diabetes with lifestyle intervention or metformin. *N Engl J Med* 346:393–403, 2002

45. Tessier D, Dawson K, Tetrault JP, Bravo G, Meneilly GS: Glibenclamide versus gliclazide in type 2 diabetes of the elderly. *Diabet Med* 11:974–980, 1994

46. Holstein A, Plaschke A, Egberts E-H: Lower incidence of severe hypoglycemia in patients with type 2 diabetes treated with glimepiride versus glibenclamide. *Diabetes Metab Res Rev* 17:467–473, 2001

47. Klimt CR, Knatterud GL, Meinert CL, Prout TE: The University Group Diabetes Program: a study of the effect of hypoglycemic agents on vascular complications in patients with adult-onset diabetes. I. Design, methods and baseline characteristics. II. Mortality results. *Diabetes* 19 (Suppl. 2): 747–830, 1970

48. Rosenstock J, Hassman DR, Madder RD, Brazinsky SA, Farrell J, Khutoryansky N, Hale PM: Repaglinide versus nateglinide monotherapy: a randomized, multicenter study. *Diabetes Care* 27:1265–1270, 2004

49. Gerich J, Raskin P, Jean-Louis L, Purkayastha D, Baron A: PRESERVE-β: twoyear efficacy and safety of initial combination therapy with nateglinide or glyburide plus metformin. *Diabetes Care* 28:2093–2100, 2005

50. Kristensen JS, Frandsen KB, Bayer T, Müller PG: Compared with repaglinide, sulfonylurea treatment in type 2 diabetes is associated with a 2.5 fold increase in symptomatic hypoglycemia with blood glucose levels ≤45 mg/dl (Abstract). *Diabetes* 49 (Suppl. 1):A131, 2000

51. Chiasson JL, Josse RG, Gomis R, Hanefeld M, Karasik A, Laakso M: Acarbose treatment and the risk of cardiovascular disease and hypertension in patients with impaired glucose tolerance: the STOPNIDDM Trial. *JAMA* 290:486–494, 2003

52. Khan MA, St. Peter JV, Xue JL: A prospective, randomized comparison of the metabolic effects of pioglitazone or rosiglitazone in patients with type 2 diabetes who were previously treated with troglitazone. *Diabetes Care* 25:708– 711, 2002

53. Goldberg RB, Kendall DM, Deeg MA, Buse JB, Zagar AJ, Pinaire JA, Tan MH, Khan MA, Perez AT, Jacober SJ, GLAI Study Investigators: A comparison of lipid and glycemic effects of pioglitazone and rosiglitazone in patients with type 2 diabetes and dyslipidemia. *Diabetes Care* 28: 1547–1554, 2005

54. Dormandy JA, Charbonnel B, Eckland DJA, Erdmann E, Massi-Benedetti M, Moules IK, Skene AM, Tan MH, Lefebvre PJ, Murray GD, Standl E, Wilcox RG, Wilhelmsen L, Betteridge J, Birkeland K, Golay A, Heine RJ, Koranyi L, Laakso M, Mokan M, Norkus A, Pirags V, Podar T, Scheen A, Scherbaum W, Schernthaner G, Schmitz O, Skrha J, Smith U, Taton J, PROactive Investigators: Secondary prevention of macrovascular events in patients with type 2 diabetes in the PROactive (PROspective pioglitAzone *Clinical Trial* in macroVascular Events): a randomized controlled trial. *Lancet* 366: 1279–1289, 2005

55. Himsworth HP, Kerr RB: Insulin-sensitive and insulin-insensitive types of diabetes mellitus. *Clin Sci* 4:119–152, 1939

56. Nathan DM, Roussell A, Godine JE: Glyburide or insulin for metabolic control in non-insulin-dependent diabetes mellitus: a randomized double-blind study. *Ann Intern Med* 108:334–340, 1988

57. Abraira C, Johnson N, Colwell J, VA CSDM Group: VA Cooperative study on glycemic control and complications in type II diabetes. *Diabetes Care* 18:1113– 1123, 1995

58. Zammitt NN, Frier BM: Hypoglycemia in type 2 diabetes. *Diabetes Care* 28:2948–2961, 2005

59. Miller CD, Phillips LS, Ziemer DC, Gallina DL, Cook CB, El-Kebbi IM: Hypoglycemia in patients with type 2 diabetes mellitus. *Arch Intern Med* 161:1653–1659, 2005

60. Raskin P, Allen E, Hollander P, Lewin A, Gabbay RA, Hu P, Bode B, Garber A: Initiating insulin therapy in type 2 diabetes. *Diabetes Care* 28:260–265, 2005

61. Dailey G, Rosenstock J, Moses RG, Ways K: Insulin glulisine provides improved glycemic control in patients with type 2 diabetes. *Diabetes Care* 27:2363–2368, 2004

62. Hollander PA, Blonde L, Rowe R, Mehta AE, Milburn JL, Hershon KS, Chiasson J-L, Levin SR: Efficacy and safety of inhaled insulin (Exubera) compared with subcutaneous insulin therapy in patients with type 2 diabetes. *Diabetes Care* 27: 256–2363, 2004

63. Rosenstock J, Zinman B, Murphy LJ, Clement SC, Moore P, Bowering CK, Hendler R, Lan S-P, Cefalu WT: Inhaled insulin improves glycemic control when substituted for or added to oral combination therapy in type 2 diabetes. *Ann Intern Med* 143:549–558, 2005

64. Cefalu WT, Skyler JS, Kourides IA, Landschulz WH, Balagtas CC, Cheng S-L, Gelfand RA, Inhaled Insulin Study Group: Inhaled human insulin treatment in patients with type 2 diabetes mellitus. *Ann Intern Med* 134:203–207, 2001

65. Kendall DM, Riddle MC, Rosenstock J, Zhuang D, Kim DD, Fineman MS, Baron AD: Effects of exenatide (exendin-4) on glycemic control and weight over 30 weeks in patients with type 2 diabetes treated with metformin and a sulfonylurea. *Diabetes Care* 28:1083–1091, 2005

66. DeFronzo R, Ratner RE, Han J, Kim DD, Fineman MS, Baron AD: Effects of exenatide on glycemic control and weight over 30 weeks in metformin-treated patients with type 2 diabetes. *Diabetes Care* 28:1092–1100, 2005

67. Buse JB, Henry RR, Han J, Kim DD, Fineman MS, Baron AD, Exenatide-113 Clinical Study Group: Effects of exenatide on glycemic control over 30 weeks in sulfonylurea- treated patients with type 2 diabetes. *Diabetes Care* 27:2628–2635, 2004

68. Heine RJ, Van Gaal LF, Johns D, Mihm MJ, Widel MH, Brodows RG: Exenatide versus insulin glargine in patients with suboptimally controlled type 2 diabetes. *Ann Intern Med* 143:559–569, 2005

69. Hollander PA, Levy P, Fineman MS, Maggs DG, Shen LZ, Strobel SA, Weyer C, Kolterman OG: Pramlintide as an adjunct to insulin therapy improves long-term glycemic and weight control in patients with type 2 diabetes. *Diabetes Care* 26: 784–790, 2003

70. Welschen LMC, Bloemendal E, Nijpels G, Dekker JM, Heine RJ, Stalman WAB, Bouter LM: Self-monitoring of blood glucose in patients with type 2 diabetes who are not using insulin: a systematic review. *Diabetes Care* 28: 1510–1517, 2005

71. Hirsch IB, Bergenstal RM, Parkin CG, Wright E, Buse JB: A real-world approach to insulin therapy in primary care practice. *Clin Diabetes* 23:78–86, 2005

72. Schwartz S, Sievers R, Strange P, Lyness WH, Hollander P: Insulin 70/30 mix plus metformin versus triple oral therapy in the treatment of type 2 diabetes after failure of two oral drugs. *Diabetes Care* 26: 2238–2243, 2003.

73. Yki-Jarvinen H, Ryysy L, Nikkila K, Tulokas T, Vanamo R, Heikkila M: Comparison of bedtime insulin regimens in patients with type 2 diabetes mellitus. *Ann Intern Med* 130:389–396, 1999

74. Strowig S, Aviles-Santa ML, Raskin P: Improved glycemic control without weight gain using triple therapy in type 2 diabetes. *Diabetes Care* 27:1577–1583, 2004

75. Fonseca V, Rosenstock J, Patwardhan R, Salzman A: Effect of metformin and rosiglitazone combination therapy in patients with type 2 diabetes mellitus. *JAMA* 283:1695–1702, 2000

76. Bailey CJ, Bagdonas A, Rubes J, McMorn SO, Donaldson J, Biswas N, Stewart MW: Rosiglitazone/metformin fixed dose combination compared with uptitrated metformin alone in type 2 diabetes mellitus: a 24 week, multicenter, randomized, double blind, parallel group study. *Clin Ther* 27:1548–1561, 2005

Management of Hyperglycemia in Type 2 Diabetes:

A Consensus Algorithm for the Initiation and Adjustment of Therapy

David M. Nathan, MD[1,2,] John B. Buse, MD, PhD[3], Mayer B. Davidson, MD[4],
Ele Ferrannini, MD[5], Rury R. Holman, FRCP[6], Robert Sherwin, MD[7] and
Bernard Zinman, MD[8]

Update regarding thiazolidinediones: a consensus statement from the American Diabetes Association and the European Association for the Study of Diabetes

The consensus algorithm for the management of type 2 diabetes was developed on behalf of the American Diabetes Association and the European Association for the Study of Diabetes approximately 1 year ago (1,2). This evidence-based algorithm was developed to help guide health care providers to choose the most appropriate treatment regimens from an ever-expanding list of approved medications. The authors continue to endorse the major features of the algorithm, including the need to achieve and maintain glycemia within or as close to the nondiabetic range as is safely possible, the initiation of lifestyle interventions and treatment with metformin at the time of diagnosis, the rapid addition of medications and transition to new regimens when target glycemia is not achieved, and the early addition of insulin therapy in patients who do not meet target A1C levels.

The availability of newly approved medications and the accrual of new clinical trial and other data should inform the algorithm. In this update, we primarily address one important issue that has received much recent attention: our current understanding of the advantages and disadvantages of the thiazolidinediones. In addition, we have revised the original **Table 1** to include the dipeptidylpeptidase-4 inhibitor sitagliptin, which was not approved by the U.S. Food

[1]*Diabetes Center, Massachusetts General Hospital, Boston, Massachusetts* [2]*Harvard Medical School, Boston, Massachusetts* [3]*University of North Carolina School of Medicine, Chapel Hill, North Carolina* [4]*Charles R. Drew University, Los Angeles, California* [5]*Department of Internal Medicine, University of Pisa, Pisa, Italy* [6]*Diabetes Trials Unit, Oxford Centre for Diabetes, Endocrinology and Metabolism, Oxford University, Oxford, U.K* [7]*Yale University School of Medicine, New Haven, Connecticut* [8]*Samuel Lunenfeld Research Institute, Mount Sinai Hospital, University of Toronto, Toronto, Ontario, Canada*

Abbreviations: CHF, congestive heart failure

Table 1. Summary of Glucose-Lowering Interventions as Monotherapy

Interventions	Expected decrease in A1C (%)	Advantages	Disadvantages
Step 1: Initial			
Lifestyle to decrease weight and increase activity	1–2	Low cost, many benefits	Fails for most in first year
Metformin	1–2	Weight neutral, inexpensive	GI side effects, rare lactic acidosis
Step 2: Additional therapy			
Insulin	1.5–3.5	No dose limit, inexpensive, improved lipid profile	Injections, monitoring, hypoglycemia, weight gain
Sulfonylureas	1–2	Inexpensive	Weight gain, hypoglycemia*
Thiazolidinediones (glitazones)	0.5–1.4	Improved lipid profile† Potential decreased risk of MI†	Fluid retention, twofold increased risk of CHF, potential increased risk of MI‡, atherogenic lipid profile, weight gain, expensive
Other drugs α-Glucosidase inhibitors	0.5–0.8	Weight neutral	Frequent GI side effects, three times/day dosing, expensive
Exenatide	0.5–1.0	Weight loss	Injections, frequent GI side effects, expensive, little experience
Glinides	1–1.5§	Short duration	Three times/day dosing, expensive, hypoglycemia
Pramlintide	0.5–1.0	Weight loss	Injections, three times/day dosing, frequent GI side effects, expensive, little experience
Sitagliptin	0.5–0.8	Weight neutral	Little experience, expensive

* Severe hypoglycemia is relatively infrequent with sulfonylurea therapy. The longer-acting agents (e.g. chlorpropamide and glibenclamide [glyburide]) are more likely to cause hypoglycemia than glipizide, extended-release glipizide, glimepiride, or gliclazide.

†Pioglitazone.

‡Rosiglitazone.

§Repaglinide is more effective at lowering A1C than nateglinide.

GI, gastrointestinal; MI, myocardial infarction.

and Drug Administration at the time of our original publication (see **Table 1**).

We are mindful of the importance of not changing this consensus guideline in the absence of definitive or compelling new data. Future updates are planned to consider further revisions of the algorithm, guided by the evidence base and clinical experience with the newer classes of glucose-lowering medications.

Figure 1. Algorithm for the Metabolic Management of Type 2 Diabetes.

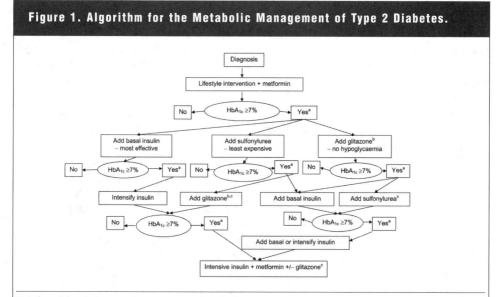

Reinforce lifestyle intervention at every visit. [a]Check A1C every 3 months until <7% and then at least every 6 months. [b]Associated with increased risk of fluid retention, CHF, and fractures. Rosiglitazone, but probably not pioglitazone, may be associated with an increased risk of myocardial infarction. [c]Although three oral agents can be used, initiation and intensification of insulin therapy is preferred based on effectiveness and lower expense.

The original consensus algorithm included the thiazolidinediones as one of three possible choices (insulin and sulfonylurea were the other two) that should be added to metformin and lifestyle intervention if target A1C levels (<7%) were not being achieved (**Figure 1**). Several recent meta-analyses (3,4), together with one performed by the manufacturer (5) and one by regulatory authorities (6), have called into question the safety of rosiglitazone with regard to the risk of myocardial infarction. The putative 30%–40% relative increase in risk of myocardial infarctions is based on data that are widely viewed as less than definitive; still, these data have led to the recommendation that clinicians exercise increased caution in prescribing rosiglitazone (7–10). Another recent meta-analysis of essentially the same dataset found no significantly increased risk of cardiovascular mortality owing to either rosiglitazone or pioglitazone (11). An interim analysis of the Rosiglitazone Evaluated for Cardiac Outcomes and Regulation of Glycemia

in Diabetes (RECORD) study, designed specifically to examine cardio-vascular outcomes of rosiglitazone therapy, revealed no statistically significant effects on myocardial infarction (hazard ratio 1.17 [95% CI 0.75–1.82]) but confirmed the risk for congestive heart failure (CHF) with rosiglitazone (2.15 [1.30–3.57]) (12). Furthermore, a meta-analysis of the clinical trial data regarding cardio-vascular disease risk and pioglitazone has suggested that the drug exerts a protective effect (13).

In addition to the concern raised regarding the potential risk of myocardial infarction with rosiglitazone, the previously recognized risk of fluid retention and resultant CHF, which applies to both pioglitazone and rosiglitazone, has now been quantified as an approximate twofold increase (11,14). These findings have led to a "black box" warning in the prescribing information for rosiglitazone regarding the risk for myocardial infarction and for both thiazolidinediones regarding the risk for CHF (15).

Both thiazolidinediones have been associated with an increased risk for fractures, particularly in women (16,17). Of note, the majority of these fractures were in the distal upper (forearm, hand, or wrist) or lower (foot, ankle, fibula, or tibia) limb, as opposed to the classic sites of osteoporotic fractures.

At this time, we do not view as definitive the clinical trial data regarding increased or decreased risk of myocardial infarctions with rosiglitazone or pioglitazone, respectively. Nor do we think that the increased risk of CHF or fractures with either of the available thiazolidinediones is of a magnitude to warrant their removal as one of the possible second-step medications in our algorithm, given that they cause hypoglycemia less frequently than other second-step drugs.

On the other hand, we do believe that the weight of the new information outlined above should prompt clinicians to consider more carefully whether to use this class of drugs versus insulin or sulfonylureas as the second step in the algorithm (**Figure 1**). As with other drug classes, there may well be clinically important differences between the two drugs in this class. The current decision not to remove either or both of the thiazolidinediones from the algorithm represents a balance between the preservation of options to treat a challenging and progressive serious disease and the recent unfavorable evidence.

In conclusion, new information suggests additional hazards associated with the use of either thiazolidinedione, and rosiglitazone in particular, may result in an increased frequency of myocardial infarctions. We therefore recommend greater caution in using the thiazolidinediones, especially in patients at risk of, or with, CHF.

FOOTNOTES

*Simultaneous publication: This article was simultaneously published in 2008 in *Diabetes Care* and *Diabetologia* by the American Diabetes Association and the European Association for the Study of Diabetes.

D.M.N. has received research grants from sanofi-aventis and support for educational programs from GlaxoSmithKline and Pfizer. J.B.B. conducts research and/or serves on advisory boards under contract between the University of North Carolina and Amylin, Bristol-Myers Squibb, GlaxoSmithKline, Hoffman-LaRoche, Eli Lilly, Novo Nordisk, Merck, Novartis, Pfizer, and sanofi-aventis. M.B.D. has received research support from Eli Lilly, Merck, and Pfizer; serves on advisory boards to Amylin, GlaxoSmithKline, Merck, and sanofi-aventis; and is on speakers bureaus for Amylin, Eli Lilly, GlaxoSmithKline, and Pfizer. E.F. has received research support from AstraZeneca, Merck Sharp & Dohme, and Novartis and serves on scientific advisory boards for Amylin, AstraZeneca, GlaxoSmithKline, Roche, Merck Sharp & Dohme, Novartis, Servier, sanofi-aventis, Boehringer Ingelheim, and Takeda. R.R.H. has received grant support from Novartis, Bristol-Myers Squibb, Novo Nordisk, Pfizer, GlaxoSmithKline, and Merck and serves on scientific advisory boards for Amylin, Novartis, Eli Lilly, Merck, and sanofi-aventis. R.S. serves on advisory boards for Amylin, Bristol-Myers Squibb, Eli Lilly, Merck, and Takeda. B.Z. has received research support from Eli Lilly, GlaxoSmithKline, Novartis, and Novo Nordisk and is a member of scientific advisory boards and/or has received honoraria for speaking from Amylin, Eli Lilly, GlaxoSmithKline, Johnson & Johnson, Merck, Novartis, Pfizer, sanofi-aventis, and Smiths Medical.

Copyright © 2008 American Diabetes Association and Springer. From *Diabetes Care*, Vol. 31, 2008;173-175. Reprinted with permission. Address reprint requests to David M. Nathan, Diabetes Center, Mass. General Hospital, Boston, MA 02114. E-mail: dnathan@partners.org

REFERENCES

1. Nathan DM, Buse JB, Davidson MB, Heine RJ, Holman RR, Sherwin R, Zinman B: Management of hyperglycemia in type 2 diabetes: a consensus algorithm for the initiation and adjustment of therapy: a consensus statement from the American Diabetes Association and the European Association for the Study of Diabetes. *Diabetes Care* 29:1963–1972, 2006

2. Nathan DM, Buse JB, Davidson MB, Heine RJ, Holman RR, Sherwin R, Zinman B; Professional Practice Committee, American Diabetes Association; European Association for the Study of Diabetes: Management of hyperglycaemia in type 2 diabetes: a consensus algorithm for the initiation and adjustment of therapy: a consensus statement from the American Diabetes Association and the European Association for the Study of Diabetes. *Diabetologia* 49:1711–1721, 2006

3. Nissen SE, Wolski K: Effect of rosiglitazone on the risk of myocardial infarction and death from cardiovascular causes. *N Engl J Med* 356:2457–2471, 2007

4. Singh S, Loke YK, Furberg CD: Long-term risk of cardiovascular events with rosiglitazone: a meta-analysis. *JAMA* 298:1189–1195, 2007

5. GalaxoSmithKline Advisory Committee Briefing Document: Cardiovascular Safety of Rosiglitazone, 2007. Philadelphia, GalaxoSmithKline, p. 40–45. Available from http://www.fda.gov/ohrms/dockets/ac/07/briefing/2007-4308b1-01-sponsor-backgrounder.pdf Accessed 25 October 2007

6. U.S. Food and Drug Administration FDA Briefing Document, 2007. Rockville, MD, Food and Drug Administration, p. 13–bp105. Available from http://www.fda.gov/ohrms/dockets/ac/07/briefing/2007-4308b1-02-fda-backgrounder.pdf. Accessed 25 October 2007

7. Psaty BM, Furberg CD: Rosiglitazone and cardiovascular risk. *N Engl J Med* 356:2522–2524, 2007

8. Drazen JM, Morrissey S, Curfman GD: Rosiglitazone—continued uncertainty about safety. *N Engl J Med* 357:63–64, 2007

9. Nathan DM: Rosiglitazone and cardiotoxicity—weighing the evidence. *N Engl J Med* 357:64–66, 2007

10. Psaty BM, Furberg CD: The record on rosiglitazone and the risk of myocardial infarction. *N Engl J Med* 357:67–69, 2007

11. Lago RM, Singh PP, Nesto RW: Congestive heart failure and cardiovascular death in patients with prediabetes and type 2 diabetes given thiazolidinediones: a meta-analysis of randomized clinical trials. *Lancet* 370:1129–1136, 2007

12. Home PD, Pocock SJ, Beck-Nielsen H, Gomis R, Hanefeld M, Jones NP, Komajda M, McMurray JJ; RECORD Study Group: Rosiglitazone evaluated for cardiovascular outcomes: an interim analysis. *N Engl J Med* 357:28–38, 2007

13. Lincoff AM, Wolski K, Nicholls SJ, Nissen SE: Pioglitazone and risk of cardiovascular events in patients with type 2 diabetes mellitus: a meta-analysis of randomized trials. *JAMA* 298:1180–1188, 2007

14. Singh S, Loke YK, Furberg CD: Thiazolidinediones and heart failure: a teleo-analysis. *Diabetes Care* 30:2248–2253, 2007

15. U.S. Food and Drug Administration: Rosiglitazone maleate (marketed as Avandia, Avandamet, and Avandaryl) information, 2007. Available from http://www.fda.gov/cder/drug/infopage/rosiglitazone/default.htm. Accessed 17 November 2007

16. Schwartz AV, Sellmeyer DE, Vittinghoff E, Palermo L, Lecka-Czernik B, Feingold KR, Strotmeyer ES, Resnick HE, Carbone L, Beamer BA, Park SW, Lane NE, Harris TB, Cummings SR.: Thiazolidinedione use and bone loss in older diabetic adults. *J Clin Endocrinol Metab* 91:3349–3354, 2006

17. Kahn SE, Haffner SM, Heise MA, Herman WH, Holman RR, Jones NP, Kravitz BG, Lachin JM, O'Neill MC, Zinman B, Viberti G; ADOPT Study Group: Glycemic durability of rosiglitazone, metformin, or glyburide monotherapy. *N Engl J Med* 355:2427–2443, 2006

Chapter 3

Insulins

R. Keith Campbell, PharmB, MBA, CDE
Joshua J. Neumiller, PharmD, CGP, FASCP

INTRODUCTION

The insulin most in use today is recombinant human insulin. It is produced in virtually unlimited quantities of highest purity in either the exact amino acid sequence of native human insulin or as rapid- or long-acting human analogs, in which the amino acid sequence is intentionally altered to enhance a specific, desired pharmacokinetic characteristic. Until the development of recombinant insulins, insulin was manufactured by processing the pancreases of cattle and hogs, resulting in the production of impure insulins structurally different from human insulin.

Concerns for a worldwide shortage of animal-derived insulin resulted in the development of the first recombinant DNA-derived commercial product, human insulin. Experiments were undertaken to change the amino acid sequence to develop rapid-acting insulins that allowed for the conversion of hexamers to dimers to monomers of insulin, resulting in quicker absorption and a more rapid onset of action. Other manipulations of the amino acids produced analog insulins having a longer duration of action with less pronounced insulin peaks. The development of these "designer" insulins has made it easier for health care practitioners and patients to use the basal/bolus concept of insulin injections to better simulate a normal physiologic insulin profile in managing both fasting and postprandial blood glucose. In comparison to 20 years ago, we now have an unlimited supply of pure insulin with unique characteristics in terms of onset, peak, and duration of action.

RAPID-ACTING INSULIN ANALOGS

Insulin Lispro, Insulin Aspart, and Insulin Glulisine

These rapid-acting insulin analogs are intended to mimic meal-stimulated insulin secretion, which occurs when the healthy pancreas responds to food by releasing a bolus of insulin. Their rapid onset enhances the ability to match insulin dose to carbohydrate (CHO) intake, ensuring that insulin and glucose reach the blood at approximately the same time. Rapid-acting insulins should be taken no more than 15 minutes before the start of a meal, but may also be given after the meal to children in whom caloric intake is often difficult to predict or to diabetes patients with gastroparesis who have unpredictable CHO absorption. The short duration of action of these insulins may lead to hyperglycemia before the next meal unless adequate basal insulin is provided. There have not been head-to-head studies to determine clinical differences in the rapid-acting insulin analogs. The manufacturers may claim minor differences based on studies comparing them to regular short-acting insulins in terms of incidence of hypoglycemia and other outcomes, but there do not seem to be any significant clinical differences. Insulin that was administered by inhalation into the lungs, once available as a dried powder, is no longer on the market. Its onset of action was similar to that of the rapid-acting insulins. Technosphere, a coated insulin with a very rapid onset and a short duration of action, is still being studied. The currently available insulins have been well accepted by the medical community and are liked by patients since they are more convenient to use in terms of timing administration with meals. All of the rapid-acting insulins are used effectively in insulin pumps and are available as insulin pens for ease of use.

SHORT-ACTING INSULIN

Regular Human Insulin

Although intended to allow matching of CHO and insulin absorption, the slower onset of regular insulin, which is generally taken 45 minutes before the start of a meal, produces a longer and less predictable lag time (time between injection and noticeable glucose-lowering effects). Regardless, regular human insulin can be used as the short-acting insulin in a multiple-injection regimen and is used in many hospitals when insulin is administered intravenously. It is equally rapid in intravenous effect and less expensive than the rapid-acting analogs. Regular insulin can also be incorporated into outpatient regimens as follows:

- It can be given with rapid-acting insulin to provide a bridge between meals, e.g., the pre-breakfast injection of rapid-acting insulin will not necessarily cover a mid-morning snack.

- Because the effects of regular insulin can last up to 6 hours, regular insulin contributes to the basal insulin and can keep glucose levels from rising when the time between meals is long.
- When a high-fat meal delays CHO digestion, adding or substituting regular insulin to the pre-meal rapid-acting insulin will ensure insulin availability when needed.

INTERMEDIATE-ACTING INSULIN

Natural Protamine Hagedorn (NPH)

For many years, NPH insulin was the most commonly prescribed longer-acting insulin in the world. NPH was developed to have a long duration of action. When derived from animal pancreas, the duration was nearly 24 hours. After it was manufactured through recombinant technology, the duration of action was shorted to around 16 hours. NPH also had the advantage of being compatible for combination with regular insulin to form a stable mixture that patients can take twice daily and derive adequate, although not ideal, management of blood glucose levels. This insulin effectively treats the hyperglycemia due to "dawn phenomenon," a condition that occurs in some patients who experience elevated early-morning blood glucose levels. Because the peak activity of NPH is at 4-10 hours, NPH taken at bedtime will work during the early morning (4:00-8:00 a.m.), when the glucose increase can be quite significant in patients with a strong dawn phenomenon. Also, NPH taken before breakfast keeps glucose levels normalized between late morning—when the effects of insulin lispro, insulin aspart, or insulin glulisine diminish—and lunch, and provides some coverage to the midday meal due to its afternoon peak. The popularity of NPH has diminished as the preference for long-acting insulin analogs has grown.

LONG-ACTING INSULIN ANALOGS

Insulin Glargine

This true basal insulin analog provides a relatively flat, smooth action over 20-24 hours. It has become the most prescribed insulin in the world. The absorption from the subcutaneous depot is very predictable and controlled by glargine's altered solubility at neutral pH. After injection in subcutaneous tissue, crystals form that dissolve slowly over time, giving glargine a long duration of action. Glargine was the first longer-acting insulin that was clear in the vial; the others were suspensions and thus cloudy in appearance. **Insulin glargine cannot be mixed with other insulin preparations in the same syringe.** Glargine is dosed once daily in most patients, either in the evening or in the morning. Glargine is often used in conjunction with oral agents, such as metformin, or as a component of a basal/bolus regimen in conjunction with a rapid-acting insulin analog.

Insulin Detemir

Insulin detemir is a basal insulin analog that is injected once or twice a day. The duration of action of insulin detemir is dose dependent, although many patients are able to inject it just once daily to get the needed basal insulin. Like glargine, detemir is usually added to oral agents in type 2 diabetes or used in conjunction with a rapid-acting insulin that is taken before meals as part of a basal/bolus regimen. Insulin detemir achieves a longer duration through binding of the insulin with albumin, both at the site of injection and within the bloodstream. Its absorption does not differ from one injection site to another. It is reported that patients gain less weight when using it as a basal insulin. **Like insulin glargine, insulin detemir should not be mixed with other insulins.**

INSULIN ABSORPTION

Perhaps the trickiest aspect of insulin therapy is the variability in insulin absorption between patients and also within a single patient from one day, or time of day, to the next. Note that the action times for the various insulin preparations discussed in this chapter are generalized.

The reality is that rates of absorption vary as much as 20-40% from one day to the next in any patient due to local tissue reactions and changes in insulin sensitivity, blood flow, depth of injection, and amount of insulin injected. Changes in insulin sensitivity also occur over weeks to months. The patient's records of SMBG are, in most cases, reliable indicators on which to base insulin therapy adjustments.

To facilitate more predictable absorption, the following factors should be taken into consideration:

- **Injection site:** Potential subcutaneous injection sites include the abdomen (avoiding 1-2 inches around the navel), upper thighs, hips/buttocks, and backs of the upper arms. However, injections into the abdomen, with its larger overall blood circulation and higher body heat, provide the quickest and most predictable absorption of rapid-acting and regular insulin. Note that injections of long-acting insulin add to the basal insulin supply, so the injection site usually has no discernible influence on rate of absorption.
- **Injection site rotation:** Patients can either choose one body area for injection and rotate within that area or rotate between body areas. Systematic rotation prevents lipohypertrophy, a result of insulin stimulation of fat cell growth, which delays insulin absorption.
- **Injection size:** Use rapid- and fast-acting insulins in small-dose injections.
- **Injection depth:** Patients should practice injecting at a consistent depth into the subcutaneous tissue.

- **Needle length:** Shorter needles, while increasing comfort, may compromise absorption, depending on the thickness of subcutaneous tissues or body composition of the patient.
- **Blood flow:** Practices that increase regional blood flow (e.g., exercise, local massage/friction, hot showers, or soaks/saunas) speed absorption and lessen predictability of insulin action.

MIXING INSULINS

Lente and ultralente insulins are no longer available, but when they were, mixing with regular or rapid-acting insulins was tricky. **Also, as mentioned previously, insulin glargine and insulin detemir should not be mixed with other insulins.**

Most insulin mixtures today are between NPH (or NPH-type insulin) and either regular or rapid-acting insulins. Insulin manufacturers now premix NPH or NPH-like insulin with their regular or rapid-acting insulin to make it more convenient for the patient. For example, Lilly has Humulin Mix 70/30 and Humalog Mix 75/25 or Humalog Mix 50/50. Novo Nordisk has Novolin 70/30 or Novolog 50/50 and 70/30 mixtures.

A table at the end of this chapter shows the insulin mixtures commonly used. When mixing insulins in one syringe, the rapid- or short-acting insulin should be drawn up first. Only insulins from the same manufacturer should be mixed. The acidic nature of insulin glargine and the unique formulation of insulin detemir preclude them from being mixed with other insulins.

Commercially prepared mixtures of NPH and regular insulin (70/30 or 50/50 NPH/regular) or of protamine suspensions of rapid-acting analogs and the respective rapid-acting analog (75/25 NPL/lispro; 50/50 NPL/lispro; and 50/50 or 70/30 aspart protamine/aspart) are very stable. These premixed insulins are less useful when there is a need to vary the dose of only one of the insulin components. Their primary advantages are convenience and accuracy, particularly for patients with visual impairment or problems with manual dexterity for whom mixing insulin would be difficult or unreliable.

For patient convenience, almost all available insulins are now available in insulin pens. Even though pens are accurate and easy to use and carry, they have been slow to catch on in the U.S., perhaps due to the fact that it takes time for busy health care practitioners to train patients to use pens. Also, there is not a satisfactory reimbursement process for the time it takes to train the patient. Despite the perceived price increase of pens, they are being used by more and more diabetes patients.

INSULIN REGIMENS

Ideally, the insulin regimen mimics physiologic insulin secretory patterns that occur in people without diabetes to the greatest extent possible, containing basal and meal-stimulated (bolus) release of insulin. Insulin pump therapy or multiple daily insulin injections are the two methods that most closely mimic natural insulin secretion in response to meals or hepatic glucose release.

The first step in choosing an insulin regimen is to establish glycemic goals. For most patients, this means that more than half of SMBG results fall within the following ranges:

- **Preprandial:** 70-130 mg/dL
- **Bedtime:** 100-140 mg/dL
- **Postprandial (1-2 hours):** <140 to 180 mg/dL

Note that blood glucose measurements are for plasma values. Most glucose meters now display plasma values, which are about 10-15% higher than those for whole blood and for which different goals were given in older publications.

It is very important to individualize blood glucose goals for the patient's age, health status, history of significant hypoglycemia, lifestyle, and personal goals. For example, it would be reasonable to modify the preprandial goal to 100-140 mg/dL or higher for a type 1 diabetes patient with severe or asymptomatic hypoglycemia. Pregnant women with either type 1 or type 2 diabetes require meticulous glycemic control; whole blood goals should be modified to <95 mg/dL fasting, <140 mg/dL 1 hour postprandial, and <120 mg/dL 2 hours postprandial. Plasma blood glucose goals should be <105 mg/dL fasting, <155 mg/dL 1 hour postprandial, and <130 mg/dL 2 hours postprandial.

Insulin for Type 1 Patients

Patients with type 1 diabetes generally need a routine of at least three injections per day. Patients should be encouraged to find injection schedules that best meet their lifestyles. This will require collaboration between the patient and the health care practitioner. Those willing to perform four injections per day would use a rapid- or short-acting insulin (lispro, aspart, glulisine, or regular) before each meal with a longer-acting component usually added at bedtime (glargine or detemir) or at both breakfast and bedtime (NPH). For prescribing information on specific insulin products, see **Table 3.4**; for drug interactions, see **Table 3.5**.

Many patients will likely be put on one of the following sample injection regimens.

Two injections/day of an insulin mixture

Theory: Postprandial glucose levels for breakfast and supper are covered by short- or rapid-acting insulin; lunch and overnight glucose levels are covered by the NPH component.
Advantage: Two injections per day.
Disadvantages: 1) NPH given at supper peaks during the night and often does not last overnight until breakfast, leading to nocturnal hypoglycemia and/or high pre-breakfast glucose levels. 2) Inflexibility in dealing with

midday glucose levels. (The NPH dose is determined before breakfast, based on expectations of food and activity for the day. However, life is often unpredictable.)

Three injections/day using NPH and a rapid-acting analog before breakfast, rapid-acting insulin at supper, and NPH at bedtime

Theory: Same as for two injections/day, except that giving NPH at bedtime rather than at supper controls blood glucose better through the night and helps prevent the dawn phenomenon.
Advantage: Better overnight glucose control.
Disadvantage: Still inflexible at midday.

Four injections/day using rapid-acting insulin

Theory: Two doses of NPH or one dose of long-acting insulin provides basal coverage during the day and overnight. Rapid-acting insulin covers postprandial glucose increases.
Advantage: Allows meal-to-meal adjustments of insulin based on preprandial blood glucose levels, CHO intake, and activity.

Four injections/day using short-acting insulin

Theory: Short-acting insulin provides day-time/meal glucose control, and two doses of NPH or one dose of long-acting insulin provides basal coverage during the day and overnight.
Advantage: Allows meal-to-meal adjustments of insulin based on preprandial blood glucose levels, CHO intake, and activity.
Disadvantage: The long duration of regular insulin may lead to delayed hypoglycemia (especially at night), compelling most health care practitioners to select rapid-acting rather than short-acting regular insulin.
Note that rapid-acting insulin can be used to make correction doses when blood glucose levels are elevated and patients should be taught how to use correction doses.

Determining Total Daily Insulin Dose

About one-half to two-thirds of the total daily insulin dose is given to cover basal needs, necessitating a longer-acting insulin. The other one-third to one-half of the total daily insulin dose should be divided and given before meals as a rapid- or short-acting insulin to control postprandial glycemia, with the dose given in proportion to meal size.

When initiating insulin therapy, baseline total daily insulin dose is often calculated as 0.6 units of insulin multiplied by the patient's body weight in kilograms. For the average 70-kg patient, baseline daily insulin dose would be 42 units/day (range 35-50 units/day), one-half to two-thirds of which is basal and the other one-third to one-half of which covers meals. Modify this calculation based on the patient's activity level and physical condition. Refer to **Table 3.1** for general guidelines.

The initial daily insulin doses may be higher in the first week because many patients are initially insulin resistant. **These are simply useful starting points**, with subsequent insulin adjustments made on the basis of the patient's SMBG results. It is important to remember that there is no one good algorithm that suits all patients.

As stated in the Introduction, there is no consensus about how to best institute and maintain insulin therapy.

- A traditional approach is to begin with a three-injection regimen (pre-breakfast, pre-supper, and bedtime injections) where the total daily dose is calculated as 0.6 units of insulin per kilogram body weight. Two-thirds of the total daily dose is given in the morning, and the remaining one-third is split between the two evening doses. The morning dose consists of two-thirds longer-acting insulin and one-third rapid- or short-acting insulin. The evening dose consists of one-half longer-acting insulin and one-half rapid- or short-acting insulin.

Example:
80-kg male, total daily dose 48 units (80 X 0.6)
Morning dose: 32 units divided as 20 units NPH and 12 units rapid- or short-acting insulin
Pre-supper dose: 8 units rapid- or short-acting insulin
Bedtime dose: 8 units NPH

- Another approach to determining total daily dose is to determine basal and bolus doses separately, as follows:
Basal insulin dose can be calculated as:

NPH: 0.2 multiplied by the patient's weight in kilograms before breakfast plus

Table 3.1. Initial Insulin Doses for Type 1 Patients

Dose (U/kg/day)	Patient's physical condition and activity level
0.5	Conditioned athlete
0.6	Motivated exerciser, woman in first phase (follicular) of menstrual cycle
0.7	Woman in last week (luteal phase) of menstrual cycle or in first trimester of pregnancy, adult mildly ill with a virus, child starting puberty
0.8	Woman in second trimester of pregnancy, child in mid-puberty, adult with a severe or localized viral infection
0.9	Woman in third trimester of pregnancy, adult ill with bacterial infection
1.0	Woman at term of pregnancy, adult with a severe bacterial infection or illness, child at peak pubescence
1.5-2.0	Child at peak pubescence who is ill

0.1 multiplied by the patient's weight in kilograms at bedtime, or

0.1 multiplied by the patient's weight in kilograms three times per day (if given every 8 hours to make it work as a basal insulin)

Insulin glargine: 0.3 multiplied by the patient's weight in kilograms given at bedtime or before breakfast (once every 24 hours)

Insulin detemir: 0.3 multiplied by the patient's weight in kilograms given at bedtime or before breakfast (once every 24 hours)

Optimal basal therapy results in blood glucose levels in the fasting state between 70 and 130 mg/dL. If desired, patients can further test whether basal therapy is optimal by following these steps:

1) Start with a meal in which blood glucose is in the target range.
2) Take only the long-acting component (glargine at bedtime or detemir once or twice a day).
3) Skip the meal for which mealtime insulin is omitted.
4) Test every 2-4 hours until the next meal.

If testing reveals levels out of the target range, increasing the amount of basal insulin is required.

Bolus insulin is given to:
1) Counteract the postprandial glucose increase, and
2) Correct pre-meal glucose levels out of the 70-130 mg/dL target range

Most of the postprandial blood glucose increase is due to the meal's CHO content. Patients can count grams of total CHO provided on food labels. In general, 1 unit of short-acting insulin covers 10-15 g CHO for most patients with type 1 diabetes. However, it is important to calculate each patient's individual insulin-to-CHO ratio (see "Determining Insulin-to-CHO Ratio" on page 50) so that patients can learn to adjust their insulin dose to CHO intake. Note that if meals include a large amount of fat, glucose absorption and availability will be delayed.

If the pre-meal glucose level is in the normal range, bolus insulin covers food only. Low pre-meal glucose levels require less bolus insulin, and high pre-meal levels require enough insulin to bring glucose back to normal, in addition to insulin to cover food (see "Correction Insulin Doses" below). Note the periods covered by each insulin dose in **Table 3.2**.

Correction Insulin Doses

There are several methods for making occasional corrections to the pre-meal rapid- or short-acting insulin dose in response to out-of-target glucose levels. (Persistent out-of-target fasting glucose levels require an adjustment of insulin given at night to cover basal needs.) The methods are based on consideration of patterns discerned in the patient's glucose monitoring records; the patient's previous experience with insulin dose, food intake, and exercise; and the patient's projections for food intake and exercise during the period to be covered by the corrected dose. It will take several

Table 3.2. Checking Insulin Adequacy

If glucose levels are out-of-target at	Check coverage provided by
Post-breakfast/pre-lunch	Pre-breakfast rapid/short insulin
Post-lunch/pre-supper	Pre-lunch rapid/short insulin and/or morning NPH
Post-supper/bedtime	Pre-supper rapid/short insulin
Mid-afternoon	Morning NPH, or long-acting insulin analog
Early morning	Evening NPH, or long-acting insulin analog

Table 3.3. Sample Sliding Scale Dose Calculation for a 60-kg Patient

PRE-MEAL BG (mg/dL)	COMPENSATORY INSULIN (UNITS)	CARBOHYDRATE (g) IN FOOD	INSULIN FOR FOOD (UNITS)	TOTAL DOSE (UNITS)
<70	-1	40	4	3
70-120	—	50	5	5
70-120	—	30	3	3
120-200	+1	50	5	6
>200	+2	40	4	6

ALERT: Insulin doses vary by patient needs and sensitivity to insulin; thus, have patients frequently monitor blood glucose levels.

similar-situation corrections for the patient and physician to create an individualized list of "standard" corrective responses. As with glucose monitoring records and records of insulin dose, food intake, and activity, encourage patients to record insulin adjustments and resulting glucose levels.

- Corrections are usually made in increments of 1-2 units rapid- or short-acting insulin. Some calculate correction doses as 3% of total daily insulin requirement. These represent starting points; insulin corrections must be individualized.

- A second correction method is based on the patient's body weight (see **Table 3.3**). For a 60-kg patient, corrections would be made in increments of ~1 unit of insulin (60 x 0.6 = 36 units total daily dose; 36 x 0.03 = 1 unit). For this individual, each unit of rapid-acting insulin covers 10 g CHO.

- Another correction method uses the following formula:

$$\frac{1500}{weight\ (kg)} = X$$

$$\frac{(glucose\ level\ -\ desired\ glucose\ level)}{X} = insulin\ supplement$$

Example:
80-kg patient who is 60 mg/dL above target glucose level would require a 3-unit supplement based on the following calculations:

$$\frac{1500}{80\ kg} = 18.75 \qquad \frac{(200-140\ mg/dL)}{18.75} = 3\ units$$

The above formula was not based on a controlled clinical trial but has made its way into the literature and is often used as a way to determine an approximate correction dose. When using rapid-acting insulin analogs, some educators and physicians use 1800 rather than 1500 in the formula.

- Another correction method focuses on timing the pre-meal insulin to compensate for out-of-target pre-meal glucose levels (see "Timing Insulin" below).

Timing Insulin

To prevent excessively high postprandial glucose levels, lag time (time between injection and noticeable glucose-lowering effects) should be consistent for every insulin injection given to cover meals. Patients have differing absorption rates and may calculate their personal lag time as follows:
1. Start with normal blood glucose (70-130 mg/dL).
2. Inject insulin. Measure blood glucose every 15 minutes.
3. The time it takes for glucose to decrease by 15 mg/dL is the patient's individual lag time.

When blood glucose values are higher than the pre-meal target, increase lag time and allow the insulin to decrease pre-meal values before eating. When blood glucose values are lower than the pre-meal target range, prevent hypoglycemia by delaying the injection until just before eating or until eating has begun.

Many type 1 diabetes patients now use insulin pumps, which are programmed to continuously provide a basal rate of insulin, allowing the patient to bolus insulin to handle CHO intake or adjust blood glucose levels. Rapid-acting insulins are almost always the desired insulin for use in insulin pumps.

Adjustments for Exercise

Encourage patients with type 1 diabetes to exercise at the same time every day, for the same duration, and at the same intensity to facilitate consistent therapy adjustments that will reduce the chances of severe hypoglycemia. In addition, SMBG before and after exercise will help identify necessary changes in food or insulin intake and educate the patient about his or her individual glycemic response to exercise.

The following guidelines apply primarily to patients with type 1 diabetes. Patients with type 2 diabetes are less likely to experience exercise-induced hypoglycemia or need supplementary CHO, which, if given, counteracts weight loss efforts.

- When the patient plans to exercise after a meal, begin by cutting the meal-related rapid- or short-acting insulin dose in half. Use SMBG results to determine whether the lowered dose resulted in hyperglycemia, glucose within the target range (70-130 mg/dL), or hypoglycemia. If needed, adjust up or down by 3% of total daily insulin requirements to prepare for a similar (timing, duration, intensity) bout of exercise.
- When the patient plans to exercise before eating, he or she may need to eat supplementary CHO. This is a simpler option than reducing the basal insulin dose active preprandially.

INSULIN FOR TYPE 2 PATIENTS

Patients with type 2 diabetes may lie anywhere on the continuum of predominant insulin resistance with relative insulin deficiency to a predominant secretory defect and insulin deficiency with insulin resistance. Diet and exercise constitute the first course of therapy for type 2 diabetes and remain central to therapy, even with the addition of pharmacologic treatments. Nutrition therapy should include calorie restriction for weight loss.

Use of oral agents, combinations of oral agents, and new injectable drugs, such as exenatide, may postpone the need for insulin treatment for many years. This period may produce acceptable A_{1c} levels, but the disease usually progresses. Insulin, if given in sufficient doses, is often capable of restoring glycemia to near normal in most patients with type 2 diabetes. For prescribing information on specific insulin products, see **Table 3.4**; for drug interactions, see **Table 3.5**.

Adding Insulin to Oral Agent Therapy

Adding a simple insulin regimen to treatment with a sulfonylurea, metformin, thiazolidinedione, dipeptidyl peptidase-4 inhibitor (sitagliptin), or combination of oral agents will improve glycemic levels in patients unable to reach glycemic goals with oral agents alone or with exenatide, and is convenient for the patient, thus improving compliance and acceptance.

- **Fasting levels above target:** The oral agent can be used to control glucose levels during the day, and the insulin can be used to better control fasting (pre-breakfast) levels.

A single bedtime injection of insulin glargine, detemir, or NPH can be added to the current dose of the oral agent. To prevent hypoglycemia, a conservative starting dose is 0.15 units/kg, titrating up in increments of 2 units every 5-7 days based on fasting blood glucose levels. Patients may be instructed to titrate their own dose upward every 5-7 days while fasting glucose is above a predetermined target until fasting goals are achieved. Results must be carefully monitored with SMBG done at least twice daily, before breakfast and before supper. More frequent SMBG is recommended.

- **Fasting levels at target; values during day above target:** If, once the fasting level is normal, glucose levels during the day are out of the target range, consider:
  - if using bedtime NPH, adding a second injection of NPH before breakfast at a dose of 0.15 X body weight in kilograms, while continuing the bedtime dose;
  - adding regular or a rapid-acting insulin pre-meal. As a starting point, calculate the dose as 1 unit/10 g CHO in the meal (see "Determining Insulin-to-CHO Ratio" on page 50); or
  - following an insulin protocol as for type 1 diabetes (using an insulin pump also produces good blood glucose outcomes). Note that most insulin pumps now sold are to patients with type 2 diabetes who use insulin.

Insulin-Only Therapy

Typically, patients with type 2 diabetes begin an insulin regimen with one bedtime injection of insulin glargine, detemir, or NPH to control fasting hyperglycemia while beginning or continuing therapy with oral medications to control meal-related glycemic increases and/or reduce insulin resistance. However, when the daytime glucose levels are frequently >250 mg/dL (uncontrolled by maximal doses of oral

medications), insulin deficiency may be profound, and many patients benefit from treatment that is similar to that for type 1 diabetes, using a rapid-acting insulin before meals in conjunction with the basal insulin.

Troubleshooting

Patient Resistance to Starting Insulin
Many type 2 diabetes patients would be better controlled on insulin but resist beginning injections despite rising glycemic levels. Education is the key to gaining patient acceptance when insulin therapy is indicated.

- Reinforce the short-term benefits of improved glycemia, including decreased nocturia and improved energy level.
- Reinforce or reintroduce information about the importance of controlling glucose levels and how it relates to the health of kidneys, eyes, and nerves and to overall well-being.
- Teach patients with type 2 diabetes that the disease course includes progressive β-cell failure and that insulin therapy is a normal part of the treatment of the condition, not a sign of failure on the part of the patient.
- Avoid using the prospect of insulin therapy as a threat to increase adherence to lifestyle change or other therapies.
- Suggest that the patient try a bedtime injection routine of insulin glargine, detemir, or NPH for 1-2 months, then plan to discuss whether the patient feels better and has more energy.
- Point out that the newer, sharper, better beveled and lubricated needles make insulin therapy essentially painless and much more convenient than before, and offer alternatives to syringes, such as pen injectors.
- Provide or refer the patient for diabetes self-management education on handling and filling syringes and making injections as comfortable as possible.

Weight Gain

Minimizing weight gain, or promoting weight loss, in patients with type 2 diabetes is vital. Weight loss of even a modest amount reduces insulin resistance and improves glycemic control. Instituting insulin, sulfonylurea, or thiazolidinedione therapy is associated with weight gain in part because, as glycemic control improves, glucose is captured by the body instead of being lost in the urine and promotes growth of adipose tissue.

A single injection of insulin glargine, detemir, or NPH before bedtime can be associated with modest weight gain. Metformin plus bedtime insulin glargine, detemir, or NPH seems to blunt this effect. Patients beginning insulin therapy should be advised to decrease calorie intake and increase exercise to avoid weight gain. Slow and careful titration of the insulin to prevent hypoglycemic events can also help in minimizing weight gain with insulin therapy.

Fasting (Morning) Hyperglycemia

Fasting (morning) hyperglycemia is common when the evening basal dose of insulin is inadequate or when NPH is given with the evening meal instead of at bedtime. The early morning rise in glycemic levels due to the dawn phenomenon combined with waning NPH insulin creates high pre-breakfast glucose levels. The solution is to delay injection of the NPH insulin until bedtime or to substitute longer-acting insulin glargine or detemir for NPH. If NPH is being given at bedtime or insulin glargine or detemir is being used, the dose may need to be increased until target levels are achieved.

A strong dawn phenomenon response that cannot be accommodated with these maneuvers may be resolved with an insulin pump. The pump can be programmed to provide a lower basal dose between midnight and 4 a.m. and an increased basal amount between 4 a.m. and 8 a.m.

Hypoglycemia

Hypoglycemia is defined as blood glucose values <70 mg/dL in most patients. Patient symptoms vary; patients with hypoglycemia unawareness—primarily those with type 1 diabetes who have had frequent bouts of hypoglycemia—may have no symptoms and are at particular risk for severe hypoglycemia (see "Hypoglycemia Unawareness" at the end of this section). Each individual must learn to recognize when to perform SMBG to confirm suspected lows.

Patients with type 1 diabetes can learn to avoid exercise-related hypoglycemia with careful planning that includes adjusting either the pre-meal rapid- or short-acting insulin dose or CHO intake (see "Adjustments for Exercise" on page 9). Patients with type 2 diabetes generally do not experience exercise-induced hypoglycemia or need supplementary CHO, which can counteract weight loss efforts.

Mild hypoglycemia can be treated by the "rule of 15": Treat with 15 g fat-free CHO, wait 15 minutes, and then repeat SMBG. Levels still below target range warrant repeating the treatment. Once normal blood glucose is achieved, a snack may be necessary when a meal is not imminent.

Patients should be encouraged to always carry glucose/dextrose tablets with them to rapidly treat low blood glucose levels (see Chapter 20 on Hypoglycemia). When the patient has severe hypoglycemia and glucose cannot be given orally, subcutaneous or intramuscular glucagon is indicated.

Hypoglycemia Unawareness

Some patients lose their ability to recognize normal warning symptoms of hypoglycemia, or their symptoms are absent or blunted. These patients are at high risk to progress to severe hypoglycemia. Hypoglycemia unawareness develops more commonly in type 1 diabetes patients who have frequent hypoglycemic episodes and have had diabetes for a long time. Preventing hypoglycemia can reverse hypoglycemia unawareness. Hypoglycemia awareness training can also improve patient recognition of early manifestations of hypoglycemia and prevent episodes of severe hypoglycemia.

For more information on these and other professional titles published by the ADA:
- Visit the ADA online bookstore at http://store.diabetes.org.
- Call 1-800-232-3472.
- Visit any nationwide bookseller.

PATIENT EDUCATION

Perhaps the most important aspect of diabetes care is the patient-health care provider relationship. The essential element of this partnership is patient education. Encourage your patients to learn all they can about how to control their glucose levels, including making appropriate insulin dose adjustments in response to SMBG.

Stress to your patients that testing, record keeping, healthy eating, and exercise are for their benefit. Healthy living with diabetes is directly due to their success at diabetes self-management.

A wide variety of patient education materials is available from the American Diabetes Association. Your patients can reach the American Diabetes Association Call Center at 1-800-DIABETES and visit the ADA website at www.diabetes.org.

The American Diabetes Association has a wide variety of medical management publications for health care professionals, such as these books:

Medical Management of Type 1 Diabetes
Medical Management of Type 2 Diabetes
Medical Management of Pregnancy
  Complicated by Diabetes
Therapy for Diabetes Mellitus and
  Related Disorders
Intensive Diabetes Management
Clinical Care of the Diabetic Foot
Complementary and Alternative Medicine
  Supplement Use in People with Diabetes:
A Clinician's Guide

ADDITIONAL INFORMATION

Additives

All insulin preparations contain spoilage retardants. In addition, NPH (neutral protamine Hagedorn) contains an absorption-inhibiting substance that prolongs the action and contributes to the uniformly cloudy appearance. Regular insulin, insulin lispro, insulin aspart, insulin glulisine, insulin detemir, and insulin glargine preparations are clear.

Because of component precipitation, NPH and insulin combinations should be rolled gently between the hands to mix the components before drawing up the dose. Shaking incorporates air, creating the problem of air bubbles in the syringe.

Determining Insulin-to-CHO Ratio

For many patients, a 1:10 or 1:15 insulin-to-CHO ratio holds true. However, other patients have a different ratio or may have a 1:10 ratio except when eating certain foods. Insulin-resistant patients may have much lower ratios. Ratios at breakfast may be lower than at other meals if the relative percentage of calories from CHO is higher, which is common.

If glucose levels 1-2 hours after eating exceed 160 mg/dL, the insulin-to-CHO ratio requires recalculation. In general, each unit of short- or rapid-acting insulin reduces blood glucose by 20 mg/dL; however, this should be individually determined in each patient by SMBG.

The following two examples show insulin-to-CHO ratio calculations. Encourage your patients to perform this calculation after different meals and different foods to understand their typical insulin-to-CHO ratio.

Example 1:
A patient with pre-meal glucose levels in the target range consumed 50 g CHO at lunch and took 5 units short-acting insulin to cover the meal. One-hour postprandial glucose was 200 mg/dL (40 mg/dL too high) indicating that: 1) the total pre-lunch insulin dose was 2 units too small (if each unit reduces the patient's glucose level by 20 mg/dL), and 2) the patient has a larger insulin-to-CHO ratio. To recalculate the ratio:

Insulin taken for food	5 units
Additional insulin needed	2 units
Total dose should have been	7 units

If 7 units would have been correct for 50 g CHO, then:

$$\frac{7 \text{ units}}{1 \text{ unit}} \times \frac{50 \text{ CHO}}{X} = \frac{50}{7X} = 7.14, \text{ a 1:7 insulin: CHO ratio}$$

This patient would better match insulin to CHO using 1 unit of insulin for every 7 g CHO in meals.

Example 2:
Same meal composition, different patient, within target pre-meal glucose level but a 1-hour postprandial glucose level of 240 mg/dL. Therefore, 4 extra units should have been added to the 5 units for food. This ratio is calculated as:

$$\frac{9 \text{ units}}{1 \text{ unit}} \times \frac{50 \text{ CHO}}{X} = \frac{50}{9X} = 5.56, \text{ a 1:6 insulin: CHO ratio}$$

This patient would better match insulin to CHO using 1 unit of insulin for every 6 g CHO in meals.

Please note that all of these ratios are rough estimates of what a patient might do. Many variables are in place that can change the scenario, and it is best for patients to keep good records and remember that when and where they inject, what they have consumed in terms of CHO, how much and when they have exercised, their degree of stress and other factors can impact the need for insulin.

Endogenous Insulin Action
Insulin is produced in the islets of Langerhans by β-cells and secreted in response to rising blood glucose levels. β-cells sense glycemic levels and maintain euglycemia by 1) basal release of insulin, and 2) postprandial bolus release of insulin.

Insulin Delivery
Options, in order of increasing cost of use, include syringes, pens with disposable cartridges, prefilled disposable pens, and the insulin pump. Consider the patient's ability to prepare and inject each insulin dose when recommending a delivery method. The use of an insulin pump requires considerable patient education and office staff support until mastered. Patients using a pump must be motivated and committed to tight glycemic control.

Insulin Potency
Insulin potency is measured in units. All preparations sold in the U.S. are available in unit-100 strength, indicating 100 units/mL. Lilly manufactures a regular human insulin that is available by prescription only in a U-500 strength (500 units/mL), which is reserved for special circumstances, such as severe insulin resistance.

Insulin Pumps
Motivated patients who are performing multiple injections and SMBG per day and who desire flexibility to compensate for unsched-

uled activities may be candidates for an insulin pump. Also, patients with a strong dawn phenomenon or with severe hypoglycemia may have better control of these problems with pumps. Any patient starting insulin pump therapy needs education and support above and beyond the usual until he or she becomes skilled at pump use and troubleshooting. Consider referring patients for education sessions with a diabetologist or diabetes educator trained and experienced in pump therapy.

Note that in 2006 the FDA approved some continuous glucose monitors that send real-time interstitial fluid values to the insulin pump for viewing. Because interstitial fluid glucose correlates highly with blood glucose, this allows patients to evaluate their blood glucose values in real time. Such devices may be a welcome addition to pump therapy.

Rapid-acting insulins—lispro, aspart, and glulisine—are well suited for use in pumps. In general, the basal infusion rate for a pump is calculated as 0.3 units/kg body weight divided over 24 hours. Pumps are generally programmed by dividing the day into four parts, although each patient's program will need to be refined to fit individual requirements.

Bolus doses are given to cover CHO content of food in meals. A starting point is to assume that 1 unit of rapid- or short-acting insulin covers 10 g CHO. However, fine-tuning requires calculation of the individual's insulin-to-CHO ratio (see "Determining Insulin-to-CHO Ratio" on page 50).

Insulin Storage

Unopened vials, cartridges, and pens of insulin should be refrigerated at 36-46°F and used before the expiration date. Vial stoppers will maintain a sufficient seal for about 100 punctures, and once opened, insulin vials can be stored at room temperature for about a month. Injecting cold insulin can be uncomfortable. Follow the manufacturer's recommendations for storing open insulin pens or cartridges.

Freezing, exposure to direct sunlight, or high temperatures (>86°F) will decrease insulin potency. Instruct patients to examine insulin appearance before drawing up the injection. NPH insulin should appear uniformly cloudy without clumping or sediment after gentle resuspension; rapid- and short-acting insulins, insulin glargine, and insulin detemir are always clear.

SUGGESTED READING

Bode B. *Medical Management of Type 1 Diabetes, 4th Edition*. American Diabetes Association. Alexandria, VA, 2003.

DeWitt DE, Hirsch IB. Outpatient insulin therapy in type 1 and type 2 diabetes mellitus. *JAMA*. 2003;289:2254-2264.

Mooradian AD, Bernbaum M, Albert SG. Narrative review: a rational approach to starting insulin therapy. *Ann Intern Med*. 2006;145(2):125-134.

Oiknine R, Bernbaum M, Mooradian AD. A critical appraisal of the role of insulin analogues in the management of diabetes mellitus. *Drugs*. 2005;65(3):325-340.

Campbell RK. *Practical Insulin, 2nd Edition*. American Diabetes Association. Alexandria, VA, 2007.

Walsh J, Roberts R, Varma C, et al. *Using Insulin*. San Diego: Torrey Pines Press, 2003.

Table 3.4: Prescribing Information for Insulins

BRAND (GENERIC)	FORM/ STRENGTH	DOSAGE	WARNINGS/PRECAUTIONS & CONTRAINDICATIONS	ADVERSE REACTIONS
RAPID-ACTING				
Apidra (insulin glulisine)	**Inj:** 100 U/mL	***Adults:*** Individualize dose. Inject SQ within 15 min before a meal or within 20 min after starting a meal. Rotate inj site (abdomen, thigh, or deltoid).	**W/P:** Hypoglycemia and hypokalemia may occur; monitor glucose and potassium levels. Rapid onset and short duration of action; follow dosage directions. Adjust dose if change in physical activity or usual meal plan. Longer-acting insulin or insulin infusion pump may be required to maintain glucose control. When used in an external pump for SQ infusion, do not dilute or mix with any other insulin. Caution when changing insulin strength, manufacturer, type, or species. Concomitant antidiabetic therapy may need adjustment. As with other insulin therapy hypoglycemic reactions and local/systemic allergic reactions may occur. May be given IV under proper medical supervision. Caution in renal/hepatic impairment. **Contra:** Episodes of hypoglycemia. **P/N:** Category C, caution in nursing.	Allergic reactions, injection site reactions, lipodystrophy, pruritus, rash, hypoglycemia.
Humalog (insulin lispro)	**Cartridge:** 100 U/mL; **Inj:** 100 U/mL; **Pen:** 100 U/mL	***Adults/Pediatrics:*** ≥3 yrs: Individualize dose. Inject SQ within 15 min before or immediately after a meal. May use with external insulin pump; do not dilute or mix with other insulin when used with pump.	**W/P:** Any change of insulin should be made cautiously. Changes in strength manufacturer, type or method of manufacture may result in the need for a change in dosage. Hypoglycemia may occur with taking too much insulin, missing or delaying meals, exercising or working more than usual. An infection or illness (especially with diarrhea or vomiting) may change insulin requirements. With type 1 DM a longer-acting insulin is usually required to maintain glucose control; not required with type 2 DM if regimen includes sulfonylureas. May be diluted with sterile diluent. Caution with potassium-lowering drugs or drugs sensitive to serum potassium levels. **Contra:** Hypoglycemia. **P/N:** Category B, caution in nursing.	Hypoglycemia, hypokalemia, allergic reaction, injection site reaction, lipodystrophy, pruritus, rash.
Novolog (insulin aspart)	**Inj:** 100 U/mL; **PenFill:** 100 U/mL; **Prefilled:** 100 U/mL	***Adults/Pediatrics:*** ≥4 yrs: Individualize dose. Inject SQ within 5-10 min before a meal. Draw first when mixing with NPH human insulin; inject immediately. Do not mix with crystalline zinc insulins, animal source insulins, or other manufacturer insulins. (External Pump) Do not use or mix with any other insulin or diluent in pump.	**W/P:** Any change of insulin should be made cautiously. Changes in strength, manufacturer, type or method of manufacture may result in the need for a change in dosage. Hypoglycemia may occur with taking too much insulin, missing or delaying meals, exercising or working more than usual, diseases of adrenal, pituitary, or thyroid glands, or progression of kidney or liver disease. May cause hypokalemia. Dosage adjustments may be needed with hepatic or renal dysfunction, during any infection, illness (especially with diarrhea or vomiting) or pregnancy. A longer-acting insulin is usually required to maintain adequate glucose control. Infusion sets and the insulin in the infusion sets should be changed q48h or sooner. Do not use in quick-release infusion sets or cartridge adapters. **Contra:** Hypoglycemia. **P/N:** Category B, caution in nursing.	Hypoglycemia, hypokalemia, lipodystrophy, hypersensitivity reaction, injection site reactions, pruritus, rash.

W/P = warnings/precautions; **Contra** = contraindications; **P/N** = pregnancy category rating and nursing considerations.

Table 3.4: Prescribing Information for Insulins

BRAND (GENERIC)	FORM/ STRENGTH	DOSAGE	WARNINGS/PRECAUTIONS & CONTRAINDICATIONS	ADVERSE REACTIONS
SHORT-ACTING AND INTERMEDIATE-ACTING				
Humulin R (insulin human, regular), **Humulin N*** (NPH, isophane)	**Inj:** 100 U/mL (Humulin N, Humulin R), 500 U/mL (Humulin R U-500); **Pen:** 100 U/mL (Humulin N)	***Adults/Pediatrics:*** Individualize dose.	**W/P:** Human insulin differs from animal source insulin. Any change in insulin should be made cautiously. Changes in strength, manufacturer, type or method of manufacture may result in the need for a change in dosage. Hypoglycemia may occur with taking too much insulin, missing or delaying meals, exercising or working more than usual. An infection or illness (especially with diarrhea or vomiting) may change insulin requirements. Administration of insulin SQ can result in lipoatrophy. **Contra:** Hypoglycemia. **P/N:** Pregnancy category is not known.	Hypoglycemia, sweating, dizziness, palpitation, tremor, hunger, restlessness, lightheadedness, inability to concentrate, headache, injection site reaction, allergic reaction.
Novolin R (insulin human, regular), **Novolin N*** (NPH, isophane)	**Inj:** 100 U/mL (Novolin N, Novolin R); **PenFill:** 100 U/mL (Novolin N, Novolin R); **Prefilled:** 100 U/mL (Novolin N, Novolin R)	***Adults/Pediatrics:*** Individualize dose.	**W/P:** Human insulin differs from animal source insulin. Any change in insulin should be made cautiously. Changes in strength, manufacturer, type or method of manufacture may result in the need for a change in dosage. Hypoglycemia may occur with taking too much insulin, missing or delaying meals, exercising or working more than usual. An infection or illness (especially if accompanied by diarrhea or vomiting) may change insulin requirements. Administration of insulin SQ can result in lipoatrophy. Novolin R is not recommended for use in insulin pumps. **P/N:** Pregnancy category is not known.	Hypoglycemia, sweating, dizziness, palpitations, tremor, hunger, restlessness, lightheadedness, inability to concentrate, headache, injection-site reaction, allergic reaction.
LONG-ACTING				
Lantus (insulin glargine)	**Inj:** 100 U/mL; **OptiClik:** 100 U/mL	***Adults/Pediatrics:*** ≥6 yrs: Individualize dose. For SQ injection only. Administer qd at same time each day. Insulin naive patients on oral antidiabetic drugs, start with 10 U qd. Switching from once-daily NPH or Ultralente does not require initial dose change. Switching from bid NPH, reduce initial dose by 20%. Maint: 2-100 U/day.	**W/P:** Human insulin differs from animal source insulin. Any change in insulin should be made cautiously. Changes in strength, manufacturer, type or method of manufacture may result in the need for a change in dosage. Hypoglycemia may occur with taking too much insulin, missing or delaying meals, exercising or working more than usual. An infection or illness (especially with diarrhea or vomiting) may change insulin requirements. Administration of insulin SQ can result in lipodystrophy. Not for IV use. Do not mix with other insulins. May cause sodium retention and edema. Caution in patients with renal and hepatic dysfunction. **P/N:** Category C, caution in nursing.	Hypoglycemia, allergic reactions, injection site reactions, lipodystrophy, pruritus, rash.
Levmir (insulin detemir)	**Inj:** 100 U/mL [3mL, 10mL]	***Adults:*** Individualize dose. Administer SQ qd or bid. **Once-Daily Dosing:** Administer with evening meal or bedtime. **Twice-Daily Dosing:** Administer evening dose with evening meal, at bedtime, or 12 hrs after morning dose. **Type 1/Type 2 Diabetes on Basal-Bolus Treatment or Patients Only on Basal Insulin:** Change on a unit-to-unit basis. **Insulin-Naive with Type 2 Diabetes Inadequately Controlled on Oral Antidiabetics:** Initial: 0.1-0.2 U/kg in evening or 10 U qd or bid. ***Pediatrics:*** Individualize dose. Administer SQ qd or bid. **Once-Daily Dosing:** Administer with evening meal or bedtime. **Twice-Daily Dosing:** Administer evening dose with evening meal, at bedtime, or 12 hrs after morning dose. **Type 1 Diabetes on Basal-Bolus Treatment or Patients Only on Basal Insulin:** Change on a unit-to-unit basis.	**W/P:** Monitor glucose; may cause hypoglycemia. Not for use in an insulin infusion pump. Should not be diluted or mixed with any other insulin preparations. May cause lipodystrophy or hypersensitivity. Dose adjustment may be needed in renal or hepatic impairment and during intercurrent conditions such as illness, emotional disturbances, or other stresses. **P/N:** Category C, caution in nursing.	Allergic reactions, injection site reactions, lipodystrophy, pruritus, rash, hypoglycemia, weight gain.

*Intermediate-acting insulin.
W/P = warnings/precautions; **Contra** = contraindications; **P/N** = pregnancy category rating and nursing considerations.

Table 3.4: Prescribing Information for Insulins

BRAND (GENERIC)	FORM/ STRENGTH	DOSAGE	WARNINGS/PRECAUTIONS & CONTRAINDICATIONS	ADVERSE REACTIONS
COMBINATION PRODUCTS				
Humalog Mix 75/25 (insulin lispro protamine/insulin lispro)	(Insulin Lispro Protamine, Human-Insulin Lispro, Human) **Inj:** 75 U-25 U/mL; **Pen:** 75 U-25 U/mL	***Adults:*** Individualize dose. Inject SQ within 15 min before a meal. May need to reduce/adjust dose with renal/hepatic impairment.	**W/P:** Any change of insulin should be made cautiously. Changes in strength, manufacturer, type or method of manufacture may result in the need for a change in dosage. Hypoglycemia may occur with taking too much insulin, missing or delaying meals, exercising or working more than usual. An infection or illness (especially with diarrhea or vomiting) may change insulin requirements. **Contra:** Hypoglycemia. **P/N:** Category B, caution in nursing.	Hypoglycemia, hypokalemia, allergic reaction, injection site reaction, lipodystrophy, pruritus, rash.
Humulin 50/50 Humulin 70/30 (isophane/regular insulin)	(Isophane/Regular) **Inj:** (Humulin 70/30) 70 U-30 U/mL (Humulin 50/50) 50 U-50 U/mL	***Adults/Pediatrics:*** Individualize dose. Administer SQ.	**W/P:** Human insulin differs from animal source insulin. Make any change of insulin cautiously. Changes in strength, manufacturer, type, or method of manufacture may result in the need for a change in dosage. Hypoglycemia may occur with too much insulin, missing or delaying meals, exercising, or working more than usual. Infection or illness (especially with diarrhea or vomiting) may change insulin requirements. Administration of insulin SQ can result in lipoatrophy. **P/N:** Pregnancy category is not known.	Hypoglycemia, sweating, dizziness, palpitation, tremor, hunger, restlessness, lightheadedness, inability to concentrate, headache, injection site reaction, allergic reaction.
Novolin 70/30 (isophane/ regular insulin)	(Isophane/Regular) **Inj:** 70 U-30 U/mL; **PenFill:** 70 U-30 U/mL; **Prefilled:** 70 U-30 U/mL	***Adults/Pediatrics:*** Individualize dose. Administer SQ.	**W/P:** Human insulin differs from animal source insulin. Any change of insulin should be made cautiously. Changes in strength, manufacturer, type or method of manufacture may result in the need for a change in dosage. Hypoglycemia may occur with taking too much insulin, missing or delaying meals, exercising or working more than usual. An infection or illness (especially with diarrhea or vomiting) may change insulin requirements. Caution with diseases of adrenal, pituitary, or thyroid glands, or progression of kidney or liver disease. Administration of insulin SQ can result in lipoatrophy. **P/N:** Pregnancy category is not known.	Hypoglycemia, sweating, dizziness, palpitation, tremor, hunger, restlessness, lightheadedness, inability to concentrate, headache, injection site reaction, allergic reaction.
Novolog Mix 50/50 (nsulin aspart protamine/ insulin aspart injection)	Insulin Aspart Protamine/Insulin Aspart) **Inj:** 100 U/mL	***Adults:*** For SQ inj only. Inject tid within 15 min of meal.	**W/P:** Exhibits peak pharmacodynamic activity between 1 and 4 hrs; administer with meals. Should not be administered IV and not for use with insulin infusion pumps. Should not be mixed with any other insulin product. Possible hypoglycemia, hypokalemia, sodium retention, and edema. Caution with fasting, autonomic neuropathy, on potassium-lowering drugs, and drugs sensitive to serum potassium levels. Administration of insulin SQ can result in lipoatrophy. Requirements may be reduced in patients with renal and/or hepatic impairment. Illness, stress, change in meals, and exercise may change insulin requirements. **Contra:** Hypoglycemia. **P/N:** Category C, safety in nursing not known.	Hypoglycemia, hypokalemia, lipoatrophy, hypersensitivity reactions, injection site reactions, pruritus, rash.
Novolog Mix 70/30 (insulin aspart protamine/insulin aspart)	(Insulin Aspart Protamine/Insulin Aspart) **Inj:** 70 U-30 U/mL; **PenFill:** 70 U-30 U/mL; **Prefilled:** 70 U-30 U/mL	***Adults:*** Individualize dose. For SQ inj only. Inject SQ bid within 15 min before breakfast and dinner. Do not mix with other insulins or use in insulin pumps.	**W/P:** Any change of insulin should be made cautiously. Changes in strength, manufacturer, type or method of manufacture may result in the need for a change in dosage. Hypoglycemia and hypokalemia may occur; caution with fasting and autonomic neuropathy. Illness, stress, change in meals and exercise may	Hypoglycemia, hypokalemia, lipodystrophy, hypersensitivity reaction, injection site reactions, pruritus, rash.

W/P = warnings/precautions; **Contra** = contraindications; **P/N** = pregnancy category rating and nursing considerations.

Table 3.4: Prescribing Information for Insulins

BRAND (GENERIC)	FORM/ STRENGTH	DOSAGE	WARNINGS/PRECAUTIONS & CONTRAINDICATIONS	ADVERSE REACTIONS
COMBINATION PRODUCTS *(Cont.)*				
Novolog Mix 70/30 (insulin aspart protamine/insulin aspart) *(Cont.)*			change insulin requirements. Smoking, temperature, and exercise affect insulin absorption. Caution with liver or kidney disease. Administration of insulin SQ can result in lipoatrophy. **Contra:** Hypoglycemia. **P/N:** Category C, safety in nursing not known.	

W/P = warnings/precautions; **Contra** = contraindications; **P/N** = pregnancy category rating and nursing considerations.

Table 3.5. Drug Interactions for Insulins

RAPID-ACTING

Apidra (insulin glulisine)

ACE inhibitors	Increases insulin effect.
Alcohol	May decrease or increase insulin effect.
Antidiabetics, oral	Increases insulin effect.
Antipsychotics, atypical (eg, olanzapine, clozapine)	Decreases insulin effect.
Beta-blockers	May decrease or increase insulin effects; may reduce or mask signs of hypoglycemia.
Clonidine	May decrease or increase insulin effects; may reduce or mask signs of hypoglycemia.
Corticosteroids	Decreases insulin effect.
Danazol	Decreases insulin effect.
Diazoxide	Decreases insulin effect.
Disopyramide	Increases insulin effect.
Diuretics	Decreases insulin effect.
Estrogens	Decreases insulin effect.
Fibrates	Increases insulin effect.
Fluoxetine	Increases insulin effect.
Glucagon	Decreases insulin effect.
Guanethidine	May reduce or mask signs of hypoglycemia.
Isoniazid	Decreases insulin effect.
Lithium salts	Decreases or increases insulin effect.
MAO inhibitors	Increases insulin effect.
Pentamidine	May initially cause hypoglycemia followed by hyperglycemia.
Pentoxifylline	Increases insulin effect.
Phenothiazine derivatives	Decreases insulin effect.
Progestogens	Decreases insulin effect.
Propoxyphene	Increases insulin effect.
Protease inhibitors	Decreases insulin effect.
Reserpine	May reduce or mask signs of hypoglycemia.
Salicylates	Increases insulin effect.
Somatropin	Decreases insulin effect.
Sulfonamides	Increases insulin effect.
Sympathomimetic agents (eg, epinephrine, albuterol, terbutaline)	Decreases insulin effect.
Thyroid hormones	Decreases insulin effect.

Table 3.5. Drug Interactions for Insulins

Humalog (insulin lispro)

ACE inhibitors	Decreases insulin requirements.
Alcohol	Decreases insulin requirements.
Angiotensin Receptor Blockers (ARBs)	Decreases insulin requirements.
Beta-blockers	Decreases insulin requirements; may mask the symptoms of hypoglycemia.
Contraceptives, oral	Increases insulin requirements.
Corticosteroids	Increases insulin requirements.
Estrogens	Increases insulin requirements.
Hypoglycemic agents, oral	Decreases insulin requirements.
Isoniazid	Increases insulin requirements.
MAO inhibitors	Decreases insulin requirements.
Niacin	Increases insulin requirements.
Octreotide	Decreases insulin requirements.
Phenothiazines	Increases insulin requirements.
Salicylates	Decreases insulin requirements.
Sulfonamides	Decreases insulin requirements.
Thyroid replacement therapy	Increases insulin requirements.

Novolog (insulin aspart)

ACE inhibitors	Increases glucose-lowering effects.
Alcohol	May potentiate or weaken blood glucose-lowering effect.
Antidiabetic agents, other	Increases glucose-lowering effects.
Beta-blockers	May potentiate or weaken blood glucose-lowering effect; causes masked or reduced hypoglycemic symptoms.
Clonidine	May potentiate or weaken blood glucose-lowering effect; causes masked or reduced hypoglycemic symptoms.
Corticosteroids	Decreases glucose-lowering effects.
Danazol	Decreases glucose-lowering effects.
Disopyramide	Increases glucose-lowering effects.
Diuretics	Decreases blood glucose-lowering effects.
Estrogens	Decreases blood glucose-lowering effects.
Fibrates	Increase glucose-lowering effects.
Fluoxetine	Increases glucose-lowering effects.
Guanethidine	Masks or reduces hypoglycemic symptoms.
Isoniazid	Decreases blood glucose-lowering effects.
Lithium salts	May potentiate or weaken blood glucose-lowering effect.
MAO inhibitors	Increases glucose-lowering effects.

Table 3.5. Drug Interactions for Insulins

Niacin	Decreases glucose-lowering effects.
Pentamidine	May initially cause hypoglycemia followed by hyperglycemia.
Phenothiazine derivatives	Decreases glucose-lowering effects.
Progesterones	Decreases glucose-lowering effects.
Propoxyphene	Increases glucose-lowering effects.
Reserpine	Masks or reduces hypoglycemic symptoms.
Salicylates	Increases glucose-lowering effects.
Somatostatin analog	Increases glucose-lowering effects.
Somatropin	Decreases glucose-lowering effects.
Sulfonamides	Increases glucose-lowering effects.
Sympathomimetic agents	Decreases glucose-lowering effects.
Thyroid hormones	Decreases glucose-lowering effects.

SHORT-ACTING AND INTERMEDIATE-ACTING
Humulin R, Novolin R; Humulin N*, Novolin N*
(insulin human-rDNA origin; insulin human-isophane* [NPH])

Alcohol	May cause changes in insulin requirements.
Antidepressants	Reduces insulin requirements.
Beta-blockers	May mask symptoms of hypoglycemia.
Contraceptives, oral	Increases insulin requirements.
Corticosteroids	Increases insulin requirements.
Hypoglycemic agents, oral	Reduces insulin requirements.
Salicylates	Reduces insulin requirements.
Sulfonamides	Reduces insulin requirements.
Thyroid replacement therapy	Increases insulin requirements.

LONG-ACTING
Lantus (insulin glargine)

ACE inhibitors	Increases glucose-lowering effects.
Alcohol	May potentiate or weaken glucose-lowering effect.
Antidiabetic agents, other	Increases glucose-lowering effects.
Antipsychotics, atypical	Decreases glucose-lowering effects.
Beta-blockers	May potentiate or weaken glucose-lowering effect; may reduce or mask signs of hypoglycemia.
Clonidine	May potentiate or weaken glucose-lowering effect; may reduce or mask signs of hypoglycemia.
Corticosteroids	Decreases glucose-lowering effects.
Danazol	Decreases glucose-lowering effects.

*Intermediate-acting insulin.

Table 3.5. Drug Interactions for Insulins

Disopyramide	Increases glucose-lowering effects.
Diuretics	Decreases glucose-lowering effects.
Estrogens	Decreases glucose-lowering effects.
Fibrates	Increases glucose-lowering effects.
Fluoxetine	Increases glucose-lowering effects.
Guanethidine	May reduce or mask signs of hypoglycemia.
Isoniazid	Decreased blood glucose-lowering effects.
Lithium salts	May potentiate or weaken glucose-lowering effect.
MAO inhibitors	Increases glucose-lowering effects.
Pentamidine	May initially cause hypoglycemia followed by hyperglycemia.
Phenothiazine derivatives	Decreases glucose-lowering effects.
Progestogens	Decreases glucose-lowering effects.
Propoxyphene	Increases glucose-lowering effects.
Protease inhibitors	Decreases glucose-lowering effects.
Reserpine	May reduce or mask signs of hypoglycemia.
Salicylates	Increases glucose-lowering effects.
Somatostatin analog	Increases glucose-lowering effects.
Somatropin	Decreases glucose-lowering effects.
Sulfonamides	Increases glucose-lowering effects.
Sympathomimetic amines	Decreases glucose-lowering effects.
Thyroid hormones	Decreases blood glucose-lowering effects.
Levemir (insulin detemir)	
ACE inhibitors	Increases glucose-lowering effects.
Alcohol	May potentiate or weaken glucose-lowering effect.
Antidiabetic agents, other	Increases glucose-lowering effects.
Beta-blockers	May potentiate or weaken glucose-lowering effect; may reduce or mask signs of hypoglycemia.
Clonidine	May potentiate or weaken glucose-lowering effect; may reduce or mask signs of hypoglycemia.
Corticosteroids	Decreases glucose-lowering effects.
Danazol	Decreases glucose-lowering effects.
Disopyramide	Increases glucose-lowering effects.
Diuretics	Decreases glucose-lowering effects.
Estrogens	Decreases glucose-lowering effects.
Fibrates	Increases glucose-lowering effects.
Fluoxetine	Increases glucose-lowering effects.
Guanethidine	May reduce or mask signs of hypoglycemia.

Table 3.5. Drug Interactions for Insulins

Insulins, other	Caution, avoid mixing with other insulins.
Isoniazid	Decreased blood glucose-lowering effects.
Lithium salts	May potentiate or weaken glucose-lowering effect.
MAO inhibitors	Increases glucose-lowering effects.
Pentamidine	May initially cause hypoglycemia followed by hyperglycemia.
Phenothiazine derivates	Decreases glucose-lowering effects.
Progestogens	Decreases glucose-lowering effects.
Propoxyphene	Increases glucose-lowering effects.
Reserpine	May reduce or mask signs of hypoglycemia.
Salicylates	Increases glucose-lowering effects.
Somatostatin analog	Increases glucose-lowering effects.
Somatotropin	Decreases glucose-lowering effects.
Sulfonamides	Increases glucose-lowering effects.
Sympathomimetic agents	Decreases glucose-lowering effects.
Thyroid hormones	Decreases glucose-lowering effects.

COMBINATION PRODUCTS

Humalog Mix 75/25 (insulin lispro-insulin lispro protamine)

ACE inhibitors	Decreases insulin requirements.
Alcohol	Decreases insulin requirements.
Angiotensin receptor blockers (ARBs)	Decreases insulin requirements.
Beta-blockers	Decreases insulin requirements; may mask signs of hypoglycemia.
Contraceptives, oral	Increases insulin requirements.
Corticosteroids	Increases insulin requirements.
Estrogens	Increases insulin requirements.
Hypoglycemic agents, oral	Decreases insulin requirements.
Isoniazid	Increases insulin requirements.
MAO inhibitors	Decreases insulin requirements.
Niacin	Increases insulin requirements.
Ocreotide	Decreases insulin requirements.
Phenothiazines	Increases insulin requirements.
Salicylates	Decreases insulin requirements.
Sulfonamides	Decreases insulin requirements.
Thyroid replacement therapy	Increases insulin requirements.

Table 3.5. Drug Interactions for Insulins

Humulin 50/50, Humulin 70/30, Novolin 70/30 (isophane insulin regular)

Alcohol	May change insulin requirements.
Antidepressants	May reduce insulin requirements.
Beta-blockers	May mask symptoms of hypoglycemia.
Contraceptives, oral	Increases insulin requirements.
Corticosteroids	Increases insulin requirements.
Hypoglycemic agents, oral	Reduces insulin requirements.
Salicylates	Reduces insulin requirements.
Sulfonamides	Reduces insulin requirements.
Thyroid replacement therapy	Increases insulin requirements.

Novolog Mix 50/50, Novolog Mix 70/30 (insulin aspart protamine-insulin aspart)

ACE inhibitors	Increases glucose-lowering effects.
Alcohol	May potentiate or weaken glucose-lowering effect.
Antidiabetic agents, other	Increases glucose-lowering effects.
Beta-blockers	May potentiate or weaken glucose-lowering effect; may reduce or mask signs of hypoglycemia.
Clonidine	May potentiate or weaken glucose-lowering effect; may reduce or mask signs of hypoglycemia.
Corticosteroids	Decreases glucose-lowering effects.
Danazol	Decreases glucose-lowering effects.
Disopyramide	Increases glucose-lowering effects.
Diuretics	Decreases glucose-lowering effects.
Estrogens	Decreases glucose-lowering effects.
Fibrates	Increases glucose-lowering effects.
Fluoxetine	Increases glucose-lowering effects.
Guanethidine	May reduce or mask signs of hypoglycemia.
Insulin products, other	Caution, do not mix with other insulins.
Isoniazid	Decreases glucose-lowering effects.
Lithium salts	May potentiate or weaken glucose-lowering effect.
MAO inhibitors	Increases glucose-lowering effects.
Niacin	Decreases glucose-lowering effects.
Pentamidine	May initally cause hypoglycemia followed by hyperglycemia.
Phenothiazine derivatives	Decreases glucose-lowering effects.
Potassium-lowering drugs (drugs sensitive to serum potassium levels)	May affect potassium levels, may cause hypoglycemia and hypokalemia.
Progesterones	Decreases glucose-lowering effects.

Table 3.5. Drug Interactions for Insulins

Propoxyphene	Increases glucose-lowering effects.
Reserpine	May reduce or mask signs of hypoglycemia.
Salicylates	Increases glucose-lowering effects.
Somatostatin analog (eg, octreotide)	Increases glucose-lowering effects.
Somatropin	Decreases glucose-lowering effects.
Sulfonamides	Increases glucose-lowering effects.
Sympathomimetics	Decreases glucose-lowering effects.
Thyroid hormones	Decreases glucose-lowering effects.

Chapter 4

Biguanides

John R. White, Jr., PharmD, PA

INTRODUCTION

Biguanides, in some form, have been used since medieval times. French lilac, or goat's rue (*Galega officinalis*) was used as a folk treatment for diabetes in southern and eastern Europe. Later, *G officinalis* was found to be rich in the compound guanidine. In 1918, the hypoglycemic activity of guanidine was confirmed. Unfortunately, guanidine was too toxic for human clinical use, but its chemical congeners, such as the alkyldiguanide synthalin A, were introduced in the early 1920s. Further analysis continued with the biguanide group in the 1920s. Clinical use of these compounds was not pursued as they fell into disfavor because of the discovery and availability of insulin products.

With the advent of sulfonylureas in the 1950s, biguanides were re-investigated for possible use in the treatment of diabetes. Metformin and phenformin were introduced in 1957, followed by buformin in 1958. No other active compounds in the biguanide category have been discovered, even though significant work on the structure-activity relationship has taken place. Clinical use of buformin was limited, but phenformin was used widely in the 1960s and 1970s. An association between phenformin and lactic acidosis resulted in the withdrawal of this compound from use in many countries. In the past decade, metformin has become the most relevant drug of the biguanide category, and perhaps the most widely used oral antihyperglycemic agent.

Metformin hydrochloride is indicated for monotherapeutic management of type 2 diabetes as an adjunct to nutrition and exercise in patients whose hyperglycemia cannot be satisfactorily managed by nutrition therapy alone. Additionally, metformin may be used concomitantly with other oral agents or with insulin.

PHARMACOLOGY

Mechanism of Action

Metformin causes a plethora of metabolic effects, including changes in carbohydrate and lipid metabolism. The effects of metformin on carbohydrate metabolism occur primarily in the liver. Metformin's main effect is associated with a reduction in basal hepatic glucose output in patients with type 2 diabetes. Approximately 75% of the reduction in hepatic glucose production occurs via blunting of gluconeogenesis while about 25% of the reduction occurs secondary to a modulation of glycogenolysis. Metformin also has been shown to enhance insulin-stimulated glucose transport in skeletal muscle. This effect is not as significant as the reduction in hepatic glucose production.

Pharmacokinetics

The absolute bioavailability of metformin ranges from 50%-60%. The compound is absorbed mainly from the small intestine, with an estimated absorption half-life of between 0.09 and 2.6 hours. The maximum concentration (C_{max}) of 1-2 mcg/mL is reached ~1-2 hours after an oral dose of between 500 and 1,000 mg. The drug undergoes negligible binding to plasma proteins. The half-life of metformin in individuals with normal renal function ranges from 1.5-4.9 hours. No measurable metabolism of metformin occurs.

In terms of elimination, ~90% of the compound is excreted via the urine within 12 hours of administration of the dose. The elimination is multiexponential, with drug loss via glomerular filtration and tubular secretion. Tubular secretion is thought to be a major route of metformin elimination because the renal clearance of this compound is ~3.5 times greater than creatinine clearance. The drug is widely distributed into most tissues in concentrations similar to those found in peripheral plasma. However, the highest concentrations are found in the salivary glands and in the intestinal wall. Relatively high concentrations are found in the liver and the kidney.

TREATMENT ADVANTAGES AND DISADVANTAGES

Metformin should arguably be the drug of first choice in the management of hyperglycemia in most obese patients with type 2 diabetes. Metformin therapy, unlike sulfonlyureas or thiazolidinediones, is not related to an increase in weight. In fact, many patients experience a mild degree of weight loss when treated with metformin. Additionally, metformin therapy may also result in a modest reduction in plasma triglyceride and low-density lipoprotein concentrations. Metformin

may also be used effectively with other oral agents and insulin. Metformin therapy can be expected to cause about a 1.5% reduction in HbA_{1c} levels.

Metformin is not tolerated by all patients, however, and also carries with it a number of relative and absolute contraindications.

THERAPEUTIC CONSIDERATIONS

Contraindications

Metformin is contraindicated in patients with:
- acute or chronic metabolic acidosis
- known hypersensitivity to metformin hydrochloride
- congestive heart failure Class 3 or 4
- renal disease or dysfunction (serum creatinine levels ≥1.5 mg/dL in male or ≥1.4 mg/dL in female patients) or abnormal creatinine clearance that may result from medical conditions such as cardiovascular collapse, acute myocardial infarction, or septicemia
- age >80 years, unless measurement of creatinine clearance demonstrates adequate renal function

Metformin should be discontinued temporarily in patients requiring radiological studies involving the use of iodinated contrast media because these agents are known to cause renal dysfunction in some individuals.

Precautions

Monitoring Renal Function

Metformin is known to be excreted via the kidneys; thus, the risk of accumulation of the medication is greater in patients with reduced renal function. The risk of lactic acidosis is increased in these patients as well. Therefore, patients with serum creatinine levels above the upper limit of normal for their age should not be treated with metformin. In elderly patients, renal function should be monitored periodically. This medication should *not* be used in patients >80 years of age unless measurement of creatinine clearance demonstrates that renal function is not reduced. It should be noted that these patients are more susceptible to the development of lactic acidosis.

Radiological Studies

Radiological studies involving the use of iodinated contrast media should be undertaken only after metformin has been discontinued. The drug should be withheld for at least 48 hours after the procedure and reinstituted only after serum creatinine levels have been shown to be normal.

Hypoxic States

Lactic acidosis is associated with cardiovascular collapse, acute congestive heart failure, acute myocardial infarction, and other conditions that cause hypoxemia. Therefore, metformin should be discontinued in patients with these medical conditions.

Surgical Procedures

Metformin therapy should be discontinued temporarily for any major surgical procedure and should be restarted only after the patient's oral intake has been resumed and renal function has shown to be normal.

Alcohol Intake

Metformin should be used cautiously in patients who are known to consume excessive alcohol, since this may lead to acidosis.

Impaired Hepatic Function

Impaired hepatic function has been associated with some cases of lactic acidosis; therefore, it is recommended that metformin not be used in patients with impaired hepatic function.

Vitamin B_{12} Levels

Seven percent of patients who are treated with metformin experience a reduction in vitamin B_{12} to subnormal levels. However, this is rarely associated with anemia and appears to be rapidly reversible with discontinuation of the medication or with vitamin B_{12} supplementation. Patients treated with metformin should therefore undergo measurement of hematological parameters annually. Hematological evaluation is also advised in any patient with apparent abnormalities. Routine serum vitamin B_{12} measurements approximately every 2-3 years may be useful in individuals with inadequate B_{12} or calcium intake and/or absorption.

Hypoglycemia

Hypoglycemia does not occur with metformin monotherapy under normal conditions. However, it may occur in patients in whom caloric intake is deficient; in patients who undertake strenuous exercise; in patients who are treated with other glucose-lowering agents, such as sulfonylureas; or in patients who consume alcohol.

SPECIAL POPULATIONS

Renal Insufficiency

In patients with reduced renal function, the plasma half-life of metformin is prolonged and the renal clearance is reduced in proportion to the decrease in creatinine clearance. For example, the renal clearance in a healthy nondiabetic patient with normal renal function given a dose of 850 mg is 552 mL/min, in comparison with patients with mildly (61-90 mL/min), moderately (31-60 mL/min), or severely (10-30 mL/min) impaired renal function, who demonstrate metformin clearances of 384, 108, and 130 mL/min, respectively.

Hepatic Insufficiency

No pharmacokinetic data are available in patients with hepatic insufficiency.

Geriatrics

Limited data are available in controlled pharmacokinetic studies evaluating the effects of age on metformin kinetics. However, it is known that total plasma clearance is lower, half-life is longer, and C_{max} is higher than in healthy young subjects. It appears that the change in metformin pharmacokinetics with aging is secondary to the changes in renal function that occur in the geriatric population.

Pediatrics

The safety and efficacy of metformin in pediatric patients between the ages of 10 and 16 has been established. Extended-release metformin has been evaluated in this population.

Gender

No pharmacokinetic differences have been observed between the sexes. Clinically, in controlled trials in patients with type 2 diabetes, no differences have been observed between male and female patients.

Ethnicity

Although no pharmacokinetic studies have been carried out evaluating differences among ethnic groups in controlled clinical trials, the effects of metformin have been shown to be comparable in non-Hispanic white, black, and Hispanic subjects.

ADVERSE EFFECTS AND MONITORING

Lactic Acidosis

Lactic acidosis is a very rare but extremely serious condition that can occur secondary to the accumulation of metformin. Lactic acidosis is fatal in ~50% of cases. Currently, the reported incidence of lactic acidosis in patients receiving metformin is extremely low (~0.03 cases per 1,000 patient-years), with a fatality rate of ~0.015 fatal cases per 1,000 patient-years. The majority of these cases have occurred in patients with significant renal insufficiency. The risk of lactic acidosis can be reduced by observing the aforementioned contraindications and precautions. Recent studies have demonstrated that if contraindications are adhered to, the rates of lactic acidosis in patients treated with metformin are no greater than background rates observed in similar patients not treated with metformin.

Gastrointestinal Reactions

Gastrointestinal symptoms, such as abdominal bloating, flatulence, anorexia, diarrhea, nausea, and vomiting, are the most common side effects observed in patients treated with metformin. Gastrointestinal complaints are ~30% more frequent in patients on metformin monotherapy than in patients treated with placebo, particularly during the initial phases of therapy. These complaints are generally transient and may resolve with continued treatment. In some cases, however, temporary dose reduction may be prudent. Gastrointestinal symptoms during initial therapy may be mitigated if patients are treated via gradual dose escalation and counseled to take their medication with meals. If significant diarrhea and/or vomiting occur, metformin should be temporarily discontinued.

Dysgeusia

Approximately 3% of patients treated with metformin will complain of an unpleasant or metallic taste in their mouths. This usually resolves spontaneously.

Dermatological Reactions

In controlled trials, the incidence of rash or dermatitis in patients treated with metformin monotherapy was comparable to that with placebo.

Hematological Reactions

As mentioned above, metformin therapy may result in a small reduction in vitamin B_{12}

levels; however, reports of megaloblastic anemia secondary to metformin are exceedingly rare. Annual monitoring of hematological parameters has been suggested.

DRUG INTERACTIONS

Sulfonylureas

In a single-dose interaction study of type 2 diabetic patients, administration of metformin with glyburide did not result in changes in metformin pharmacokinetics or pharmacodynamics. Reductions in glyburide area under the curve (AUC) and C_{max} were observed but were extremely variable. Because this was a single-dose study and there is a lack of correlation between glyburide, serum concentrations, and pharmacokinetic effect, the clinical significance of this interaction is uncertain.

Furosemide

Metformin/furosemide interaction was studied in healthy subjects in a single-dose trial. This trial demonstrated that the pharmacokinetic parameters of both medications were affected by coadministration. Furosemide caused an increase in metformin's C_{max} and AUC (22% and 15%, respectively) without altering metformin's renal clearance. Furosemide's C_{max} and AUC were reduced by 31% and 12%, respectively. The terminal half-life of furosemide was reduced by 32%, without any significant alteration in renal clearance.

Nifedipine

Nifedipine apparently enhances the absorption of metformin. In a coadministration study with nifedipine, plasma metformin C_{max} and AUC were increased by 20% and 9%, respectively, while the time to maximum concentration (T_{max}) and the half-life were unchanged.

Cationic Drugs

An interaction between metformin and cimetidine has been observed in normal healthy subjects, with a 60% increase in peak metformin concentrations and a 40% increase in metformin AUC. However, in one single-dose study, the elimination half-life of metformin was unchanged. Metformin apparently has no effect on cimetidine kinetics. Other compounds that are eliminated via renal tubular secretion have the potential for causing an interaction with metformin by competing for renal tubular transport systems; therefore, these drugs should be used with caution. Examples include amiloride, digoxin, morphine, procainamide, quinidine, quinine, ranitidine, triamterene, trimethoprim, and vancomycin.

Other

Metformin should be used cautiously with compounds that may lead to loss of glycemic control.

See **Table 4.2**, or refer to the full prescribing information, for more drug interaction guidance.

DOSAGE AND ADMINISTRATION

The usual starting dose of 500-mg metformin tablets is once a day, given with the largest meal of the day. Doses may be titrated in increments of one tablet every week up to a maximum of 2,500 mg per day. Metformin is often administered at a dose of 1,000 mg twice a day with the morning and evening meals. If a dose of 2,500 mg is required, the patient may tolerate it better if it is given three times a day with meals.

The usual starting dose of 850-mg metformin tablets is once daily, given with the largest meal of the day. Dosage increases are usually made in increments of one tablet every other week given in divided doses up to a maximum of 2,550 mg per day. The most common maintenance dose is 850 mg given twice a day with the morning and evening meals. However, if necessary, patients may be given 850 mg three times a day with meals.

The usual starting dose of the extended-release form is 500 mg once a day, given with the largest meal of the day. Doses may be titrated in increments of one tablet every week up to a maximum of 2,000 mg given with the evening meal. Patients previously treated with conventional metformin may be safely switched to the extended-release form at the same total daily dose (up to 2,000 mg) given as one daily dose of the extended-release form.

See **Table 4.1**, or refer to the full prescribing information, for more dosing guidance.

SUGGESTED READING

Bailey CJ. Biguanides and NIDDM. *Diabetes Care*. 15:755-772, 1992.

Bailey CJ. Metformin, an update. *Gen Pharmacol*. 24:1299-1309, 1993.

Bailey CJ, Path MRC, Turner RC. Metformin. *N Engl J Med*. 334:574-578, 1996.

Cryer DR, Mills DJ, Nicholas SP, Stadel BV, Henry DH. Comparative outcomes study of metformin intervention versus conventional approach. *Diabetes Care*. 28;3:539-543, 2005.

DeFronzo RA, Goodman AM. The Multicenter Metformin Study Group: Efficacy of metformin in patients with NIDDM. *N Engl J Med*. 333:541-549, 1995.

Fowler M. Diabetes treatment, part 2: oral agents for glycemic management. *Clinical Diabetes*. 25;4:131-139, 2007.

Garber AJ, Duncan TG, Goodman AM, Mills DJ, Rohlf JL. Efficacy of metformin in type II diabetes: results of a double-blind placebo-controlled, dose-response trial. *Am J Med*. 102:491-497, 1997.

Gugliano D, Quantraro A, Consoli G, Minei A, Ceriello A, DeRosa N, Onofrio ED. Metformin for obese, insulin-treated diabetic patients: improvements in glycaemic control and reduction of metabolic risk factors. *Eur J Clin Pharmacol*. 44:107-112, 1993.

Kirpichnikov D, McFarlane SI, Sowers JR. Metformin: an update. *Ann Intern Med*. 137:25-33, 2002.

Kosi RR. Practical review of oral antihyperglycemic agents for type 2 diabetes mellitus. *The Diabetes Educator*. 32;6:869-876, 2006.

Salpeter SR, Greyber E, Pasternik GA, Salpeter EE. Risk of fatal and nonfatal lactic acidosis with metformin use in type 2 diabetes mellitus. *Arch Intern Med*. 163:2594-2602, 2003.

Table 4.1. Prescribing Information for Biguanides

GENERIC (BRAND)	FORM/ STRENGTH	DOSAGE	WARNINGS/PRECAUTIONS & CONTRAINDICATIONS	ADVERSE REACTIONS
Metformin HCl (Fortamet)	Tab, Extended-Release: 500mg, 1000mg	*Adults:* ≥17 yrs: Take with evening meal. Initial: 500-1000mg qd. With Insulin: Initial: 500mg qd. Titrate: May increase by 500mg/week. Max: 2500mg/day. Decrease insulin dose by 10-25% if FPG <120mg/dL. Elderly/Debilitated/Malnourished: Conservative dosing; do not titrate to max.	W/P: Lactic acidosis reported (rare); increased risk with renal dysfunction, increased age, DM, CHF, and other conditions with risk of hypoperfusion and hypoxemia. Avoid use in patients ≥80 yrs unless renal function is normal. Monitor renal function and for ketoacidosis and metabolic acidosis. Avoid in renal/hepatic impairment. D/C in hypoxic states (eg, CHF, shock, acute MI), loss of blood glucose control due to stress (give insulin), acidosis, dehydration, sepsis. Temporarily d/c prior to surgery (due to restricted food intake) and procedures requiring intravascular iodinated contrast materials. May decrease serum vitamin B_{12} levels. Increased risk of hypoglycemia in elderly, debilitated/malnourished, adrenal or pituitary insufficiency, or alcohol intoxication. Contra: Renal disease/ dysfunction (SrCr ≥1.5mg/dL [males], ≥1.4mg/dL [females], or abnormal CrCl), CHF, metabolic acidosis, diabetic ketoacidosis. D/C temporarily (48 hrs) for radiologic studies with intravascular iodinated contrast materials. P/N: Category B, not for use in nursing.	Diarrhea, nausea, dyspepsia, flatulence, abdominal pain, headache.
Metformin HCl (Glucophage, Glucophage XR, Riomet)	Sol: (Riomet) 500mg/5mL; Tab: 500mg, 850mg, 1000mg*; Tab, Extended-Release: 500mg, 750mg *scored	*Adults:* (Sol, Tab) Initial: 500mg bid or 850mg qd with meals. Titrate: Increase by 500mg/week, or 850mg every 2 weeks, or may increase from 500mg bid to 850mg bid after 2 weeks. Max: 2550mg/day. Give in 3 divided doses with meals if dose is >2g/day. (Tab, Extended-Release) Initial: ≥17 yrs: 500mg qd with evening meal. Increase by 500mg/week. Max: 2000mg/day. With Insulin: Initial: 500mg qd. Titrate: Increase by 500mg/week. Max: 2500mg/day and 2000mg/day (XR). Decrease insulin dose by 10-25% when FPG <120mg/dL. Swallow whole; do not crush or chew. Elderly/Debilitated/Malnourished: Conservative dosing; do not titrate to Max. *Pediatrics:* 10-16 yrs: (Sol, Tab) Initial: 500mg bid with meals. Titrate: Increase by 500mg/week. Max: 2000mg/day.	W/P: Lactic acidosis reported (rare); increased risk with renal dysfunction, increased age, DM, CHF, and other conditions with risk of hypoperfusion and hypoxemia. Avoid use in patients ≥80 yrs unless renal function is normal. Monitor renal function and for ketoacidosis and metabolic acidosis. Avoid in renal/hepatic impairment. D/C in hypoxic states (eg, CHF, shock, acute MI), loss of blood glucose control due to stress (give insulin), acidosis, dehydration, sepsis. Temporarily d/c prior to surgery (due to restricted food intake) and procedures requiring intravascular iodinated contrast materials. May decrease serum vitamin B_{12} levels. Increased risk of hypoglycemia in elderly, debilitated/malnourished, adrenal or pituitary insufficiency, or alcohol intoxication. Monitor renal function. Contra: Renal disease/dysfunction (SrCr ≥1.5mg/dL [males], ≥1.4mg/dL [females], or abnormal CrCl), CHF, metabolic acidosis, diabetic ketoacidosis. D/C temporarily (48 hrs) for radiologic studies with intravascular iodinated contrast materials. P/N: Category B, not for use in nursing.	Lactic acidosis, diarrhea, nausea, vomiting, flatulence, abdominal discomfort, abnormal stools, hypoglycemia, myalgia, dizziness, dyspnea, nail disorder, rash, sweating, taste disorder, chest discomfort, chills, flu syndrome, palpitations, asthenia, indigestion, headache.
Metformin HCl (Glumetza)	Tab, Extended-Release: 500mg, 1000mg	*Adults:* ≥18 yrs: Take with evening meal. Initial: 1000mg qd. With Insulin: Initial: 500mg qd. Titrate: May increase by 500mg/week. Max: 2000mg/day. Decrease insulin dose by 10-25% if FPG <120mg/dL. Elderly/Debilitated/Malnourished: Conservative dosing; do not titrate to max. Swallow whole; do not crush or chew.	W/P: Lactic acidosis reported (rare); increased risk with renal dysfunction, increased age, DM, CHF, and other conditions with risk of hypoperfusion and hypoxemia. Avoid use in patients ≥80 yrs unless renal function is normal. Monitor renal function and for ketoacidosis and metabolic acidosis. Avoid in renal/hepatic impairment. D/C in hypoxic states (eg, CHF, shock, acute MI), loss of blood glucose control due to stress (give insulin), acidosis, dehydration, sepsis. Temporarily d/c prior to surgery (due to restricted food/fluid intake) or procedures requiring intravascular iodinated contrast materials. May decrease	Hypoglycemia, diarrhea, nausea.

W/P = warnings/precautions; Contra = contraindications; P/N = pregnancy category rating and nursing considerations.

Table 4.1. Prescribing Information for Biguanides

GENERIC (BRAND)	FORM/ STRENGTH	DOSAGE	WARNINGS/PRECAUTIONS & CONTRAINDICATIONS	ADVERSE REACTIONS
Metformin HCl (Glumetza) *(Cont.)*			serum vitamin B_{12} levels. Increased risk of hypoglycemia in elderly, debilitated/ malnourished, adrenal or pituitary insufficiency, or alcohol intoxication. **Contra:** Renal disease or dysfunction (SrCr ≥1.5mg/dL [males], ≥1.4mg/dL [females], or abnormal CrCl), CHF, metabolic acidosis, including diabetic ketoacidosis. D/C temporarily (48 hrs) for radiologic studies with intravascular iodinated contrast materials. **P/N:** Category B, not for use in nursing.	
COMBINATION DRUGS				
Metformin HCl/ Glipizide (Metaglip)	Tab: (Glipizide-Metformin) 2.5mg-250mg, 2.5mg-500mg, 5mg-500mg	*Adults:* Initial: 2.5mg-250mg qd. If FBG 280-320mg/dL, give 2.5mg-500mg bid. Titrate: Increase by 1 tab/day every 2 weeks. Max: 10mg-1g/day or 10mg-2g/day given in divided doses. **Second-Line Therapy:** Initial: 2.5mg-500mg or 5mg-500mg bid (with morning and evening meals). Starting dose should not exceed daily dose of metformin or glipizide already being taken. Titrate: Increase by no more than 5mg-500mg/day. Max: 20mg-2g/day. **Elderly/Debilitated/ Malnourished:** Do not titrate to max dose. Take with meals.	**W/P:** Lactic acidosis reported (rare); increased risk with renal dysfunction, increased age, DM, CHF, and other conditions with risk of hypoperfusion and hypoxemia. Avoid use in patients ≥80 yrs unless renal function is normal. Increased risk of cardiovascular mortality. Increased risk of hypoglycemia in elderly, debilitated/ malnourished, adrenal or pituitary insufficiency, or alcohol intoxication. D/C in hypoxic states (eg, CHF, shock, acute MI) and prior to surgical procedures (due to restricted food intake). Avoid in renal/ hepatic impairment. May decrease serum vitamin B_{12} levels. Impaired renal and/or hepatic function may slow glipizide excretion. Withhold treatment with any condition associated with dehydration or sepsis. Monitor renal function. **Contra:** Renal disease/dysfunction (SrCr ≥1.5mg/ dL [males], ≥1.4mg/dL [females], abnormal CrCl), metabolic acidosis, diabetic ketoacidosis. D/C temporarily (48 hrs) for radiologic studies with intravascular iodinated contrast materials. **P/N:** Category C, not for use in nursing.	Upper respiratory tract infection, HTN, headache, diarrhea, dizziness, musculoskeletal pain, nausea, vomiting, abdominal pain.
Metformin HCl/ Glyburide (Glucovance)	Tab: (Glyburide-Metformin) 1.25mg-250mg, 2.5mg-500mg, 5mg-500mg	*Adults:* Take with meals. Initial: 1.25mg-250mg qd. If HbA$_1$c >9% or FPG >200mg/dL, give 1.25mg-250mg bid. Titrate: Increase by 1.25mg-250mg/day every 2 weeks. Do not use 50mg-500mg tab for initial therapy. **Second-Line Therapy:** Initial: 2.5mg-500mg or 5mg-500mg bid. Starting dose should not exceed daily doses of glyburide (or sulfonylurea equivalent) or metformin already being taken. Titrate: Increase by no more than 5mg-500mg/day. Max: 20mg-2000mg/day. **With Concomitant TZD:** Initiate and titrate TZD as recommended. If hypoglycemia occurs, reduce glyburide component. **Elderly/ Debilitated/Malnourished:** Conservative dosing; do not titrate to max.	**W/P:** Lactic acidosis reported (rare); increased risk with renal dysfunction, increased age, DM, CHF, and other conditions with risk of hypoperfusion and hypoxemia. Avoid use in patients ≥80 yrs unless renal function is normal. Increased risk of cardiovascular mortality. Increased risk of hypoglycemia in elderly, debilitated/ malnourished, adrenal or pituitary insufficiency, or alcohol intoxication. D/C in hypoxic states (eg, CHF, shock, acute MI), loss of blood glucose control due to stress (give insulin), acidosis and prior to surgical procedures (due to restricted food intake). Monitor renal function and for ketoacidosis and metabolic acidosis. Avoid in renal/hepatic impairment. May decrease serum vitamin B12 levels. When used with a TZD, monitor LFTs and for weight gain. Withhold treatment with any condition associated with hypoxemia, dehydration, or sepsis. **Contra:** Renal disease or dysfunction (SrCr ≥1.5mg/dL [males], ≥1.4mg/dL [females], or abnormal CrCl), CHF, metabolic acidosis, including diabetic ketoacidosis. D/C temporarily (48 hrs) for radiologic studies with intravascular iodinated contrast materials. **P/N:** Category B, not for use in nursing.	Hypoglycemia, nausea, vomiting, abdominal pain, upper respiratory infection, headache, dizziness, diarrhea.

BB = black box warning; **W/P** = warnings/precautions; **Contra** = contraindications; **P/N** = pregnancy category rating and nursing considerations.

Table 4.1. Prescribing Information for Biguanides

GENERIC (BRAND)	FORM/ STRENGTH	DOSAGE	WARNINGS/PRECAUTIONS & CONTRAINDICATIONS	ADVERSE REACTIONS
Metformin HCl/ Pioglitazone (ActoPlus Met)	Tab: (Pioglitazone-Metformin) 15mg-500mg, 15mg-850mg	***Adults:*** Individualize dose. **Prior Pioglitazone/Metformin:** Base on current regimen. **Prior Metformin Monotherapy or Pioglitazone Monotherapy:** Initial: 15mg-500mg or 15mg-850mg qd-bid. Titrate: Gradually increase after assessing adequacy of therapeutic response. Max: (Pioglitazone) 45mg, (Metformin) 2550mg. **Elderly/Debilitated/Malnourished:** Conservative dosing; do not titrate to max dose.	**BB:** Thiazolidinediones may cause or exacerbate CHF in some patients. Actoplus Met is not recommended in patients with symptomatic heart failure. **W/P:** (Metformin) Lactic acidosis reported (rare); increased risk with renal dysfunction, increased age, DM, CHF, and other conditions with risk of hypoperfusion and hypoxemia. Avoid in patients ≥80 yrs unless normal renal function. Monitor renal function and for ketoacidosis and metabolic acidosis. Avoid in renal/hepatic impairment. D/C in hypoxic states (eg, CHF, shock, acute MI), loss of blood glucose control due to stress (give insulin), acidosis, dehydration, sepsis. Temporarily d/c prior to surgery (due to restricted food intake) and procedures requiring IV iodinated contrast materials. May decrease serum B_{12} levels. Increased risk of hypoglycemia in elderly, debilitated/ malnourished, adrenal or pituitary insufficiency, or alcohol intoxication. Monitor renal function. Alcohol known to potentiate effect of metformin on lactate metabolism. (Pioglitazone) May cause fluid retention and exacerbation/initiation of heart failure; d/c if cardiac status deteriorates. Avoid if NYHA Class III of IV cardiac status. Use lowest approved dose if systolic heart failure (NYHA Class II). Not for use in type 1 diabetes or for diabetic ketoacidosis treatment. Caution with edema. Dose-related weight gain reported. Ovulation in premenopausal anovulatory patients may occur; risk of pregnancy with inadequate contraception. May decrease Hgb and Hct. Avoid with active liver disease, if ALT levels >2.5x ULN. D/C if jaundice occurs or ALT >3x ULN on therapy. Macular edema reported. **Contra:** Established NYHA Class III or IV heart failure, renal disease or dysfunction (eg, SrCr ≥1.5mg/dL [males], ≥1.4mg/dL [females], or abnormal CrCl) and metabolic acidosis, including diabetic ketoacidosis. Temporarily d/c in patients undergoing radiologic studies involving intravascular iodinated contrast materials. **P/N:** Category C, not for use in nursing.	Upper respiratory tract infection, diarrhea, nausea, edema, headache, UTI, sinusitis, dizziness, weight increase, new onset or worsening diabetic macular edema.
Metformin HCl/ Repaglinide (PrandiMet)	Tab: (Repaglinide-Metformin) 1mg-500mg, 2mg-500mg	***Adults:*** Individualize dose. Administer 2 to 3 times a day up to 4mg-1000mg per meal. Max daily dose: 10mg-2500mg. **Patients Inadequately Controlled with Metformin HCl Monotherapy:** 1mg-500mg bid with meals. Gradual dose escalation required. **Patients Inadequately Controlled with Meglitinide Monotherapy:** 500mg of metformin bid. Gradual dose escalation required. **Concomitant Use of Repaglinide/ Metformin:** Initiate at the dose similar to (but not exceeding) the current dose. Titrate to maximum daily dose as necessary.	**BB:** Lactic acidosis may occur due to metformin accumulation. If suspected, d/c PrandiMet and hospitalize patient. **W/P:** Lactic acidosis reported (rare), increased risk with sepsis, dehydration, excess alcohol intake, hepatic impairment, renal impairment, and acute CHF. Assess renal function prior to initiation and annually thereafter. Not indicated for use in combination with NPH insulin. Avoid in hepatic impairment and excess alcohol intake. D/C in hypoxic states (eg, CHF, shock, acute MI), prior to surgical procedures, procedures requiring use of intravascular iodinated contrast materials, and ketoacidosis. May cause vitamin B_{12} deficiency and hypoglycemia. **Contra:** Renal impairment (SrCr ≥1.5mg/dL [males], ≥1.4mg/dL [females], or abnormal CrCl). Acute or chronic metabolic acidosis, including diabetic ketoacidosis. Patients receiving both gemfibrozil and itraconazole. **P/N:** Category C, not for use in nursing.	Hypoglycemia, headache, diarrhea, nausea, upper respiratory tract infection.

BB = black box warning; **W/P** = warnings/precautions; **Contra** = contraindications; **P/N** = pregnancy category rating and nursing considerations.

Table 4.1. Prescribing Information for Biguanides

GENERIC (BRAND)	FORM/ STRENGTH	DOSAGE	WARNINGS/PRECAUTIONS & CONTRAINDICATIONS	ADVERSE REACTIONS
Metformin HCl/ Rosiglitazone maleate (Avandamet)	Tab: (Rosiglitazone-Metformin) 2mg-500mg, 4mg-500mg, 2mg-1000mg, 4mg-1000mg	**Adults:** **Prior Metformin Therapy of 1000mg/day:** Initial: 2mg-500mg tab bid. **Prior Metformin Therapy of 2000mg/day:** Initial: 2mg-1000mg tab bid. **Prior Rosiglitazone Therapy of 4mg/day:** Initial: 2mg-500mg tab bid. **Prior Rosiglitazone Therapy of 8mg/day:** 4mg-500mg tab bid. Titrate: May increase by increments of 4mg rosiglitazone and/or 500mg metformin. Max: 8mg-2000mg/day. **Drug-Naive Patients:** Initial: 2mg-500mg qd-bid. If HbA$_{1c}$ >11% and FPG >270mg/dL: Initial: 2mg-500mg bid. Titrate: After 4 weeks, may increase by increments of 2mg-500mg per day. Max: 8mg-2000mg per day. **Elderly/ Debilitated/Malnourished:** Conservative dosing; do not titrate to max dose. Take with meals.	**BB:** Thiazolidinediones may cause or exacerbate CHF in some patients. Avandamet is not recommended in patients with symptomatic heart failure. **W/P:** Lactic acidosis reported (rare); increased risk with renal dysfunction, increased age, DM, CHF, and other conditions with risk of hypoperfusion and hypoxemia. Avoid use in patients ≥80 yrs unless renal function is normal. Monitor renal function and for ketoacidosis and metabolic acidosis. D/C in hypoxic states (eg, CHF, shock, acute MI), loss of blood glucose control due to stress, acidosis and prior to surgical procedures (due to restricted food intake). May decrease serum vitamin B$_{12}$ levels. Increased risk of hypoglycemia with concomitant use with other hypoglycemic agents, elderly, debilitated/malnourished, adrenal or pituitary insufficiency, or alcohol intoxication. May cause fluid retention and exacerbation/initiation of heart failure; d/c if cardiac status deteriorates. Avoid with NYHA Class III or IV cardiac status. Not for use in type 1 diabetes or for diabetic ketoacidosis treatment. Caution with edema. Dose-related weight gain reported. Ovulation in premenopausal anovulatory patients may occur; risk of pregnancy with inadequate contraception. May decrease Hgb and Hct. Avoid with active liver disease, if ALT levels >2.5x ULN, or if jaundice occurred with troglitazone. Check LFTs before therapy, every 2 months for 1 year, and periodically thereafter, or if hepatic dysfunction symptoms occur. D/C if ALT >3x ULN on therapy. Not for use with insulin. Increased incidence of bone fracture was noted in female patients **Contra:** Established NYHA Class III or IV heart failure, renal disease/ dysfunction (SrCr ≥1.5mg/dL [males], ≥1.4mg/dL [females], or abnormal CrCl), metabolic acidosis, including diabetic ketoacidosis. D/C temporarily (48 hrs) for radiologic studies with intravascular iodinated contrast materials. **P/N:** Category C, not for use in nursing.	Upper respiratory tract infection, headache, back pain, hyperglycemia, fatigue, sinusitis, diarrhea, dizziness, abdominal pain, viral infection, arthralgia, anemia, dyspepsia, nausea, vomiting.
Metformin HCl/ Sitagliptin phosphate (Janumet)	Tab: (Sitagliptin-Metformin) 50mg-500mg, 50mg-1000mg	**Adults:** Individualize dosing. **Patient Not Controlled on Metformin Monotherapy:** Initial: 100mg/day (50mg bid) of sitagliptin + metformin dose. **Patient on Metformin 850mg BID:** Initial: 50mg-1000mg tab bid. **Patient Not Controlled on Sitagliptin Monotherapy:** Initial: 50mg-500mg tab bid. Titrate: Gradual increase to 50mg-1000mg tab bid. Max: 100mg of sitagliptin and 2000mg of metformin. Take with meals.	**BB:** Lactic acidosis may occur due to metformin accumulation. If acidosis suspected, d/c drug and hospitalize patient immediately. **W/P:** Lactic acidosis reported (rare), increased risk with renal dysfunction. Assess renal function prior to initiation and during treatment; caution in elderly. Avoid in renal/hepatic impairment. May decrease vitamin B$_{12}$ levels; monitor hematologic parameters. May cause hypoglycemia in elderly, debilitated/malnourished, adrenal or pituitary insufficiency, or alcohol intoxication. D/C in hypoxic states (eg, CHF, shock, acute MI), prior to surgical procedures (due to restricted food and fluid intake), and procedures requiring use of intravascular iodinated contrast materials. **Contra:** Renal disease (SrCR ≥1.5mg/dL [males], ≥1.4mg/dL [females], or abnormal CrCl), metabolic acidosis, including diabetic ketoacidosis. D/C for 48 hrs in patients undergoing radiologic studies with intravascular iodinated contrast materials. **P/N:** Category B, caution in nursing.	(Metformin) Diarrhea, nausea/vomiting, flatulence, abdominal discomfort, indigestion, asthenia, and headache. (Sitagliptin) Nasopharyngitis.

BB = black box warning; **W/P** = warnings/precautions; **Contra** = contraindications; **P/N** = pregnancy category rating and nursing considerations.

Table 4.2. Drug Interactions for Biguanides

Metformin HCl (Fortamet, Glucophage, Glucophage XR, Glumetza, Riomet)

Alcohol	Potentiates effects of metformin on lactate metabolism; potentiates hypoglycemia; avoid excessive alcohol intake.
Calcium channel blockers	May cause hyperglycemia.
Cationic drugs (eg, digoxin, amiloride, procainamide, quinidine, quinine, ranitidine, trimethoprim, vancomycin, triamterene, morphine)	May increase metformin levels.
Cimetidine	May increase metformin levels.
Contraceptives, oral	May cause hyperglycemia.
Corticosteroids	May cause hyperglycemia.
Diuretics	May cause hyperglycemia.
Estrogens	May cause hyperglycemia.
Furosemide	May increase metformin levels; may decrease furosemide levels.
Isoniazid	May cause hyperglycemia.
Nicotinic acid	May cause hyperglycemia.
Nifedipine	May increase metformin levels.
Phenothiazines	May cause hyperglycemia.
Phenytoin	May cause hyperglycemia.
Sympathomimetics	May cause hyperglycemia.
Thiazides	May cause hyperglycemia.
Thyroid products	May cause hyperglycemia.

COMBINATION DRUGS

Glipizide-Metformin HCl (Metaglip)

Alcohol	Potentiates effect of metformin on lactate metabolism; potentiates hypoglycemia; avoid excessive alcohol intake.
Azoles	Potentiates hypoglycemia.
Beta-blockers	Potentiates hypoglycemia.
Calcium channel blockers	May cause hyperglycemia.
Cationic drugs (eg, digoxin, amiloride, procainamide, quinidine, quinine, ranitidine, trimethoprim, vancomycin, triamterene, morphine)	May increase metformin levels.
Chloramphenicol	Potentiates hypoglycemia.
Cimetidine	May increase metformin levels.

Table 4.2. Drug Interactions for Biguanides

Contraceptives, oral	May cause hyperglycemia.
Corticosteroids	May cause hyperglycemia.
Coumarins	Potentiates hypoglycemia.
Diuretics	May cause hyperglycemia.
Estrogens	May cause hyperglycemia.
Furosemide	May increase metformin levels; may decrease furosemide levels.
Isoniazid	May cause hyperglycemia.
MAO inhibitors	Potentiates hypoglycemia.
Miconazole	Severe hypoglycemia reported with oral miconazole.
Nicotinic acid	May cause hyperglycemia.
Nifedipine	May increase metformin levels.
NSAIDs	Potentiates hypoglycemia.
Phenothiazines	May cause hyperglycemia.
Phenytoin	May cause hyperglycemia.
Probenecid	Potentiates hypoglycemia.
Protein bound drugs (highly)	Potentiates hypoglycemia.
Salicylates	Potentiates hypoglycemia.
Sulfonamides	Potentiates hypoglycemia.
Sympathomimetics	May cause hyperglycemia.
Thiazides	May cause hyperglycemia.
Thyroid products	May cause hyperglycemia.
Glyburide-Metformin HCI (Glucovance)	
Alcohol	Potentiates effects of metformin on lactate metabolism; potentiates hypoglycemia; avoid excessive alcohol intake.
Beta-blockers	Potentiates hypoglycemia.
Calcium channel blockers	May cause hyperglycemia.
Cationic drugs (eg, digoxin, amiloride, procainamide, quinidine, quinine, ranitidine, trimethoprim, vancomycin, triamterene, morphine)	May increase metformin levels.
Chloramphenicol	Potentiates hypoglycemia.
Cimetidine	May increase metformin levels.
Ciprofloxacin	Potentiates hypoglycemia.
Contraceptives, oral	May cause hyperglycemia.
Corticosteroids	May cause hyperglycemia.
Coumarins	Potentiates hypoglycemia.

Table 4.2. Drug Interactions for Biguanides

Estrogens	May cause hyperglycemia.
Furosemide	May increase metformin levels; may decrease furosemide levels.
Isoniazid	May cause hyperglycemia.
MAO inhibitors	Potentiates hypoglycemia.
Miconazole	Severe hypoglycemia reported with oral miconazole.
Nicotinic acid	May cause hyperglycemia.
Nifedipine	May increase metformin levels.
NSAIDs	Potentiates hypoglycemia.
Phenothiazines	May cause hyperglycemia.
Phenytoin	May cause hyperglycemia.
Probenecid	Potentiates hypoglycemia.
Salicylates	Potentiates hypoglycemia.
Sulfonamides	Potentiates hypoglycemia.
Sympathomimetics	May cause hyperglycemia.
Thiazides	May cause hyperglycemia.
Thiazolidinediones (eg, rosiglitazone)	Potentiates hypoglycemia.
Thyroid products	May cause hyperglycemia.

Pioglitazone HCl-Metformin HCl (Actoplus Met)

Alcohol	Potentiates effects of metformin on lactate metabolism; potentiates hypoglycemia; avoid excessive alcohol intake.
Calcium channel blockers	May cause hyperglycemia.
Cationic drugs (eg, digoxin, amiloride, procainamide, quinidine, quinine, ranitidine, trimethoprim, vancomycin, triamterene, morphine)	May increase metformin levels.
Cimetidine	May increase metformin levels.
Contraceptives, oral (eg, ethinyl estradiol, norethindrone)	Caution when coadministering, may decrease effectiveness, may cause hyperglycemia.
Corticosteroids	May cause hyperglycemia.
CYP2C8 inducers (eg, rifampin)	May significantly decrease AUC of pioglitazone.
CYP2C8 inhibitors (eg, gemfibrozil)	May significantly increase AUC of pioglitazone.
Diuretics	May cause hyperglycemia.
Estrogens	May cause hyperglycemia.
Furosemide	May increase metformin levels, may decrease furosemide levels.

Table 4.2. Drug Interactions for Biguanides

Hypoglycemic agents, oral	Caution, risk of hypoglycemia.
Insulin	Caution, risk of hypoglycemia.
Isoniazid	May cause hyperglycemia.
Ketoconazole	May inhibit pioglitazone metabolism; perform more frequent monitoring of glycemic control.
Midazolam	May cause a reduction in midazolam levels.
Nicotinic acid	May cause hyperglycemia.
Nifedipine	May increase metformin levels.
Phenothiazines	May cause hyperglycemia.
Phenytoin	May cause hyperglycemia.
Sympathomimetics	May cause hyperglycemia.
Thiazides	May cause hyperglycemia.
Thyroid products	May cause hyperglycemia.
Metformin HCl-Repaglinide (PrandiMet)	
Cationic drugs (eg, amiloride, digoxin, morphine, procainamide, quinidine, quinine, ranitidine, triamterene, trimethoprim, vancomycin)	Potential interaction with metformin by competing for common renal tubular secretion.
Cimetidine	May increase the AUC of metformin.
Clarithromycin	May increase the AUC of repaglinide.
CYP2C8 inhibitors (eg, trimethoprim)	May increase the AUC of repaglinide.
CYP2C8/3A4 enzyme inducers (eg, rifampin)	May decrease the AUC of repaglinide.
CYP3A4 inhibitors (eg, itraconazole, ketoconazole)	May increase the AUC of repaglinide.
Furosemide	May increase the AUC of metformin; may decrease the AUC of furosemide.
Gemfibrozil	Potentiates repaglinide; may potentiate hypoglycemia.
Ibuprofen	May increase the AUC of metformin.
Levonorgestrel/ethinyl estradiol	May decrease the AUC of repaglinide; may increase the AUC of ethinyl estradiol.
Nifedipine	May increase the AUC of metformin; may decrease the AUC of repaglinide.
Propranolol	May decrease the AUC of metformin.
Simvastatin	May decrease the AUC of repaglinide.
Rosiglitazone maleate-Metformin HCl (Avandamet)	
Alcohol	Potentiates effects of metformin on lactate metabolism; potentiates hypoglycemia; avoid excessive alcohol intake.

Table 4.2. Drug Interactions for Biguanides

Calcium channel blockers	May cause hyperglycemia.
Cationic drugs (eg, digoxin, amiloride, procainamide, quinidine, quinine, ranitidine, trimethoprim, vancomycin, triamterene, morphine)	May increase metformin levels.
Cimetidine	May increase metformin levels.
Contraceptives, oral	May cause hyperglycemia.
Corticosteroids	May cause hyperglycemia.
CYP2C8 inducers (eg, rifampin)	May decrease AUC of rosiglitazone.
CYP2C8 inhibitors (eg, gemfibrozil)	May increase AUC of rosiglitazone.
Diuretics	May cause hyperglycemia.
Estrogens	May cause hyperglycemia.
Furosemide	May increase metformin levels, may decrease furosemide levels.
Isoniazid	May cause hyperglycemia.
Nicotinic acid	May cause hyperglycemia.
Nifedipine	May increase metformin levels.
Phenothiazines	May cause hyperglycemia.
Phenytoin	May cause hyperglycemia.
Sympathomimetics	May cause hyperglycemia.
Thiazides	May cause hyperglycemia.
Thyroid products	May cause hyperglycemia.
Sitagliptin-Metformin HCl (Janumet)	
Alcohol	Potentiates effects of metformin on lactate metabolism; potentiates hypoglycemia; avoid excessive alcohol intake.
Calcium channel blockers	May cause hyperglycemia.
Cationic drugs (eg, digoxin, amiloride, procainamide, quinidine, quinine, rantidine, trimethoprim, vancomycin, triamterene, morphine)	May increase metformin levels.
Contraceptives, oral	May cause hyperglycemia.
Corticosteroids	May cause hyperglycemia.
Digoxin	Monitor digoxin levels.
Diuretics	May cause hyperglycemia.
Estrogens	May cause hyperglycemia.
Furosemide	May increase metformin levels; may decrease furosemide levels.

Table 4.2. Drug Interactions for Biguanides

Isoniazid	May cause hyperglycemia.
Nicotinic acid	May cause hyperglycemia.
Nifedipine	May increase metformin levels.
Phenothiazines	May cause hyperglycemia.
Phenytoin	May cause hyperglycemia.
Sympathomimetics	May cause hyperglycemia.
Thiazides	May cause hyperglycemia.
Thyroid products	May cause hyperglycemia.

Chapter 5

Thiazolidinediones

John R. White, Jr., PharmD, PA

INTRODUCTION

The first thiazolidinedione (TZD), ciglitazone, was synthesized in 1982. It was soon thereafter discovered that ciglitazone reduced insulin resistance in obese and diabetic animals. Because of their effects on insulin resistance, TZDs have been developed as pharmacological agents for the management of type 2 diabetes, although they were initially synthesized as potential lipid-reducing agents. Since their discovery, three TZDs have been introduced to the market in the U.S.: troglitazone (Rezulin), rosiglitazone (Avandia), and pioglitazone (Actos); the latter two agents are currently on the market.

These compounds are orally active and are unrelated to the other oral anti-hyper-glycemic agents either chemically or by mechanism of action. A thiazolidine-2-4-dione structure is common to all three of these drugs, with differences in potency, receptor binding, metabolic effects, pharmacokinetics, and side effects being governed by modifications in the side chain (see **Figure 1**).

TZDs have been used in the management of type 2 diabetes as monotherapeutic agents and in combination with insulin, metformin, DPP-IV inhibitors, and sulfonylureas. Additionally, they have been studied and found to be effective in treating insulin-resistant women with polycystic ovarian syndrome. TZDs are sometimes referred to as "insulin sensitizers."

Figure 1. Thiazolidine-2-4-Dione Structure

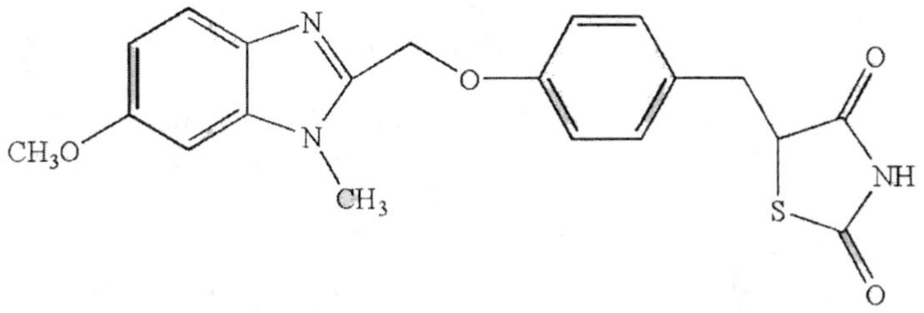

PHARMACOLOGY

Mechanism of Action

The precise mechanism of action or relative importance of various mechanisms of action of the thiazolidinediones is not completely understood. These drugs improve glycemic control by increasing insulin sensitivity. The primary mechanism of action appears to be the direct stimulation of a family of receptors on the nuclear surface of cells that are responsible for the modulation of lipid homeostasis, adipocyte differentiation, and insulin action. TZDs are potent and highly selective agonists for one of the isoforms in this family of receptors, known as peroxisome-proliferator-activated receptor-gamma (PPARγ). The TZDs also display some cross reactivity with other isoforms in the PPAR family, PPAR-α and PPAR-$\triangle$. Different relative affinities of various TZDs for these three receptor types may explain the different effects these three agents have on lipid profiles.

PPARγ is probably the most important of these three receptors in terms of the antidiabetic action of TZDs. A relationship between ability to stimulate PPARγ and antihyperglycemic activity has been reported. TZDs stimulate the expression of genes responsible for the production of glucose transporters (GLUT1 and GLUT4). PPARγ stimulation has also been shown to reduce TNF-α (tumor necrosis factor-alpha) and hepatic glucokinase expression. TZDs may cause a reduction in the number of large adipocytes and an increase in the number of small adipocytes, leading to lower free fatty acid and triglyceride levels and improved insulin sensitivity. The relative importance of each of these mechanisms or potential mechanisms is not currently understood.

Pharmacokinetics

Pioglitazone

Following the administration of pioglitazone, maximum concentration (C_{max}) occurs within 2 hours. Food may delay the absorption rate, but not the extent of absorption. Pioglitazone may be taken without regard to meals. Pioglitazone is extensively bound to serum protein (>99%), whereas its metabolites M-III and M-IV are >98% bound. The apparent volume of distribution (V_d) is a mean of 0.63 L/kg. Pioglitazone is extensively metabolized via oxidation and hydroxylation, with metabolites being partially converted to glucoronide or sulfate conjugates. Metabolites M-III (keto derivatives) and M-IV (hydroxy derivatives), along with parent pioglitazone, are the predominant species found in human serum at steady state. Approximately 15%-30% of pioglitazone can be recovered in the urine following oral administration. The mean serum half-lives of pioglitazone and total pioglitazone are 3-7 hours and 16-24 hours, respectively. Pioglitazone clearance is 5-7 L/hour.

Rosiglitazone

Following the administration of rosiglitazone, C_{max} occurs within 1 hour. Food may delay the absorption rate, but the extent of absorption is not clinically significantly changed. Rosiglitazone may be taken without regard to meals. It is extensively bound to serum protein (>99.8%), primarily albumin. The apparent volume of distribution (V_d) was a mean of 17.6 L/kg in the population studied. Rosiglitazone is extensively metabolized via N-demethylation and hydroxylation, followed by conjugation with glucoronic acid or sulfate. No unchanged drug is found in the urine. The metabolites of rosiglitazone are less potent than the parent compound and are not thought to contribute to the insulin-sensitizing effects of the drug. After administration of labeled rosiglitazone, ~64% is eliminated via the urine and 23% is eliminated via the feces. The mean serum half-life for labeled rosiglitzone material ranges from 103 to 158 hours. Rosiglitazone clearance is ~3 L/hour.

TREATMENT ADVANTAGES AND DISADVANTAGES

As a class, the TZDs are effective in reducing hyperglycemia in patients with type 2 diabetes. Reductions in hyperglycemia vary significantly between patients. Some researchers have even suggested the terms "responders" and "nonresponders" in the population of patients treated with TZDs. HbA_{1C} lowering can be expected to be somewhere between 0.5%-1.5% in most patients. Significant differences between the two available agents, in terms of glycemic lowering, are not obvious; however, the TZDs are slightly less effective than metformin or sulfonlyureas. In most cases, the later agents would probably be used initially.

Because of the association between the first TZD marketed (troglitazone) and fulminate hepatic failure, patients treated with TZDs should have their liver function tested prior to initiation of therapy and periodically thereafter. Troglitazone was removed from the market, leaving behind the concern that the hepatotoxic reaction might be a class effect. While this concern has not been supported by data from the legion of patients treated with pioglitazone and rosiglitazone, testing is still recommended.

Several studies have suggested a link between the use of TZDs and reduced bone density and fractures. While it has been demonstrated that patients with type 2 diabetes mellitus are at increased risk of fracture compared with their euglycemic peers, recent evidence has been suggested that use of TZDs in patients at risk for osteoporosis may result in a higher fracture rate.

Clinicians should be mindful of this possibility when prescribing oral antihyperglycemic agents. The most salient suggested mechanism for TZD-induced osteoporosis is via inhibition of bone formation by PPAR-mediated diversion of mesenchymal progenitor cells into the adipocytes rather than osteoblasts.

TZDs have also been associated with mild to moderate weight gain (1-5 kg) in some patients. Initially, this weight gain was thought to be due primarily to edema but has since been shown to be nonedema weight gain.

Rosiglitazone and pioglitazone have different effects on lipid profiles. This difference may be related to relative effect of these agents on the PPARα nuclear receptor. Pioglitazone has a higher affinity for PPARα and is associated with mild improvements in lipid profiles (reduction of TG and increases in HDL). Both agents may cause an increase in LDL. Indirect comparisons of pioglitazone and rosiglitazone suggest that rosiglitazone probably causes more LDL elevation than pioglitazone.

As stated above, both agents can cause edema. This may in turn increase the incidence of exacerbations of CHF in patients who have underlying disease. This effect seems to be more pronounced in patients who are also treated with insulin. Edema, if it occurs, can sometimes be mitigated via the use of diuretics. However, TZDs are contraindicated in patients with NYHA class III or IV failure.

The published conclusions regarding the impact of TZDs on overall cardiovascular mortality are conflicting. A handful of contradictory manuscripts and a plethora of opposing opinions and editorials on this subject have been published. While it is clear that untreated hyperglycemia is a major risk factor for cardiovascular mortality, it is not clear that treating hyperglycemia in patients with TZDs results in significantly more cardiovascular mortality than is encountered in patients treated with other modalities.

THERAPEUTIC CONSIDERATIONS

Significant Warnings and Precautions

Diabetes
These agents should not be used to treat patients with type 1 diabetes or to manage patients in diabetic ketoacidosis.

Hypoglycemia
Patients whose diabetes is being managed with a TZD in combination with insulin or oral hypoglycemic agents may be at risk for hypoglycemia. In some cases a reduction in the dose of the hypoglycemic agent may be warranted.

Ovulation
The TZDs may cause resumption of ovulation in premenopausal women with anovulation secondary to insulin resistance. These patients may be at risk for pregnancy if adequate contraception is not used. TZDs have been studied as a treatment for anovulation in women with polycystic ovarian syndrome and have been shown to be effective.

Hematology
Reductions in hemoglobin and hematocrit have been observed in patients treated with pioglitazone and rosiglitazone. Reductions in hemoglobin and hematocrit with the TZDs are ≤4% and ≤1 g/dL, respectively. These changes are possibly due to volume expansion and have not been associated with significant hematological effects. They occur within the first 4-8 weeks of therapy and have been shown to persist for at least 2 years.

Edema
Rosiglitazone and pioglitazone have been associated with mild to moderate edema in some patients.

Cardiac
TZDs are contraindicated in patients with NYHA class III and IV failure because their use is associated with increased rates of hospitalization for CHF exacerbations.

Hepatic Toxicity
Serum transaminase elevations
No evidence of hepatotoxicity has been observed with either rosiglitazone or pioglitazone. In the phase III trials of rosiglitazone, 0.2% of patients treated with rosiglitazone had reversible elevations in ALT greater than three times the upper limit of normal, compared with 0.2% of patients treated with placebo. In the phase III trials of pioglitazone, 0.26% of patients treated with pioglitazone had reversible elevations in ALT greater than three times the upper limit of normal, compared with 0.25% of patients treated with placebo.

Fulminant hepatic failure
Troglitazone was associated with several cases of fulminant hepatic failure resulting in the need for liver transplant or in death and was removed from the market.

Pregnancy and Nursing
Pioglitazone and rosiglitazone are classified as pregnancy category C. The currently available TZDs should not be administered to breast-feeding women.

SPECIAL POPULATIONS

Renal Dysfunction
Dose adjustments for rosiglitazone or pioglitazone are not required in patients with renal

dysfunction. However, use of some of the other antihyperglycemic agents is not recommended in patients with renal dysfunction, thereby eliminating the possibility of combination therapy with those agents (combination metformin/TZD therapy, for example) in this population.

Hepatic Dysfunction

Patients with impaired hepatic function (Child-Pugh grade B/C) have a 45% reduction in pioglitazone and total pioglitazone mean peak concentrations, but no change in mean area under the curve (AUC) when compared with normal subjects. In patients with impaired hepatic function (Child-Pugh grade B/C), C_{max} and AUC values for rosiglitazone were increased two- and threefold, respectively, and elimination half-life was increased by 2 hours. Rosiglitazone and pioglitazone should not be used in patients with clinical evidence of active liver disease or with serum ALT concentrations >2.5 times the upper limit of normal.

Elderly

Age does not result in clinically significant changes in the effects or pharmacokinetics of rosiglitazone or pioglitazone. No dosage adjustments are needed in this population.

Pediatrics

No pharmacokinetic, safety, or efficacy data for the TZDs are available in children.

Ethnicity

No differences in the effects of these agents has been observed in any ethnic group.

Gender

Rosiglitazone clearance was reported to be 6% lower in males of comparable body weight. In monotherapeutic trials with rosiglitazone, a slightly greater therapeutic response (quantitative differences were not reported) was observed in female patients, while no such difference was reported in metformin/rosiglitazone combination trials. Interestingly, sex-related differences were less marked in more obese patients. Women tend to have a greater fat mass than men for a given body mass index. The gender-related differences in effect may be due to this difference in fat mass because the molecular target PPARγ is highly expressed in lipid tissue. Although there are slight differences in the effects of both rosiglitazone and pioglitazone in women, no dose adjustment is recommended and, as in men, treatment in women must be individualized.

ADVERSE EFFECTS AND MONITORING

Weight Gain

As mentioned above, weight gain appears to be a class effect of the TZDs.

Pioglitazone

In Phase III trials, the following was reported: Pioglitazone monotherapy was associated with a 1.1- to 6.2-lb weight increase, compared with a 2.86- to 4.18-lb weight loss in patients treated with placebo. In combination with sulfonylureas, pioglitazone was associated with a 4.2- and 6.4-lb weight gain (15- and 30-mg doses, respectively), compared with a 1.8-lb weight loss in those managed with placebo. Pioglitazone/insulin combination therapy was associated with a mean 5- and 8.2-lb weight increase (15- and 30-mg doses, respectively), compared with no weight change in placebo-treated patients. Pioglitazone/metformin therapy was associated with a 2.2-lb weight increase, compared with a 3-lb weight loss in those treated with placebo.

Rosiglitazone

In Phase III trials the following was reported: Rosiglitazone monotherapy was associated with a 2.6-lb and 7.7-lb (4- and 8-mg doses respectively) weight gain. Rosiglitazone/metformin combination therapy was associated with weight gain of 1.5 and 5 lb (4- and 8-mg doses, respectively). A mean weight loss of 2.2 lb was observed in the placebo and placebo/metformin arms of these studies. Rosiglitazone/sulfonylurea combination therapy was associated with 3.9- and 6.5-lb weight gain (4- and 8-mg doses, respectively), compared with a 4.3-lb weight gain in patients treated with sulfonylurea alone.

Anemia

Reductions in hemoglobin and hematocrit ($\leq 4\%$ and ≤ 1 g, respectively) have been observed in patients treated with pioglitazone or rosiglitazone. These changes are possibly due to volume expansion and have not been associated with significant hematological effects. They occur within the first 4-8 weeks of therapy and have been shown to persist for at least 2 years. These effects are usually mild and no routine monitoring for anemia has been recommended.

Liver Function Abnormalities

Currently, it is recommended that patients treated with rosiglitazone or pioglitazone undergo serum transaminase monitoring at the initiation of therapy and periodically thereafter, based on the judgment of the clinician. Patients treated with rosiglitazone or pioglitazone who present with ALT levels ≥ 2.5 times the upper limit of normal should have their ALT levels assessed with some frequency. Patients treated with rosiglitazone or pioglitazone who present with ALT levels ≥ 3 times the upper limit of normal should have the level rechecked and should discontinue the drug if the elevation persists.

DRUG INTERACTIONS

Cytochrome P450 enzymes play a role in the metabolism of the thiazolidinediones. Rosiglitazone is metabolized predominantly by CYP2C8 and to a lesser degree by CYP2C9. In vitro drug metabolism studies have suggested that rosiglitazone does not inhibit the major CYP450 enzymes at clinically relevant concentrations. CYP3A4 is partially responsible for the metabolism of pioglitazone.

Glyburide

No interaction between glyburide or rosiglitazone was found in one study, while yet another small study in Japanese patients reported a slight increase in glyburide AUC and C_{max} when glyburide and rosiglitazone were coadministered.

Glimepiride

No interaction has been found between glimepiride and rosiglitazone.

Glipizide

No interaction has been found between glipizide and pioglitazone.

Warfarin

No significant effect has been found between warfarin and pioglitazone or rosiglitazone.

Ethanol

No significant effect has been found between moderate amounts of ethanol and pioglitazone or rosiglitazone.

Metformin

The pharmacokinetics of metformin when used in combination with rosiglitazone or pioglitazone are unchanged.

Digoxin

Rosiglitazone and pioglitazone do not alter the pharmacokinetics of digoxin.

Oral Contraceptives

When pioglitazone was coadministered with a combination oral contraceptive (ethinyl estradiol/norethindrone) for 21 days, an 11% reduction in ethinyl estradiol AUC and an 11%-14% reduction in ethinyl estradiol C_{max} values were reported. The clinical significance of this is unknown. Rosiglitazone has been shown to have no clinically significant effect on the pharmacokinetics of ethinyl estradiol or norethindrone.

Ranitidine

Administration of ranitidine did not alter the pharmacokinetics of either rosiglitazone or pioglitazone, suggesting that the absorption of these compounds is not significantly altered by increases in gastrointestinal pH.

Acarbose

Administration of acarbose had no clinically significant effect on the single dose pharmacokinetics of rosiglitazone.

Ketoconazole

The administration of ketoconazole in vitro appears to significantly inhibit the metabolism of pioglitazone.

See **Table 5.2,** or the full prescribing information, for more drug interaction guidance.

DOSAGE AND ADMINISTRATION

Pioglitazone is available in 15-, 30-, and 45-mg tablets. Pioglitazone can always be given just once daily in doses of 15, 30, or 45 mg. Usual initial doses are either 15 or 30 mg. Dose escalation should in most cases be based on re-evaluation of HbA_{1c} after 3 months of therapy at a given dose unless rapid deterioration of glycemic control dictates otherwise. Pioglitazone may be given without regard to meals.

Rosiglitazone is given either once or twice daily and is available in a 2-, 4-, and 8-mg tablet. The typical starting dose is 4 mg daily as a single or as a divided dose. Dose escalations should be made at 8-12 week intervals. In phase III trials, the greatest response was observed in patients treated with 4 mg twice daily. The maximum daily dose is 8 mg.

See **Table 5.1,** or the full prescribing information, for more dosing guidance.

SUGGESTED READING

Vasudevan AR, Balasubramanyam, A. Thiazolidinediones: A review of their mechanisms of insulin sensitization, therapeutic potential, clinical efficacy, and tolerability. *Diab Tech & Thera.* 2004; 6(6): 850-863.

Chilcott J, Tappenden P, Jones ML, Wight JP, A systematic review of the clinical effectiveness of pioglitazone in the treatment of type 2 diabetes mellitus. *Clin Ther.* 2001;23(11):1792-1823.

Chiquette E, Ramirez G, Defronzo R. A meta-analysis comparing the effect of thiazolidinediones on cardiovascular risk factors. *Arch Intern Med.* 2004;164:2097-2104.

Fowler M. Diabetes treatment, part 2: oral agents for glycemic management. *Clin Diabetes.* 2007; 25;4:131-139.

Grey AB, Skeletal toxicity of thiazolidinediones. *Ann Intern* Med. 2008; 148(7): 563-563.

Inzucchi SE. Oral antihyperglycemic therapy for type 2 diabetes: scientific review. *JAMA*. 2002;287:360-372.

Kahn SE, Haffner SM, Heise MA, Herman WH, Holman RR, Jones NP et al; ADOPT Study Group. Glycemic durability of rosiglitazone, metformin, or glyburide monotherapy. *N Engl J Med*. 2006;355:2427-2443.

Kosi RR. Practical review of oral antihyperglycemic agents for type 2 diabetes mellitus. *Diabetes Educator*. 2006; 32;6:869-876.

Nissen SE, Wolski K. Effect of rosiglitazone on the risk of myocardial infarction and death from cardiovascular causes. *N Engl J Med*. 2007;356:2457-2571.

Nissen SE, Nicholls SJ, Wolski K, Nesto R, Kupfer S, Perez A, Jure H, et al. Comparison of pioglitazone vs glimepiride on progression of coronary atherosclerosis in patients with Type 2 diabetes: The PERISCOPE Randomized Controlled Trial. *JAMA*, 2008; 299(13): 1561-1573.

van Wijk JP, de Koning EJ, Martens EP, Rabelink TJ. Thiazolidinediones and blood lipids in type 2 diabetes. *Arterioscler Thromb Vasc Biol*. 2003;23:1744-1749.

Table 5.1. Prescribing Information for Thiazolidinediones

GENERIC (BRAND)	FORM/ STRENGTH	DOSAGE	WARNINGS/PRECAUTIONS & CONTRAINDICATIONS	ADVERSE REACTIONS
Pioglitazone HCl (Actos)	Tab: 15mg, 30mg, 45mg	*Adults:* **Monotherapy:** Initial: 15-30mg qd. Max: 45mg/day. **Combination Therapy:** Initial: 15-30mg qd. Max: 30mg/day. Decrease insulin dose by 10-25% if hypoglycemia occurs or if plasma glucose is <100mg/dL. Decrease sulfonylurea dose with hypoglycemia also.	**BB:** Thiazolidinediones may cause or exacerbate CHF in some patients. Pioglitazone is not recommended in patients with symptomatic heart failure. **W/P:** May cause fluid retention and exacerbation/initiation of heart failure; d/c if cardiac status deteriorates. Avoid if NYHA Class III or IV cardiac status. Use lowest approved dose if systolic heart failure (NYHA Class II). Not for use in type 1 diabetes or for diabetic ketoacidosis treatment. Caution with edema. Dose-related weight gain reported. Ovulation in premenopausal anovulatory patients may occur; risk of pregnancy with inadequate contraception. May decrease Hgb and Hct. Avoid with active liver disease, if ALT levels >2.5x ULN, or if jaundice occurred with troglitazone. Check LFTs before therapy, every 2 months for 1 yr, and periodically thereafter, or if hepatic dysfunction symptoms occur. D/C if jaundice occurs or ALT >3x ULN on therapy. Macular edema reported. Increased incidence of bone fracture was noted in female patients. **Contra:** Established NYHA Class III or IV heart failure. **P/N:** Category C, not for use in nursing.	Upper respiratory tract infection, myalgia, tooth disorder, headache, sinusitis, pharyngitis, transient CPK level elevations, CHF, weight gain, aggravated DM, edema, dyspnea, new onset or worsening of diabetic macular edema.
Rosiglitazone maleate (Avandia)	Tab: 2mg, 4mg, 8mg	*Adults:* ≥18 yrs: Initial: 2mg bid or 4mg qd. Titrate: May increase after 8-12 weeks to 4mg bid or 8mg qd. Max: 8mg/day as monotherapy or with metformin; 4mg/day in combination with sulfonylureas or insulin. Decrease insulin by 10-25% if hypoglycemic or FPG <100mg/dL; individualize further adjustments based on glucose-lowering response.	**BB:** Thiazolidinediones may cause or exacerbate CHF in some patients. Rosiglitazone is not recommended in patients with symptomatic heart failure. Studies have shown rosiglitazone to be associated with an increased risk of myocardial ischemic events, such as angina or MI. **W/P:** May cause fluid retention and exacerbation/initiation of heart failure; d/c if cardiac status deteriorates. Increased risk of CV events with NYHA Class I or II cardiac status; avoid with NYHA Class III or IV cardiac status. Not for use in type 1 diabetes or diabetic ketoacidosis treatment. Caution with edema. Macular edema reported. Dose-related weight gain reported. Ovulation in premenopausal anovulatory patients may occur; risk of pregnancy with inadequate contraception. May decrease Hgb and Hct. Avoid with active liver disease, if ALT levels >2.5x ULN, or if jaundice occurred with troglitazone. Check LFTs before therapy, every 2 months for 1 year, and periodically thereafter, or if hepatic dysfunction symptoms occur. D/C if ALT >3x ULN on therapy. Increased incidence of bone fracture in female patients. Increased risk of myocardial ischemic events observed. Risk for hypoglycemia. Monitor blood glucose and HbA_{1c} measurements. CHF and MI during coadministration with insulin. Increased incidence of bone fractures in female patients. **Contra:** Established NYHA Class III or IV heart failure. Coadministration with insulin or nitrates. **P/N:** Category C, not for use in nursing.	Upper respiratory tract infection, injury, headache, back pain, hyperglycemia, fatigue, sinusitis, anemia, edema.

BB = black box warning; **W/P** = warnings/precautions; **Contra** = contraindications; **P/N** = pregnancy category rating and nursing considerations.

Table 5.1. Prescribing Information for Thiazolidinediones

GENERIC (BRAND)	FORM/ STRENGTH	DOSAGE	WARNINGS/PRECAUTIONS & CONTRAINDICATIONS	ADVERSE REACTIONS
COMBINATION DRUGS				
Pioglitazone HCl/Glimepiride (Duetact)	Tab: (Pioglitazone-Glimepiride) 30mg-2mg, 30mg-4mg	***Adults:*** Base recommended starting dose on current regimen of pioglitazone and/or sulfonylurea. Give with 1st meal of day. **Current Glimepiride Monotherapy or Prior Pioglitazone plus Glimepiride Separately:** Initial: 30mg-2mg or 30mg-4mg qd. **Current Pioglitazone or Different Sulfonylurea Monotherapy or Combination of Both:** Initial: 30mg-2mg qd. Adjust dose based on response. Max: Once daily at any strength. **Elderly/Debilitated/Malnourished/Renal or Hepatic Insufficiency (ALT ≤2.5x ULN):** Initial: 1mg glimepiride prior to prescribing Duetact. **Systolic Dysfunction:** Initial: 15-30mg of pioglitazone; titrate carefully to lowest Duetact dose.	**BB:** Thiazolidinediones may cause or exacerbate CHF in some patients. Duetact is not recommended in patients with symptomatic heart failure. **W/P:** (Glimepiride): Increased CV mortality. Hypoglycemia risk if debilitated, malnourished, or with adrenal, pituitary, renal or hepatic insufficiency. Hypoglycemia may be masked in elderly. May lose blood glucose control with stress. Secondary failure may occur. D/C if skin reactions persist or worsen. (Pioglitazone): May cause fluid retention and exacerbation/initiation of heart failure; d/c if cardiac status deteriorates. Avoid if NYHA Class III or IV cardiac status. Not for use in type 1 DM or diabetic ketoacidosis treatment. Caution with edema. Dose-related weight gain reported. Ovulation in premenopausal anovulatory patient may occur; risk of pregnancy with inadequate contraception. May decrease Hgb and Hct. Avoid with active liver disease, if ALT levels >2.5x ULN, or if jaundice occurred. Check LFTs before therapy, every 2 months for 1 yr, and periodically thereafter, or if hepatic dysfunction symptoms occur. D/C if ALT >3x ULN on therapy. Macular edema and fractures reported. **Contra:** Established NYHA Class III or IV heart failure, diabetic ketoacidosis. **P/N:** Category C, not for use in nursing.	Hypoglycemia, upper respiratory tract infection, increased weight, lower limb edema/pain, headache, UTI, diarrhea, nausea, new onset or worsening diabetic macular edema with decreased visual acuity.
Pioglitazone/ Metformin HCl (ActoPlus Met)	Tab: (Pioglitazone-Metformin) 15mg-500mg, 15mg-850mg	***Adults:*** Individualize dose. **Prior Pioglitazone/Metformin:** Base on current regimen. **Prior Metformin Monotherapy or Pioglitazone Monotherapy:** Initial: 15mg-500mg or 15mg-850mg qd-bid. Titrate: Gradually increase after assessing adequacy of therapeutic response. Max: (Pioglitazone) 45mg, (Metformin) 2550mg. **Elderly/Debilitated/Malnourished:** Conservative dosing; do not titrate to max dose.	**BB:** Thiazolidinediones may cause or exacerbate CHF in some patients. Actoplus Met is not recommended in patients with symptomatic heart failure. **W/P:** (Metformin) Lactic acidosis reported (rare); increased risk with renal dysfunction, increased age, DM, CHF, and other conditions with risk of hypoperfusion and hypoxemia. Avoid in patients ≥80 yrs unless normal renal function. Monitor renal function and for ketoacidosis and metabolic acidosis. Avoid in renal/hepatic impairment. D/C in hypoxic states (eg, CHF, shock, acute MI), loss of blood glucose control due to stress (give insulin), acidosis, dehydration, sepsis. Temporarily d/c prior to surgery (due to restricted food intake) and procedures requiring IV iodinated contrast materials. May decrease serum B_{12} levels. Increased risk of hypoglycemia in elderly, debilitated/ malnourished, adrenal or pituitary insufficiency, or alcohol intoxication. Monitor renal function. Alcohol known to potentiate effect of metformin on lactate metabolism. (Pioglitazone) May cause fluid retention and exacerbation/initiation of heart failure; d/c if cardiac status deteriorates. Avoid if NYHA Class III of IV cardiac status. Use lowest approved dose if systolic heart failure (NYHA Class II). Not for use in type 1 diabetes or for diabetic ketoacidosis treatment. Caution with edema. Dose-related weight gain reported. Ovulation in premenopausal anovulatory patients may occur; risk of pregnancy with inadequate contraception.	Upper respiratory tract infection, diarrhea, nausea, edema, headache, UTI, sinusitis, dizziness, weight increase, new onset or worsening diabetic macular edema.

BB = black box warning; **W/P** = warnings/precautions; **Contra** = contraindications; **P/N** = pregnancy category rating and nursing considerations.

Table 5.1. Prescribing Information for Thiazolidinediones

GENERIC (BRAND)	FORM/ STRENGTH	DOSAGE	WARNINGS/PRECAUTIONS & CONTRAINDICATIONS	ADVERSE REACTIONS
Pioglitazone/ Metformin HCl (ActoPlus Met) (Cont.)			May decrease Hgb and Hct. Avoid with active liver disease, if ALT levels >2.5x ULN. D/C if jaundice occurs or ALT >3x ULN on therapy. Macular edema reported. **Contra:** Established NYHA Class III or IV heart failure, renal disease or dysfunction (eg, SrCr ≥1.5mg/dL [males], ≥1.4mg/dL [females], or abnormal CrCl) and metabolic acidosis, including diabetic ketoacidosis. Temporarily d/c in patients undergoing radiologic studies involving intravascular iodinated contrast materials. **P/N:** Category C, not for use in nursing.	
Rosiglitazone maleate/ Glimepiride (Avandaryl)	**Tab: (Rosiglitazone-Glimepiride)** 4mg-1mg, 4mg-2mg, 4mg-4mg, 8mg-2mg, 8mg-4mg	***Adults:*** Initial: 4mg-1mg qd with 1st meal of day. **With Sulfonylurea or Thiazolidinedione:** Initial: 4mg-2mg qd. **Switching From Prior Combination Therapy:** Same dose of each component already being taken. **Prior Thiazolidinedione Monotherapy:** Titrate dose. After 1-2 weeks with inadequate control, increase glimepiride component in no more than 2mg increments at 1-2 week intervals. Max: 8mg-4mg qd. **Prior Sulfonylurea Monotherapy:** May take 2-3 months for full effect of rosiglitazone; do not exceed 8mg of rosiglitazone daily. Titrate: May increase glimepiride component. **Elderly/Debilitated/ Malnourished/Renal, Hepatic or Adrenal Insufficiency:** Initial: 4mg-1mg qd. Titrate carefully.	**BB:** Thiazolidinediones may cause or exacerbate CHF in some patients. Avandaryl is not recommended in patients with symptomatic heart failure. **W/P:** (Glimepiride) Increased cardiovascular mortality. Hypoglycemia risk if debilitated, malnourished, or with adrenal, pituitary, renal or hepatic insufficiency. Hypoglycemia may be masked in elderly. May lose blood glucose control with stress. Secondary failure may occur. D/C if skin reactions persist or worsen. (Rosiglitazone) May cause fluid retention and exacerbation/initiation of heart failure; d/c if cardiac status deteriorates. Increased risk of CV events with NYHA Class I and II heart failure. Not for use in type 1 DM or diabetic ketoacidosis treatment. Caution with edema. May cause macular edema. Dose-related weight gain reported. Ovulation in premenopausal anovulatory patient may occur; risk of pregnancy with inadequate contraception. May decrease Hgb and Hct. Avoid with active liver disease, if ALT levels >2.5x ULN, or if jaundice occurred with rosiglitazone. Check LFTs before therapy, every 2 months for 1 yr, and periodically thereafter, or if hepatic dysfunction symptoms occur. D/C if ALT >3x ULN on therapy. Increased incidence of bone fracture was noted in female patients. Combination use with insulin not recommended. **Contra:** Established NYHA Class III or IV heart failure, diabetic ketoacidosis. **P/N:** Category C, not for use in nursing.	Upper respiratory tract infection, injury, headache, hypoglycemia, anemia, edema.
Rosiglitazone/ Metformin HCl maleate (Avandamet)	**Tab: (Rosiglitazone-Metformin)** 2mg-500mg, 4mg-500mg, 2mg-1000mg, 4mg-1000mg	***Adults:*** **Prior Metformin Therapy of 1000mg/day:** Initial: 2mg-500mg tab bid. **Prior Metformin Therapy of 2000mg/day:** Initial: 2mg-1000mg tab bid. **Prior Rosiglitazone Therapy of 4mg/day:** Initial: 2mg-500mg tab bid. **Prior Rosiglitazone Therapy of 8mg/day:** 4mg-500mg tab bid. Titrate: May increase by increments of 4mg rosiglitazone and/or 500mg metformin. Max: 8mg-2000mg/day. **Drug-Naïve Patients:** Initial: 2mg-500mg qd-bid. If **HbA₁c >11% and FPG >270mg/dL:** Initial: 2mg-500mg bid. Titrate: After 4 weeks, may increase by increments of 2mg-500mg per day. Max: 8mg-2000mg per day. **Elderly/ Debilitated/Malnourished:** Conservative dosing; do not titrate to max dose. Take with meals.	**BB:** Thiazolidinediones may cause or exacerbate CHF in some patients. Avandamet is not recommended in patients with symptomatic heart failure. **W/P:** Lactic acidosis reported (rare); increased risk with renal dysfunction, increased age, DM, CHF, and other conditions with risk of hypoperfusion and hypoxemia. Avoid use in patients ≥80 yrs unless renal function is normal. Monitor renal function and for ketoacidosis and metabolic acidosis. D/C in hypoxic states (eg, CHF, shock, acute MI), loss of blood glucose control due to stress, acidosis and prior to surgical procedures (due to restricted food intake). May decrease serum vitamin B₁₂ levels. Increased risk of hypoglycemia with concomitant use with other hypoglycemic agents, elderly, debilitated/malnourished, adrenal or pituitary insufficiency, or alcohol	Upper respiratory tract infection, headache, back pain, hyperglycemia, fatigue, sinusitis, diarrhea, dizziness, abdominal pain, viral infection, arthralgia, anemia, dyspepsia, nausea, vomiting.

BB = black box warning; **W/P** = warnings/precautions; **Contra** = contraindications; **P/N** = pregnancy category rating and nursing considerations.

Table 5.1. Prescribing Information for Thiazolidinediones

GENERIC (BRAND)	FORM/ STRENGTH	DOSAGE	WARNINGS/PRECAUTIONS & CONTRAINDICATIONS	ADVERSE REACTIONS
COMBINATION DRUGS *(Cont.)*				
Rosiglitazone/ Metformin HCl maleate (Avandamet) *(Cont.)*			intoxication. May cause fluid retention and exacerbation/initiation of heart failure; d/c if cardiac status deteriorates. Avoid with NYHA Class III or IV cardiac status. Not for use in type 1 diabetes or for diabetic ketoacidosis treatment. Caution with edema. Dose-related weight gain reported. Ovulation in premenopausal anovulatory patients may occur; risk of pregnancy with inadequate contraception. May decrease Hgb and Hct. Avoid with active liver disease, if ALT levels >2.5x ULN, or if jaundice occurred with troglitazone. Check LFTs before therapy, every 2 months for 1 year, and periodically thereafter, or if hepatic dysfunction symptoms occur. D/C if ALT >3x ULN on therapy. Not for use with insulin. Increased incidence of bone fracture was noted in female patients **Contra:** Established NYHA Class III or IV heart failure, renal disease/ dysfunction (SrCr ≥1.5mg/dL [males], ≥1.4mg/dL [females], or abnormal CrCl), metabolic acidosis, including diabetic ketoacidosis. D/C temporarily (48 hrs) for radiologic studies with intravascular iodinated contrast materials. **P/N:** Category C, not for use in nursing.	

BB = black box warning; **W/P** = warnings/precautions; **Contra** = contraindications; **P/N** = pregnancy category rating and nursing considerations.

Table 5.2. Drug Interactions for Thiazolidinediones

Pioglitazone (Actos)

CYP2C8 inducers (eg, rifampin)	May significantly decrease the AUC of pioglitazone.
CYP2C8 inhibitors (eg, gemfibrozil)	May significantly increase the AUC of pioglitazone.
Ethinyl estradiol	Caution, may reduce contraceptive efficacy.
Hypoglycemic agents, oral	Caution, risk of hypoglycemia.
Insulin	Caution, risk of hypoglycemia.
Ketoconazole	May inhibit pioglitazone metabolism; perform more frequent monitoring of glycemic control.
Midazolam	May cause reduction in midazolam levels.
Norethindrone	Caution, may reduce contraceptive efficacy.

Rosiglitazone (Avandia)

CYP2C8 inducers (eg, rifampin)	May decrease AUC of rosiglitazone.
CYP2C8 inhibitors (eg, gemfibrozil)	May increase AUC of rosiglitazone.
Hypoglycemic agents, oral	Caution, risk of hypoglycemia.

COMBINATION DRUGS

Pioglitazone HCl-Glimepiride (Duetact)

Beta-blockers	May potentiate hypoglycemia.
Contraceptives, oral	Caution, risk of hyperglycemia.
Corticosteroids	Caution, risk of hyperglycemia.
Coumarins	May potentiate hypoglycemia.
CYP2C8 enzyme inducers (eg, rifampin)	May significantly decrease the AUC of pioglitazone.
CYP2C8 enzyme inhibitors (eg, gemfibrozil)	May significantly increase the AUC of pioglitazone.
CYP3A4 substrate	May be a weak inducer of CYP3A4 substrate.
Estrogens	Caution, risk of hyperglycemia.
Ethinyl estradiol	May decrease levels of ethinyl estradiol.
Isoniazid	Caution, risk of hyperglycemia.
MAO inhibitors	May potentiate hypoglycemia.
Miconazole	Warning, severe hypoglycemia reported with oral miconazole.
Midazolam	May decrease levels of midazolam.
Nicotinic acid	Caution, risk of hyperglycemia.
Phenothiazines	Caution, risk of hyperglycemia.
Phenytoin	Caution, risk of hyperglycemia.

Table 5.2. Drug Interactions for Thiazolidinediones

Salicylates	May potentiate hypoglycemia.
Sulfonamides	May potentiate hypoglycemia.
Sympathomimetics	Caution, risk of hyperglycemia.
Thiazides	Caution, risk of hyperglycemia.
Thyroid products	Caution, risk of hyperglycemia.
Pioglitazone HCl-Metformin HCl (Actoplus Met)	
Alcohol	Potentiates effects of metformin on lactate metabolism; potentiates hypoglycemia; avoid excessive alcohol intake.
Calcium channel blockers	May cause hyperglycemia.
Cationic drugs (eg, digoxin, amiloride, procainamide, quinidine, quinine, ranitidine, trimethoprim, vancomycin, triamterene, morphine)	May increase metformin levels.
Cimetidine	May increase metformin levels.
Contraceptives, oral (containing ethinyl estradiol and norethindrone)	Caution when coadministering, may decrease effectiveness, may cause hyperglycemia.
Corticosteroids	May cause hyperglycemia.
CYP2C8 enzyme inducers (eg, rifampin)	May significantly decrease AUC of pioglitazone.
CYP2C8 enzyme inhibitors (eg, gemfibrozil)	May significantly increase AUC of pioglitazone.
Diuretics	May cause hyperglycemia.
Estrogens	May cause hyperglycemia.
Furosemide	May increase metformin levels, may decrease furosemide levels.
Hypoglycemic agents, oral	Warning, risk of hypoglycemia.
Insulin	Warning, risk of hypoglycemia.
Isoniazid	May cause hyperglycemia.
Ketoconazole	May inhibit pioglitazone metabolism; perform more frequent monitoring of glycemic control.
Midazolam	May cause a reduction in midazolam levels.
Nicotinic acid	May cause hyperglycemia.
Nifedipine	May increase metformin levels.
Phenothiazines	May cause hyperglycemia.
Phenytoin	May cause hyperglycemia.
Sympathomimetics	May cause hyperglycemia.
Thiazides	May cause hyperglycemia.
Thyroid products	May cause hyperglycemia.

Table 5.2. Drug Interactions for Thiazolidinediones

Rosiglitazone maleate-Glimepiride (Avandaryl)

Beta-blockers	May mask symptoms of hypoglycemia.
Contraceptives, oral	Caution, risk of hyperglycemia.
Corticosteroids	Caution, risk of hyperglycemia.
CYP2C8 inducers (eg, rifampin)	May decrease the AUC of rosiglitazone.
CYP2C8 inhibitors (eg, gemfibrozil)	May increase the AUC of rosiglitazone.
Estrogens	Caution, risk of hyperglycemia.
Isoniazid	Caution, risk of hyperglycemia.
Miconazole	Warning, severe hypoglycemia reported with oral miconazole.
Nicotinic acid	Caution, risk of hyperglycemia.
Phenothiazines	Caution, risk of hyperglycemia.
Phenytoin	Caution, risk of hyperglycemia.
Sympathomimetics	Caution, risk of hyperglycemia.
Thiazides	Caution, risk of hyperglycemia.
Thyroid products	Caution, risk of hyperglycemia.

Rosiglitazone maleate-Metformin HCl (Avandamet)

Alcohol	Potentiates effects of metformin on lactate metabolism; potentiates hypoglycemia; avoid excessive alcohol intake.
Calcium channel blockers	May cause hyperglycemia.
Cationic drugs (eg, digoxin, amiloride, procainamide, quinidine, quinine, ranitidine, trimethoprim, vancomycin, triamterene, morphine)	May increase metformin levels.
Cimetidine	May increase metformin levels.
Contraceptives, oral	May cause hyperglycemia.
Corticosteroids	May cause hyperglycemia.
CYP2C8 inducers (eg, rifampin)	May decrease AUC of rosiglitazone.
CYP2C8 inhibitors (eg, gemfibrozil)	May increase AUC of rosiglitazone.
Diuretics	May cause hyperglycemia.
Estrogens	May cause hyperglycemia.
Furosemide	May increase metformin levels, may decrease furosemide levels.
Isoniazid	May cause hyperglycemia.
Nicotinic acid	May cause hyperglycemia.
Nifedipine	May increase metformin levels.

Table 5.2. Drug Interactions for Thiazolidinediones

Phenothiazines	May cause hyperglycemia.
Phenytoin	May cause hyperglycemia.
Sympathomimetics	May cause hyperglycemia.
Thiazides	May cause hyperglycemia.
Thyroid products	May cause hyperglycemia.

Chapter 6

Sulfonylureas

John R. White, Jr., PharmD, PA

INTRODUCTION

Sulfonylureas have been used in the management of type 2 diabetes for almost 50 years. Their mechanism of action in reducing hyperglycemia is complex, but essentially, they act on the pancreatic β-cell to increase both basal and meal-stimulated insulin secretion. Some studies have suggested sulfonylureas exert minor effects through extrapancreatic mechanisms. Long-term glycemic control with sulfonylurea treatment can cause improvement in several metabolic pathways in type 2 diabetes, including decreased overproduction of hepatic glucose, improved insulin action in skeletal muscle and adipose tissue, and increased efficiency of meal-stimulated insulin secretion.

Six sulfonylurea agents are currently available in the U.S.: the first-generation agents chlorpropamide, tolbutamide, and tolazamide; and the second-generation agents glyburide (glibenclamide), glipizide, and glimepiride.

PHARMACOLOGY

Mechanism of Action

Sulfonylureas exert their antihyperglycemic effect by stimulating insulin secretion in the pancreas. Insulin secretion is regulated by ATP-dependent potassium channels in the plasma membrane of the pancreatic β-cell. The ATP-dependent potassium channel consists of two subunits, one containing a sulfonylurea receptor and the other containing the channel itself. In patients with type 2 diabetes who retain some degree of β-cell function, sulfonylureas bind to the sulfonylurea receptor and close the ATP-dependent potassium channel. As potassium accumulates within the β-cell membrane, the β-cell depolarizes, leading to an influx of calcium. The increased concentration of calcium causes insulin granules to migrate to the cell surface, where the granules fuse with the membrane and release the insulin.

Sulfonylureas are also thought to exert extrapancreatic effects on the liver, peripheral tissues, and skeletal muscle. Although the precise mechanisms by which these effects improve hyperglycemia have not been demonstrated, it is likely that the direct effect of insulin secretion by the pancreas results in portal hyperinsulinemia that suppresses hepatic glucose production and causes a decrease in fasting plasma glucose. The improved glycemic state ameliorates glucose toxicity, thereby enhancing insulin sensitivity in skeletal muscle and adipose tissue. Patients with type 2 diabetes characteristically have defects in both insulin secretion and insulin action; therefore, regardless of the mechanism of action of the sulfonylurea drugs, they are effective in controlling hyperglycemia in these patients.

Pharmacokinetics

The sulfonylureas display marked differences in absorption, metabolism, and elimination. The first-generation sulfonylureas (chlorpropamide, tolbutamide, and tolazamide) are extensively protein bound, whereas the second-generation agents (glyburide or glibenclamide, glipizide, and glimepiride) do not bind to circulating plasma proteins.

All sulfonylureas are nearly completely absorbed; however, the onset and the duration of action are determined by the unique pharmacokinetic features of each agent and its specific formulation. Most sulfonylureas have a relatively short plasma half-life, usually in the range of 4-10 hours; only chlorpropamide has a half-life longer than 24 hours (see **Table 6.1**). Because most sulfonylureas maintain glycemic control effectively with twice-daily dosing, the tissue half-life on the β-cell receptor or the hypoglycemic effect itself must be considerably longer than the plasma half-life.

All sulfonylureas are metabolized in the liver, some to weakly active or inactive metabolites, others, such as chlorpropamide, only partially. The first-generation sulfonylureas are excreted exclusively by the kidney, whereas the second-generation agents and their metabolites are excreted in differing proportions in the urine and feces. A higher proportion of biliary excretion occurs with glyburide and glimepiride than with glipizide.

Advantages/Disadvantages

As initial treatment in patients with type 2 diabetes, sulfonylureas can induce a mean decrease in HbA_{1c} of 1%-2% and can reduce fasting plasma glucose by 60-70 mg/dL (3.3-3.8 mmol/L). The improvement in glycemic control that occurs with sulfonylureas, as with other antidiabetic agents, is somewhat greater in patients with poorer initial glycemic control and somewhat less in patients with only moderate hyperglycemia.

Sulfonylureas are indicated as an adjunct to nutrition therapy and exercise to lower blood glucose levels in patients with type 2 diabetes whose hyperglycemia has not been controlled adequately by nutrition therapy alone. The ideal candidates for treatment with sulfonylureas are patients with type 2 diabetes who have significant insulin deficiency but sufficient residual β-cell function to respond to stimulation. Patients are likely to demonstrate a good glycemic response to sulfonylureas if they:

- had onset of hyperglycemia after age 30 years
- have been diagnosed with hyperglycemia for <5 years
- have a fasting glucose level <300 mg/dL (16.7 mmol/L)

Table 6.1. Comparative Pharmacokinetics of Sulfonylureas

NAME	DOSE/RANGE (MG)	PEAK LEVEL (HR)	DURATION OF EFFECT (HR)	HALF-LIFE (HR)	METABOLITES	EXCRETION
SULFONYLUREA						
Tolbutamide	500-3,000	3-4	6-10	5-7	Inactive	Urine
Chlorpropamide	100-500	2-4	36-48	24-48	Active or unchanged	Urine
Tolazamide	100-1,000	3-4	16-24	7	Weakly active	Urine
Glipizide	2.5-40	1-3	12-14	2-4	Inactive	Urine 80% Feces 20%
Glyburide (*Glibenclamide*)	1.25-20	~4	12-24	10	Inactive and weakly active	Urine 50% Feces 50%
Glimepiride	1-8	2-3	16-24	9	Active	Urine 60% Feces 40%

Source: Campbell RK, White J. *Diabetes and Medications*. American Diabetes Association. Alexandria, VA. 2000.

- are normal weight or obese
- are willing to comply with a reasonable nutrition and exercise program
- are not totally insulin deficient

Approximately 20%-25% of patients with newly diagnosed type 2 diabetes fail to respond to initial sulfonylurea therapy (primary failures) and are best treated with another oral antihyperglycemic agent. Of the 75%-80% of patients who initially achieved good glycemic control, 3%-5% lose their responsiveness each year (secondary failures), most likely because of progressive β-cell failure, tachyphylaxis to the sulfonylurea, and weight gain.

With the progressive decline in β-cell function, the response to sulfonylurea treatment diminishes over time, and changes in treatment strategy will be necessary. The decrease in β-cell function is not the only possible cause of a lack of effectiveness, however. An increase in insulin resistance may play a role. There are also patient-related factors, including weight gain, poor compliance, inactivity, and stress or intercurrent illness. Therapy-related factors are another possible reason for a lack of response; for example, inadequate dosage, impaired absorption due to hyperglycemia, and concomitant treatment with diabetogenic drugs.

While in some cases sulfonlyureas may be the first oral medication used to bring a newly diagnosed patient's blood glucose under control, it is commonly the second agent used (after metformin). The combination of a sulfonylurea and metformin is very commonly used and is arguably the most frequently encountered combination of oral antidiabetic drugs.

Data from several studies have suggested that the second-generation sulfonylurea glimepiride (Amaryl) may be associated with a lower incidence of hypoglycemia and less weight gain and may improve insulin sensitivity compared to other sulfonylureas.

THERAPEUTIC CONSIDERATIONS

Significant Warnings and Precautions

The sulfonylureas are contraindicated in patients with a known hypersensitivity to the drug and in those with diabetic ketoacidosis (DKA), with or without coma. DKA should be treated with insulin.

The product information for the sulfonylurea drugs contains a special warning that the administration of oral antidiabetic agents has been reported to be associated with increased risk of cardiovascular mortality compared with treatment with nutrition therapy alone or nutrition therapy plus insulin. This warning is based on the results of a long-term, prospective clinical trial, the University Group Diabetes Program. Although only one sulfonylurea, tolbutamide, was included in this study, this warning may also apply to other agents of this class, considering their similar mechanism of action and chemical structures. The validity of this finding has been questioned, however; the UK Prospective Diabetes Study (UKPDS) found no increased cardiovascular mortality with sulfonylureas. The validity of this warning has been called into question.

Hypoglycemia

The most serious complication of sulfonylurea therapy is hypoglycemia, and all sulfonylureas are capable of producing severe hypoglycemia. Appropriate patient selection, dosage, and instructions are important to avoid hypoglycemic episodes. Debilitated or malnourished patients and those with adrenal, pituitary, or hepatic insufficiency are particularly susceptible to the hypoglycemic action of sulfonylureas. Hypoglycemia may be difficult to recognize in the elderly and in people taking β-adrenergic blocking agents or other sympatholytic drugs. Hypoglycemia is more likely to occur when caloric intake is deficient, after severe or prolonged exercise, when alcohol is ingested, or when more than one glucose-lowering drug is used.

Loss of Blood Glucose Control

A loss of blood glucose control may occur if a patient experiences stress through fever, trauma, infection, or surgery. It may be necessary to institute insulin therapy in combination with the sulfonylurea. However, the combined use of a sulfonylurea and insulin may increase the risk of hypoglycemia.

Pregnancy and Nursing

The sulfonylureas are pregnancy category C. Chlorpropamide has not been evaluated for teratogenic effects. Glipizide and glimepiride have been found to be fetotoxic in rats at doses that produced maternal hypoglycemia. In some studies in rats, non-teratogenic skeletal deformities were observed after exposure during gestation and lactation. There are no adequate and well-controlled studies of sulfonylureas in pregnant women. On the basis of animal studies, sulfonylureas should not be used during pregnancy. Because a higher incidence of congenital abnormalities is associated with abnormal maternal blood glucose levels during pregnancy, insulin therapy is recommended during pregnancy to maintain blood glucose levels as close to normal as possible.

Pediatric Use

The safety and effectiveness of sulfonylureas in pediatric patients have not been established.

Special Populations

Patients with Hepatic or Renal Dysfunction

Because sulfonylureas are metabolized in the liver, they are, as a class, contraindicated in patients with hepatic dysfunction. Chlorpropamide is contraindicated in patients with diminished renal function because the kidney is the primary mode of excretion.

Elderly Patients

Hypoglycemia is the most significant risk of the use of sulfonylureas and other oral agents in elderly patients. Both renal and hepatic insufficiency are substantial risk factors for the development of severe hypoglycemia during sulfonylurea treatment in the elderly. Chlorpropamide is contraindicated in elderly patients (>60-65 years) because of the normal age-related decline in glomerular filtration rate.

ADVERSE EFFECTS AND MONITORING

Sulfonylureas are usually well tolerated and the frequency of side effects, other than hypoglycemia, is low. The most common adverse events associated with sulfonylurea treatment other than hypoglycemia, are dizziness, headache, asthenia, and nausea. In comparative clinical trials, common adverse events occurred at similar rates with glimepiride and glipizide but were less likely to occur with glimepiride than glyburide. Hematological complications, including thrombocytopenia, agranulocytosis, and hemolytic anemia have been described with tolbutamide and chlorpropamide, but appear to be very rare with the second-generation sulfonylureas. Skin reactions are nonspecific and rare. Abnormal liver function tests and icterus are uncommon.

Certain side effects are unique to the specific agents because of their individual chemical structures. For example, chlorpropamide has antidiuretic properties that can lead to water retention and hyponatremia. In predisposed individuals, chlorpropamide frequently causes an alcohol-induced flush; this phenomenon also occurs occasionally with tolbutamide.

DRUG INTERACTIONS

The hypoglycemic action of sulfonylureas may be potentiated by certain drugs, including nonsteroidal anti-inflammatory drugs (NSAIDs) and other drugs that are highly bound to protein, such as salicylates, sulfonamides, chloramphenicol, coumarins, probenecid, monoamine oxidase inhibitors, and β-adrenergic blocking agents. Patients given these drugs concomitantly with a sulfonylurea should be monitored closely for hypoglycemia. Similarly, when these drugs are withdrawn, patients on sulfonylurea therapy should be observed closely for loss of glycemic control.

Other drugs tend to produce hyperglycemia and may lead to loss of glycemic control in patients taking sulfonylureas. These drugs include the thiazides and other diuretics, corticosteroids, phenothiazines, thyroid products, estrogens, oral contraceptives, phenytoin, nicotinic acid, sympathomimetics, and isoniazid. When these drugs are withdrawn, patients should be observed closely for hypoglycemia.

See **Table 6.3**, or refer to the full prescribing information for more drug interaction guidance.

DOSAGE AND ADMINISTRATION

Treatment with sulfonylureas is typically instituted at a low dose and increased at four- to seven-day intervals until the maximal benefit is achieved. In patients with good dietary compliance and in those who lose weight, sulfonylurea therapy may be reduced or discontinued; however, some data suggest that maintenance therapy with low doses of a sulfonylurea can better provide long-term glycemic control. See **Table 6.2** for more dosing information.

Most patients will achieve the maximal benefit in improved glycemic control with one-half to two-thirds of the recommended maximal dose. When sulfonylurea therapy fails to meet target blood glucose levels, a second oral antihyperglycemic agent or insulin can be added to the regimen.

A number of factors influence the choice of a sulfonylurea, including its intrinsic potency, onset of action, duration of action, patterns of metabolism and excretion, and beneficial and detrimental side effects. The intrinsic potency of a sulfonylurea is a function of its binding affinity to the receptor. Glyburide and glimepiride are the most potent drugs in this class; tolbutamide the least potent. Glimepiride does not affect potassium channels in cardiac tissue.

The duration of action of a sulfonylurea is an important consideration (see **Table 6.1**). Of the first-generation agents, chlorpropamide has a very long half-life and duration of action and needs to be given only once daily; tolbutamide, on the other hand, has a very short duration of action and needs to be administered two or three times a day. Most of the second-generation agents, which have a duration of 16-24 hours, can be administered once a day at the usual therapeutic doses, but maximal doses may need to be divided into two daily doses. A newer second-generation agent, glimepiride, may be administered before or with breakfast, with equivalent blood glucose-lowering effect.

The patterns of metabolism and excretion are also important to the risk of side effects. Because sulfonylureas are metabolized—and therefore inactivated—in the liver, the risk of hypoglycemia is significantly increased in patients with hepatic impairment. Similarly, sulfonylureas that are excreted primarily in the urine are more likely to cause hypoglycemia in patients with renal dysfunction than are those that are excreted in large part via the biliary tract.

When a particular sulfonylurea fails as monotherapy to maintain acceptable glycemic control, combining a sulfonylurea with other forms of antihyperglycemic therapy is indicated. Sulfonylureas may be combined with most other forms of antihyperglycemic agents in patients with type 2 diabetes except the other oral secretagogues.

The rationale for combination therapy lies in the mechanism of action of sulfonylureas, to increase insulin secretion. As insulin secretory function declines because of progressive β-cell failure, a sulfonylurea has a diminished effect on insulin secretion. The mechanisms by which other oral antihyperglycemic agents reduce blood glucose levels can complement the action of sulfonylureas to achieve glycemic control.

For example, the combination of a sulfonylurea and metformin is effective because metformin does not affect β-cell function; rather, it reduces hepatic glucose production and improves insulin resistance in skeletal muscle, providing an additive glucose-lowering effect. Sulfonylurea/metformin combinations are the most commonly used oral combination therapy for type 2 diabetes.

When added to a sulfonylurea, an α-glucosidase inhibitor, which delays the absorption of glucose in the small intestine, provides an additive effect by lowering postprandial glucose levels and improving the action of endogenous insulin.

The thiazolidinediones also enhance insulin sensitivity in skeletal muscle and glucose utilization in the liver, and several clinical trials have demonstrated their effectiveness as combination therapy with a sulfonylurea.

Sulfonylureas and insulin have been used extensively in combination therapy. Glycemic control can usually be achieved with this combination by the addition of insulin in a relatively low dose administered in a simple regimen. The extrahepatic effects of the sulfonylurea are thought to increase the efficacy of the insulin. One of the more successful regimens involves the administration of bedtime insulin glargine or NPH in combination with daytime sulfonylurea, sometimes referred to as BIDS therapy.

SUGGESTED READING

Fowler M. Diabetes Treatment, Part 2: Oral Agents for Glycemic Management. *Clin Diabetes.* 25;4:131-139, 2007.

Kahn SE, Haffner SM, Heise MA, Herman WH, Holman RR, Jones NP, et al; ADOPT Study Group: Glycemic durability of rosiglitazone, metformin, or glyburide monotherapy. *N Engl J Med.* 355 : 2427-2443,2006.

Kosi RR. Practical review of oral antihyperglycemic agents for type 2 diabetes mellitus. *The Diabetes Educator.* 32;6:869-876, 2006.

Langtry HD, Balfour JA. Glimepiride: a review of its use in the management of type 2 diabetes mellitus. *Drugs.* 55:563-584, 1998.

UK Prospective Diabetes Study Group: Intensive blood glucose control with sulphonylureas or insulin compared with conventional treatment and risk of complications in patients with type 2 diabetes (UKPDS 33). *Lancet.* 352:837-853, 1998.

White, J., Campbell RK. Recent developments in the pharmacological reduction of blood glucose in patients with type 2 diabetes. *Clin. Diabetes.* 2001 19: 153-159.

Table 6.2. Prescribing Information for Sulfonylureas

GENERIC (BRAND)	FORM/ STRENGTH	DOSAGE	WARNINGS/PRECAUTIONS & CONTRAINDICATIONS	ADVERSE REACTIONS
Chlorpropamide (Diabinese)	Tab: 100mg*, 250mg* *scored	*Adults:* Initial: 250mg qd. Titrate: After 5-7 days, adjust by 50-125mg/day every 3-5 days for control. Maint: 100-500 qd. Max: 750mg qd. Elderly/Debilitated/ Malnourished/Renal or Hepatic Dysfunction: Initial: 100-125mg qd. Maint: Conservative dosing. Take with breakfast. Divide dose with GI intolerance. If <40U/day insulin, discontinue therapy. If ≥40 U/day insulin, decrease dose by 50% and start chlorpropamide therapy. Adjust insulin dose depending on response.	W/P: Increased risk of cardiovascular mortality. Hypoglycemia risk especially with renal/hepatic insufficiency, elderly, debilitated, malnourished, and adrenal/ pituitary insufficiency. Loss of blood glucose control when exposed to stress (fever, trauma, infection or surgery); d/c therapy and start insulin. Secondary failure can occur over a period of time. Contra: Diabetic ketoacidosis and Type I diabetes. P/N: Category C, not for use in nursing.	Hypoglycemia, cholestatic jaundice, diarrhea, nausea, vomiting, anorexia, pruritus, photosensitivity reactions, skin eruptions, blood dyscrasias, hepatic porphyria, disulfiram-like reactions.
Glimepiride (Amaryl)	Tab: 1mg*, 2mg*, 4mg* *scored	*Adults:* Initial: 1-2mg qd with breakfast or 1st main meal. Titrate: After 2mg, may increase by up to 2mg every 1-2 weeks. Maint: 1-4mg qd. Max: 8mg qd. Amaryl/ Metformin: Add Metformin to 8mg qd for better glucose control. Amaryl/Insulin Therapy: If FBG >150mg/dL on 8mg qd, add low-dose insulin; increase insulin weekly as needed. Renal Insufficiency: Initial: 1mg qd. Elderly/Debilitated/ Malnourished/Hepatic Insufficiency: Dose conservatively to avoid hypoglycemia.	W/P: Increased cardiovascular mortality. Hypoglycemia risk if debilitated, malnourished, or with adrenal, pituitary, renal or hepatic insufficiency. Hypoglycemia may be masked in elderly. May lose blood glucose control with stress. Secondary failure may occur. D/C if skin reactions persist or worsen. Contra: Diabetic ketoacidosis. P/N: Category C, not for use in nursing.	Dizziness, nausea, asthenia, headache, hypoglycemia.
Glipizide (Glucotrol, Glucotrol XL)	Tab: (Glucotrol) 5mg*, 10mg*; Tab, Extended- Release: (Glucotrol XL) 2.5mg, 5mg, 10mg *scored	*Adults:* (Glucotrol XL) Do not chew, divide, or crush. Initial: 5mg qd with breakfast. Use lower doses if sensitive to hypoglycemics. Usual: 5-10mg qd. Max: 20mg/day. Combination Therapy: Initial: 5mg qd. (Glucotrol): Initial: 5mg qd 30 min before breakfast. Geriatric/Hepatic Impairment: Initial 2.5mg qd. Titrate: Increase by 2.5-5mg after several days. Max: 40mg/day. Divide doses >15mg and give 30 min before a meal. (Glucotrol XL, Glucotrol) Switch From Insulin: If on ≤20 U/day: Stop insulin; start Glucotrol XL or Glucotrol 5mg qd. If on >20 U/day: Reduce insulin dose by 50% and add Glucotrol XL or Glucotrol 5mg qd. Further insulin reductions depend on response.	W/P: Increased risk of hypoglycemia with the elderly, debilitated, malnourished, renal and hepatic disease, adrenal or pituitary insufficiency. Increased risk of cardiovascular mortality. Loss of blood glucose control when exposed to stress (fever, trauma, infection, or surgery); d/c therapy and start insulin. Secondary failure can occur over a period of time. (Glucotrol XL) GI disease will reduce retention time of the drug. Caution with pre-existing severe GI narrowing. Contra: Diabetic ketoacidosis. P/N: Category C, not for use in nursing.	Hypoglycemia, nausea, diarrhea, allergic skin reactions, disulfiram-like reactions, dizziness, drowsiness, asthenia, headache.
Glyburide (DiaBeta)	Tab: 1.25mg*, 2.5mg*, 5mg* *scored	*Adults:* Initial: 2.5-5mg qd with breakfast or first main meal; give 1.25mg if sensitive to hypoglycemia. Titrate: Increase by no more than 2.5mg/day at weekly intervals. Maint: 1.25-20mg given qd or in divided doses. Max: 20mg/day. May give bid with >10mg/day. Renal/ Hepatic Disease, Elderly, Debilitated, Malnourished, Adrenal or Pituitary Insufficiency: Initial: 1.25mg qd. Transfer From Other Oral Antidiabetic Agents: Initial: 2.5-5mg/day. Switch From Insulin: If <20 U/day: 2.5-5mg qd. If 20-40 U/day: 5mg qd. If >40 U/day: Decrease insulin dose by 50% and give 5mg qd. Titrate: Progressive withdrawal of insulin and increase by 1.25-2.5mg/day every 2-10 days.	W/P: Increased risk of cardiovascular mortality. Risk of hypoglycemia, especially with renal and hepatic disease, elderly, debilitated or malnourished patients, and those with adrenal or pituitary insufficiency. May need to d/c and give insulin with stress (eg, fever, trauma). Secondary failure may occur. D/C if jaundice, hepatitis, or persistent skin reaction occur. Hematologic reactions and hyponatremia reported. Contra: Diabetic ketoacidosis. P/N: Category C, not for use in nursing.	Hypoglycemia, nausea, epigastric fullness, heartburn, allergic skin reactions, disulfiram-like reactions (rarely), hyponatremia, liver function abnormalities, photosensitivity reactions.
Glyburide (Glynase PresTab)	Tab: 1.5mg*, 3mg*, 6mg* *scored	*Adults:* Initial: 1.5-3mg qd with breakfast or 1st main meal. Renal/Hepatic Disease/Elderly/Debilitated/Malnourished/ Adrenal or Pituitary Insufficiency: Initial: 0.75mg qd. Titrate: Increase by no more than 1.5mg/day at weekly intervals. Maint: 0.75-12mg qd or in divided doses. Max: 12mg/day given qd or bid. Transfer from Other Sulfonylureas: Starting dose should not exceed 3mg/day. Switch from	W/P: Increased risk of cardiovascular mortality. Risk of hypoglycemia, especially with renal and hepatic disease, elderly, debilitated, malnourished, and adrenal or pituitary insufficiency. Loss of blood glucose control when exposed to stress (eg, fever, trauma, infection or surgery); d/c therapy and start insulin. Secondary failure can occur over a period of time. D/C if cholestatic jaundice or hepatitis	Hypoglycemia, nausea, epigastric fullness, heartburn, allergic skin reactions, disulfiram-like reactions (rarely), hyponatremia, blood dyscrasias, LFT abnormalities, photosensitivity reactions.

W/P = warnings/precautions; Contra = contraindications; P/N = pregnancy category rating and nursing considerations.

Table 6.2. Prescribing Information for Sulfonylureas

GENERIC (BRAND)	FORM/ STRENGTH	DOSAGE	WARNINGS/PRECAUTIONS & CONTRAINDICATIONS	ADVERSE REACTIONS
Glyburide (Glynase PresTab) *(Cont.)*		**Insulin:** If <20 U/day, substitute with 1.5-3mg qd. If 20-40 U/day, give 3mg qd. If >40 U/day, decrease insulin dose by 50% and give 3mg qd. Titrate: Progressive withdrawal of insulin and increase by 0.75-1.5mg every 2-10 days.	occur. Retitrate when transferring from other glyburide products. Contra: Diabetic ketoacidosis, and as sole therapy of type 1 DM. **P/N:** Category B, not for use in nursing.	
Glyburide (Micronase)	**Tab:** 1.25mg*, 2.5mg*, 5mg* *scored	**Adults:** Initial: 2.5-5mg qd with breakfast or 1st main meal; give 1.25mg if sensitive to hypoglycemia. Titrate: Increase by no more than 2.5mg/day at weekly intervals. Maint: 1.25-20mg given qd or in divided doses. Max: 20mg/day. May give bid with >10mg/day. **Renal or Hepatic Disease/ Elderly/Debilitated/Malnourished/Adrenal or Pituitary Insufficiency:** Initial: 1.25mg qd. **Transfer From Other Oral Antidiabetic Agents:** Initial: 2.5-5mg/day. **Switch From Insulin:** If <20 U/day: 2.5-5mg qd. If 20-40 U/day: 5mg qd. If >40 U/day, decrease dose by 50% and give 5mg qd. Titrate: Progressive withdrawal of insulin, and increase by 1.25-2.5mg/day every 2-10 days. **Concomitant Metformin:** Add glyburide gradually to max dose of metformin monotherapy after 4 weeks if needed.	**W/P:** Increased risk of cardiovascular mortality. Risk of hypoglycemia, especially with renal and hepatic disease, elderly, debilitated or malnourished patients, and those with adrenal or pituitary insufficiency. May need to d/c and give insulin with stress (eg, fever, trauma). Secondary failure may occur. D/C if jaundice, hepatitis, or persistent skin reaction occur. Hematologic reactions and hyponatremia reported. **Contra:** Diabetic ketoacidosis, and as sole therapy for type 1 DM. **P/N:** Category B, not for use in nursing.	Hypoglycemia, nausea, epigastric fullness, heartburn, allergic skin reactions, disulfiram-like reactions (rarely), hyponatremia, liver function abnormalities, photosensitivity reactions.
Tolazamide (Tolinase**)	**Tab:** 250mg*, 500mg* *scored	**Adults:** Initial: 100-250mg qd with breakfast. If FBG <200mg/dL, start at 100mg qd. If FBG >200mg/dL, start at 250mg qd. Titrate: 100-250mg every week. Maint: 250-500mg qd. Max: 1000mg qd. **Elderly/Debilitated/ Malnourished/Renal or Hepatic Insufficiency:** Conservative dosing to avoid hypoglycemia.	**W/P:** Increased cardiovascular mortality. Hypoglycemia risk if debilitated, elderly, malnourished, or with adrenal, pituitary, renal or hepatic insufficiency. Hypoglycemia may be masked in elderly. May lose blood glucose control with stress. Primary and secondary failure may occur. **Contra:** Diabetic ketoacidosis and type 1 DM. **P/N:** Category C, not for use in nursing.	Nausea, epigastric fullness, heartburn, hypglycemia, allergic skin reactions, blood dyscrasias, hepatic porphyria, disulfiram-like reactions (rarely).
Tolbutamide (Orinase**)	**Tab:** 500 mg* *scored	**Adults:** Initial: 1-2g qd. Titrate: increase or decrease according to response. Maint: 0.25-3g qd. Max 3g qd. **Elderly/ Debilitated/Malnourished/Renal or Heptatic Insufficiency:** Conservative dosing to avoid hypoglycemia.	**W/P:** Increased cardiovascular mortality. Hypoglycemia risk if debilitated, elderly, malnourished, or with adrenal, pituitary, renal or hepatic insufficiency. Hypoglycemia may be masked in elderly. May lose blood glucose control with stress. Primary and secondary failure may occur. **Contra:** Diabetic ketoacidosis and type 1 DM. **P/N:** Category C, not for use in nursing.	Hypoglycemia, nausea, epigastric fullness, heartburn, allergic skin reactions, blood dyscrasias, hepatic porphyria, disulfiram-like reactions (rarely), hyponatremia, headache, taste disturbances.
COMBINATION DRUGS				
Glimepiride/ Pioglitazone HCl (Duetact)	**Tab:** (Pioglitazone- Glimepiride) 30mg- 2mg, 30mg-4mg	**Adults:** Base recommended starting dose on current regimen of pioglitazone and/or sulfonylurea. Give with 1st meal of day. **Current Glimepiride Monotherapy or Prior Pioglitazone plus Glimepiride Separately:** Initial: 30mg-2mg or 30mg-4mg qd. **Current Pioglitazone or Different Sulfonylurea Monotherapy or Combination of Both:** Initial: 30mg-2mg qd. Adjust dose based on response. Max: Once daily at any strength. **Elderly/Debilitated/ Malnourished/Renal or Hepatic Insufficiency (ALT ≤2.5x ULN):** Initial: 1mg glimepiride prior to prescribing Duetact. **Systolic Dysfunction:** Initial: 15-30mg of pioglitazone; titrate carefully to lowest Duetact dose.	**BB:** Thiazolidinediones may cause or exacerbate CHF in some patients. Duetact is not recommended in patients with symptomatic heart failure. **W/P:** (Glimepiride): Increased CV mortality. Hypoglycemia risk if debilitated, malnourished, or with adrenal, pituitary, renal or hepatic insufficiency. Hypoglycemia may be masked in elderly. May lose blood glucose control with stress. Secondary failure may occur. D/C if skin reactions persist or worsen. (Pioglitazone): May cause fluid retention and exacerbation/initiation of heart failure; d/c if cardiac status deteriorates. Avoid if NYHA Class III or IV cardiac status. Not for use in type 1 DM or diabetic ketoacidosis treatment. Caution with edema. Dose-related weight gain reported. Ovulation in premenopausal anovulatory patient may occur; risk of pregnancy with inadequate	Hypoglycemia, upper respiratory tract infection, increased weight, lower limb edema/pain, headache, UTI, diarrhea, nausea, new onset or worsening diabetic macular edema with decreased visual acuity.

**Brand name not available in the U.S.
BB = black box warning; **W/P** = warnings/precautions; **Contra** = contraindications; **P/N** = pregnancy category rating and nursing considerations.

Table 6.2. Prescribing Information for Sulfonylureas

GENERIC (BRAND)	FORM/ STRENGTH	DOSAGE	WARNINGS/PRECAUTIONS & CONTRAINDICATIONS	ADVERSE REACTIONS
Glimepiride/ Pioglitazone HCl (Duetact) (Cont.)			contraception. May decrease Hgb and Hct. Avoid with active liver disease, if ALT levels >2.5x ULN, or if jaundice occurred. Check LFTs before therapy, every 2 months for 1 yr, and periodically thereafter, or if hepatic dysfunction symptoms occur. D/C if ALT >3x ULN on therapy. Macular edema and fractures reported. **Contra:** Established NYHA Class III or IV heart failure, diabetic ketoacidosis. **P/N:** Category C, not for use in nursing.	
Glimepiride/ Rosiglitazone maleate (Avandaryl)	Tab: (Rosiglitazone-Glimepiride) 4mg-1mg, 4mg-2mg, 4mg-4mg, 8mg-2mg, 8mg-4mg	*Adults:* Initial: 4mg-1mg qd with 1st meal of day. **With Sulfonylurea or Thiazolidinedione:** Initial: 4mg-2mg qd. **Switching From Prior Combination Therapy:** Same dose of each component already being taken. **Prior Thiazolidinedione Monotherapy:** Titrate dose. After 1-2 weeks with inadequate control, increase glimepiride component in no more than 2mg increments at 1-2 week intervals. Max: 8mg-4mg qd. **Prior Sulfonylurea Monotherapy:** May take 2-3 months for full effect of rosiglitazone; do not exceed 8mg of rosiglitazone daily. Titrate: May increase glimepiride component. **Elderly/Debilitated/ Malnourished/Renal, Hepatic or Adrenal Insufficiency:** Initial: 4mg-1mg qd. Titrate carefully.	**BB:** Thiazolidinediones may cause or exacerbate CHF in some patients. Avandaryl is not recommended in patients with symptomatic heart failure. **W/P:** (Glimepiride) Increased cardiovascular mortality. Hypoglycemia risk if debilitated, malnourished, or with adrenal, pituitary, renal or hepatic insufficiency. Hypoglycemia may be masked in elderly. May lose blood glucose control with stress. Secondary failure may occur. D/C if skin reactions persist or worsen. (Rosiglitazone) May cause fluid retention and exacerbation/initiation of heart failure; d/c if cardiac status deteriorates. Increased risk of CV events with NYHA Class I and II heart failure. Not for use in type 1 DM or diabetic ketoacidosis treatment. Caution with edema. May cause macular edema. Dose-related weight gain reported. Ovulation in premenopausal anovulatory patient may occur; risk of pregnancy with inadequate contraception. May decrease Hgb and Hct. Avoid with active liver disease, if ALT levels >2.5x ULN, or if jaundice occurred with rosiglitazone. Check LFTs before therapy, every 2 months for 1 yr, and periodically thereafter, or if hepatic dysfunction symptoms occur. D/C if ALT >3x ULN on therapy. Increased incidence of bone fracture was noted in female patients. Combination use with insulin not recommended. **Contra:** Established NYHA Class III or IV heart failure, diabetic ketoacidosis. **P/N:** Category C, not for use in nursing.	Upper respiratory tract infection, headache, hypoglycemia, anemia, edema.
Glipizide/ Metformin HCl (Metaglip)	Tab: (Glipizide-Metformin) 2.5mg-250mg, 2.5mg-500mg, 5mg-500mg	*Adults:* Initial: 2.5mg-250mg qd. If FBG 280-320mg/dL, give 2.5mg-500mg bid. Titrate: Increase by 1 tab/day every 2 weeks. Max: 10mg-1g/day or 10mg-2g/day given in divided doses. **Second-Line Therapy:** Initial: 2.5mg-500mg or 5mg-500mg bid (with morning and evening meals). Starting dose should not exceed daily dose of metformin or glipizide already being taken. Titrate: Increase by no more than 5mg-500mg/day. Max: 20mg-2g/day. **Elderly/Debilitated/ Malnourished:** Do not titrate to max dose. Take with meals.	**W/P:** Lactic acidosis reported (rare); increased risk with renal dysfunction, increased age, DM, CHF, and other conditions with risk of hypoperfusion and hypoxemia. Avoid use in patients ≥80 yrs unless renal function is normal. Increased risk of cardiovascular mortality. Increased risk of hypoglycemia in elderly, debilitated/ malnourished, adrenal or pituitary insufficiency, or alcohol intoxication. D/C in hypoxic states (eg, CHF, shock, acute MI) and prior to surgical procedures (due to restricted food intake). Avoid in renal/ hepatic impairment. May decrease serum vitamin B$_{12}$ levels. Impaired renal and/or hepatic function may slow glipizide excretion. Withhold treatment with any condition associated with dehydration or sepsis. Monitor renal function. **Contra:** Renal disease/dysfunction (SrCr ≥1.5mg/ dL [males], ≥1.4mg/dL [females], abnormal CrCl), metabolic acidosis, diabetic ketoacidosis. D/C temporarily (48 hrs) for radiologic studies with intravascular iodinated contrast materials. **P/N:** Category C, not for use in nursing.	Upper respiratory tract infection, HTN, headache, diarrhea, dizziness, musculoskeletal pain, nausea, vomiting, abdominal pain.

BB = black box warning; **W/P** = warnings/precautions; **Contra** = contraindications; **P/N** = pregnancy category rating and nursing considerations.

Table 6.2. Prescribing Information for Sulfonylureas

GENERIC (BRAND)	FORM/ STRENGTH	DOSAGE	WARNINGS/PRECAUTIONS & CONTRAINDICATIONS	ADVERSE REACTIONS
COMBINATION DRUGS *(Cont.)*				
Glyburide/ Metformin HCl (Glucovance)	Tab: (Glyburide-Metformin) 1.25mg-250mg, 2.5mg-500mg, 5mg-500mg	*Adults:* Take with meals. Initial: 1.25mg-250mg qd. If HbA$_{1C}$ >9% or FPG >200mg/dL, give 1.25mg-250mg bid. Titrate: Increase by 1.25mg-250mg/day every 2 weeks. Do not use 50mg-500mg tab for initial therapy. **Second-Line Therapy:** Initial: 2.5mg-500mg or 5mg-500mg bid. Starting dose should not exceed daily doses of glyburide (or sulfonylurea equivalent) or metformin already being taken. Titrate: Increase by no more than 5mg-500mg/day. Max: 20mg-2000mg/day. **With Concomitant TZD:** Initiate and titrate TZD as recommended. If hypoglycemia occurs, reduce glyburide component. **Elderly/Debilitated/ Malnourished:** Conservative dosing; do not titrate to max.	**W/P:** Lactic acidosis reported (rare); increased risk with renal dysfunction, increased age, DM, CHF, and other conditions with risk of hypoperfusion and hypoxemia. Avoid use in patients ≥80 yrs unless renal function is normal. Increased risk of cardiovascular mortality. Increased risk of hypoglycemia in elderly, debilitated/ malnourished, adrenal or pituitary insufficiency, or alcohol intoxication. D/C in hypoxic states (eg, CHF, shock, acute MI), loss of blood glucose control due to stress (give insulin), acidosis and prior to surgical procedures (due to restricted food intake). Monitor renal function and for ketoacidosis and metabolic acidosis. Avoid in renal/hepatic impairment. May decrease serum vitamin B$_{12}$ levels. When used with a TZD, monitor LFTs and for weight gain. Withhold treatment with any condition associated with hypoxemia, dehydration, or sepsis. **Contra:** Renal disease or dysfunction (SrCr ≥1.5mg/dL [males], ≥1.4mg/dL [females], or abnormal CrCl), CHF, metabolic acidosis, including diabetic ketoacidosis. D/C temporarily (48 hrs) for radiologic studies with intravascular iodinated contrast materials. **P/N:** Category B, not for use in nursing.	Hypoglycemia, nausea, vomiting, abdominal pain, upper respiratory infection, headache, dizziness, diarrhea.

W/P = warnings/precautions; **Contra** = contraindications; **P/N** = pregnancy category rating and nursing considerations.

Table 6.3. Drug Interactions for Sulfonylureas

Chlorpropamide (Diabinese)

Alcohol	Moderate to large amounts may increase risk of hypoglycemia; may produce disulfiram-like reaction.
Barbiturates	Caution with use.
Beta-blockers	Potentiates hypoglycemia; may mask symptoms of hypoglycemia.
Calcium channel blockers	Caution, risk of hyperglycemia.
Chloramphenicol	Potentiates hypoglycemia.
Contraceptives, oral	Caution, risk of hyperglycemia.
Corticosteroids	Caution, risk of hyperglycemia.
Coumarins	Potentiates hypoglycemia.
Diuretics	Caution, risk of hyperglycemia.
Estrogens	Caution, risk of hyperglycemia.
Isoniazid	Caution, risk of hyperglycemia.
MAO Inhibitors	Potentiates hypoglycemia.
Miconazole	Warning, severe hypoglycemia with oral miconazole has been reported.
Nicotinic acid	Caution, risk of hyperglycemia.
NSAIDs	Potentiates hypoglycemia.
Phenothiazines	Caution, risk of hyperglycemia.
Phenytoin	Caution, risk of hyperglycemia.
Probenecid	Potentiates hypoglycemia.
Protein-bound drugs (highly)	Potentiates hypoglycemia.
Salicylates	Potentiates hypoglycemia.
Sulfonamides	Potentiates hypoglycemia.
Sympathomimetics	Caution, risk of hyperglycemia.
Thyroid products	Caution, risk of hyperglycemia.

Glimepiride (Amaryl)

Alcohol	Potentiates hypoglycemia.
Beta-blockers	Potentiates hypoglycemia; may mask symptoms of hypoglycemia.
Chloramphenicol	May potentiate hypoglycemia.
Contraceptives, oral	Caution, risk of hyperglycemia.
Corticosteroids	Caution, risk of hyperglycemia.
Coumarins	Potentiates hypoglycemia.
Diuretics	Caution, risk of hyperglycemia.
Estrogens	Caution, risk of hyperglycemia.
Insulin	Caution, monitor for hypoglycemia.
Isoniazid	Caution, risk of hyperglycemia.

Table 6.3. Drug Interactions for Sulfonylureas

MAO inhibitors	Potentiates hypoglycemia.
Metformin	Caution, monitor for hypoglycemia.
Miconazole	Warning, severe hypoglycemia has been reported with oral miconazole.
Nicotinic acid	Caution, risk of hyperglycemia.
NSAIDs	Potentiates hypoglycemia.
Phenothiazines	Caution, risk of hyperglycemia.
Phenytoin	Caution, risk of hyperglycemia.
Probenecid	Potentiates hypoglycemia.
Protein-bound drugs (highly)	Potentiates hypoglycemia.
Salicylates	Potentiates hypoglycemia.
Sulfonamides	Potentiates hypoglycemia.
Sulfonylureas (long-acting)	Caution, monitor for hypoglycemia when switching from a long-acting sulfonylurea.
Sympatholytic agents	Caution, may mask hypoglycemia.
Sympathomimetics	Caution, risk of hyperglycemia.
Thyroid products	Caution, risk of hyperglycemia.
Glipizide (Glipizide ER, Glucotrol XL, Glucotrol)	
Alcohol	Potentiates hypoglycemia; may produce disulfiram-like reaction.
Beta-blockers	Potentiates hypoglycemia; may mask symptoms of hypoglycemia.
Calcium channel blockers	Caution, risk of hyperglycemia.
Chloramphenicol	Potentiates hypoglycemia.
Contraceptives, oral	Caution, risk of hyperglycemia.
Corticosteroids	Caution, risk of hyperglycemia.
Coumarins	Potentiates hypoglycemia.
Diuretics	Caution, risk of hyperglycemia.
Estrogens	Caution, risk of hyperglycemia.
Fluconazole	Potentiates hypoglycemia.
Isoniazid	Caution, risk of hyperglycemia.
MAO inhibitors	Potentiates hypoglycemia.
Miconazole	Warning, severe hypoglycemia reported with oral miconazole.
Nicotinic acid	Caution, risk of hyperglycemia.
NSAIDs	Potentiates hypoglycemia.
Phenothiazines	Caution, risk of hyperglycemia.
Phenytoin	Caution, risk of hyperglycemia.
Probenecid	Potentiates hypoglycemia.
Protein-bound drugs (highly)	Potentiates hypoglycemia.
Salicylates	Potentiates hypoglycemia.

Table 6.3. Drug Interactions for Sulfonylureas

Sulfonamides	Potentiates hypoglycemia.
Sympathomimetics	Caution, risk of hyperglycemia.
Thyroid products	Caution, risk of hyperglycemia.
Glyburide (Diabeta, Glynase Pres-Tab, Micronase)	
Alcohol	Potentiates hypoglycemia; may produce disulfiram-like reaction.
Beta-blockers	Potentiates hypoglycemia; may mask symptoms of hypoglycemia.
Calcium channel blockers	Caution, risk of hyperglycemia.
Chloramphenicol	Potentiates hypoglycemia.
Contraceptives, oral	Caution, risk of hyperglycemia.
Corticosteroids	Caution, risk of hyperglycemia.
Coumarin	May increase or decrease coumarin effects.
Coumarins	Potentiates hypoglycemia.
Diuretics	Caution, risk of hyperglycemia.
Estrogens	Caution, risk of hyperglycemia.
Fluoroquinolones	Potentiates hypoglycemia.
Isoniazid	Caution, risk of hyperglycemia.
MAO inhibitors	Potentiates hypoglycemia.
Miconazole	Warning, severe hypoglycemia has been reported with oral miconazole.
Nicotinic acid	Caution, risk of hyperglycemia.
NSAIDs	Potentiates hypoglycemia.
Phenothiazines	Caution, risk of hyperglycemia.
Phenytoin	Caution, risk of hyperglycemia.
Probenecid	Potentiates hypoglycemia.
Protein-bound drugs (highly)	Potentiates hypoglycemia.
Salicylates	Potentiates hypoglycemia.
Sulfonamides	Potentiates hypoglycemia.
Sympathomimetics	Caution, risk of hyperglycemia.
Thyroid products	Caution, risk of hyperglycemia.
Tolazamide (Tolinase*)	
Alcohol	Potentiates hypoglycemia
Beta blockers	Potentiates hypoglycemia; may mask signs of hypoglycemia
Calcium channel blockers	Risk of hyperglycemia
Chloramphenicol	Potentiates hypoglycemia
Contraceptives, oral	Risk of hyperglycemia
Corticosteroids	Risk of hyperglycemia
Coumarins	Potentiates hypoglycemia

*Brand name not available in the U.S.

Table 6.3. Drug Interactions for Sulfonylureas

Diuretics	Risk of hyperglycemia
Estrogens	Risk of hyperglycemia
Isoniazid	Risk of hyperglycemia
MAOIs	Potentiates hypoglycemia
Miconazole	Severe hypoglycemia
Nicotinic Acid	Risk of hyperglycemia
NSAIDs	Potentiates hypoglycemia
Phenothiazines	Risk of hyperglycemia
Phenytoin	Risk of hyperglycemia
Probenecid	Potentiates hypoglycemia
Protein-bound drugs (highly)	Potentiates hypoglycemia
Salicylates	Potentiates hypoglycemia
Sulfonamides	Potentiates hypoglycemia
Sympathomimetics	Risk of hyperglycemia
Thyroid products	Risk of hyperglycemia
Tolbutamide (Orinase*)	
Alcohol	Potentiates hypoglycemia
Beta blockers	Potentiates hypoglycemia, may mask signs of hypoglycemia
Calcium channel blockers	Risk of hyperglycemia
Chloramphenicol	Potentiates hypoglycemia
Contraceptives, oral	Risk of hyperglycemia
Corticosteroids	Risk of hyperglycemia
Coumarins	Potentiates hypoglycemia
Diuretics	Risk of hyperglycemia
Estrogens	Risk of hyperglycemia
Isoniazid	Risk of hyperglycemia
MAOIs	Potentiates hypoglycemia
Miconazole	Severe hypoglycemia
Nicotinic Acid	Risk of hyperglycemia
NSAIDs	Potentiates hypoglycemia
Phenothiazines	Risk of hyperglycemia
Phenytoin	Risk of hyperglycemia
Probenecid	Potentiates hypoglycemia
Protein-bound drugs (highly)	Potentiates hypoglycemia
Salicylates	Potentiates hypoglycemia

*Brand name not available in the U.S.

Table 6.3. Drug Interactions for Sulfonylureas

Sulfonamides	Potentiates hypoglycemia
Sympathomimetics	Risk of hyperglycemia
Thyroid products	Risk of hyperglycemia

COMBINATION DRUGS

Glimepiride-Pioglitazone HCl (Duetact)

Beta-blockers	May potentiate hypoglycemia.
Contraceptives, oral	Caution, risk of hyperglycemia.
Corticosteroids	Caution, risk of hyperglycemia.
Coumarins	May potentiate hypoglycemia.
CYP2C8 enzyme inducers (eg, rifampin)	May significantly decrease the AUC of pioglitazone.
CYP2C8 enzyme inhibitors (eg, gemfibrozil)	May significantly increase the AUC of pioglitazone.
CYP3A4 substrate	May be a weak inducer of CYP3A4 substrate.
Estrogens	Caution, risk of hyperglycemia.
Ethinyl estradiol	May decrease levels of ethinyl estradiol.
Isoniazid	Caution, risk of hyperglycemia.
MAO inhibitors	May potentiate hypoglycemia.
Miconazole	Warning, severe hypoglycemia reported with oral miconazole.
Midazolam	May decrease levels of midazolam.
Nicotinic acid	Caution, risk of hyperglycemia.
Phenothiazines	Caution, risk of hyperglycemia.
Phenytoin	Caution, risk of hyperglycemia.
Salicylates	May potentiate hypoglycemia.
Sulfonamides	May potentiate hypoglycemia.
Sympathomimetics	Caution, risk of hyperglycemia.
Thiazides	Caution, risk of hyperglycemia.
Thyroid products	Caution, risk of hyperglycemia.

Glimepiride-Rosiglitazone maleate (Avandaryl)

Beta-blockers	May mask symptoms of hypoglycemia.
Contraceptives, oral	Caution, risk of hyperglycemia.
Corticosteroids	Caution, risk of hyperglycemia.
CYP 2C8 inducers (eg, rifampin)	May decrease the AUC of rosiglitazone.
CYP 2C8 inhibitors (eg, gemfibrozil)	May increase the AUC of rosiglitazone.
Estrogens	Caution, risk of hyperglycemia.
Isoniazid	Caution, risk of hyperglycemia.

Table 6.3. Drug Interactions for Sulfonylureas

Miconazole	Warning, severe hypoglycemia reported with oral miconazole.
Nicotinic acid	Caution, risk of hyperglycemia.
Phenothiazines	Caution, risk of hyperglycemia.
Phenytoin	Caution, risk of hyperglycemia.
Sympathomimetics	Caution, risk of hyperglycemia.
Thiazides	Caution, risk of hyperglycemia.
Thyroid products	Caution, risk of hyperglycemia.
Glipizide-Metformin HCl (Metaglip)	
Alcohol	Potentiates effect of metformin on lactate metabolism; potentiates hypoglycemia; avoid excessive alcohol intake.
Azoles, some	Potentiates hypoglycemia.
Beta-blockers	Potentiates hypoglycemia.
Calcium channel blockers	May cause hyperglycemia.
Cationic drugs (eg, digoxin, amiloride, procainamide, quinidine, quinine, ranitidine, trimethoprim, vancomycin, triamterene, morphine)	May increase metformin levels.
Chloramphenicol	Potentiates hypoglycemia.
Cimetidine	May increase metformin levels.
Contraceptives, oral	May cause hyperglycemia.
Corticosteroids	May cause hyperglycemia.
Coumarins	Potentiates hypoglycemia.
Diuretics	May cause hyperglycemia.
Estrogens	May cause hyperglycemia.
Furosemide	May increase metformin levels; may decrease furosemide levels.
Isoniazid	May cause hyperglycemia.
MAO inhibitors	Potentiates hypoglycemia.
Miconazole	Warning, severe hypoglycemia reported with oral miconazole.
Nicotinic acid	May cause hyperglycemia.
Nifedipine	May increase metformin levels.
NSAIDs	Potentiates hypoglycemia.
Phenothiazines	May cause hyperglycemia.
Phenytoin	May cause hyperglycemia.
Probenecid	Potentiates hypoglycemia.
Protein-bound drugs (highly)	Potentiates hypoglycemia.
Salicylates	Potentiates hypoglycemia.

Table 6.3. Drug Interactions for Sulfonylureas

Sulfonamides	Potentiates hypoglycemia.
Sympathomimetics	May cause hyperglycemia.
Thiazides	May cause hyperglycemia.
Thyroid products	May cause hyperglycemia.
Glyburide-Metformin HCl (Glucovance)	
Alcohol	Potentiates effects of metformin on lactate metabolism; potentiates hypoglycemia; avoid excessive alcohol intake.
Beta-blockers	Potentiates hypoglycemia.
Calcium channel blockers	May cause hyperglycemia.
Cationic drugs (eg, digoxin, amiloride, procainamide, quinidine, quinine, ranitidine, trimethoprim, vancomycin, triamterene, morphine)	May increase metformin levels.
Chloramphenicol	Potentiates hypoglycemia.
Cimetidine	May increase metformin levels.
Ciprofloxacin	Potentiates hypoglycemia.
Contraceptives, oral	May cause hyperglycemia.
Corticosteroids	May cause hyperglycemia.
Coumarins	Potentiates hypoglycemia.
Estrogens	May cause hyperglycemia.
Furosemide	May increase metformin levels; may decrease furosemide levels.
Isoniazid	May cause hyperglycemia.
MAO inhibitors	Potentiates hypoglycemia.
Miconazole	Warning, severe hypoglycemia reported with oral miconazole.
Nicotinic acid	May cause hyperglycemia.
Nifedipine	May increase metformin levels.
NSAIDs	Potentiates hypoglycemia.
Phenothiazines	May cause hyperglycemia.
Phenytoin	May cause hyperglycemia.
Probenecid	Potentiates hypoglycemia.
Salicylates	Potentiates hypoglycemia.
Sulfonamides	Potentiates hypoglycemia.
Sympathomimetics	May cause hyperglycemia.
Thiazides	May cause hyperglycemia.
Thiazolidinediones (eg, rosiglitazone)	Potentiates hypoglycemia.
Thyroid products	May cause hyperglycemia.

α-Glucosidase Inhibitors

Lance K. Campbell, PharmD, MHA

INTRODUCTION

The gold standard for measuring glycemia over a period of time is the glycated hemoglobin (HbA_{1c}) level. The primary components that affect HbA_{1c} are fasting plasma glucose (FPG) and postprandial plasma glucose (PPG) levels. In patients in whom control of PPG levels is difficult, HbA_{1c} levels will continue to be higher despite well-controlled FPG levels. More recent evidence suggests that poorly controlled PPG levels are a risk factor for coronary heart disease. Whether this risk is increased by high PPG levels, the resultant increase in postprandial insulin (PPI) levels, or a combination of both is not known, but the need to control high PPG levels in patient with diabetes is evident.

The α-glucosidase inhibitors offer one possible treatment alternative to decrease PPG, and subsequent PPI, levels. They act by delaying the absorption of simple carbohydrates in the small intestine, thereby blunting the PPG peak normally associated with the ingestion of a meal. Two of these medications, acarbose (Precose) and miglitol (Glyset), are approved for use in the U.S. A third medication, voglibose (Volix), is available in Japan and India, but not in the U.S. Only acarbose and miglitol will be discussed here.

The use of α-glucosidase inhibitors in the U.S. is minimal at best. In many ways, this is unfortunate since the drugs are effective in reducing PPG. One of the barriers to their use is that the patient needs to start with low doses and have the doses increased over 10-12 weeks to get maximum effectiveness and lowered GI side effects. Patients do not like to suffer from flatulence. Most practitioners seldom select these drugs from the now large tool box of medications available to try to normalize blood glucose. Other classes of drugs are better at reducing HbA_{1c} and we have newer drugs that also lower postprandial blood glucose excursions with fewer annoying side effects. This class of drugs is, at best, a second- or third-line choice for treating type 2 diabetes.

PHARMACOLOGY

Mechanism of Action

α-glucosidase inhibitors are named for their ability to reversibly bind α-glucosidase enzymes in the brush border of the small intestine. These enzymes include sucrase, maltase, isomaltase, and glucoamylase. α-glucosidase enzymes assist in the digestion of dietary carbohydrates by breaking down disaccharides and oligosaccharides (ie, sugar and starch) into glucose and other monosaccharides that can be absorbed in the small intestine. The competitive, reversible binding by the α-glucosidase inhibitors delays the absorption of carbohydrates from the gastrointestinal tract, which results in more even absorption of simple sugars throughout the gut. This results in the blunting of the normally sharp rise in PPG levels associated with the digestion of a meal.

The affinity that acarbose and miglitol have for α-glucosidase enzymes differs somewhat. Miglitol does not have an inhibitory effect on lactase, whereas acarbose inhibits a small percentage (~10%); however, this percentage is small enough that lactose absorption is not affected. Acarbose also inhibits pancreatic amylase, whereas miglitol does not. In addition, miglitol appears to be a more potent inhibitor than acarbose on a milligram-to-milligram basis. There is no evidence that these differences in affinity or potency have any significant clinical effects.

There has been some speculation in the clinical literature of a second mechanism of action for miglitol. Unlike acarbose, miglitol is almost completely absorbed by the small intestine, leading researchers to consider an additional, extraintestinal effect of the drug. Specifically, miglitol has been shown to have a suppressive activity on hepatic glycogenolysis in vitro, which is theorized to occur in vivo as well. Several studies have been conducted to explore the possibility of an extraintestinal effect of miglitol that could lower FPG levels secondary to suppressing glycogenolysis. The results are contradictory, so it is not possible to draw any conclusions about the clinical significance of this alternative mechanism of action. It should be noted, however, that the manufacturer of miglitol states that "there is no evidence that systemic absorption of miglitol contributes to its therapeutic effect."

Pharmacokinetics

Following oral administration of acarbose, very little of the drug is absorbed by the small intestine. The bioavailability of the active drug is ~1%-2%, and peak plasma concentrations occur in ~1 h. In addition, metabolites formed from intestinal bacteria and gut enzymes breaking down the drug have a bioavailability of ~34%, with absorption occurring ~14-24 hours after drug administration. Metabolism of acarbose occurs exclusively in the intestines. The natural bacterial flora and digestive enzymes break acarbose down into at least 13 different metabolites. Only one metabolite appears to have α-glucosidase-inhibiting behavior. The small amount of unchanged drug that is absorbed is completely excreted via the kidneys.

Following oral administration of miglitol, peak plasma concentrations normally occur in ~3 hours. Miglitol is absorbed from the small intestine via an active transport mechanism that represents a rate-limiting step and can affect both the bioavailability of the drug and the timing of its onset of action. Both vary in accordance with the amount of the drug administered. At a dose of 25 mg, the absorption is rapid and complete, with a bioavailability of ~100%. At higher doses, such as the maximum recommended dose of 100 mg, complete absorption can take up to 7 hours, with bioavailability values ranging from 50%-70%. Because the site of action of miglitol is the brush border of the small intestine, the absorption rate of the drug does not affect its clinical efficacy.

Miglitol is primarily distributed into extracellular fluids, with minimal tissue penetration. This results in the relatively small volume of distribution of 0.18 L/kg. Miglitol has very low permeation of the blood-brain barrier. Protein binding of miglitol is <4%. Miglitol is renally excreted unchanged, with any drug not initially absorbed in the small intestine being eliminated in the feces. No metabolism of miglitol is observed. The amount excreted in the urine is directly affected by the amount absorbed via the active transport mechanism in the small intestines. As such, the amount of renal excretion is correlated with the initial dosage administered. At lower doses, such as 25 mg, the amount excreted unchanged in the urine is 95%. At higher doses, such as 100 mg, the amount excreted unchanged in the urine is less, representing ~95% of the incompletely absorbed drug. The elimination half-life is 2-3 hours.

TREATMENT ADVANTAGES AND DISADVANTAGES

Acarbose has been approved by the FDA as monotherapy for type 2 diabetes in patients whose diabetes is not well controlled with nutrition therapy alone. Acarbose has also been approved for combination therapy with sulfonylureas, insulin, or metformin. Miglitol has been approved by the FDA as monotherapy for type 2 diabetes in patients whose diabetes is not well controlled with nutrition therapy alone or in combination with oral sulfonylureas.

There have been over 200 clinical trials performed measuring the clinical efficacy of acarbose. Acarbose was used extensively in Europe long before its FDA approval in the U.S. Miglitol boasts a somewhat more modest number of studies. Several large clinical trials with acarbose, including the large postmarketing PROTECT (Precose Resolution of Optimal Titration to Enhance Current Therapies) study, which enrolled over 6,000 patients, have shown a decrease in HbA_{1c} values of ~0.5%-0.7%, or ~0.6%-1.1% when changes from baseline in placebo-treated patients are subtracted from changes from baseline in acarbose-treated patients. PPG levels tend to decrease in the range of 40-50 mg/dL (2.2-2.8 mmol/L), and FPG decreases in the range of 25-30 mg/dL (1.4-1.7 mmol/L).

Small short-term studies and larger clinical trials have shown the primary clinical effects of miglitol to be a modest decrease in HbA_{1c} levels, a significant decrease in PPG levels, and a subsequent small decrease in PPI levels. Mean placebo-subtracted changes in HbA_{1c} from baseline range from 0.4%-1.2% in the larger trials, with the notable exception of one study that measured a change of 1.3%. PPG levels have a large range of change, decreasing by ~20-60 mg/dL (1.1-3.3 mmol/L).

The clinical efficacies of acarbose and miglitol appear to be similar; however, no comparative clinical trials have been conducted, so it is difficult to judge whether there is any clinical advantage to using one product versus the other.

The use of α-glucosidase inhibitors in the U.S. is minimal, despite their effectiveness in reducing postprandial hyperglycemia. One of the barriers to their use is the need to titrate the dose of the medication over 10-12 weeks to decrease the probability of GI adverse effects. Other classes of drugs, such as the biguanides, the sulfonylureas, and the thiazolidinediones reduce HbA_{1c} more significantly and have become the preferred agents for achieving euglycemic blood levels in patients with diabetes.

THERAPEUTIC CONSIDERATIONS

Significant Warnings and Precautions

α-glucosidase inhibitors do not cause hypoglycemia, but when used in combination with oral sulfonylureas or insulin, hypoglycemia may result. Because α-glucosidase inhibitors block the absorption of dietary carbohydrates, patients experiencing hypoglycemia must use glucose tablets instead of foods containing complex carbohydrates to raise blood glucose levels. In the case of severe hypoglycemia, a glucagon injection or intravenous glucose injections may be necessary. Patients must remember to monitor blood glucose levels, particularly in stressful situations such as fever, infection, trauma, or surgery, all of which can raise blood glucose levels regardless of treatment with α-glucosidase inhibitors. Treatment with insulin may be necessary in these situations to avoid diabetic ketoacidosis.

Systemically absorbed α-glucosidase inhibitors are almost exclusively eliminated renally. Therefore, drug accumulation can occur in patients with renal dysfunction, particularly with miglitol, given its high amount of systemic absorption compared with acarbose. α-glucosidase inhibitors should not be used in patients with renal impairment or insufficiency (ie, creatinine clearance <25 mL/min). There is no need for dose adjustments of α-glucosidase inhibitors for patients with hepatic dysfunction. α-glucosidase inhibitors are not hepatically metabolized, although acarbose should not be used in patients with cirrhosis.

Acarbose and miglitol are both pregnancy category B, indicating that the safety of the drug has not been established in pregnant women. Both drugs are excreted in small amounts in breast milk, so neither is recommended as treatment in nursing mothers.

Acarbose and miglitol are both contraindicated in patients with the following conditions:
• Diabetic ketoacidosis
• Gastrointestinal problems
  – Inflammatory bowel disease
  – Colonic ulceration
  – Partial intestinal obstruction
  – Chronic intestinal diseases associated with marked disorders of digestion or absorption or with conditions that may deteriorate as a result of increased gas formation in the intestine
• Hypersensitivity to acarbose or miglitol or any of their components
  In addition, acarbose is contraindicated in patients with cirrhosis or with a plasma creatinine concentration of >2.0 mg/dL

(176.8 mmol/L). Although miglitol is not specifically contraindicated in patients with renal dysfunction, its use is not recommended because renal dysfunction can result in a high systemic accumulation of the drug.

Special Populations
There is a unique collection of studies in the miglitol clinical literature that address specific patient populations with a high prevalence of diabetes: Hispanic-American, African-American, and elderly patients. Results of these studies are similar to non-specialized patient populations. No information on the pharmacokinetics of acarbose in different ethnic groups is available. One U.S. clinical study showed similar clinical efficacy in European-American and African-American patients, with a slightly better trend in Hispanic-American patients. The pharmacokinetics of acarbose are similar in Caucasian and Japanese patients, and its pharmacodynamics are similar in Caucasian and African-American patients.

There is no need for dose adjustments of α-glucosidase inhibitors for elderly patients. No significant differences in pharmacokinetics have been observed in elderly patients versus younger patients for either drug. No information regarding the treatment of children with α-glucosidase inhibitors is available.

Adverse Effects and Monitoring
The adverse effects of α-glucosidase inhibitors occur secondary to their innate mechanism of action. Both acarbose and miglitol exert their action locally in the small intestine, blocking the breakdown and absorption of complex carbohydrates. The delayed absorption results in the complex sugars moving to the large intestine. The natural flora of the large intestine ferment the carbohydrates, resulting in the production of gas, which leads to the most common side effects of α-glucosidase inhibitors: flatulence, abdominal distention and pain, and

diarrhea. The gastrointestinal effects are by far the most common problem associated with α-glucosidase inhibitors, occurring in one-third to two-thirds of patients receiving acarbose in clinical trials. The incidence of similar problems in patients treated with miglitol tends to be a bit lower, but this could be due to using lower initial doses and appropriate dose titration in these trials.

The gastrointestinal symptoms of α-glucosidase inhibitors tend to be transient in nature. Redistribution of the digestive enzymes in the gut usually occurs several weeks after therapy is initiated, resolving the common adverse effects. The delayed carbohydrate absorption caused by α-glucosidase inhibitors does not result in significant weight loss or malnutrition problems in patients taking the drug on a long-term basis.

Elevated liver function tests (ie, transaminases) have been observed in clinical trials with patients taking acarbose at dosages of 200-300 mg tid. All enzyme elevations resolved with the discontinuation of therapy. Elevated liver function tests have only been observed in patients receiving dosages of acarbose that exceed the manufacturer's recommended maximum dose of 100 mg tid. The manufacturer of acarbose recommends monitoring liver functions tests every 3 months during the first year of treatment and periodically thereafter. Dose reductions or discontinuation may be necessary if elevation of liver function tests occurs.

Drug Interactions

As described in the Significant Warnings and Precautions section earlier, an additive hypoglycemic effect may occur when α-glucosidase inhibitors are used in combination with sulfonylureas or insulin. Several studies of combination therapy with α-glucosidase inhibitors and insulin have shown a decreased need for insulin, sometimes requiring a reduction in insulin dosage to avoid a hypoglycemic event. Any medications that elevate glucose levels, including thiazide diuretics, corticosteroids, oral contraceptives and estrogen, niacin, phenothiazides, thyroid supplements, and calcium channel blockers, may reduce the efficacy of α-glucosidase inhibitors.

Miglitol has been shown to reduce the AUC (area under the curve) and peak concentrations of glyburide, but the clinical significance of this interaction is unknown. A similar interaction occurs with metformin, but the reduction is minimal. Acarbose has no effect on the absorption and distribution of glyburide. Acarbose does cause a significant reduction in the acute bioavailability of metformin, but overall bioavailability is not affected, so there is most likely no clinical significance to this interaction.

Acarbose has no interactions with digoxin, nifedipine, propanolol, or ranitidine. Acarbose has been shown to elevate liver function tests at very high doses, so it might be prudent to avoid acetaminophen, a well known hepatic toxin, especially if a patient drinks alcohol regularly. Results from studying interactions between digoxin and miglitol have been contradictory, showing a reduction of digoxin levels in healthy volunteers but not in patients with diabetes. The reason for this discrepancy is unknown, but providers may wish to consider monitoring digoxin levels periodically in patients taking these two drugs concomitantly. Miglitol also significantly reduces the bioavailability of propanolol and ranitidine, but has no drug interactions with nifedipine, antacids, or warfarin. Activated charcoal and digestive enzyme preparations, such as amylase and pancreatin, may interfere with the local activity of α-glucosidase inhibitors in the gut.

See **Table 7.2,** or refer to the full prescribing information for more drug interaction guidance.

Dosage and Administration

Treatment for diabetes must be individualized for each patient to assure maximal clinical efficacy with minimal adverse effects. See **Table 7.1**, or refer to the full prescribing information for more dosing guidance. Note that some patients may need to begin with once-daily dosing to decrease the likelihood of adverse effects.

The incidence of gastrointestinal side effects can be significantly reduced for patients receiving α-glucosidase inhibitors by starting with a small initial daily dose and titrating slowly to an appropriate maintenance dose. All doses should be given with the first bite of each meal, since α-glucosidase inhibitors can only exert their effects in the presence of dietary carbohydrates in the small intestine.

Many patients may experience reduced gastrointestinal side effects by using an acarbose dosing regimen that starts with an initial dose of 25 mg qd for 2 weeks, followed by 25 mg bid for 2 weeks, and then 25 mg tid. Once a patient is tolerating 25 mg tid, the titration schedule for acarbose is to increase the dose by 50 mg tid every 4-8 weeks, depending on 1-hour PPG levels, HbA_{1c}, and adverse effects. The titration schedule for miglitol is 25 mg tid for 4-8 weeks, followed by 50 mg tid for 3 months, at which time efficacy should be assessed with an HbA_{1c} measurement. Patients who are not adequately responding to miglitol therapy and who are tolerant of a higher dose can then be increased to 100 mg tid.

SUGGESTED READING

Buse J, Hart K, Minasi L. The PROTECT study: final results of a large multicenter postmarketing study in patients with type 2 diabetes: Precose Resolution of Optimal Titration to Enhance Current Therapies. *Clin Ther.* 1998;20:257-269.

Campbell LK, White JR, Campbell RK. Acarbose: Its role in the treatment of diabetes mellitus. *Ann Pharmacother.* 1996; 30:1255-1262.

Campbell LK, Baker DE, Campbell RK. Miglitol: Assessment of its role in the treatment of patients with diabetes mellitus. *Ann Pharmacother.* 2000;34:1291-1301.

Scott LJ, Spencer CM: Miglitol. A review of its therapeutic potential in type 2 diabetes mellitus. *Drugs.* 2000;59(3):521-549.

Scheen AJ. IS there a role for α-glucosidase inhibitors in the prevention of type 2 diabetes mellitus. *Drugs.* 2003;63(10):933-51.

Van de Laar FA, Lucassen PL, Addermans RP, Van de Lisdonk EH, Rutten GE, Van Weel C. α-glucosidase inhibitors for patients with type 2 diabetes. *Diabetes Care.* 2005;28:166-175.

Table 7.1. Prescribing Information for α-Glucosidase Inhibitors

GENERIC (BRAND)	FORM/ STRENGTH	DOSAGE	WARNINGS/PRECAUTIONS & CONTRAINDICATIONS	ADVERSE REACTIONS
Acarbose (Precose)	**Tab:** 25mg, 50mg, 100mg	***Adults:*** Initial: 25mg tid with first bite of each main meal. To minimize GI effects: 25mg qd, increase gradually to 25mg tid. Titrate: After reaching 25mg tid, may increase at 4-8 week intervals. Maint: 50-100mg tid. Max: ≤60kg: 50mg tid. >60kg: 100mg tid. If no further reduction in post prandial or HbA$_{1C}$ with 100mg tid, consider reducing dose.	**W/P:** Avoid with significant renal dysfunction (SrCr >2mg/dL). May need to d/c and give insulin with stress (eg, fever, trauma). Dose-related elevated serum transaminase levels reported. Monitor serum transaminases every 3 months for first year then periodically. Reduce dose or d/c if elevated serum transaminases persist. Use glucose (dextrose) instead of sucrose (sugar cane) to treat mild to moderate hypoglycemia. **Contra:** Diabetic ketoacidosis, cirrhosis, inflammatory bowel disease, colonic ulceration, partial or predisposition to intestinal obstruction, chronic intestinal disease with marked disorders of digestion or absorption, and conditions that may deteriorate from increased intestinal gas formation. **P/N:** Category B, not for use in nursing.	Transient flatulence, diarrhea, abdominal pain.
Miglitol (Glyset)	**Tab:** 25mg, 50mg, 100mg	***Adults:*** Initial: 25mg tid. May give 25mg qd (to minimize GI side effects) and gradually increase to tid. Titrate: After 4-8 weeks, increase to 50mg tid. Maint: 50mg tid. After 3 months may increase to 100mg tid if needed. Max: 100mg tid. Take with first bite of each main meal.	**W/P:** Use glucose (dextrose) not sucrose (cane sugar) to treat mild-moderate hypoglycemia. Temporary insulin therapy may be necessary at times of stress such as fever, trauma, infection, or surgery. Not recommended with renal impairment (SrCr >2mg/dL). **Contra:** Ketoacidosis, inflammatory bowel disease, colonic ulceration, partial intestinal obstruction or if predisposed to intestinal obstruction. Chronic intestinal diseases with digestion or absorption disorders/conditions may deteriorate with increased gas formation in the intestine. **P/N:** Category B, not for use in nursing.	Flatulence, diarrhea, abdominal pain, skin rash, decreased serum iron.

W/P = warnings/precautions; **Contra** = contraindications; **P/N** = pregnancy category rating and nursing considerations.

Table 7.2. Drug Interactions for α-Glucosidase Inhibitors

Acarbose (Precose)

Amylase	May reduce the effect of acarbose; avoid concomitant use.
Calcium channel blockers	Caution, risk of hyperglycemia.
Charcoal	May reduce the effect of acarbose; avoid concomitant use.
Contraceptives, oral	Caution, risk of hyperglycemia.
Corticosteroids	Caution, risk of hyperglycemia.
Digoxin	May effect bioavailability of digoxin; may require dose adjustment of digoxin.
Diuretics	Caution, risk of hyperglycemia.
Estrogens	Caution, risk of hyperglycemia.
Insulin	Monitor for hypoglycemia.
Isoniazid	Caution, risk of hyperglycemia.
Nicotinic acid	Caution, risk of hyperglycemia.
Pancreatin	May reduce the effect of acarbose; avoid concomitant use.
Phenothiazines	Caution, risk of hyperglycemia.
Phenytoin	Caution, risk of hyperglycemia.
Sulfonylureas	Monitor for hypoglycemia.
Sympathomimetics	Caution, risk of hyperglycemia.
Thyroid products	Caution, risk of hyperglycemia.

Miglitol (Glyset)

Amylase	May reduce effect of miglitol.
Charcoal	May reduce effect of miglitol.
Digoxin	May interact.
Glyburide	May interact.
Metformin	May interact.
Pancreatin	May reduce effect of miglitol.
Propranolol	May reduce the bioavailability of propranolol.
Ranitidine	May reduce the bioavailability of ranitidine.

Chapter 8

Glinides (Meglitinides)

John R. White, Jr., PharmD, PA

INTRODUCTION

The glinide agents are secretagogues that were developed to be structurally and pharmacologically unrelated to the sulfonylureas (SUs). These agents were designed to promote an insulin release profile similar to physiological, glucose-stimulated insulin release. The glinide agents are intended to be taken only when the patient eats, thus allowing the patient more freedom in the timing of meals. They were also designed to have a short half-life to reduce the risk of hypoglycemia. Currently, two compounds are available in this category, nateglinide and repaglinide.

PHARMACOLOGY

Mechanism of Action

The glinide class is structurally unrelated to the SUs, but like that class, lowers blood glucose levels by stimulating insulin release from the pancreas. As with the SUs, release of insulin is dependent on functioning β-cells in the pancreatic islets; it is glucose dependent and diminishes at low glucose concentrations. Like the SUs, the glinides bind to receptors in the pancreas, the configuration of the binding is different. Also like the SUs, the glinides close ATP-dependent potassium channels in the pancreatic islet β-cell membrane.

Potassium channel blockade depolarizes the β-cell, which leads to an opening of calcium channels; this results in an increased calcium influx, which induces insulin secretion. The glinides have a more rapid onset and a shorter duration of action than the SUs.

Pharmacokinetics

Peak plasma concentrations of repaglinide are reached within 1 hour following oral administration. The mean absolute bioavailability is 56%. Administration with food does not affect the time to peak, but it reduces the mean peak concentration by 20% and the area under the plasma time concentration curve (AUC) is reduced by 12.4%. The volume of distribution is 31 liters, and protein binding is >98%.

The elimination half-life is ~1 hour. Repaglinide is metabolized via oxidative biotransformation and conjugation to inactive metabolites. The metabolites are primarily excreted in the feces (90%). Only 0.1% of the repaglinide dose is excreted unchanged in the urine, and <2% is excreted unchanged in the feces.

Nateglinide is rapidly and almost completely absorbed with a T_{max} of between $^1/_2$ hour and 2 hours. Peak levels of nateglinide are lower when the medication is taken after a meal, than when taken shortly before a meal or on an empty stomach. The absolute bioavailability of nateglinide has consistently been reported to be between 72%-75%. The volume of distribution of nateglinide in humans has been reported to be approximately 10 liters. Nateglinide is highly bound to albumin and to a lesser degree to α-1 acid glycoprotein, with an overall protein binding of 98%-99%).

Nateglinide is extensively metabolized by the cytochrome P450 enzyme system prior to excretion. Nateglinide is metabolized via dual cytochrome P450 isoenzyme systems, CYP3A4 (30%) and CYP2C9 (70%). Approximately 16% of nateglinide is excreted unchanged in the urine.

TREATMENT ADVANTAGES AND DISADVANTAGES

The glinides are indicated as an adjunct to nutrition and exercise to lower blood glucose in patients with type 2 diabetes whose hyperglycemia cannot be controlled satisfactorily by nutrition and exercise alone. The expected HbA$_{1c}$ lowering effect of the glinides is generally less than that of the SUs. Typical HgbA$_{1c}$ lowering is usually in the range of 0.7%-1.5% in a responding patient.

Glinides are also potentially useful with other forms of antihyperglycemic therapy, with the exception of sulfonlyureas. They also have very little if any efficacy when substituted for SUs in patients who are not responding adequately to SUs.

Glinides carry with them a relatively low incidence of hypoglycemia and may be attractive for use in patients who are predisposed to hypoglycemia, such as the elderly. They may also be useful in cases where patients consume one or two large meals daily and require glycemic coverage at those particular times.

Since glinides do not contain the sulfa moiety, they may be preferred to SUs in patients with a history of sulfa allergy.

The major disadvantages of the glinides are the need for multiple daily doses, less HgbA$_{1c}$-lowering capacity than the SUs, and cost.

THERAPEUTIC CONSIDERATIONS

Significant Warnings and Precautions

The glinides are contraindicated in patients with diabetic ketoacidosis, type 1 diabetes, or known hypersensitivity to either nateglinide or repaglinide.

Hypoglycemia

The glinides are capable of producing hypoglycemia. Patients with hepatic, adrenal, or pituitary insufficiency, as well as elderly, debilitated, or malnourished patients, may be more susceptible. While the frequency of hypoglycemia is less with the glinides than with the SUs, the frequency of hypoglycemia is greatest in patients who have not been previously treated with oral blood glucose-lowering agents and those with an HbA$_{1c}$ <8%.

Loss of Control of Blood Glucose

If the patient experiences stress, such as fever, trauma, infection, or surgery, it may be necessary to temporarily replace a glinide with insulin therapy.

Pregnancy and Nursing

Repaglinide is categorized in pregnancy category C. Repaglinide was nonteratogenic in animal studies. However, nonteratogenic skeletal deformities were observed following exposure during gestation and lactation. Abnormal blood glucose levels during pregnancy are associated with a higher incidence of congenital abnormalities; therefore, insulin therapy is recommended during pregnancy to maintain blood glucose levels as close to normal as possible.

The manufacturer recommends that repaglinide not be administered to nursing mothers. It is not known whether repaglinide is excreted in human milk, but it is excreted in the milk of some animals. This recommendation is based on the risk of hypoglycemia and the concern that skeletal deformities, such as those observed in the animal studies, may occur.

Nateglinide is also categorized as pregnancy category C. Until more data in this population are available, it is not recommended that nateglinide be used during pregnancy.

While it is not known whether or not nateglinide is excreted in the human milk, some animal studies suggest secretion into the milk of lactating animals. At this time, the manufacturer recommends that nateglinide not be administered to nursing women.

Pediatrics

The safety and effectiveness of repaglinide and nateglinide have not been established in children. Therefore its use in this population is not currently recommended.

Special Populations

Renal Dysfunction

Patients with renal dysfunction may have increased AUC and peak serum repaglinide levels. However, no adjustment in the initial dose of repaglinide is necessary.

No dosage adjustment is needed for nateglinide in patients with mild to severe renal dysfunction.

Hepatic Dysfunction

Patients with moderate to severe impairment of liver function will have higher serum concentrations and more unbound repaglinide and metabolites than will patients with normal hepatic function. However, the altered serum concentrations and unbound fraction have not been shown to alter the response to the repaglinide. It

may be possible that some patients with hepatic dysfunction will respond differently and may require longer dosing intervals and/or lower doses of repaglinide.

Increases in peak concentration and overall drug exposure to nateglinide were increased by about 30% in nondiabetic subjects with mild hepatic dysfunction when compared with healthy volunteers. No dosage adjustment is recommended in patients with mild to moderate hepatic dysfunction; nateglinide should be used with caution in patients with severe hepatic failure.

Geriatrics

The pharmacokinetics of neither repaglinide nor nateglinide are significantly affected by age, and no dose adjustment is recommended.

Ethnic Groups

Ethnicity does not appear to affect the pharmacokinetics of repaglinide or nateglinide.

Gender

Women treated with repaglinide may have a higher AUC (15%-70%) than men, but the frequency of adverse events or hypoglycemia is not increased. Adjustments in dose should be based on clinical response and not on gender.

No differences in pharmacokinetics of nateglinide between males and females have been reported.

Adverse Effects and Monitoring

The adverse effects most commonly reported during repaglinide therapy have included hypoglycemia, upper respiratory infections, sinusitis, nausea, diarrhea, constipation, arthralgia, weight gain, and headache. The adverse effect profile of nateglinide is similar. Monitoring blood glucose levels and only taking a glinide if a meal is to be consumed can help to reduce the risk of hypoglycemia.

Drug Interactions

Repaglinide metabolism may be inhibited by inhibitors of CYP3A4, such as ketoconazole, miconazole, and erythromycin. Agents that induce CYP3A4 metabolism, such as rifampin, barbiturates, and carbamazepine, may reduce repaglinide levels.

Coadministration of repaglinide with the CYP450 inhibitor clarithromycin resulted in significantly higher concentrations of repaglinide. This increase may necessitate a dosage reduction of repaglinide in cases where both medications are prescribed.

Gemfibrozil causes a significant rise in repaglinide serum levels and in hypoglycemic effect. Thus, gemfibrozil should not be started in patients treated with repaglinide and repaglinide should not be started in patients treated with gemfibrozil. Gemfibrozil has a synergistic inhibitory effect on the metabolism of repaglinide when administered with itraconazole, and therefore itraconazole should be avoided in the rare situation where a patient might be treated with both gemfibrozil and repaglinide.

Repaglinide does not interact with digoxin, theophylline, warfarin, or cimetidine.

The hypoglycemic action of repaglinide may be potentiated by nonsteroidal anti-inflammatory drugs (NSAIDs) and other agents that are highly plasma-protein bound, salicylates, sulfonamides, chloramphenicol, coumarins, probenecid, monoamine oxidase inhibitors (MAOIs), and β-blockers. Loss of glycemic control may occur with concomitant administration with agents that may produce hyperglycemia, such as thiazides and other diuretics, corticosteroids, phenothiazines, thyroid products, estrogens, oral contraceptives, phenytoin, nicotinic acid, sympathomimetics, calcium channel blockers, and isoniazid.

Since nateglinide is highly protein bound, there is a possibility that it may undergo drug interactions via changes in protein binding with other highly bound drugs. However, in-vitro displacement studies evaluating the possibility of other drugs displacing nateglinide have revealed no interaction with furosemide, propranolol, captropril, nicardipine, pravastatin, glyburide, warfarin, phenytoin, acetylsalicylic acid, tolbutamide, or metformin. Additionally, nateglinide appeared not to influence the protein binding of propranolol, glyburide, nicardipine, warfarin, phenytoin, acetylsalicylic acid, and tolbutamide.

Certain drugs such as NSAIDs, salicylates, MAOIs, and nonselective β-blockers may potentiate the blood glucose-lowering effect of nateglinide. Conversely, the pharmacologic effect of nateglinide may be reduced by sympathomimetics, thyroid products, corticosteroids, and thiazide diuretics.

See **Table 8.2**, or refer to the full prescribing information for the drug in question for more drug interaction guidance.

Dosage and Administration

Repaglinide is available in 0.5-, 1-, and 2-mg tablets; it is also available as a combination drug with metformin. Nateglinide is available in 60-mg and 120-mg tablets.

For patients not previously treated or whose HbA$_{1c}$ is <8%, the starting dose of repaglinide should be 0.5 mg. For patients previously treated with blood glucose-lowering drugs and whose HbA$_{1c}$ is ≥8%, the initial dose is 1 or 2 mg before each meal. Dosage adjustments should be determined by blood glucose response. The preprandial dose should be increased until satisfactory blood glucose control is achieved or until a maximum dose of 4 mg/dose or 16 mg/day is reached. Most dosage adjustments should be done at weekly intervals or longer, but dosage adjustments in patients with hepatic insufficiency should be less frequent.

Glycemic control with repaglinide has been shown to be maintained with administration before meals when two, three, or four meals per day are eaten (corresponding to two, three, or four doses per day) and repaglinide is administered at the start of the meal or 15 or 30 minutes before the meal. Doses are usually taken within 15 minutes of the meal, but may be taken any time from immediately before to as long as 30 minutes before the meal. Patients who skip a meal or add an extra meal should be instructed to skip or add a dose for that meal respectively.

When repaglinide replaces another oral hypoglycemic agent, the first repaglinide dose may be administered on the day after the final dose of the other agent is given. After conversion to repaglinide, patients should be monitored closely for hypoglycemia. In particular, when a patient is switched from a longer half-life SU, close monitoring for up to 1 week or longer may be indicated.

Nateglinide should be given in most instances at a dose of 120 mg, three times daily, 1 to 30 minutes before a meal. Nateglinide should not be taken if a meal is skipped. However, it has been suggested that nateglinide has a very low potential for causing hypoglycemia even in a missed meal situation. The 120-mg dose of nateglinide should be used in most monotherapeutic and most combination regimens. A 60-mg dose is available, however, and should be used in cases where patients are very near their HbA_{1c} goal at the time that nateglinide is added.

See **Table 8.1**, or refer to the full prescribing information for more dosing guidance.

SUGGESTED READING

Blicklé, JF. Meglitinide analogues: a review of clinical data focused on recent trials. *Diabetes & Metabolism*. Volume 32, Issue 2, April 2006;113-120.

Hirschberg Y, Pietri AO, Karara AH, McLeod JF. Improved control of mealtime glucose excursions with coadministration of nateglinide and metformin. *Diabetes Care*. 2000;23:349-53.

Horton ES, Clinkingbeard C, Gatlin M, Foley J, Mallows S, Shen S. Nateglinide alone and in combination with metformin improves glycemic control by reducing mealtime glucose levels in type 2 diabetes. *Diabetes Care*. 2000;23:1660-1665.

Jijakli H, Ulusoy S, Malaisse WJ: Dissociation between the potency and reversibility of the insulinotropic action of two glinide analogues. *Pharmacol Res*. 1996; 34:105-108.

Kalbag JB, Nedelman JR, Walter YH, McLeod JF. Mealtime glucose regulation with nateglinide in healthy volunteers: comparison with repaglinide and placebo. *Diabetes Care*. 2001;24:73-77.

Landgraf R, Bilo HJ, Muller PG: A comparison of repaglinide and glibenclamide in the treatment of type 2 diabetic patients previously treated with sulphonylureas. *Eur J Clin. Pharmacol* 1999; 55:165-171.

Malaisse WJ: Stimulation of insulin release by non-sulfonylurea hypoglycemic agents: the glinide family. *Horm Metab Res*. 1995; 27:263-266.

SUGGESTED READING *(continued)*

Malaisse WJ: Insulinotropic action of glinide analogues: modulation by an activator of ATP-sensitive K+ channels and high extracellular KHH1 concentrations. *Pharmacol Res.* 1995; 32:111-114.

Moses R, Slobodniuk R, Boyages S, Colagiuri S, Kidson W, Carter J, Donnelly T, Moffitt P, Hopkins H: Effect of repaglinide addition to metformin monotherapy on glycemic control in patients with type 2 diabetes. *Diabetes Care.* 1999;22:119-124.

Scheen AJ. Drug-drug and food-drug pharmacokinetic interactions with new insulinotropic agents repaglinide and nateglinide. *Clin Pharmacokinet.* 2007;46(2):93-108.

Wolffenbuttel BH, Landgraf R, Dutch and German Repaglinide Study Group: A 1-year multicenter randomized double-blind comparison of repaglinide and glyburide for the treatment of type 2 diabetes. *Diabetes Care* 1999; 22:463-467.

Table 8.1. Prescribing Information for Glinides (Meglitinides)

GENERIC (BRAND)	FORM/ STRENGTH	DOSAGE	WARNINGS/PRECAUTIONS & CONTRAINDICATIONS	ADVERSE REACTIONS
Nateglinide (Starlix)	**Tab:** 60mg, 120mg	***Adults:*** Initial/Maint: 120mg tid before meals (with or without metformin or TZD). Take 1-30 min before meals. May use 60mg tid (with or without metformin or TZD) in patients near goal HbA$_{1c}$. Skip dose if meal is skipped.	**W/P:** Caution in moderate to severe hepatic impairment. Transient loss of glucose control with trauma, surgery, fever, and infection; may need insulin therapy. Secondary failure may occur in prolonged therapy. Hypoglycemia risk in elderly, debilitated, malnourished, strenuous exercise, and with adrenal or pituitary insufficiency. Autonomic neuropathy may mask hypoglycemia. **Contra:** Diabetic ketoacidosis and type 1 diabetes, **P/N:** Category C, not for use in nursing.	URI, flu symptoms, dizziness, arthropathy, diarrhea, hypoglycemia, back pain, jaundice, cholestatic hepatitis, elevated liver enzymes.
Repaglinide (Prandin)	**Tab:** 0.5mg, 1mg, 2mg	***Adults:*** Take within 15-30 min before meals. Skip dose if skipping meal and add dose if adding meal. Initial: **Treatment-Naive or HbA$_{1c}$ <8%:** 0.5mg with each meal. **Previous Oral Therapy/Combination Therapy and HbA$_{1c}$ ≥8%:** 1-2mg with each meal. Titrate: May double preprandial dose up to 4mg (bid-qid) at no less than 1-week intervals. Maint: 0.5-4mg with meals. Max: 16mg/day. If hypoglycemia with combination metformin or TZD occurs, reduce repaglinide dose. **Renal Dysfunction: CrCl 20-40mg/dL:** Initial: 0.5mg with each meal; titrate carefully. **Hepatic Dysfunction:** Increase intervals between dose adjustments.	**W/P:** Hypoglycemia risk, especially with renal/hepatic insufficiency, elderly, malnourished, and adrenal/pituitary insufficiency. Loss of blood glucose control when exposed to stress (fever, trauma, infection, or surgery); d/c therapy, and start insulin. Secondary failure can occur over a period of time. Caution with hepatic and renal dysfunction. Not indicated for use in combination with NPH insulin. **Contra:** Diabetic ketoacidosis and type 1 diabetes. **P/N:** Category C, not for use in nursing.	Hypoglycemia, cardiovascular effects, respiratory infections, URI, bronchitis, sinusitis, rhinitis, paresthesia, nausea, diarrhea, constipation, vomiting, dyspepsia, arthralgia, back pain, headache, chest pain.
COMBINATION DRUG				
Repaglinide/ Metformin HCl (PrandiMet)	**Tab: (Repaglinide-Metformin)** 1mg-500mg, 2mg-500mg	***Adults:*** Individualize dose. Administer 2 to 3 times a day up to 4mg-1000mg per meal. Max daily dose: 10mg-2500mg. **Patients Inadequately Controlled with Metformin HCl Monotherapy:** 1mg-500mg bid with meals. Gradual dose escalation required. **Patients Inadequately Controlled with Meglitinide Monotherapy:** 500mg of metformin bid. Gradual dose escalation required. **Concomitant Use of Repaglinide/ Metformin:** Initiate at the dose similar to (but not exceeding) the current dose. Titrate to maximum daily dose as necessary.	**BB:** Lactic acidosis may occur due to metformin accumulation. If suspected, d/c PrandiMet and hospitalize patient. **W/P:** Lactic acidosis reported (rare), increased risk with sepsis, dehydration, excess alcohol intake, hepatic impairment, renal impairment, and acute CHF. Assess renal function prior to initiation and annually thereafter. Not indicated for use in combination with NPH insulin. Avoid in hepatic impairment and excess alcohol intake. D/C in hypoxic states (eg, CHF, shock, acute MI), prior to surgical procedures, procedures requiring use of intravascular iodinated contrast materials, and ketoacidosis. May cause vitamin B$_{12}$ deficiency and hypoglycemia. **Contra:** Renal impairment (SrCr ≥1.5mg/dL [males], ≥1.4mg/dL [females], or abnormal CrCl). Acute or chronic metabolic acidosis, including diabetic ketoacidosis. Patients receiving both gemfibrozil and itraconazole. **P/N:** Category C, not for use in nursing.	Hypoglycemia, headache, diarrhea, nausea, upper respiratory tract infection.

BB = black box warning; **W/P** = warnings/precautions; **Contra** = contraindications; **P/N** = pregnancy category rating and nursing considerations.

Table 8.2. Drug Interactions for Glinides (Meglitinides)

Nateglinide (Starlix)

Alcohol	Potentiates hypoglycemia.
Beta-blockers	May mask symptoms of hypoglycemia.
Beta-blockers, nonselective	Potentiates hypoglycemia.
Corticosteroids	Caution, risk of hyperglycemia.
Liquid meals	Reduces peak plasma levels of nateglinide.
MAO inhibitors	Potentiates hypoglycemia.
NSAIDs	Potentiates hypoglycemia.
Protein-bound drugs (high)	Use with caution.
Salicylates	Potentiates hypoglycemia.
Sympathomimetics	Caution, risk of hyperglycemia.
Thiazides	Caution, risk of hyperglycemia.
Thyroid products	Caution, risk of hyperglycemia.
Tolbutamide	May potentiate tolbutamide.

Repaglinide (Prandin)

Alcohol	Potentiates hypoglycemia.
Beta-blockers	Potentiates hypoglycemia; may mask symptoms of hypoglycemia.
Calcium channel blockers	Caution, risk of hyperglycemia.
Chloramphenicol	Potentiates hypoglycemia.
Corticosteroids	Caution, risk of hyperglycemia.
Coumarins	Potentiates hypoglycemia.
CYP2C8 inhibitors	May inhibit repaglinide metabolism.
CYP3A4 inducers (eg, rifampin, barbiturates, carbamazepine)	May increase repaglinide metabolism.
CYP3A4 inhibitors	May inhibit repaglinide metabolism.
Diuretics	Caution, risk of hyperglycemia.
Erythromycin	May inhibit repaglinide metabolism.
Estrogens	Caution, risk of hyperglycemia.
Ethinyl estradiol	Increases ethinyl estradiol levels; increased repaglinide levels.
Gemfibrozil	May inhibit repaglinide metabolism; may increase blood glucose levels; monitor levels if using concomitantly; avoid concomitant use.
Isoniazid	Caution, risk of hyperglycemia.
Protein-bound drugs (high)	Potentiates hypoglycemia.

Table 8.2. Drug Interactions for Glinides (Meglitinides)

Itraconazole	Avoid itraconazole use if on concomitant therapy with gemfibrozil and repaglinide; may cause a synergistic effect.
Ketoconazole	May inhibit repaglinide metabolism.
Levonorgestrel	Increases levonorgestrel levels; increases repaglinide levels.
MAO inhibitors	Potentiates hypoglycemia.
Miconazole	May inhibit repaglinide metabolism.
Montelukast	May inhibit repaglinide metabolism.
Nicotinic acid	Caution, risk of hyperglycemia.
NSAIDs	Potentiates hypoglycemia.
Phenothiazines	Caution, risk of hyperglycemia.
Phenytoin	Caution, risk of hyperglycemia.
Probenecid	Potentiates hypoglycemia.
Salicylates	Potentiates hypoglycemia.
Simvastatin	Increases repaglinide levels.
Sulfonamides	Potentiates hypoglycemia.
Sympathomimetics	Caution, risk of hyperglycemia.
Thyroid products	Caution, risk of hyperglycemia.
Trimethoprim	May inhibit repaglinide metabolism.

COMBINATION DRUG

Repaglinide-Metformin HCl (PrandiMet)

Cationic drugs	Potential interaction with metformin by competing for common renal tubular secretion. Examples of cationic drugs include amiloride, digoxin, morphine, procainamide, quinidine, quinine, ranitidine, triamterene, trimethoprim, vancomycin.
Cimetidine	May increase the AUC of metformin.
Clarithromycin	May increase the AUC of repaglinide.
CYP2C8 inhibitors	May increase the AUC of repaglinide (eg, trimethoprim).
CYP3A4 inhibitors	May increase the AUC of repaglinide (eg, itraconazole, ketoconazole).
CYP2C8/3A4 inducers	May decrease the AUC of repaglinide (eg, rifampin).
Furosemide	May increase the AUC of metformin; may decrease the AUC of furosemide.
Gemfibrozil	Potentiates repaglinide; may potentiate hypoglycemia.
Ibuprofen	May increase the AUC of metformin.
Levonorgestrel/ ethinyl estradiol	May decrease the AUC of repaglinide; may increase the AUC of ethinyl estradiol.
Nifedipine	May increase the AUC of metformin; may decrease the AUC of repaglinide.
Propranolol	May decrease the AUC of metformin.
Simvastatin	May decrease the AUC of repaglinide.

Chapter 9

Dipeptidyl Peptidase-4 (DPP-4) Inhibitors

Joshua J. Neumiller, PharmD, CGP, FASCP

INTRODUCTION

Increased understanding within the scientific community regarding the actions of endogenous glucoregulatory peptides, namely glucose-dependent insulinotropic polypeptide (GIP) and glucagon-like peptide-1 (GLP-1), produced new and novel targets for drug therapy to treat type 2 diabetes. Sitagliptin—an inhibitor of dipeptidyl peptidase-4 (DPP-4)—prevents the proteolytic degradation of endogenous incretin molecules, effectively prolonging the action of natural incretin molecules within the body. Sitagliptin was approved for the treatment of type 2 diabetes as monotherapy or as add-on therapy to metformin or a thiazolidinedione in October of 2006, and is the first DPP-4 inhibitor approved by the FDA. In October of 2007, sitagliptin's indications were expanded to include use as initial combination therapy with metformin in drug-naive patients, as add-on therapy to a sulfonylurea, and as add-on therapy to a sulfonylurea plus metformin. Sitagliptin is also available in combination with metformin, as Janumet, which is being promoted by the manufacturer as first-line therapy in patients with type 2 diabetes. This section will review the pharmacology of sitagliptin and other DPP-4 inhibitors currently in development, as well as the properties, considerations, and role for sitagliptin in the treatment of type 2 diabetes.

PHARMACOLOGY

Mechanism of Action

Insulin secretion and utilization is important in terms of glucose metabolism and homeostasis. Observations that insulin secretion varies depending on the route of glucose administration prompted vigorous research in the area of incretin hormone function and the potential therapeutic role of these hormones in the treatment of diabetes. When identical plasma glucose elevations are induced in people via different routes of glucose administration, oral glucose intake results in greater insulin secretion than intravenous glucose administration. This phenomenon is known as the incretin effect. The incretin effect is mediated via gut hormones that induce insulin secretion from the β-cells of the pancreas in response to oral glucose administration. GIP and GLP-1 were the first two incretin hormones to be purified and studied. Both GIP and GLP-1 exhibit multiple actions that aid in glucose regulation, making these molecules viable drug targets in the treatment of type 2 diabetes.

DPP-4 inhibitors were developed to take advantage of the incretin effect in the treatment of type 2 diabetes. DPP-4 inhibitors exert their pharmacological effects by inhibiting the degradation of GLP-1. By inhibiting the enzymatic breakdown of GLP-1, sitagliptin (as well as other DPP-4 inhibitors currently in development) augments the effects of endogenous GLP-1 by prolonging its effects within the body. These beneficial effects include: 1) stimulation of insulin secretion, 2) inhibition of glucagon secretion, and 3) stimulation of β-cell proliferation. Endogenous DPP-4 enzyme is widely distributed, and is located in many tissues including liver, lung, kidney, GI tract, and endothelial cells. **Figure 1** provides a diagram of the physiological effects of endogenous GLP-1 that are augmented with the use of DPP-4 inhibitors. Recent evidence indicates that GLP-1 agonists and DPP-4 inhibitors may be associated with inhibition of β-cell apoptosis, or cell death, and may thus possess β-cell–protective properties. While sitagliptin is theorized to be β-cell protective, most data stem from in vitro studies, and further research is needed to identify the role of sitagliptin in β-cell protection. However, unlike GLP-1 agonists (eg, exenatide), DPP-4 inhibitors are not generally associated with a slowing of gastric empty-ing or the induction of weight loss. This difference is thought to be because DPP-4 inhibitors stabilize GLP-1 levels rather than induce a super-physiological GLP-1 action as is the case with exenatide and other GLP-1 agonists in development. An additional advantage of DPP-4 inhibitors when compared to GLP analogs is the route of administration. GLP analogs, such as exenatide, are polypeptide molecules that are susceptible to degradation within the digestive tract, thus necessitating the administration of these agents via injection. DPP-4 inhibitors, in contrast, can be administered orally and convey many of the same benefits as GLP analogs with increased ease of use and patient acceptability.

Pharmacokinetics

Sitagliptin is rapidly absorbed upon oral administration, with a bioavailability of approximately 87%. The pharmacokinetic properties of sitagliptin appear unaffected by age, gender, race, and body mass index,

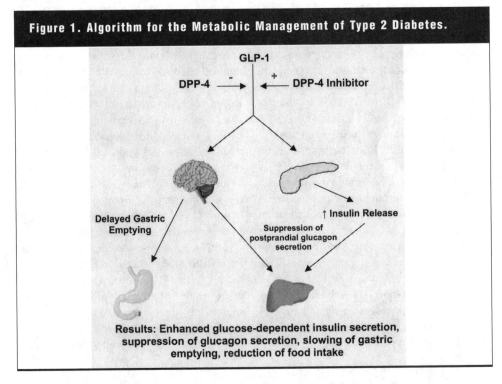

Figure 1. Algorithm for the Metabolic Management of Type 2 Diabetes.

GLP-1

DPP-4 —⁻→ ←₊— DPP-4 Inhibitor

Delayed Gastric Emptying

↑ Insulin Release

Suppression of postprandial glucagon secretion

Results: Enhanced glucose-dependent insulin secretion, suppression of glucagon secretion, slowing of gastric emptying, reduction of food intake as reported in data from clinical trials. Following administration of a single oral 100-mg dose of sitagliptin in healthy volunteers, peak serum levels were achieved in approximately 1-4 hours. The mean volume of distribution at steady state is 198 L after a single dose of sitagliptin, with approximately 38% of sitagliptin reversibly bound to plasma proteins.

Sitagliptin is estimated to be 79% excreted unchanged in the urine via active tubular secretion. In vitro studies indicate that sitagliptin is modestly metabolized via CYP3A4 with some contribution from the 2C8 isoenzyme. Because sitagliptin is largely eliminated via renal excretion, dosage adjustments are recommended in those with moderate to severe renal impairment. The terminal half-life of a single dose of 100 mg of sitagliptin was found to be 12.4 hours on average in healthy volunteers. When examined, moderate hepatic impairment did not show significant alterations in the pharmacokinetic profile of sitagliptin.

diabetes. Combination therapy with sulfonylureas has been associated with a slightly increased risk of hypoglycemia. In one study, the risk of hypoglycemia was 12.2% in patients taking sitagliptin plus glimepiride with or without metformin versus 1.8% in those taking glimepiride with or without metformin. Overall, sitagliptin has demonstrated acceptable efficacy and tolerability standards in clinical trials. In addition to A_{1C} reduction, improvements in fasting and postprandial glucose levels and a lack of weight gain were also seen with sitagliptin treatment, thus strengthening the case for sitagliptin as add-on therapy in patients with type 2 diabetes. The fact that this class of drugs is weight neutral is one of its main promotional points. Sitagliptin is available in combination with metformin, as Janumet. It is believed that future drugs in this class will also be made available as fixed-dose combinations with metformin. The combination products are being promoted as first-line therapy for patients with type 2 diabetes.

TREATMENT ADVANTAGES AND DISADVANTAGES

Treatment with sitagliptin generally results in a modest A_{1C} reduction, with a reduction range of 0.48-0.85% from baseline in clinical trials. While it is not associated with a large A_{1C} lowering ability, sitagliptin does possess a number of characteristics that make it desirable for use as adjunct therapy to diet and exercise, or as add-on therapy to metformin, a thiazolidinedione, a sulfonylurea, or metformin plus a sulfonylurea. Sitagliptin is dosed once daily, making its use favorable in those desiring to minimize pill burden. The use of sitagliptin also poses a minimal risk of hypoglycemia when given as monotherapy, and sitagliptin has a relatively mild side-effect profile when compared with other agents used in the treatment of type 2

THERAPEUTIC CONSIDERATIONS

Warnings and Precautions

Sitagliptin is eliminated largely via the kidneys. Thus, caution and dose reduction is warranted in patients with renal disease. Furthermore, renal function should be assessed in patients under consideration for sitagliptin therapy prior to drug initiation. Vildagliptin, another DPP-4 inhibitor currently in phase III clinical trials, was associated with the development of necrotic skin lesions during primate studies (at relatively high doses), and postmarketing reports of serious allergic and hypersensitivity reactions have been reported in patients taking sitagliptin. These reactions included cases of anaphylaxis; angioedema; and exfoliative skin conditions, including Stevens-Johnson syndrome. While the occurrence of these drug reactions are rare, patients should be aware of any abnormal skin lesions or changes upon initiation of sitagliptin and report any unusual reactions to their health care provider. Sitagliptin is contraindicated in patients with type 1 diabetes and is not intended for use in the treatment of diabetic ketoacidosis. Patients with a documented hypersensitivity to sitagliptin or any of its components should not initiate therapy with sitagliptin.

Special Populations

Little clinical information is available regarding sitagliptin use in older adults with type 2 diabetes; however, dose adjustment is recommended for patients with renal compromise. Of note, patients with moderate renal insufficiency receiving 50 mg/day of sitagliptin experienced a mean increase in serum creatinine of 0.12 mg/dL versus an increase of 0.07 mg/dL in matched controls with the same degree of renal impairment receiving placebo. The clinical relevance of the observed increase in serum creatinine is not known at this time. Dosage adjustments are not recommended for patients with mild to moderate hepatic impairment; however, sitagliptin has not been formally evaluated in patients with advanced hepatic disease.

Sitagliptin is rated as a pregnancy Category B agent by the FDA, and should only be used during pregnancy if deemed necessary. Caution is advised in women who are nursing, as it is currently unknown if sitagliptin is secreted into human breast milk. Safety and efficacy in patients under 18 years of age has not been studied.

Adverse Effects and Monitoring

During clinical trials with sitagliptin, the incidence of adverse events and discontinuation of therapy were similar for sitagliptin and placebo controls. Clinical trial adverse event data identified three common side effects occurring with more frequency than events seen in control subjects, namely nasopharyngitis, upper respiratory tract infection, and headache. Additionally, the overall incidence of hypoglycemia in subjects receiving sitagliptin monotherapy was similar to that of placebo controls. The occurrence of hypoglycemia not increased when sitagliptin treatment was administered in combination with metformin or pioglitazone, but an increase in the rate of hypoglycemia was noted when sitagliptin was studied in combination with glimepiride. In some clinical trials, treatment with sitagliptin also resulted in an increase in white blood cell count (approximately 200 cells/μL) compared to placebo; this increase was attributed to an increase in neutrophil numbers. It is unknown at this time if this finding is clinically significant.

Therapeutic monitoring recommendations for patients receiving sitagliptin include periodic monitoring of hemoglobin A_{1C} and self-monitoring of blood glucose. Patients under consideration for sitagliptin therapy should receive renal function testing prior to therapy as well as periodically during treatment, and the dose of sitagliptin should be adjusted accordingly to prevent drug accumulation.

Drug Interactions

Despite the limited metabolism of sitagliptin by CYP450 enzymes 3A4 and 2C8, it is considered unlikely that any clinically relevant interactions exist with other drugs that utilize the CYP450 system. While sitagliptin is also a p-glycoprotein substrate, sitagliptin does not appear to inhibit p-glycoprotein transport of other drugs that utilize this pathway.

When studied in combination with concomitant drugs in clinical trials, sitagliptin did not meaningfully alter the pharmacokinetic profiles of metformin, glyburide, simvastatin, rosiglitazone, warfarin, or oral contraceptives. When coadministered with a

600-mg dose of cyclosporine, a potent inhibitor of p-glycoprotein activity, peak serum concentrations of sitagliptin were increased by approximately 68%. The renal clearance of sitagliptin was not altered, however, and the observed change in the peak concentration of sitagliptin was not considered clinically meaningful.

For digoxin, 100 mg of sitagliptin in combination with 0.25 mg daily of digoxin for 10 days resulted in an 11% increase in the area under the curve (AUC) and an 18% increase in peak plasma levels of digoxin. While digoxin dosage adjustments are not recommended when the drug is given in combination with sitagliptin, patients receiving these agents in combination should receive periodic monitoring of serum digoxin levels to prevent toxicity.

See **Table 9.2**, or refer to the full prescribing information for more drug interaction guidance.

Dosage and Administration

Sitagliptin is available commercially in 25-mg (pink), 50-mg (light beige) and 100-mg (beige) tablets. For type 2 diabetes patients with normal renal function, sitagliptin is dosed at 100 mg once daily as monotherapy or in combination with metformin, a thiazolidinedione, a sulfonylurea, or metformin plus a sulfonylurea. Sitagliptin can be taken with or without food, and because sitagliptin is eliminated via renal excretion, dosage adjustments are required for patients with moderate to severe renal impairment. For patients with a creatinine clearance (CrCl) ≥30 to <50 mL/min, the recommended dose of sitagliptin is 50 mg once daily. For patients with CrCl <30 mL/min or with end-stage renal disease requiring dialysis, the recommended dose of sitagliptin is 25 mg once daily. Sitagliptin is also available in combination with metformin. This combination pill, Janumet, is available in 50/500 mg and 50/1000 mg of sitagliptin and metformin, respectively. It is recommended that Janumet be taken twice daily with meals and titrated slowly to minimize the gastrointestinal side effects associated with metformin use.

See **Table 9.1**, or refer to the full prescribing information for more dosing guidance.

SUGGESTED READING

Ahrén B. Dipeptidyl peptidase-4 inhibitors: clinical data and clinical implications. *Diabetes Care*. 2007;30(6):1344-1350.

Campbell RK. Rationale for dipeptidyl peptidase 4 inhibitors: a new class of oral agents for the treatment of type 2 diabetes mellitus. *Ann Pharmacother*. 2007;41(1):51-60.

Deacon CF. Dipeptidyl peptidase 4 inhibition with sitagliptin: a new therapy for type 2 diabetes. *Expert Opin Investig Drugs*. 2007;16(4):533-545.

Deacon CF, Holst JJ. Dipeptidyl peptidase IV inhibitors: a promising new therapeutic approach for the management of type 2 diabetes. *Int J Biochem Cell Biol*. 2006;38(5-6):831-844.

Lyseng-Williamson KA. Sitagliptin. *Drugs*. 2007;67(4):587-597.

McKennon SA. Campbell RK. The physiology of incretin hormones and the basis for DPP-4 inhibitors. *Diabetes Educ*. 2007;33(1):55-66.

Table 9.1. Prescribing Information for Dipeptidyl Peptidase-4 Inhibitors

GENERIC (BRAND)	FORM/ STRENGTH	DOSAGE	WARNINGS/PRECAUTIONS & CONTRAINDICATIONS	ADVERSE REACTIONS
Sitagliptin phosphate (Januvia)	Tab: 25mg, 50mg, 100mg	*Adults:* 100mg qd. **CrCl ≥30 to <50mL/min:** 50mg qd. **CrCl: <30mL/min:** 25mg qd.	**W/P:** Assess renal function prior to initiation of treatment. Cause hypoglycemia when used in combination with a sulfonylurea. Anaphylaxis, angioedema, and exfoliative skin conditions reported. **Contra:** Anaphylaxis or angioedema **P/N:** Category B, caution in nursing.	(Monotherapy/ Combination therapy) Upper respiratory tract infection, nasopharyngitis, headache. (Combination therapy) hypoglycemia.
COMBINATION DRUG				
Sitagliptin phosphate/ Metformin HCl (Janumet)	Tab: (Sitagliptin-Metformin) 50mg-500mg, 50mg-1000mg	*Adults:* Individualize dosing. **Patient Not Controlled on Metformin Monotherapy:** Initial: 100mg/day (50mg bid) of sitagliptin + metformin dose. **Patient on Metformin 850mg BID:** Initial: 50mg-1000mg tab bid. **Patient Not Controlled on Sitagliptin Monotherapy:** Initial: 50mg-500mg tab bid. Titrate: Gradual increase to 50mg-1000mg tab bid. Max: 100mg of sitagliptin and 2000mg of metformin. Take with meals.	**BB:** Lactic acidosis may occur due to metformin accumulation. If acidosis suspected, d/c drug and hospitalize patient immediately. **W/P:** Lactic acidosis reported (rare), increased risk with renal dysfunction. Assess renal function prior to initiation and during treatment; caution in elderly. Avoid in renal/hepatic impairment. May decrease vitamin B_{12} levels; monitor hematologic parameters. May cause hypoglycemia in elderly, debilitated/malnourished, adrenal or pituitary insufficiency, or alcohol intoxication. D/C in hypoxic states (eg, CHF, shock, acute MI), prior to surgical procedures (due to restricted food and fluid intake), and procedures requiring use of intravascular iodinated contrast materials. **Contra:** Renal disease (SrCR ≥1.5mg/dL [males], ≥1.4mg/dL [females], or abnormal CrCl), metabolic acidosis, including diabetic ketoacidosis. D/C for 48 hrs in patients undergoing radiologic studies with intravascular iodinated contrast materials. **P/N:** Category B, caution in nursing.	(Metformin) Diarrhea, nausea/vomiting, flatulence, abdominal discomfort, indigestion, asthenia, and headache. (Sitagliptin) Nasopharyngitis.

BB = black box warning; **W/P** = warnings/precautions; **Contra** = contraindications; **P/N** = pregnancy category rating and nursing considerations.

Table 9.2. Drug Interactions for Dipeptidyl Peptidase-4 Inhibitors

Sitagliptin phosphate (Januvia)

Digoxin	May slightly increase digoxin levels; monitor appropriately.
Sulfonylureas	Caution, may cause hypoglycemia when used concomitantly; may require lower dose of sulfonylurea to reduce risk.

COMBINATION DRUG

Sitagliptin phosphate-Metformin HCl (Janumet)

Alcohol	Potentiates effects of metformin on lactate metabolism; potentiates hypoglycemia; avoid excessive alcohol intake.
Calcium channel blockers	May cause hyperglycemia.
Cationic drugs (eg, digoxin, amiloride, procainamide, quinidine, quinine, rantidine, trimethoprim, vancomycin, triamterene, morphine)	May increase metformin levels.
Contraceptives, oral	May cause hyperglycemia.
Corticosteroids	May cause hyperglycemia.
Digoxin	Monitor digoxin levels.
Diuretics	May cause hyperglycemia.
Estrogens	May cause hyperglycemia.
Furosemide	May increase metformin levels, may decrease furosemide levels.
Isoniazid	May cause hyperglycemia.
Nicotinic acid	May cause hyperglycemia.
Nifedipine	May increase metformin levels.
Phenothiazines	May cause hyperglycemia.
Phenytoin	May cause hyperglycemia.
Sympathomimetics	May cause hyperglycemia.
Thiazides	May cause hyperglycemia.
Thyroid products	May cause hyperglycemia.

Chapter 10

Bile Acid Sequestrants

R. Keith Campbell, PharmB, MBA, CDE

INTRODUCTION

At the time this book was written, colesevelam (marketed as Welchol) was the latest medication approved by the FDA for the treatment of type 2 diabetes (in January 2008). It had a previous indication for lowering LDL cholesterol, but studies showed that it also significantly lowered HbA$_{1c}$ levels and could be used alone or in combination with other diabetes medications. It is not considered first-line therapy for type 2 diabetes but could become an important addition to other antidiabetes agents. Bile acid sequestrants (BAS) were initially approved to lower LDL cholesterol and were often combined with statin drugs for this purpose. Colesevelam is available in tablet form and is being promoted for type 2 diabetes patients with elevated LDL cholesterol who have not been able to achieve target blood glucose or HbA$_{1c}$ levels. It lowers HbA$_{1c}$ on average by 0.5 percent. Plasma glucose levels were decreased by 13%. Although other BAS can lower HbA$_{1c}$, colesevelam is the only one approved for this use in patients with diabetes. It is not indicated for type 1 diabetes patients.

PHARMACOLOGY

Colesevelam was specifically engineered for affinity and high-capacity bile acid binding. Studies in diabetes patients with high choles-

terol and elevated LDL-C showed that glucose levels decreased by 13% after 24 weeks of treatment. Subsequent studies evaluated colesevelam as adjunctive therapy for improving glycemic control. In patients with inadequate glycemic control on sulfonylureas and/or metformin therapy, 12 weeks of colesevelam HCl treatment significantly improved HbA$_{1c}$ and levels of fructosamine and postprandial glucose, as well as reduced levels of LDL-C, total cholesterol, and apolipoprotein B.

Mechanism of Action

The mechanism by which colesevelam improves glycemic control is unknown. Proposed mechanisms include reduction in glucose absorption or changes in the time course of glucose absorption in the gastrointestinal tract. It is also theorized that BAS cause disruption of the entero-hepatic pathway of bile metabolism. This mechanism is plausible since diabetes patients appear to have faulty regulation of bile acid metabolism, including increased bile acid synthesis, an increased bile acid pool, and alteration in bile acid composition. Bile acids are endogenous ligands of the farnesoid X receptor (FXR), a bile acid-activated nuclear receptor that plays a role in glucose metabolism. The proposed effect of this is that by preventing the reabsorption of bile acids in the intestinal lumen, BAS may deactivate the FXR and resultant pathways.

Another proposed mechanism is that BAS increase the release of incretins, lending to an increase in both first- and second-phase glucose-stimulated insulin release. It is frustrating to not know the exact mechanism by which BAS reduce glucose levels, but the simple fact is that colesevelam does so while at the same time lowering LDL-C.

Pharmacokinetics

Colesevelam hydrochloride is a hydrophilic, water-insoluble polymer that is not hydrolyzed by digestive enzymes and is not absorbed from the GI tract. Again, since it is not absorbed, its distribution is limited to the GI tract.

Colesevelam HCl is not metabolized systemically and does not interfere with systemic drug-metabolizing enzymes such as cytochrome P450.

With reference to excretion, in healthy volunteers, an average of only 0.05% of administered radioactivity from a single ^{14}C-labeled colesevelam HCl dose was excreted in the urine.

TREATMENT ADVANTAGES AND DISADVANTAGES

Colesevelam HCl is a nonabsorbed, polymeric, lipid-lowering and glucose-lowering agent intended for oral administration. Colesevelam hydrochloride is a high-capacity bile acid-binding molecule. Recently, the American Association of Clinical Endocrinologists (AACE) placed colesevelam in their Road Map to Achieve Glycemic Goals in patients naïve to therapy (type 2) at level 2 for patients with an initial HbA_{1c} between 7% and 8% and who should be using combination therapy, especially metformin. It would also seem appropriate to target type 2 patients who have not quite been able to achieve an HbA_{1c} of 7 or less who have elevated LDL-C. Lowering the HbA_{1c} of the many type 2 patients who cannot quite

achieve a target HbA_{1c} of 7 or less with an oral medication with relatively few side effects and little weight gain that drops HbA_{1c} by 0.5 % seems a reasonable alternative.

Colesevelam should not be used for the treatment of type 1 diabetes patients or for the treatment of diabetic ketoacidosis. It has not been studied in type 2 diabetes as monotherapy or in combination with a dipeptidyl peptidase-4 inhibitor and has not been extensively studied in combination with thiazolidinediones. Patients using this drug should be strongly encouraged to follow a prescribed nutrition and exercise program. Because the drug is not absorbed, it is also appealing in terms of not having systemic side effects and unlike many other treatments for type 2 diabetes it does not cause significant weight gain.

The major barriers to colesevelam's use include the fact that the patient needs to take 6 tablets a day or 3 tablets twice daily with food and plenty of fluid, and many patients develop constipation. The tablet size of colesevelam can cause dysphagia or esophageal obstruction and should be used with caution in patients with dysphagia or swallowing disorders.

In general, colesevelam is a useful addition to the tool chest of classes of drugs used to orally treat type 2 diabetes.

THERAPEUTIC CONSIDERATIONS

Since BAS can cause gastrointestinal problems including constipation; patients need to be instructed to take the tablets with food and plenty of fluid. A major concern in diabetes patients are those with gastroparesis or other malabsorption disorders or at risk for bowel obstruction that may enhance constipation problems. Readers are encouraged to closely review the package insert.

Significant Warnings/Precautions

The effect of colesevelam on cardiovascular morbidity and mortality has not been determined. It is known that in studies whereby LDL-C is decreased, cardiovascular benefits usually follow but statins are the drug of first choice to treat most lipid disorders.

It is known and is a concern that BAS can increase serum TG concentrations. The effect on TG is about 5% greater versus placebo, but larger increases have been observed when colesevelam was added to sulfonylureas or insulin patients with type 2 diabetes with increases of 18% and 22%, respectively.

Hypertriglyceridemia of sufficient severity can cause acute pancreatitis. The long-term effect of hypertriglyceridemia on the risk of coronary artery disease is uncertain. Caution should be exercised when treating patients with TG levels >300 mg/dL. Because most patients in the colesevelam clinical trials had baseline TG <300 mg/dL, it is unknown whether patients with more uncontrolled baseline hypertriglyceridemia would have greater increases in serum TG levels. In addition, the use of colesevelam is contraindicated in patients with TG levels >500 mg/dL. Lipid parameters, including TG levels and non-HDL-C, should be obtained before starting colesevelam and periodically thereafter. It should be discontinued if TG levels exceed 500 mg/dL or if the patient develops hypertriglyceridemia-induced pancreatitis.

Precautions Regarding Vitamin K or Fat-Soluble Vitamin Deficiencies

BAS may decrease the absorption of fat-soluble vitamins A, D, E, and K. No specific clinical studies have been conducted to evaluate the effects of colesevelam on the absorption of coadministered dietary or supplemental vitamin therapy. Patients on oral vitamin supplementation should take their vitamins at least 4 hours prior to colesevelam. Caution should be exercised when treating patients with a susceptibility to deficiencies of vitamin K (eg, patients on warfarin, patients with malabsorption syndromes) or other fat-soluble vitamins.

SPECIAL POPULATIONS

Pregnancy

Colesevelam is a pregnancy category B drug with inadequate studies in pregnant women and there is no reasonable reason to use it in pregnant women. Note that rat and rabbit studies did not show any fetal harm.

Nursing Mothers

Colesevelam is not expected to be excreted in human milk because colesevelam HCl is not absorbed systemically from the gastrointestinal tract.

Pediatrics

Colesevelam has not been studies in pediatric patients and the tablet size would make it difficult for most children to swallow.

Geriatrics

Colesevelam use did not differ in effectiveness or safety between older and younger patients related to primary hyperlipidemia or type 2 diabetes.

Hepatic Impairment

No special considerations or dosage adjustments are recommended when colesevelam is administered to patients with hepatic impairment.

Renal Impairment

No overall differences in safety or effectiveness were observed between patients with CrCl <50 mL/min and those with a CrCl ≥50 mL/min.

Adverse Effects and Monitoring

As stated before, the side effect profile of colesevelam is quite good. The major side effects are related to its GI effects and possible elevation of triglycerides. The three major adverse effects that were significantly higher than placebo were constipation (11% vs 7% for placebo), dyspepsia (8.3% vs 3.5%) and nausea (4.2% vs 3.9%). Hypoglycemia had an incidence of 3% compared with 2.3% for placebo with no reports of severe hypoglycemia. In summary, colesevelam HCl is considered a safe and well-tolerated treatment for type 2 diabetes.

Patients should be monitored for constipation and other GI problems. Obtain pre-levels of HbA_{1c}, plasma glucose, LDL-C, TG and then re-test after 12 weeks of therapy. Instruct patients to consume a diet that promotes bowel regularity and to stop the drug if abdominal pain or severe constipation occurs.

Drug Interactions

Drugs with a known interaction with colesevelam (eg, glyburide, levothyroxine, oral contraceptives) should be administered at least 4 hours prior to colesevelam. Drugs that have not been tested for interaction with colesevelam, especially those with a narrow therapeutic index (eg, phenytoin), should also be administered at least 4 hours prior to administration. Alternatively, monitor blood levels of the coadministered drug. Because it may impact the absorption of fat-soluble vitamins, patients receiving warfarin should be carefully monitored; vitamin supplementation may be appropriate.

See **Table 10.2**, or refer to the full prescribing information for more drug interaction guidance.

Dosing and Administration

Patients should be advised to take colesevelam with a meal and adequate fluids. It can be taken as 6 tablets once daily or 3 tablets twice daily.

See **Table 10.1**, or refer to the full prescribing information for more dosing guidance.

SUGGESTED READING

Bays HE, Cohen DE. Rationale and design of a prospective clinical trial program to evaluate the glucose-lowering effects of colesevelam HCl in patients with type 2 diabetes mellitus. *Curr Med Res Opin*. 2007;23:1673-84.

Bays HE, Goldberg RB. The 'forgotten' bile acid sequestrants: is now a good time to remember? *Am J Ther*. 2007:14;567-580.

Davidson MH. The use of colesevelam hydrochloride in the treatment of dyslipidemia: a review. *Expert Opin Pharmacother*. 2007;8(15):2569-78.

Staels B, Kuipers F. Bile acid sequestrants and the treatment of type 2 diabetes mellitus. *Drugs*. 2007;67(10):1383-92.

Zieve FJ, Kalin MF Schwartz SL, Jones MR, Bailey WL. Results of the Glucose-Lowering Effect of Welchol Study (GLOWS): A randomized, double-blind, placebo-controlled pilot study evaluating the effect of colesevelam hydrochloride on glycemic control in subjects with type 2 diabetes. *Clin Ther*. 2007;29:74-83.

Welchol Package Insert. Daiichi Sankyo, Parsippany. NJ. January 2008.

Table 10.1: Prescribing Information for Bile Acid Sequestrants

GENERIC (BRAND)	FORM/ STRENGTH	DOSAGE	WARNINGS/PRECAUTIONS & CONTRAINDICATIONS	ADVERSE REACTIONS
Colesevelam HCl (Welchol)	Tab: 625mg	*Adults:* **Hyperlipidemia/Type 2 DM:** 3 tabs bid or 6 tabs qd. Take with liquids and a meal.	**W/P:** Monitor lipids, including TG and non-HDL-cholesterol levels prior to initiation of treatment and periodically thereafter. Caution in TG levels >300mg/dL, dysphagia or swallowing disorders, gastroparesis, GI motility disorders, major GI tract surgery, bowel obstruction, and those susceptible to vitamin K or fat soluble vitamin deficiencies. Coadministered drugs should be given at least 4 hrs prior to treatment; monitor drug levels. Not for use in treatment of type 1 DM or for diabetic ketoacidosis. **Contra:** Bowel obstruction, hypertriglyceridemia-induced pancreatitis, serum TG concentrations >500mg/dL. **P/N:** Category B, caution in nursing.	Asthenia, constipation, dyspepsia, pharyngitis, myalgia, nausea, hypoglycemia, bowel obstruction, dysphagia, esophageal obstruction, fecal impaction, hypertriglyceridemia, pancreatitis, increased transaminases.

W/P = warnings/precautions; **Contra** = contraindications; **P/N** = pregnancy category rating and nursing considerations.

Table 10.2. Drug Interactions for Bile Acid Sequestrants

Colesevelam (Welchol)

Contraceptives, oral (eg, ethinyl estradiol, norethindrone)	Decreases levels of ethinyl estradiol and norethindrone.
Glyburide	Decreases levels of glyburide.
Insulin	Increases triglyceride levels.
Levothyroxine	Decreases levels of levothyroxine.
Phenytoin	Decreases phenytoin levels; monitor levels.
Sulfonylureas	Increases triglyceride levels.
Thyroid hormone replacement therapy	Elevates TSH levels; monitor levels.
Warfarin	Concomitant use decreases International Normalized Ratio (INR); monitor INR levels.

Chapter 11

Glucagon-Like Peptide-1 (GLP-1) Analog

Stephen M. Setter, PharmD, CDE, DVM

INTRODUCTION

The incretin, glucagon-like peptide - 1 (GLP-1) is synthesized and excreted from the L cells of the distal ileum and colon in response to a meal. Endogenous GLP-1 is rapidly degraded by dipeptidyl peptidase-4 (DPP-4) within minutes. Exendin-4, a 39-amino acid GLP-1 agonist, is derived from the salivary gland venom of the gila monster (*Heloderma suspectum*) and resists degradation by DPP-4. Exenatide, a synthetically derived peptide of exendin-4, is currently approved in the U.S. as Byetta in injectable form as adjunctive therapy to treat type 2 diabetes for patients currently using metformin, a sulfonylurea, a combination of metformin and sulfonylurea or a combination of metformin and a thiazolidinedione who have not reached target glycemic goals. The medical community has embraced the use of exenatide due to its having several different mechanisms of action for lowering blood glucose as well as the potential for patients to lose weight.

PHARMACOLOGY

Mechanism of Action

The incretin mimetic exenatide enhances glucose-dependent insulin secretion by pancreatic β-cells and restores first-phase insulin response. Impaired first-phase insulin secretion is an early physiological defect in patients with type 2 diabetes. In addition, during hyperglycemia, exenatide lowers serum glucagon concentrations resulting in reduced hepatic glucose release and decreased insulin need. Gastric emptying is also delayed, thereby reducing meal-related glucose excursions. Food intake is also reduced. During phase III clinical trials, exenatide resulted in a progressive decrease in body weight over 30 weeks of therapy.

Pharmacokinetics/ Pharmacodynamics

Subcutaneous administration of exenatide results in a C_{max} of 211 pg/mL, with a mean AUC of 1036 pg • h/mL and a T_{max} of 2.1 hours. Bioavailability is similar when injected into the upper arm, abdomen, or thigh. V_d is 28.3 L. Glomerular filtration is the primary route of elimination, with proteolytic degradation being secondary. Terminal half-life is 2.4 hours with a mean apparent clearance of 9.1L/h. Exenatide concentrations are detectable for approximately 10 hours postdose. Due to a 10-fold reduction in exenatide clearance in patients with end stage renal disease (ESRD), exenatide is not recommended in this patient population. Hepatic dysfunction is not expected to alter exenatide's pharmacokinetic profile.

Exenatide is associated with a dose-dependent increase in serum insulin concentrations within 3 hours of administration, resulting in marked reduction ofserum glucose concentrations. Reduction in fasting plasma glucose occurs between 3-4 hours post SC administration.

TREATMENT ADVANTAGES AND DISADVANTAGES

Injectable exenatide lowers HbA_{1C} by 0.8%-1.1% with an associated weight loss of 1.6-2.8 kg in 26-30 week trials at the 10 mcg bid dose. Exenatide does not require refrigeration after the first dose.

Disadvantages include its high rate of nausea and the potential development of anti-exenatide antibodies. Another potential disadvantage, particularly for those without insurance coverage, is its expense: 1 month supply of the 5 mcg pen costs approximately $213 (U.S.) and the one-month 10-mcg pen costs approximately $230 dollars (U.S.).

The only GLP-1 analog currently available is exenatide; however, a long-acting release (LAR) product (LAR exenatide) is in development. In addition, an oral formulation of exenatide in capsule form, utilizing enteric coated interferon nano-particles, is being developed under the name Nodexen. Another GLP-1 agonist, Liraglutide, is in phase III clinical trials.

THERAPEUTIC CONSIDERATIONS

Significant Warnings and Precautions

Patients with type 1 diabetes or those with diabetic keotacidosis should not receive exenatide. In addition, it should be apparent that exenatide is not a substitute for insulin.

Anti-exenatide antibodies do form in a small proportion of users, which may result in a poor response to therapy. If the glycemic response is suboptimal or fails to persist with time, alternatives may need to be considered. In one trial of 16 week's duration, 9% of patients had increased antibody titers at the end of the trial. Patients with elevated titers in general had an attenuated response to therapy.

Acute pancreatitis has been reported in patients using exenatide; therefore, severe abdominal distress or pain accompanied with vomiting should be appropriately evaluated.

In general, exenatide should not be used in patients with severe GI disease, **especially those with gastroparesis or a history of bowel obstruction.**

As expected, exenatide patients concurrently on a sulfonylurea are at increased risk of hypoglycemia. A common practice that decreases this risk is to decrease the dose of the sulfonylurea upon initiation of exenatide with dose titrations of each agent based on clinical response.

Patients with severe renal impairment (SCr <30 mL/min) or ESRD should not receive exenatide.

Exenatide is pregnancy category C and should only be used if its benefit clearly outweighs the potential risk. The extent and amount of exenatide that enters the breast milk is unknown; breastfeeding mothers should either discontinue breastfeeding while taking exenatide or discontinue exenatide while breastfeeding.

Special Populations

Mild to moderate renal dysfunction does not require dosage adjustment. Exenatide is not recommended for patients with severe renal impairment or those with ESRD. Because exenatide is primarily cleared via the kidneys, no dosage alterations are required in patients with impaired hepatic function. Race, age (eg, elderly patients), obesity and gender do not appreciably alter the pharmacokinetics of exenatide. Safety and efficacy have not been established nor studied in children, and therefore the drug is not recommended in this patient population.

Adverse Effects and Monitoring

Common side effects associated with exenatide include nausea, vomiting, diarrhea, dizziness, headache, feeling jittery, and dyspepsia. With initiation of exenatide, nausea is very common (~40%) but often subsides with continued use. If exenatide is used with a sulfonylurea, hypoglycemia may occur. It's recommended that sulfonylurea dose reduction be considered upon initiation of exenatide. As with all antidiabetic therapies, monitoring of daily blood glucose is warranted with periodic HbA_{1C} determinations.

Drug Interactions

As with all antidiabetic agents, exenatide can theoretically interact with other medications that can raise or lower blood glucose. Prudent use of concomitant therapies with appropriate monitoring of fasting and postprandial blood glucose is warranted.

Specifically, exenatide has been studied with the coadministration of acetaminophen, digoxin, lisinopril, lovastatin, and warfarin. Acetaminophen's AUC and Cmax decreased, while Tmax decreased. Digoxin's C_{max} and T_{max} were delayed when administered concomitantly with exenatide. Lisinopril's T_{max} was delayed 2 hours when given with exenatide, and lovastatin's AUC and C_{max} were decreased while the T_{max} was delayed by 4 hours. As illustrated by exenatide's coadministration with these oral therapies, the pharmacokinetics of orally administered drugs dependent upon normal gastric emptying time may be altered. Therefore, it is advisable to administer the aforementioned oral therapies 1 hour prior to exenatide administration; follow this practice for other orally administered therapies as well. This is also true for patients taking oral antibiotics or oral contraceptives. Specifically as regards acetaminophen, give acetaminophen at least 1 hour prior to or 4 hours post exenatide injection.

Exenatide my alter INR when given in a patient taking warfarin. Therefore, vigilant monitoring of INR upon initiation and maintenance of exenatide therapy is warranted. With regard to meals and exenatide's propensity to alter gastric emptying, exenatide should be administered at any time up to 60 minutes prior the two main meals of the day, with meals being at least 6 hours or more apart.

See **Table 11.2**, or refer to the full prescribing information for more drug interaction guidance.

Dosage and Administration

Exenatide is administered subcutaneously at any time up to 60 minutes prior to the morning and evening meals, with a minimum 6 hours between injections. Injections may be self-administered in the thigh, abdomen, or upper arm. For patients on metformin or a sulfonylurea, exenatide should be started at 5 mcg bid. If clinically warranted, and if appropriately tolerated, after 1 month the dose may be increased to 10 mcg bid. Patients should be instructed never to administer exenatide after a meal and should never make up a missed dose. Instruct patients to resume therapy with the next regularly scheduled dose.

See **Table 11.1**, or refer to the full prescribing information for more dosing guidance.

SUGGESTED READING

Buse JB, Henry RR, Han J, et al for the Exenatide-113 Clinical Study Group. Effects of exenatide (exendin-4) on glycemic control over 30 weeks in sulfonylurea-treated patients with type 2 diabetes. *Diabetes Care.* 2004;27:2628-2635.

DeFronzo RA, Ratner RE, Han J, et al. Effects of exenatide (exendin-4) on glycemic control and weight over 30 weeks in metformin-treated patients with type 2 diabetes. *Diabetes Care.* 2005;28:1092-1100.

Drucker DJ. Enhancing encretin action for the treatment of type 2 diabetes. *Diabetes Care.* 2003;26:2929-2940.

Dungan K, Buse JB. Glucagon-like peptide 1-based therapies for type 2 diabetes: a focus on exenatide. *Clin Diabetes.* 2005;23:56-62.

Fineman MS, Bicsak TA, Shen LZ, et al. Effect on glycemic control of exenatide (synthetic exendin-4) additive to existing metformin and/or sulfonylurea treatment in patients with type 2 diabetes. *Diabetes Care.* 2003;26:2370-2377.

Fineman MS, Shen LZ, Taylor K, et al. Effectiveness of progressive dose escalation of exenatide (exendin-4) in reducing dose-limiting side effects in subjects with type 2 diabetes. *Diabtes Metab Res Rev.* 2004;20:411-417.

Keating GM. Exenatide. *Drugs.* 2005;65:1681-1692.

Kendall DM, Riddle MC, Rosenstock J, et al. Effects of exenatide (exendin-4) on glycemic control over 30 weeks in patients with type 2 diabetes treated with metformin and a sulfonylurea. *Diabetes Care.* 2005;28:1083-1091.

Kim A, MacConell L, Zhuang D, et al.: Effects of once-weekly dosing of a long-acting release formulation of exenatide on glucose control and body weight in subjects with type 2 diabetes. *Diabetes Care.* 30:1487-1493, 2007

Kolterman OG, Kim DD, Shen L, et al. Pharmacokinetics, pharmacodynamics, and safety of exenatide in patients with type 2 diabetes mellitus. *Am J Health Syst Pharm.* 2005;62:173-181.

Neilson LL, Baron AD. Pharmacology of exenatide (synthetic exendin-4) for the treatment of type 2 diabetes. *Curr Opin Investig Drugs.* 2003;4:401-405.

Table 11.1: Prescribing Information for Glucagon-Like Peptide-1 Analog

GENERIC (BRAND)	FORM/ STRENGTH	DOSAGE	WARNINGS/PRECAUTIONS & CONTRAINDICATIONS	ADVERSE REACTIONS
Exenatide (Byetta)	**Inj:** 5mcg/dose, 10mcg/dose [60-dose prefilled pen]	***Adults:*** 5mcg SQ bid, 60 min before am & pm meals. Titrate: May increase to 10mcg bid after 1 month. Reduction of sulfonylurea dose may be considered to reduce risk of hypoglycemia.	**W/P:** Not a substitute for insulin. Avoid with type 1 DM, treatment of diabetic ketoacidosis, ESRD, severe renal impairment (CrCl <30mL/min), or severe GI disease. Acute pancreatitis reported. Increased incidence of hypoglycemia with sulfonylureas. Observe for signs and symptoms of hypersensitivity reactions; patients with abdominal pain should be investigated. When used with thiazolidinediones possible CP and/or chronic hypersensitivity pneumonitis. **P/N:** Category C, caution in nursing.	Nausea, vomiting, diarrhea, feeling jittery, dizziness, headache, dyspepsia, injection-site reactions; dysgeusia, somnolence, generalized pruritus and/or urticaria, macular or papular rash, angioedema, rare reports of anaphylactic reaction, abdominal pain, hypoglycemia.

W/P = warnings/precautions; **P/N** = pregnancy category rating and nursing considerations.

Table 11.2. Drug Interactions for Glucagon-Like Peptide-1 Analog

Exenatide (Byetta)

Oral Drugs	May reduce the rate and extent of absorption of orally administered drugs; use with caution if taking oral medications that require rapid GI absorption; orally administered drugs that are dependent on threshold levels (eg, **contraceptives**, **antibiotics**) should be taken 1 hr before administration of exenatide.
Warfarin	Caution with concomitant use; may lead to increased INR and possible bleeding.

Chapter 12

Pramlintide

Brian J. Gates, PharmD

INTRODUCTION

Pramlintide was approved by the FDA in March 2005. It is a synthetic analog of the naturally occurring hormone amylin, which is co-secreted with insulin from β-cells in the pancreas and works in concert with insulin to lower blood glucose. Amylin is absent in patients with type 1 diabetes and reduced in patients with type 2 diabetes. Amylin will not work as an injectable medication because it is too viscous. Pramlintide is very similar in structure to amylin, but has a proline residue substituted in positions 25, 28, and 29 of the amino acid chain. Pramlintide is indicated for use in both type 1 and type 2 diabetes as an adjunctive therapy for patients who have inadequate blood glucose control despite optimal treatment with meal-time insulin. In type 2 patients, pramlintide can be added even if the patient is already taking the mealtime insulin along with a sulfonylurea or metformin. Pramlintide has been studied as an adjunct treatment for patients taking a basal insulin without concurrent mealtime insulin, but it received a nonapprovable letter from the FDA for this indication in September 2007.

PHARMACOLOGY

Mechanism of Action

Pramlintide mimics the actions of amylin. In a patient without diabetes, amylin and insulin are both released in response to elevated blood glucose levels. Amylin has three major effects on the regulation of blood glucose. One effect is slowed gastric emptying, which allows for more gradual absorption of carbohydrates and thereby reduces post-prandial spikes in blood glucose. The total amount of carbohydrate absorbed is not altered. A second effect of amylin is to reduce release of glucagon from the pancreas. Glucagon is a regulatory hormone that counters the effect of insulin and increases blood glucose. Release of insulin does not slow release of glucagon, and amylin can help maintain appropriate balance between glucagon and insulin. The third effect of amylin is to centrally cause satiety, which may decrease the total amount of carbohydrates (and calories) consumed during a meal. The calorie reduction may ultimately promote weight loss, which may further help glucose control in some patients.

Pharmacokinetics

The absolute bioavailability of a subcutaneous dose of pramlintide is 30%-40%. Injections into the abdomen and thigh demonstrated more consistent kinetics than injections into the arm. Bioavailability was not affected by amount of adipose tissue at the injection site. Pramlintide is approximately 40% unbound in plasma and is not expected to be affected by changes in protein binding.

Pramlintide has short half-life of ~48 minutes. It is metabolized renally and has an active metabolite, des-lys pramlintide. However, no accumulation was found with the metabolite.

TREATMENT ADVANTAGES AND DISADVANTAGES

Pramlintide offers a potential advantage when a patient continues to have difficulty with post-prandial blood glucose control despite using scheduled doses of mealtime insulin. The lack of amylin and its regulatory effects may substantially hinder insulin's effectiveness in some patients. Pramlintide may help restore balance to factors regulating post-prandial blood glucose and allow insulin to work more effectively. It may also help patients to lose weight in contrast to some diabetes medications that cause weight gain. Some patients have experienced significant weight loss, as evidenced by the warnings in the prescribing guidelines regarding potential anorexia from the medication. Pramlintide therefore may be a reasonable option in patients who have had difficulty losing weight.

A potential disadvantage is that pramlintide is an injectable agent and substantially increases the number of injections since it is only used by patients who are already injecting insulin with each meal. Pramlintide and insulin cannot be mixed and must be injected into different sites. Pramlintide can substantially increase the risk of hypoglycemia, and patients must be capable of careful monitoring to avoid hypoglycemia.

At this time, pramlintide is the only agent available in its class. Though it was released approximately the same time as exenatide, these agents have different mechanisms and are utilized differently in the treatment of diabetes.

THERAPEUTIC CONSIDERATIONS

Contraindications
Pramlintide is contraindicated if:
- The patient has a hypersensitivity to pramlintide or any components, including the ingredient metacresol
- The patient has a confirmed diagnosis of gastroparesis because pramlintide may further worsen this condition
- The patient has hypoglycemic unawareness

Precautions
Prescribing information for pramlintide contains a boxed warning regarding potentially severe hypoglycemic episodes. Pramlintide itself will not cause hypoglycemia, but because it is only indicated for use in conjunction with insulin, a severe drop in blood sugar may be seen with the combination. Even patients who are capable of identifying hypoglycemia must use caution if they are involved in potentially dangerous activities requiring alertness, such as driving a car or operating heavy machinery, as the reaction will occur within up to 3 hours of injecting pramlintide. The manufacturer recommends carefully selecting patients regarding their ability to recognize and manage hypoglycemic episodes, providing education regarding the medications and its effects, and reducing insulin doses when pramlintide is initiated.

Special Populations

Geriatrics

Data available in patients up to 85 years of age found no differences in geriatric patients from younger adults, and no age-related dosage adjustments are recommended by the manufacturer. However, geriatric patients may be more sensitive to the effects of hypoglycemia. Therefore, it is important to carefully select geriatric patients for risk of and ability to manage hypoglycemia, and in geriatric patients it may be appropriate to titrate the dose more slowly than the standard adult dose. The pen injector may be easier for some geriatric patients to administer and may prevent complications. It also may be reasonable to start geriatric patients at a lower dose than the typical adult starting dose.

Pediatrics

Pramlintide is not approved for use in pediatric patients, and to date a paucity of information is available regarding pramlintide in children. Until further information is available, use is not recommended in children.

Pregnancy and Breastfeeding

Pramlintide is a pregnancy category C medication. It is not known if it is excreted into breast milk, but it could pass easily into breast milk based on its structure. Therefore, it is recommended that mothers taking pramlintide nurse only if the benefit is considered to outweigh the risk.

Renal Insufficiency

In studies of patients with moderate to severe renal impairment (creatinine clearance <50 mL/min but >20 mL/min), no effect on pramlintide clearance was found. Patients on dialysis have not been studied.

Hepatic Insufficiency

No studies have been conducted in patients with hepatic impairment. However, no changes are expected in patients with hepatic insufficiency because pramlintide is almost exclusively eliminated through the kidneys.

Gender

No differences among male and female patients were noted in studies. However, no trials have been conducted to specifically examine differences between male and female patients.

Ethnicity

Though studies have not been conducted to specifically examine the effects of ethnicity on pramlintide, no differences among different ethnic groups were found in initial trials. Studies were primarily conducted in Caucasian, African-American, and Hispanic patients.

Adverse Effects and Monitoring

The list of adverse events from pramlintide is short, but those effects that patients have experienced require attention from both health care professionals and patients to ensure appropriate management.

Hypoglycemia

Severe hypoglycemia is the adverse event of greatest concern, but in clinical trials the incidence of severe hypoglycemia was low. Patients should be screened carefully for history of difficulty with hypoglycemia, capability to recognize symptoms of hypoglycemia, and willingness and ability to monitor blood glucose carefully and adhere to patient instructions. When pramlintide is added, the dose of insulin should be decreased by 50% with continued blood glucose monitoring. The insulin dose can be increased if necessary when a stable dose of pramlintide has been reached.

Gastrointestinal Effects

Gastrointestinal events were the most common complaint by patients in clinical trials and included nausea, vomiting, and anorexia. Nausea can be managed by starting with low doses and gradually titrating the dose no more frequently than every three to seven days as long as no nausea is present. Though some beneficial weight loss has been found, patients should be monitored to ensure weight is lost at an appropriate rate and anorexia does not develop.

Injection-Site Reactions

Patients have experienced injection-site reactions while taking pramlintide. It is important to ensure that patients are using proper technique and are rotating injection sites.

Drug Interactions

The primary drug interaction concerns with pramlintide relate to its effect on gastrointestinal motility. Little data exists regarding these potential interactions. The manufacturer recommends against concurrent use of pramlintide with medications that also decrease gastrointestinal motility (eg, anticholinergics, opioids) as well as medications that affect nutrient absorption (such as the α-glucosidase inhibitors acarbose and miglitol).

Medications that need to have a rapid therapeutic effect, such as analgesics, may need to be dosed either one hour before or two hours after pramlintide. Studies with acetaminophen demonstrated that the time to peak concentration of acetaminophen was slowed when given at the same time as pramlintide.

Pramlintide must be used carefully with any other agents that lower blood glucose to avoid severe hypoglycemia. Specific studies have not been done to determine if pramlintide alters the absorption of other antihyperglycemic agents.

As noted in the Dosage and Administration section, pramlintide cannot be mixed with insulin in the same syringe because the kinetics of pramlintide will be altered. Pramlintide

and insulin must also be injected in separate sites to avoid the two medications interfering with each other's absorption.

See **Table 12.2**, or refer to the full prescribing information for more drug interaction guidance.

Dosage and Administration

Different dosing schedules are utilized in type 1 and type 2 diabetes patients. However, in both patient groups the dose of mealtime insulin must be reduced by 50% when pramlintide is initiated to avoid severe hypoglycemia. A reduction in the dose of combination products such as 70/30 is also recommended because of its rapid-acting component. Because of pramlintide's short half-life, a decrease in basal insulin is typically not necessary. Patients must conduct frequent blood glucose monitoring to avoid hypoglycemia and determine the need for further adjustments of insulin dose. The injection should be given in the thigh or abdomen rather than in the arm because of inconsistent absorption from the arm. Pramlintide cannot be mixed with insulin in the same syringe, and they should also be injected in different locations so that they will not interfere with each other's absorption.

Pramlintide now is available in a pen, which may be substantially easier for patients to use. All patients taking pramlintide should consider using the pen because the manufacturer plans to discontinue supplying the vial by 2011. When patients are switching to the vial, they must be educated that the pen dose is measured in micrograms, rather than in units, used in drawing doses from the vial.

Type 1 Diabetes Patients

The recommended starting dose is 15 mcg given with each major meal (more than 250 calories or 30 g of carbohydrates). If nausea is not bothersome after three to seven days, the dose can be increased in 15-mcg increments to a target dose of 30 to 60 mcg with each major meal. If difficulty with nausea is experienced after titration, the dose can be decreased back to the previous level to give the patient more time to tolerate the medication.

Type 2 Diabetes Patients

The recommended starting dose is 60 mcg with each major meal. If nausea is not bothersome after three to seven days, the dose can be increased to 120 mcg with each major meal (more than 250 calories or 30 g of carbohydrates). If difficulty with nausea is experienced after titration, the dose can be decreased back to 60 mcg to give the patient more time to tolerate the medication.

See **Table 12.1**, or refer to the full prescribing information for more dosing guidance.

Additional Information for All Patients

The insulin dose may need to be further decreased as pramlintide is titrated to avoid hypoglycemia. Once a stable pramlintide dose is achieved, the insulin dose can be increased if necessary for adequate glucose control. Pramlintide is stable for 30 days at room temperature, and the manufacturer recommends a new vial or pen after 30 days.

SUGGESTED READING

Edelman SV. Optimizing diabetes treatment using an amylin analogue. *Diabetes Educ.* 2008;34 Suppl 1:4S-10S.

Edelman S, Garg S, Frias J, et al. A double-blind, placebo-controlled trial assessing pramlintide treatment in the setting of intensive insulin therapy in type 1 diabetes. *Diabetes Care.* 2006 29:2189-95.

Ratner RE, Dickey R, Fineman M, et al. Amylin replacement with pramlintide as an adjunct to insulin therapy improves long-term glycaemic and weight control in Type 1 diabetes mellitus: a 1-year, randomized controlled trial. *Diabet Med.* 2004;21:1204-12.

Riddle M, Brown C, Zhang B, et al. Pramlintide improved glycemic control and reduced weight in patients with type 2 diabetes using basal insulin. *Diabetes Care.* 2 007;30:2794-2799.

Rubin RR, Peyrot M. Assessing treatment satisfaction in patients treated with pramlintide as an adjunct to insulin therapy. *Curr Med Res Opin.* 2007; 23:1919-29.

Smith SR, Blundell JE, Burns C. Pramlintide treatment reduces 24-h caloric intake and meal sizes and improves control of eating in obese subjects: a 6-wk translational research study. *Am J Physiol Endocrinol Metab.* 2007;293:E620-7.

Want LL. Optimizing treatment success with an amylin analogue. *Diabetes Educ.* 2008; 34 Suppl 1:11S-7S.

Whitehouse F, Kruger DF, Fineman M, et al. A randomized study and open-label extension evaluating the long-term efficacy of pramlintide as an adjunct to insulin therapy in type 1 diabetes. *Diabetes Care.* 2002;25:724-30.

Table 12.1. Prescribing Information for Pramlintide

GENERIC (BRAND)	FORM/ STRENGTH	DOSAGE	WARNINGS/PRECAUTIONS & CONTRAINDICATIONS	ADVERSE REACTIONS
Pramlintide acetate (Symlin, Symlin Pen)	**Inj:** 600mcg/mL [5mL]; **Pen injector:** 1000mcg/mL [1.5mL, 2.7mL]	***Adults:*** Before initiating therapy reduce insulin dose by 50%. Monitor blood glucose frequently. Adjust insulin dose once target dose of primitive is maintained. **Type 2 DM:** Initial: 60mcg SQ immediately prior to meals. Titrate: 120mcg as tolerated. **Type 1 DM:** Initial: 15mcg SQ immediately prior to meals. Titrate: Increase by 15mcg increments to 30mcg or 60mcg as tolerated.	**BB:** Use with insulin; risk of insulin-induced severe hypoglycemia, particularly with type 1 DM. Severe hypoglycemia usually occurs within 3 hrs of injection. Serious injuries may occur if severe hypoglycemia occurs while operating a motor vehicle, heavy machinery, or during other high-risk activities. Appropriate patient selection, careful patient instruction, and insulin dose adjustments are necessary to reduce this risk. **W/P:** Do not mix with insulin; administer as separate injections. **Contra:** Confirmed diagnosis of gastroparesis; hypoglycemia unawareness. **P/N:** Category C, caution in nursing.	Nausea, headache, anorexia, vomiting, abdominal pain, fatigue, dizziness, coughing, pharyngitis.

BB = black box warning; **W/P** = warnings/precautions; **Contra** = contraindications; **P/N** = pregnancy category rating and nursing considerations.

Table 12.2. Drug Interactions for Pramlintide

Pramlintide acetate (Symlin, Symlin Pen)	
Analgesics	Administer 1 hr before or 2 hrs after injection.
Gastrointestinal motility agents (eg, anticholinergic agents such as atropine)	Warning, do not administer with Symlin.
Intestinal absorption slowing agents (eg, α-glucosidase inhibitors)	Warning, do not administer with Symlin.
Rapid-acting oral agents	Administer 1 hr before or 2 hrs after injection.

Section II
Management of Macrovascular Disease

People with diabetes are at considerably higher risk for macrovascular disease and related complications when compared to people without diabetes. The prevention and management of macrovascular disease in patients with diabetes mellitus includes the individualized treatment of high blood pressure and hyperlipidemia, the use of antiplatelet therapies to minimize the risk of thrombosis, and smoking cessation counseling and treatment when appropriate to minimize cardiovascular risk. The chapters in this section will discuss treatment options and considerations for the reduction of macrovascular risk in patients with diabetes.

Chapter 13

Management of Hypertension

Joshua J. Neumiller, PharmD, CGP, FASCP

INTRODUCTION

Blood pressure management is a vital component of the treatment plan for people with diabetes for prevention of both micro- and macrovascular complications. Hypertension and diabetes are both independent risk factors for microvascular disease, peripheral vascular disease, cardiovascular disease, and cerebral vascular disease. Given the additional risk afforded to people with comorbid diabetes and hypertension, and considering that people with diabetes are twice as likely to have a diagnosis of hypertension, proper management and treatment of hypertension is critical in this at-risk population.

Reduction of blood pressure in hypertensive patients is strongly correlated with a reduction in overall cardiovascular risk. Likewise, blood pressure reduction slows or even halts the progression of microvascular complications in the diabetic patient. According to guidance from The Seventh Report of the Joint National Committee on Prevention, Detection, Evaluation, and Treatment of High Blood Pressure (JNC VII) and the American Diabetes Association, a recommended blood pressure treatment goal for people with diabetes is <130/80 mmHg. In the UK Prospective Diabetes Study (UKPDS), each 10-mmHg decrease in mean systolic blood pressure was associated with a 12% risk reduction for any complication related to diabetes, a 15% decrease for deaths related to diabetes, an 11% decrease for myocardial infarction, and a 13% decrease in risk for the development of microvascular complications. Overall, the findings from this study and others indicate that normalization of blood pressure is as important as normalization of blood glucose in reducing the risk of complications in people with diabetes. Additionally, epidemiological studies indicate that blood pressures ≥120/70 mmHg are associated with increased cardiovascular event rates and mortality in people with diabetes. A threshold value for risk reduction with improved blood pressure control has not yet been identified, with risk reduction continuing well into the "normal" blood pressure range. Achieving blood pressures below the current standard of <130/80 mmHg is difficult to achieve, however, and often requires multidrug therapies and places patients at increased risk of adverse drug events and adverse outcomes. Current studies are underway to ascertain if more aggressive hypertension treatment strategies would convey added benefit to the reduction of cardiovascular events and microvascular disease in people with diabetes without placing them at undue risk of morbidity associated with such strict blood pressure control.

Table 1. Lifestyle Modifications to Manage Hypertension

MODIFICATION	RECOMMENDATION	APPROXIMATE SYSTOLIC BLOOD PRESSURE REDUCTION (RANGE)
Weight Reduction	Maintain normal body weight (defined as a body mass index 18.5-24.9 kg/m²).	5-20 mmHg/10kg weight loss
Adopt DASH Eating Plan	Consume a diet rich in fruits, vegetables, and low-fat dairy products with a reduced content of saturated and total fat.	8-14 mmHg
Dietary Sodium Restriction	Reduce dietary sodium intake to no more than 21.4g of sodium.	2-8 mmHg
Physical Activity	Engage in regular aerobic physical activity such as brisk walking for at least 30 minutes per day, most days of the week.	4-9 mmHg
Moderation of Alcohol Consumption	Limit consumption of alcohol to no more than 2 drinks per day in most men, and to no more than 1 drink per day in women and lighter weight persons.	2-4 mmHg

Adapted from The Seventh Report of the Joint National Committee on Prevention, Detection, Evaluation, and Treatment of High Blood Pressure (JNC VII).

NONPHARMACOLOGICAL MANAGEMENT OF HYPERTENSION

Dietary management of essential hypertension with moderate sodium restriction has proved effective in lowering blood pressure in people with diabetes. Additionally, moderate weight loss has been demonstrated in several studies to have a positive relationship with blood pressure reduction. While the effects of sodium restriction on blood pressure have not been specifically studied in the diabetic population, sodium restriction studies in patients with essential hypertension have demonstrated reductions in systolic blood pressure of approximately 5 mmHg and reductions of 2-3 mmHg in diastolic values with moderate sodium restriction. The JNC VII guidelines advocate the adoption of the Dietary Approaches to Stop Hypertension (DASH) eating plan. A DASH eating plan with 1,600 mg of sodium has demonstrated effects on blood pressure similar to single-drug therapy. Additionally, moderation of alcohol consumption can

result in blood pressure reduction in those consuming large amounts of daily alcohol. Implementation of an exercise regimen has been shown to have beneficial effects on blood pressure, and is recommended by the JNC VII guidelines. Overall, lifestyle modifications such as those listed above are associated with improvements in blood pressure control, enhanced antihypertensive drug efficacy, and an overall decrease in cardiovascular risk. **Table 1** outlines lifestyle modifications recommended within the JNC VII treatment guidelines.

PHARMACOLOGICAL MANAGEMENT OF HYPERTENSION

Diuretics
Diuretics have been widely used for several decades as first-line agents in the treatment of hypertension. Diuretics reduce total body sodium through their natriuretic action, and are effective in reducing the expanded plasma volume often associated with hypertension in diabetes. **While diuretics are associated with**

adverse effects on glucose tolerance and lipids, they can be very beneficial in the treatment of hypertension and fluid overload in patients with diabetes. Some evidence suggests thiazide-type diuretics exhibit efficacy in lowering cardiovascular risk and may be beneficial in patients with impaired renal function or diabetic nephropathy.

Pharmacology
Mechanism of Action
The mechanism of action varies depending on the class of diuretic. Thiazide-type diuretics work by increasing sodium, chloride, and water excretion by inhibiting sodium ion transport across the renal tubular epithelium. Loop diuretics, such as furosemide, inhibit the reabsorption of sodium and chloride in the ascending limb of the loop of Henle by inhibiting chloride binding to the $Na^+/K^+/2Cl^-$ cotransporter, thus resulting in diuresis. Potassium-sparing diuretics, such as triamterene and amiloride, work by inhibiting the sodium-potassium ion exchange system in the distal renal tubule independent of aldosterone. Spironolactone, in contrast, inhibits the effects of aldosterone on the distal renal tubule, thus enhancing sodium, chloride, and water excretion.

Pharmacokinetics
Pharmacokinetic properties vary widely depending on the class of diuretic and agent used. Refer to full product labeling for specific pharmacokinetic information.

Treatment Advantages and Disadvantages
Reduction in cardiovascular morbidity and mortality with diuretic therapy has been demonstrated in terms of stroke and congestive heart failure (CHF) reduction in large randomized clinical trials, and thiazide diuretics have specifically demonstrated efficacy in reducing the risk of cardiovascular morbidity in elderly patients with isolated

systolic hypertension. Low-dose thiazide therapy has demonstrated a reduction of cardiovascular event rates by 34% when compared to placebo, with an absolute risk reduction twice as great for subjects with diabetes when compared to nondiabetic subjects.

Unfortunately, diuretics can cause adverse metabolic effects at higher doses, including worsening of glucose tolerance with high-dose diuretic therapy. Worsening of glucose tolerance typically occurs after two to four weeks of therapy in patients with diabetes, but these effects may not surface for months or even years in some patients. Thiazide diuretics are the most likely diuretics to cause adverse glycemic effects, followed by loop diuretics. Potassium-sparing diuretics are typically not associated with inducing glucose intolerance. Of particular concern in patients with diabetes, thiazide diuretics have also been linked to small elevations in LDL cholesterol and triglyceride levels, sexual dysfunction, and orthostatic hypotension.

Therapeutic Considerations
Warnings/Precautions
Diuretic therapy should not be initiated in patients with preexisting electrolyte abnormalities until they have been corrected. Likewise, diuretic use is contraindicated in patients with anuria. Patients with a propensity toward hypovolemia or hypotension should be treated cautiously with diuretic agents.

Special Populations
Elderly patients are particularly sensitive to the hypotensive effects of diuretics. Therapy should be initiated with low doses with careful upward titrations as tolerated to achieve the desired antihypertensive effect. Thiazide diuretics may not be effective in patients with a creatinine clearance <60mL/min, however the use of loop diuretics is recommended for patients with decreased renal function. Cautious use of diuretics in pregnant or nursing women is recommended.

Adverse Effects and Monitoring

Treatment with thiazide diuretics has been associated with hypokalemia, hyponatremia, volume depletion, hypercalcemia, and hyperuricemia. Diuresis can result in dehydration, dizziness, muscle cramps, and orthostatic hypotension. Orthostatic hypotension is more pronounced with the use of loop diuretics. Potassium supplementation may be required in patients taking loop diuretics, as well as some patients on thiazide therapy. Worsening of glucose tolerance can occur in patients with diabetes. Diuretics are also associated with small elevations in LDL cholesterol and triglyceride levels, sexual dysfunction, and orthostatic hypotension.

Drug Interactions

Drug interactions will vary depending on agents used. Refer to the full product label for specific information. In general, the hypotensive effects of diuretics can be potentiated by other antihypertensive medications. Hypokalemia resulting from diuretic therapy can increase the potential for proarrhythmic effects due to medications including cardiac glycosides and dofetilide. Additionally, nonsteroidal anti-inflammatory drugs (NSAIDs) can antagonize the effects of diuretic therapy due to fluid and sodium retention induced by this class of medication. See **Table 13.3** for more information.

Dosage and Administration

Dosage and administration guidelines vary depending on class of diuretic and agent used. See **Table 13.2**, or refer to the product information for the drug in question for specific dosing and administration information.

β-**Adrenergic Antagonists**

β-blockers have demonstrated reduction in cardiovascular morbidity and mortality in large, population-based, randomized clinical trials, however, careful consideration of the risks and benefits of β-blocker therapy is essential. Careful consideration is also warranted when choosing a specific agent for use. **While β-blockers are associated with masking the signs and symptoms of hypoglycemia, their use in patients with diabetes who have a history of myocardial infarction have demonstrated clear benefits in the prevention of subsequent cardiovascular events.**

Pharmacology

Mechanism of Action

β-adrenergic antagonists competitively compete with catecholamines for binding at sympathetic receptor sites. β-1 selective, or "cardioselective" agents, preferentially antagonize β-1 receptors in the heart and vasculature. Nonselective β-blockers, however, exert antagonist activity at both β-1 and β-2 receptor sites. β-2 blockade in bronchial and vascular smooth muscle corresponds to a less profound antihypertensive effect (due to unopposed α-vasoconstriction) and can potentially cause or exacerbate bronchospasm. β-1 receptor antagonism results in decreases in heart rate, cardiac output, diastolic blood pressure, and systolic blood pressure.

Pharmacokinetics

The pharmacokinetic properties of the various β-blockers vary greatly depending on dosage form used and route of administration. Refer to full product labeling for specific pharmacokinetic information.

Treatment Advantages and Disadvantages

β-blockers have demonstrated efficacy in patients with myocardial infarction with relative reductions in mortality reaching 25%. Because patients with diabetes and a history of myocardial infarction have an increased risk of mortality when compared to those without diabetes, the benefits of β-blocker therapy may be greater in the diabetic population. β-blockers are not without side effects. Elderly patients are particularly sensitive to the fatigue and other bothersome side effects associated with therapy. In patients with diabetes, concern exists regarding the effects of β-blockers on the perception and recovery from hypoglycemia. Of note, nonselective agents are associated with a blunted counter-regulatory response to hypoglycemia when compared to cardioselective agents. This effect appears to be particularly significant in patients using insulin therapy. Avoiding the use of β-blockers in patients with a history of severe hypoglycemia or hypoglycemic unawareness may be prudent in some cases. In post-myocardial infarction patients, however, the proven benefits of β-blocker therapy appear to outweigh the risks associated with their use.

Therapeutic Considerations
Warnings/Precautions
Abrupt discontinuation of β-blockers can result in the development of myocardial ischemia, myocardial infarction, ventricular arrhythmias, or rebound hypertension. Patients discontinuing therapy should be tapered downward to prevent such events. β-blockers are contraindicated in patients with severe bradycardia, sick sinus syndrome, or advanced AV block unless a functioning pacemaker is in place due to the potential for exacerbation of these conditions. β-blocker therapy should also be avoided in patients with decompensated systolic CHF. A contraindication for use also exists for patients with severe peripheral arterial circulatory disorders as the development of gangrene has been reported rarely in this population.

Special Populations
Elderly patients may have unpredictable responses to β-adrenergic receptor antagonists. Elderly patients may be less sensitive to the antihypertensive effects of this category

of medication, and are particularly sensitive to adverse events associated with therapy.

Adverse Effects and Monitoring
Of particular concern in patients with diabetes, β-blockers can worsen glucose tolerance with severe cases of hyperglycemia reported in some cases. This effect appears to be dose and duration related, and can be additive in nature in patients also receiving thiazide and/or loop diuretics. β-blockers, particularly nonselective agents such as propranolol, have more pronounced adverse effects on glucose tolerance than cardioselective agents. Therapy with β-blockers has also been associated with worsening of triglyceride levels and lowering of HDL levels in some patients.

Additionally, β-adrenergic antagonists are associated with intensification of hypoglycemic severity as well as delayed hypoglycemic resolution. The signs and symptoms of hypoglycemia can be masked with β-antagonists such that patients are unaware of typical sympathetic responses to hypoglycemia such as tachycardia, palpitations, hunger, tremor, irritability, and confusion. Perspiration is characteristically enhanced by β-blocker therapy, and patients should be aware of increased sweating as a symptom of low blood sugars. Again, nonselective agents tend to have more of a blunting effect on hypoglycemic symptoms when compared to β-1 selective agents.

Drug Interactions
Potential drug interactions with β-receptor antagonists are numerous and can vary depending on the agent. In general, β-blockers can augment the hypotensive effects of other antihypertensive medications, thus caution is warranted when β-blockers are added to existing antihypertensive regimens. β-blockers can also antagonize sympathomimetic therapies. Pharmacologically, β-receptor antagonists depress AV node conduction, thus additive

Figure 1. Mechanism of Action of ACE Inhibitors and ARBs.

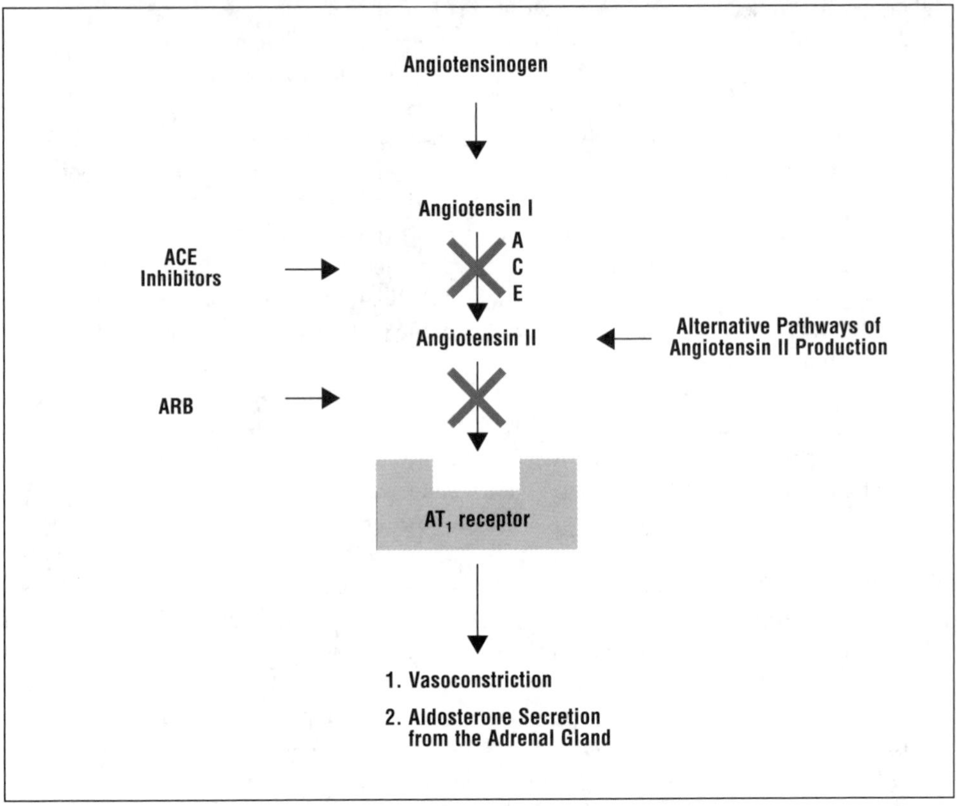

Angiotensinogen

↓

Angiotensin I

ACE
Inhibitors →

A
C
E

↓

Angiotensin II ← Alternative Pathways of
Angiotensin II Production

ARB →

AT$_1$ receptor

↓

1. Vasoconstriction
2. Aldosterone Secretion
   from the Adrenal Gland

effects are possible when given with other antiarrhythmic medications that exert significant effects on AV node conduction. See **Table 13.3** for more information.

Dosage and Administration
Doses and frequency of administration will vary depending on the agent and dosage form used. See **Table 13.2**, or refer to the product information for the drug in question for specific dosing information.

Angiotensin Converting Enzyme (ACE) Inhibitors

Angiotensin converting enzyme (ACE) inhibitors are a class of medication widely used in the treatment of hypertension in patients with and without diabetes. **ACE inhibitors have been promoted as the drug category of choice for the treatment of hypertension in people with diabetes due to their beneficial effects on the prevention of diabetic nephropathy, and should be considered as first-line agents for the treatment of hypertension in patients with diabetes that do not have a contraindication to therapy.**

Pharmacology
Mechanism of Action
ACE inhibitors compete with angiotensin I for its binding site on the angiotensin-converting enzyme (ACE). The result of ACE inhibition is prevention of the conversion of angiotensin I to angiotensin II. Angiotensin II is a potent inducer of vasoconstriction, and acts as a negative feedback mediator for renin

activity. Ultimately, with lowered angiotensin II levels, blood pressure is decreased and plasma renin activity is increased. **Figure 1** outlines the mechanism of action of ACE inhibitors as well as angiotensin receptor blockers (ARBs).

Pharmacokinetics
Pharmacokinetic properties vary depending on the ACE inhibitor used. Most ACE inhibitors are typically dosed once daily, however twice-daily dosing can be used for some products. Refer to full product labeling for specific pharmacokinetic information.

Treatment Advantages and Disadvantages
ACE inhibitors have assumed a valuable role in the treatment of hypertension in patients with diabetes with or without diabetic nephropathy. The UK Prospective Diabetes Study/Hypertension in Diabetes Study (UKPDS-HDS) demonstrated similar efficacy regarding mortality associated with microvascular and cardiovascular complications in patients with type 2 diabetes when comparing the ACE inhibitor captopril to atenolol. ACE inhibitors have been extensively studied in terms of treatment in patients with diabetic nephropathy, demonstrating positive effects in this population. Studies indicate that ACE inhibitors are not only effective in the treatment of hypertension in patients with type 2 diabetes and nephropathy, but use of these agents can also be beneficial in terms of management of proteinuria and the progression of renal damage in these patients. The Heart Outcomes Prevention Evaluation (HOPE) study with ramipril demonstrated a decrease in cardiovascular risk despite minor changes in blood pressure, thus indicating benefits in patients with diabetes that are independent of the antihypertensive effects of ACE inhibitors. Additionally, ACE inhibitor therapy has demonstrated benefit in preventing the progression of diabetic retinopathy.

Therapeutic Considerations
Warnings/Precautions
Important contraindications to ACE inhibitor therapy include ACE inhibitor hypersensitivity, history of angioedema, and renal artery stenosis. ACE inhibitors should be used cautiously in patients with a history of or current hyperkalemia due to their potassium-sparing effects.

Special Populations
ACE inhibitors are pregnancy category D drugs due to an association with fetal and neonatal morbidity and mortality with administration to pregnant women. Use during the first trimester has been associated with a potential to induce birth defects. ACE inhibitors should be avoided in women planning to become pregnant, and women taking ACE inhibitors should discontinue use as soon as possible following the detection of pregnancy. Cautious use is warranted in elderly patients due to their increased susceptibility to the hypotensive effects of ACE inhibitors and an increased likelihood of decreased renal function in this population.

Adverse Effects and Monitoring
One problematic side effect associated with ACE inhibitor therapy is drug-induced cough. Occasional acute decreases in renal function can also occur. ACE inhibitors are potassium-sparing agents, and hyperkalemia can occur in some patients, especially those with renal insufficiency. Common side effects encountered with therapy include dizziness, hypotension, peripheral edema, and fatigue. Serious cases of angioedema have been associated with ACE inhibitor therapy.

Drug Interactions
Because ACE inhibitors decrease aldosterone secretion, which leads to small increases in serum potassium levels, the risk of hyperkalemia can be increased when coadminis-

tered with other drugs that increase serum potassium levels such as potassium-sparing diuretics, potassium supplements, and heparin. NSAIDs may attenuate the antihypertensive effects of ACE inhibitors by inhibiting the synthesis of vasodilatory prostaglandins. Additionally, in patients with compromised renal function, the coadministration of ACE inhibitors and NSAIDs may lead to deterioration of renal function. Aspirin has also been implicated in attenuating the effects of ACE inhibitors, however the benefits of using aspirin in combination with ACE inhibitors in patients with CAD and left ventricular dysfunction tend to outweigh the risk. See **Table 13.3** for more information.

Dosage and Administration
Dosage and administration guidelines vary depending on specific agent used. See **Table 13.2**, or refer to the product information for the drug in question for specific dosing information. Dosage adjustments may be necessary in patients with renal impairment.

Angiotensin II Receptor Blockers (ARBs)
Angiotensin II receptor antagonists are generally well-tolerated agents used in the treatment of hypertension. ARBs efficacy in terms of cardiovascular risk reduction in patients with CHF has been demonstrated in a variety of clinical trials. **ARBs may be a viable treatment option in diabetic patients with hypertension who have contraindications or those who cannot tolerate ACE inhibitor therapy.**

Pharmacology
Mechanism of Action
ARBs antagonize angiotensin II at the angiotensin$_1$ (AT$_1$) receptor subtype. Angiotensin II binding at the AT$_1$ receptor results in vasoconstriction and stimulation of the synthesis and release of aldosterone.

By selectively blocking an AT$_1$ receptor in vascular smooth muscle and the adrenal gland, ARBs inhibit vasoconstriction and aldosterone secretion, thus decreasing blood pressure. The mechanism of action of ARBs is outlined in **Figure 1** within the ACE inhibitor section.

Pharmacokinetics
Pharmacokinetic parameters of the ARBs vary depending on the particular agent in question. ARBs are dosed once to twice daily depending on the agent and patient specific variables. Refer to full product labeling for specific pharmacokinetic information.

Treatment Advantages and Disadvantages
In general, ARBs are well tolerated, appear to not cause deleterious metabolic effects that may be problematic in patients with diabetes, and should be considered for patients with diabetic proteinuria who are intolerant to ACE inhibitor therapy. Limited data with valsartan indicate that it reduces proteinuria in patients with hypertension and renal disease; however further study is warranted to determine comparative renoprotective efficacy and long-term cardiovascular benefits compared to ACE inhibitor therapy.

Therapeutic Considerations
Warnings/Precautions
ARBs should be used cautiously in patients with impaired renal or hepatic function. Due to similarities in the pharmacology of ACE inhibitors and ARBs, caution is recommended in patients with a history of angioedema or renal artery stenosis (RAS). ARBs should be used cautiously in patients with a history of or current hyperkalemia due to the potassium-sparing effects of ARBs as a function of their effects on aldosterone.

Special Populations
Elderly patients are more susceptible to the hypotensive effects of ARBs, and are more

likely to have impaired renal and hepatic function, thus the half-life of ARBs can be considerably longer in geriatric patients. ARBs are rated pregnancy category D during the second and third trimesters of pregnancy. Spontaneous abortions and newborn renal dysfunction have been reported in cases where pregnant women have taken valsartan.

Adverse Effects and Monitoring
Common side effects associated with ARB therapy include dizziness, diarrhea, peripheral edema, and myalgia. Serious adverse events include hypotension and hyperkalemia. Decreases in renal function have been noted in some patients. In contrast to ACE inhibitors, cough is rarely induced by ARB use.

Drug Interactions
Because ARBs can induce small increases in serum potassium levels, the risk of hyperkalemia can be increased when coadministered with other drugs that increase serum potassium levels such as potassium-sparing diuretics, potassium supplements, and heparin. NSAIDs may attenuate the antihypertensive effects of ARBs by inhibiting the synthesis of vasodilatory prostaglandins. Additionally, in patients with compromised renal function, the coadministration of ARBs and NSAIDs may lead to deterioration of renal function. ARBs should be used with caution or avoided in patients on lithium therapy due to an increased risk of lithium toxicity when taken together. See **Table 13.3** for more information.

Dosage and Administration
Dosage and administration guidelines vary depending on specific agent used. See **Table 13.2**, or refer to the product information for the drug in question for specific dosing information. Dosage adjustments may be required in patients with impaired renal or hepatic function.

Calcium Channel Blockers (CCBs)
Calcium channel blockers (CCBs) exert their pharmacological effects on the vasculature via inhibition of calcium influx via membrane-bound voltage-dependent calcium channels, resulting in decreased intracellular calcium levels within smooth muscle leading to vasodilation. CCBs are subdivided into three main categories: the dihydropyridines, the benzothiazepines (diltiazem), and the phenylalkylamines (verapamil). Diltiazem and verapamil are often referred to collectively as nondihydropyridine CCBs. Dihydropyridines primarily exhibit vasodilatory effects with minimal effects on cardiac contractility and atrioventricular conduction. Nondihydropyridines, in contrast, have significant effects on cardiac conduction, thus distinct differences exist between the various CCBs, requiring careful consideration when choosing an agent for the treatment of hypertension. **Some evidence indicates that CCBs may have positive effects on proteinuria in patients with diabetic nephropathy, however, long-term studies are lacking. CCBs appear to be viable options for add-on therapy in patients with diabetes requiring multiple antihypertensive agents to meet blood pressure goals.**

Pharmacology
Mechanism of Action
CCBs as a class inhibit the influx of extracellular calcium across vascular smooth muscle and myocardial cell membranes to induce peripheral and coronary artery vasodilation. The resulting vasodilation leads to reduction in blood pressure and increased perfusion of the myocardium. Differences exist between various CCBs in regard to selectivity for coronary versus peripheral vasodilation. In general, dihydropyridine CCBs, such as nifedipine and amlodipine, exert effects mainly on arteriolar vasculature. Verapamil, in contrast, is relatively specific to the coronary

vascular system. Diltiazem, like verapamil, is a nondihydropyridine CCB, with intermediate dilatory effects on peripheral and myocardial vasculature.

Pharmacokinetics

Pharmacokinetic parameters vary significantly depending on the class of CCB in question as well as the dosage form used. Refer to full product labeling for specific pharmacokinetic information.

Treatment Advantages and Disadvantages

While CCBs have been used in the U.S. for decades, their use and place in therapy is still a topic of debate. Short-acting dihydropyridines (such as nifedipine) have been associated with increased morbidity and mortality in some patient groups. The Established Populations for Epidemiologic Studies of the Elder (EPESE) and the Multicenter Isradipine Diuretic Atherosclerosis Study (MIDAS) both reported decreased survival and increased angina and cardiovascular events in patients treated with dihydropyridine CCBs. Additionally, studies such as the Appropriate Blood Pressure Control (ABC) study and the Fosinopril vs. Amlodipine Cardiovascular Events Randomized Trial (FACET) both demonstrated a reduction in cardiovascular events in those treated with ACE inhibitors versus those treated with CCBs.

As a group, CCBs have not demonstrated any deleterious effects on glucose control or lipid concentrations, with verapamil reported as demonstrating improvements in glucose tolerance. Some studies indicate reductions in left ventricular hypertrophy and decreased risk of myocardial infarction (MI) in patients treated with ACE inhibitor and CCB combination therapy. In regard to monotherapy, treatment with amlodipine is considered somewhat less effective than treatment with ACE inhibitors or ARBs in slowing the progression of renal disease in patients with diabetic nephropathy or hypertensive renal disease.

Therapeutic Considerations

Warnings/Precautions

CCB therapy is contraindicated in patients with a history or susceptibility to hypotension. Precautions associated with CCB use include patients with bradycardia, heart failure, cardiogenic shock, aortic stenosis, and renal or hepatic disease. Nondihydropyridine CCBs are specifically contraindicated in patients with cardiac conduction abnormalities such as sick sinus syndrome and Wolff-Parkinson-White Syndrome. CCBs can also exacerbate the symptoms of gastroesophageal reflux disease (GERD) due to relaxation of smooth muscle within the lower esophageal sphincter. See the chart at the end of this chapter, or refer to the full prescribing information for additional drug-specific precautions and warnings.

Special Populations

Elderly patients are particularly susceptible to the hypotensive effects of CCBs. Women who are pregnant or breastfeeding should be assessed by an appropriate health care provider prior to CCB use. African-American patients tend to respond better to CCB and diuretic therapy compared to β-blockers, ACE inhibitors, or ARBs.

Adverse Effects and Monitoring

Common side effects associated with CCB therapy include dizziness, peripheral edema (particularly with dihydropyridines), flushing, and headache. Dihydropyridine CCBs are associated with reflex tachycardia; however, the incidence of reflex tachycardia with amlodipine is minimal due to its gradual onset of action. Nifedipine is associated with causing gingival hyperplasia in some patients, thus proper oral hygiene is critical in patients using this agent. Nondihydropyridines are associated with the development of serious cardiac conduction abnormalities and arrhythmias. Caution is recommended with diltiazem and verapamil in patients with a history of arrhythmia. Other serious side effects associated with CCB therapy include hypotension, visual disturbances, and serious skin reactions including Stevens-Johnson syndrome.

Drug Interactions
Drug interactions involving CCBs are numerous. Patients being considered for CCB therapy should have a thorough evaluation of their drug regimen for possible drug interactions prior to CCB initiation. Diltiazem and verapamil are associated with more of a risk for drug interactions than are dihydropyridine CCBs, as diltiazem and verapamil are potent inhibitors of the CYP3A4 enzyme. See **Table 13.3** for more information.

Dosage and Administration
Dosage and administration guidelines vary depending on specific agent used. See **Table 13.2**, or refer to the full prescribing information regarding specific dosing and administration information. Dosage reductions may be required in patients with renal or hepatic dysfunction depending on the agent used.

α-**Adrenergic Antagonists**
α-adrenergic antagonists inhibit α-postsympathetic adrenergic receptors, leading to vasodilation and reduction in blood pressure. The antihypertensive effects of these agents at clinically utilized doses are similar to reductions observed with medications from other classes. Long-term trials in patients with diabetes to evaluate reductions in microvascular and cardiovascular risk have not been conducted. α-**adrenergic antagonists can be used in patients with diabetes with resistant hypertension as add-on therapy when patients are nonresponsive to other therapies with proven renal benefits.**

Pharmacology
Mechanism of Action
α-blockers competitively inhibit α-1 adrenergic receptors in the sympathetic nervous system. Use of these agents results in peripheral vasodilation and associated decreases in peripheral vascular resistance and blood pressure.

Pharmacokinetics
Pharmacokinetic parameters will vary depending on the agent used. Refer to full product labeling for specific pharmacokinetic information.

Treatment Advantages and Disadvantages
While long-term trials in patients with diabetes to evaluate reductions in microvascular and cardiovascular risk have not been conducted, α-antagonists have been associated with improved insulin sensitivity in patients with significant insulin resistance. Additionally, slight benefits have been observed in reductions of LDL cholesterol in small clinical trials, and doxazosin is additionally thought to have favorable effects on triglycerides, total cholesterol, and HDL concentrations. The Antihypertensive and Lipid-Lowering Treatment to Prevent Heart Attack Trial (ALLHAT) study had an arm comparing doxazosin (an α-antagonist) with a β-blocker, a calcium channel blocker, and an ACE inhibitor versus a diuretic. This portion of the trial was terminated due to an observed increase in cardiovascular events in patients receiving the α-blocker. These findings, as well as the risk for orthostatic hypotension and other adverse events, raise some concern regarding the use of these agents in the diabetic population. Of note in patients with diabetes, α-antagonists do not tend to worsen insulin resistance and exert mild to negligible effects on sexual dysfunction.

Therapeutic Considerations

Warnings/Precautions

Upon initiation of therapy, patients starting α-antagonists should be monitored closely for postural hypotension. Doxazosin should be used with caution in patients with hepatic disease because this drug is primarily metabolized by the liver.

Special Populations

Doxazosin is considered a pregnancy category B agent, and it is unknown if doxazosin concentrates in breast milk. Elderly patients are more susceptible to the hypotensive effects of α-antagonists, thus careful monitoring and slow titration is warranted in this population if α-blocker therapy is deemed necessary.

Adverse Effects and Monitoring

α-antagonists have a strong association with orthostatic hypotension, particularly upon initiation of therapy. Common side effects can include dizziness, weight gain, somnolence, peripheral edema, blurred vision, and dyspnea. Rare but serious cardiac adverse effects have been reported including angina, palpitations, and sinus tachycardia. Sinus bradycardia has also been reported.

Drug Interactions

The major concern with drug interactions with α-antagonists involves additive hypotensive effects when given with other agents. Other agents that may potentiate the hypotensive effects of α-antagonists include diuretics, monoamine oxidase inhibitors, and alcohol. Coadministration of α-antagonists with phosphodiestarase-5 (PDE-5) inhibitors, such as sildenafil, can result in symptomatic postural hypotension. Sildenafil doses above 25 mg should not be administered within four hours of α-blocker administration. See **Table 13.3** for more information.

Dosage and Administration

Dosage and administration guidelines vary depending on specific agent used. See **Table 13.2**, or refer to the full prescribing for specific dosing and administration information.

Clonidine

Clonidine is a centrally acting α-2 receptor agonist used in the management of hypertension. Clonidine is effective in lowering blood pressure by decreasing sympathetic outflow from the central nervous system. Clonidine and other centrally acting agents, however, have not been studied in detail in regard to their effects on the progression and development of microvascular complications or cardiovascular disease. **Clonidine can be used in patients with diabetes with resistant hypertension as add-on therapy when patients are nonresponsive to other therapies with proven renal benefits. However, patients must be selected carefully due to the risk of hypotension and falls with clonidine use.**

Pharmacology

Mechanism of Action

Clonidine is a central acting α-noradrenergic agonist. Stimulation of α-noradrenergic receptors in the central nervous system inhibits sympathetic outflow and tone. Suppression of sympathetic pathways decreases vascular tone in the heart, kidneys, and peripheral vasculature. The net effects of clonidine therapy are decreased peripheral vascular resistance and a reduction in blood pressure.

Pharmacokinetics

Clonidine is rapidly absorbed following oral administration with bioavailability nearing 100%. Clonidine is highly lipid soluble and readily distributes into the central nervous system, with a CSF elimination half-life of ~1.3 hours and a serum half-life of ~12 hours. Clonidine undergoes hepatic metabolism with ~50% of a given dose processed by the liver to inactive metabolites, and is ~45% renally excreted. Transdermal clonidine preparations release the drug at a constant rate for seven days, with a therapeutic plasma concentration reached within two to three days of patch therapy.

Treatment Advantages and Disadvantages

While the administration of clonidine can be very convenient for patients who utilize the transdermal patch, clonidine use is associated with a variety of side effects that limit the utility of its use. A major disadvantage of clonidine therapy is orthostatic hypotension, which is of particular concern in diabetic patients with cardiovascular autonomic neuropathy. Additionally, clonidine has not been formally evaluated in terms of microvascular and cardiovascular risk reduction in people with diabetes.

Therapeutic Considerations

Warnings/Precautions

Abrupt discontinuation of clonidine is not recommended due to the risk of severe rebound hypertension. Clonidine is also associated with sedation and drowsiness, so patients should be cautioned when performing potentially dangerous activities such as driving or operating machinery. For patients with a history of major depressive disorder, clonidine should be used cautiously due to the potential of this agent to induce depressive episodes. While clonidine has been used successfully in patients with diabetes, transient increases in blood sugar have been noted with clonidine use. Clonidine should be used cautiously in patients with renal or hepatic dysfunction.

Special Populations

Clonidine is an FDA pregnancy class C agent, and should be avoided in pregnant women. Clonidine should also be avoided in breastfeeding women as clonidine concentrations reach levels in breast milk approximately twice that achieved in maternal plasma. Elderly patients should be treated with caution because they are more likely to have decreased renal function and are more susceptible to the hypotensive and sedative effects of clonidine. If used in an elderly patient, clonidine should be initiated at a low dose and titrated slowly to desired therapeutic effect.

Adverse Effects and Monitoring

Clonidine is associated with a variety of anticholinergic side effects, and the most frequently reported side effects associated with clonidine use include dry mouth, drowsiness, dizziness, sedation, and constipation. Transdermal clonidine may decrease the severity of systemic anticholinergic side effects when compared to the oral formulation. Symptoms of fatigue and lethargy can be particularly bothersome in elderly patients, and symptomatic hypotension can occur, which is a huge concern in the elderly population. Oral clonidine therapy can result in sodium and fluid retention during the first few days of therapy, but is typically responsive to diuretic therapy. It can also cause adverse cardiovascular events including palpitations, sinus tachycardia, and sinus bradycardia. Of particular concern in patients with diabetes, clonidine use can result in transient increases in blood glucose as well as symptoms of sexual dysfunction, including impotence, decreased libido, and ejaculatory dysfunction.

Drug Interactions

Prior to initiation of clonidine, patients should receive a thorough drug interaction screen to avoid harmful drug interactions with this medication. Clonidine can potentiate the effects of concomitant CNS depressants, and can lead to symptomatic hypotension when coadministered with other antihypertensive agents. Clonidine should also be used cautiously with other medications that slow the heart rate such as amiodarone, β-blockers, and cardiac glycosides. This drug interaction overview is certainly not comprehensive, as clonidine interacts with a variety of medications. See **Table 13.3**, or refer to the full prescribing information for additional drug interaction information.

Dosage and Administration
For oral administration, clonidine is typically initiated at 0.1 mg twice daily and increased by 0.1-0.2 mg/day to desired effect. Transdermal clonidine is administered once weekly, with dose titrations recommended every one to two weeks. As with oral clonidine, transdermal clonidine is initiated with a 0.1 mg/24 hours patch. See **Table 13.2**, or refer to the full prescribing information for more guidance.

Other Centrally Acting Drugs
Similar to clonidine, other centrally acting agents used for the treatment of hypertension to lower blood pressure by decreasing sympathetic outflow from the central nervous system. Other centrally acting antihypertensive medications include methyldopa, reserpine, and guanfacine. **While not used as commonly as other antihypertensive medications, centrally acting agents are still used from time to time in patients with resistant hypertension, and can be used in patients with diabetes**

when deemed appropriate. Centrally acting agents have not been studied in terms of microvascular and cardiovascular risk reduction in patients with diabetes. Common side effects of these medications include drowsiness, impotence, and dry mouth. Less commonly, these agents can exacerbate depression, and methyldopa use is rarely associated with Coombs-positive anemia.

Combination Therapies
Management of hypertension in patients with type 2 diabetes is generally more complicated than the treatment of hypertension in people without diabetes. Because of the difficulty associated with the treatment of hypertension in this population, treatment likely requires the use of multiple medications to meet treatment goals. Fortunately, a variety of drug combinations are available to health care practitioners for use. Combinations include ACE inhibitors with CCBs, ACE inhibitors with diuretics, β-blockers with diuretics, ARBs with diuretics, centrally acting antihypertensives with diuretics, and diuretic combinations. Use of combination products can help with patient adherence and ease pill burden in patients on multidrug regimens. Some combination products are available in generic form, making them affordable for patients on fixed incomes with limited or no insurance coverage. For additional information, see **Tables 13.2** and **13.3**, or refer to the drug's specific product information.

SUGGESTED READING

Arauz-Pacheco C, Parrott MA, Raskin P. The treatment of hypertension in adult patients with diabetes. *Diabetes Care*. 2002;25(1):134-147.

Epstein M, Sowers JR. Diabetes mellitus and hypertension. *Hypertension*. 1992;19:403-418.

Hypertension Management in Adults with Diabetes. *Diabetes Care*. 2004;27 (Suppl.1):S65-67.

Joint National Committee on Prevention, Detection, Evaluation, and Treatment of High Blood Pressure: Seventh Report of the Joint National Committee on Prevention, Detection, Evaluation and Treatment of High Blood Pressure. *Hypertension*. 2003;42:1206-1252.

Sowers JR, Epstein M, Frohlich ED. Diabetes, hypertension, and cardiovascular disease: an update. *Hypertension*. 2001;37:1053-1059.

Vijan S, Hayward RA. Treatment of hypertension in type 2 diabetes mellitus: blood pressure goals, choice of agents, and setting priorities in diabetes care. *Ann Intern Med*. 2003;138:593-602.

Table 13.2. Prescribing Information for Antihypertensive Agents

GENERIC (BRAND)	FORM/ STRENGTH	DOSAGE	WARNINGS/PRECAUTIONS & CONTRAINDICATIONS	ADVERSE REACTIONS
ALPHA ANTAGONISTS				
Doxazosin mesylate (Cardura)	**Tab:** 1mg*, 2mg*, 4mg*, 8mg* *scored	***Adults:* HTN:** Initial: 1mg qd (am or pm). Monitor BP 2-6 hrs and 24 hrs after 1st dose. Titrate: Increase to 2mg qd then upwards as needed. Max: 16mg/day. **BPH:** Initial: 1mg qd (am or pm). Titrate: May double the dose every 1-2 weeks. Max: 8mg/day.	**W/P:** Monitor for orthostatic hypotension and syncope with 1st dose and dose increase. Caution with hepatic dysfunction. Rule out prostate cancer. Priapism (rare), leukopenia/neutropenia reported. **P/N:** Category C, caution with nursing.	Fatigue/malaise, hypotension, edema, dizziness, dyspnea, weight gain.
Prazosin HCl (Minipress)	**Cap:** 1mg, 2mg, 5mg	***Adults:*** Initial: 1mg bid-tid. Maint: 6-15mg/day in divided doses. Max: 40mg/day. **Concomitant Diuretic/ Antihypertensive:** Reduce to 1-2mg tid, then retitrate.	**W/P:** Syncope may occur, usually after initial dose or dose increase. Excessive postural hypotensive effects. Avoid driving for 24 hrs after 1st dose or dose increase. Always start on 1mg cap. False (+) for pheochromocytoma. **P/N:** Category C, caution in nursing.	Dizziness, headache, drowsiness, lack of energy, weakness, palpitations, nausea.
Terazosin HCl (Hytrin)	**Cap:** 1mg, 2mg, 5mg, 10mg	***Adults:* HTN:** Initial: 1mg hs, then slowly increase dose. Usual: 1-5mg/day. Max: 20mg/day. If response is substantially diminished at 24 hrs, may increase dose or give in 2 divided doses. **BPH:** Initial: 1mg qhs. Titrate: Increase stepwise as needed. Usual: 10mg/day. May increase to 20mg/day after 4-6 weeks. Max: 20mg/day. If discontinue for several days, restart at initial dose.	**W/P:** Monitor for orthostatic hypotension and syncope initially and with dose increase. Rule out prostate cancer. Priapism (rare) reported. Possibility of hemodilution. **P/N:** Category C, caution with nursing.	Asthenia, postural hypotension, headache, dizziness, dyspnea, nasal congestion/rhinitis, somnolence, impotence, blurred vision, palpitations, nausea, peripheral edema, priapism, thrombocytopenia, atrial fibrillation.
ALPHA ANTAGONIST COMBINATION				
Prazosin HCl/ Polythiazide (Minizide)	**Cap:** (Polythiazide-Prazosin) 0.5mg-1mg, 0.5mg-2mg, 0.5mg-5mg	***Adults:*** 1 cap bid-tid. Determine strength by individual component titration.	**BB:** Not for initial therapy of HTN. **W/P:** Syncope may occur, usually after initial dose or dose increase. Excessive postural hypotensive effects. Avoid driving for 24 hrs after 1st dose or dose increase. Always start on 1mg prazosin. Caution with severe renal disease, hepatic dysfunction, or progressive liver disease. Sensitivity reactions may occur with history of allergy or bronchial asthma. May exacerbate or activate SLE. Hyperuricemia, hypokalemia or frank gout may occur. Monitor electrolytes. May manifest latent DM. Enhanced effects in the post-sympathectomy patient. May decrease serum protein-bound iodine levels. False (+) for pheochromocytoma. **Contra:** Anuria, thiazide or sulfonamide sensitivity. **P/N:** Category C, not for use in nursing.	Dizziness, headache, drowsiness, lack of energy, weakness, palpitations, nausea, blood dyscrasias, rash.
ALPHA- AND BETA-BLOCKERS				
Carvedilol (Coreg, Coreg CR)	**Tab:** 3.125mg, 6.25mg, 12.5mg, 25mg; **Cap, Extended-Release:** 10mg, 20mg, 40mg, 80mg	***Adults:*** Individualize dose. Take with food. Monitor dose increases. Take extended-release capsules in am and swallow whole. **CHF: Tab:** Initial: 3.125mg bid for 2 weeks. Titrate: May double dose every 2 weeks as tolerated. Max: 50mg bid if >85kg. Reduce dose if HR <55 beats/min. **Cap, Extended-Release:** Initial: 10mg qd for 2 weeks. Titrate: May double dose every 2 weeks as tolerated. Max: 80mg/day. Reduce dose if HR <55 beats/min. **HTN: Tab:** Initial: 6.25mg bid for 7-14 days. Titrate: May double dose at 7-14 day intervals. Max: 50mg/day. **Cap, Extended-Release:** Initial: 20mg qd for 7-14 days. Titrate: May double dose every 7-14 days as tolerated. Max: 80mg/day. **LVD Post-MI: Tab:** Initial: 6.25mg bid for 3-10 days. Titrate: May double dose every	**W/P:** Avoid abrupt discontinuation; taper over 1-2 weeks. Hepatic injury reported; d/c and do not restart if develop hepatic injury. Hypotension and syncope reported, most commonly during up-titration period; avoid driving or hazardous tasks during initiation period. May mask hypoglycemia and hyperthyroidism. May potentiate insulin-induced hypoglycemia and delay recovery of serum glucose levels. Decrease dose if pulse <55 beats/min. Monitor renal function during uptitration with low BP (SBP <100mmHg), ischemic heart disease, diffuse vascular disease and/or renal insufficiency. Worsening heart failure or fluid retention may occur with uptitration. Caution in pheochromocytoma, peripheral vascular disease, major surgery with anesthesia, Prinzmetal's variant angina,	Bradycardia, fatigue, edema, hypotension, dizziness, headache, diarrhea, nausea, vomiting, hyperglycemia, weight increase, dyspnea, anemia, increased cough, arthralgia.

BB = black box warning; **W/P** = warnings/precautions; **Contra** = contraindications; **P/N** = pregnancy category rating and nursing considerations.

Table 13.2. Prescribing Information for Antihypertensive Agents

GENERIC (BRAND)	FORM/ STRENGTH	DOSAGE	WARNINGS/PRECAUTIONS & CONTRAINDICATIONS	ADVERSE REACTIONS
ALPHA- AND BETA-BLOCKERS *(Cont.)*				
Carvedilol (Coreg, Coreg CR) *(Cont.)*		3-10 days to target of 25mg bid. May begin with 3.125mg bid and slow up-titration rate if clinically indicated. **Cap, Extended-Release:** Initial: 20mg qd for 3-10 days. Titrate: May double dose every 3-10 days to target of 80mg qd.	and bronchospastic disease. Effectiveness of carvedilol in patients younger than 18 years of age has not been established. **Contra:** Bronchial asthma or related bronchospastic conditions, 2nd- or 3rd-degree AV block, sick sinus syndrome, severe bradycardia (without permanent pacemaker), cardiogenic shock, decompensated heart failure requiring IV inotropic therapy, severe hepatic impairment. **P/N:** Category C, not for use in nursing.	
Labetalol HCl (Trandate)	**Tab:** 100mg*, 200mg*, 300mg* *scored	**Adults:** PO: Initial: 100mg bid. Titrate: May increase by 100mg bid every 2-3 days. Maint: 200-400mg bid. **Severe HTN:** 1200-2400mg/day given bid-tid. Titrate: Do not increase by more than 200mg bid. **Elderly:** Initial: 100mg bid. Titrate: May increase by 100mg bid. Maint: 100-200mg bid.	**W/P:** Caution with hepatic dysfunction. Avoid abrupt withdrawal; may exacerbate ischemic heart disease. Caution with latent cardiac insufficiency, may exacerbate cardiac failure, reduce sinus HR, and slow AV conduction. Avoid in overt CHF. Avoid with bronchospastic disease. Paradoxical HTN in pheochromocytoma reported. D/C prior to surgery. Caution with DM; may mask symptoms of hypoglycemia. **Contra:** Bronchial asthma, overt cardiac failure, greater than first degree heart block, cardiogenic shock, severe bradycardia, other conditions associated with hypotension, history of obstructive airway disease. **P/N:** Category C, caution in nursing.	Dizziness, fatigue, nausea, vomiting, dyspepsia, paresthesia, nasal stuffiness, ejaculation failure, impotence, edema, dyspnea, headache, vertigo, postural hypotension, increased sweating.
ANGIOTENSIN CONVERTING ENZYME (ACE) INHIBITORS				
Benazepril HCl (Lotensin)	**Tab:** 5mg, 10mg, 20mg, 40mg	**Adults:** If possible, d/c diuretic 2-3 days prior to initiation of therapy. Initial: 10mg qd or 5mg with concomitant diuretic. Maint: 20-40mg/day given qd-bid. Resume diuretic if BP not controlled. Max: 80mg/day. **CrCl <30mL/min/1.73m²:** Initial: 5mg qd. Max: 40mg/day. **Pediatrics:** ≥6 yrs: Initial: 0.2mg/kg qd. Max: 0.6mg/kg.	**BB:** When used in pregnancy, ACE inhibitors can cause injury and even death to the developing fetus during 2nd and 3rd trimesters. D/C therapy when pregnancy detected. **W/P:** D/C if angioedema, jaundice, or if marked LFT elevation occurs. Risk of hyperkalemia with DM, renal dysfunction. Persistent nonproductive cough reported. Monitor WBCs in renal and collagen vascular disease. Anaphylactoid reactions reported. Fetal/neonatal morbidity and death reported. Monitor for hypotension in high risk patients (eg, surgery/anesthesia, prolonged diuretic therapy, heart failure, volume and/or salt depletion, etc). Caution with CHF, renal dysfunction, and renal artery stenosis. Less effective on BP in blacks and more reports of angioedema than nonblacks. **Contra:** History of ACE inhibitor-associated angioedema. **P/N:** Category D, not for use in nursing.	Cough, dizziness, headache, fatigue, somnolence, postural dizziness, nausea.
Captopril (Capoten)	**Tab:** 12.5mg*, 25mg*, 50mg*, 100mg* *scored	**Adults:** Take 1 hour before meals. **HTN:** If possible, d/c recent antihypertensive drug for 1 week prior to therapy. Initial: 25mg bid-tid. Titrate: May increase to 50mg bid-tid after 1-2 weeks. Usual: 25-150mg bid-tid. Max: 450mg/day. **CHF:** Initial: 25mg tid; or 6.25-12.5mg tid with risk of hypotension or salt/volume depletion. Usual: 50-100mg tid. Max: 450mg/day. **Left Ventricular Dysfunction Post-MI:** Initial: 6.25mg single dose, then 12.5mg tid. Titrate: Increase to 25mg tid over next several days, then to 50mg tid over next several weeks. Usual: 50mg tid. **Diabetic Nephropathy:** 25mg tid. **Significant Renal Dysfunction:** Decrease initial dose and titrate slowly.	**BB:** ACE inhibitors can cause death/injury to developing fetus during 2nd and 3rd trimesters. Stop therapy if pregnancy detected. **W/P:** D/C if jaundice or marked LFT elevation occurs. Risk of hyperkalemia with DM, renal dysfunction. Persistent nonproductive cough, anaphylactoid reactions, neutropenia with myeloid hypoplasia reported. Fetal/neonatal morbidity and death reported. Monitor for hypotension in high-risk patients (surgery/ anesthesia, dialysis, heart failure, volume/ salt depletion, etc). Caution with CHF, renal dysfunction, renal artery stenosis, collagen vascular disease (especially with renal dysfunction). Monitor WBC before therapy, then every 2 weeks for 3 months, then periodically. Less effective on BP in blacks	Proteinuria, rash, hypotension, dysgeusia, cough, MI, CHF.

BB = black box warning; **W/P** = warnings/precautions; **Contra** = contraindications; **P/N** = pregnancy category rating and nursing considerations.

Table 13.2. Prescribing Information for Antihypertensive Agents

GENERIC (BRAND)	FORM/ STRENGTH	DOSAGE	WARNINGS/PRECAUTIONS & CONTRAINDICATIONS	ADVERSE REACTIONS
Captopril (Capoten) *(Cont.)*			and more reports of angioedema than nonblacks. **Contra:** History of ACE inhibitor associated angioedema. **P/N:** Category C (1st trimester) and D (2nd and 3rd trimesters), not for use in nursing.	
Enalapril maleate (Vasotec)	**Tab:** 2.5mg*, 5mg*, 10mg, 20mg *scored	***Adults:* HTN:** If possible, d/c diuretic 2-3 days prior to therapy. Initial: 5mg qd, 2.5mg qd with concomitant diuretic. Usual: 10-40mg/day given qd or bid. Resume diuretic if BP not controlled. **CrCl ≤30mL/min:** Initial: 2.5mg/day. **Dialysis:** 2.5mg/day on dialysis days. **Heart Failure:** Initial: 2.5mg/day. Usual: 2.5-20mg given bid. Max: 40mg/day. **Left Ventricular Dysfunction:** Initial: 2.5mg bid. Titrate: Increase to 20mg/ day. **Hyponatremia or SrCr 1.6mg/dL with Heart Failure:** Initial: 2.5mg qd. Titrate: Increase to 2.5mg bid, then 5mg bid. Max: 40mg/day. ***Pediatrics:* HTN: 1 month-16 yrs:** Initial: 0.08mg/kg (up to 5mg) qd. Titrate: Adjust according to response. Max: 0.58mg/kg/dose (or 40mg/dose). Avoid if GFR <30mL/min/ 1.73m2. (To prepare 200mL of 1mg/mL sus: Add 50mL of Bicitra®; to polyethylene terephthalate bottle with ten 20mg tabs and shake for at least 2 min. Let stand for 60 min, then shake again for 1 min. Add 150mL of Ora-Sweet SF™; and shake, then refrigerate. Can store up to 30 days.)	**BB:** ACE inhibitors can cause death/injury to developing fetus during 2nd and 3rd trimesters. Stop therapy if pregnancy detected. **W/P:** D/C if angioedema, jaundice, or if marked LFT elevation occurs. Risk of hyperkalemia with DM, renal dysfunction. Persistent nonproductive cough reported. Monitor WBCs in renal or collagen vascular disease. Anaphylactoid reactions reported. Fetal/neonatal morbidity and death reported. Monitor for hypotension in high-risk patients (heart failure, surgery/ anesthesia, hyponatremia, high-dose diuretic therapy, severe volume and/or salt depletion, etc). Caution with CHF, obstruction to left ventricle outflow tract, renal dysfunction, and renal artery stenosis. Less effective on BP in blacks and more reports of angioedema than nonblacks. Intestinal angioedema reported. **Contra:** History of ACE inhibitor associated angioedema and hereditary or idiopathic angioedema. **P/N:** Category C (1st trimester) and D (2nd and 3rd trimesters), not for use in nursing.	Fatigue, orthostatic effects, asthenia, diarrhea, nausea, headache, dizziness, cough, rash, hypotension, vomiting.
Enalaprilat (Vasotec I.V.)	**Inj:** 1.25mg/mL	***Adults:*** Administer IV over 5 min. Usual: 1.25mg q6h for no longer than 48 hrs. Max: 20mg/day. **Concomitant Diuretic/ CrCl ≤30mL/min:** Initial: 0.625mg, may repeat after 1 hr. Maint: 1.25mg q6h. **Risk of Excessive Hypotension:** Initial: 0.625mg over 5 min to 1 hr. **PO/IV Conversion:** Give 5mg/day PO for 1.25mg IV q6h and 2.5mg/day PO for 0.625mg q6h IV.	**BB:** ACE inhibitors can cause death/injury to developing fetus during 2nd and 3rd trimesters. Stop therapy if pregnancy detected. **W/P:** D/C if angioedema, jaundice, or if marked LFT elevation occurs. Risk of hyperkalemia with DM, renal dysfunction. Persistent nonproductive cough reported. Monitor WBCs in renal or collagen vascular disease. Anaphylactoid reactions reported. Fetal/neonatal morbidity and death reported. Monitor for hypotension in high risk patients (heart failure, surgery/ anesthesia, hyponatremia, high dose diuretic therapy, severe volume and/or salt depletion, etc). Caution with CHF, obstruction to left ventricle outflow tract, renal dysfunction, and renal artery stenosis. Less effective on BP in blacks and more reports of angioedema than nonblacks. **Contra:** History of ACE inhibitor associated angioedema and hereditary or idiopathic angioedema. **P/N:** Category C (1st trimester) and D (2nd and 3rd trimesters), not for use in nursing.	Hypotension, headache, angioedema, myocardial infarction, fatigue, dizziness, fever, rash, constipation, cough.
Fosinopril sodium (Monopril)	**Tab:** 10mg*, 20mg, 40mg *scored	***Adults:*** If possible, d/c diuretic 2-3 days before therapy. Initial: 10mg qd, monitor carefully if cannot d/c diuretic. Maint: 20-40mg/day. Resume diuretic if BP not controlled. Max: 80mg/day. **Heart Failure:** Initial: 10mg qd, 5mg with moderate to severe renal failure or vigorous diuresis. Titrate: Increase over several weeks. Maint: 20-40mg qd. Max: 40mg qd. **Elderly:** Start at low end of dosing range.	**BB:** ACE inhibitors can cause death/injury to developing fetus during 2nd and 3rd trimesters. Stop therapy if pregnancy detected. **W/P:** D/C if angioedema, jaundice, or if marked LFT elevation occur. Risk of hyperkalemia with DM, renal dysfunction. Persistent non-productive cough reported. Monitor WBCs in renal and collagen vascular disease. Anaphylactoid reactions reported. Fetal/neonatal morbidity and death reported. Monitor for hypotension in high-risk patients (heart failure, volume and/or salt depletion, surgery/anesthesia, etc). Less effective on BP in blacks and	Dizziness, cough, hypotension, musculoskeletal pain.

BB = black box warning; **W/P** = warnings/precautions; **Contra** = contraindications; **P/N** = pregnancy category rating and nursing considerations.

Table 13.2. Prescribing Information for Antihypertensive Agents

GENERIC (BRAND)	FORM/ STRENGTH	DOSAGE	WARNINGS/PRECAUTIONS & CONTRAINDICATIONS	ADVERSE REACTIONS
ANGIOTENSIN CONVERTING ENZYME (ACE) INHIBITORS *(cont.)*				
Fosinopril sodium (Monopril) *(Cont.)*			more reports of angioedema than nonblacks. Caution with CHF, renal or hepatic dysfunction, renal artery stenosis. May cause false low measurement of serum digoxin level. **Contra:** History of ACE inhibitor associated angioedema. **P/N:** Category C (1st trimester) and D (2nd and 3rd trimesters), not for use in nursing.	
Lisinopril (Prinivil)	**Tab:** 5mg*, 10mg*, 20mg* *scored	*Adults:* **HTN:** If possible, d/c diuretic 2-3 days prior to therapy. Initial: 10mg qd; 5mg qd with diuretic. Usual: 20-40mg qd. Resume diuretic if BP not controlled. Max: 80mg/day. **CrCl 10-30mL/min:** Initial: 5mg/day. Max: 40mg/day. **CrCl <10mL/min:** Initial: 2.5mg/day. Max: 40mg/day. **Heart Failure:** Initial: 5mg qd. Usual: 5-20mg qd. **Hyponatremia or CrCl ≤30mL/min:** Initial: 2.5mg qd. **AMI:** Initial: 5mg within 24 hrs, then 5mg after 24 hrs, then 10mg after 48 hrs, then daily. Use 2.5mg during first 3 days with low systolic BP. Maint: 10mg qd for 6 weeks, 2.5-5mg with hypotension. D/C with prolonged hypotension. **Elderly:** Caution with dose adjustment. *Pediatrics:* **≥6 yrs: HTN:** Initial: 0.07mg/kg qd (up to 5mg total). Adjust dose based on BP response. Max: 0.61mg/kg qd (40mg/day).	**BB:** ACE inhibitors can cause death/injury to developing fetus during 2nd and 3rd trimesters. Stop therapy if pregnancy detected. **W/P:** Intestinal/head/neck occurs. angioedema reported. D/C if angioedema, jaundice, or if marked LFT elevation Risk of hyperkalemia with DM, renal dysfunction. Persistent nonproductive cough reported. Monitor WBCs in renal and collagen vascular disease. Anaphylactoid reactions reported. Fetal/neonatal morbidity and death reported. Monitor for hypotension in high-risk patients (eg, heart failure with systolic BP <100mmHg, surgery/anesthesia, hyponatremia, high dose diuretic therapy, severe volume and/or salt depletion). Caution with renal artery stenosis, CHF, renal dysfunction, or if obstruction to left ventricle outflow tract. Less effective on BP in blacks and more reports of angioedema than nonblacks. Caution in hypoglycemia and leukopenia/neutropenia. Patients should report any indication of infection which may be sign of leukopenia/neutropenia. **Contra:** History of ACE inhibitor-associated angioedema and hereditary or idiopathic angioedema. **P/N:** Category C (1st trimester) and D (2nd and 3rd trimesters), not for use in nursing.	Hypotension, diarrhea, headache, dizziness, cough, chest pain.
Lisinopril (Zestril)	**Tab:** 2.5mg, 5mg, 10mg, 20mg, 30mg, 40mg	*Adults:* **HTN:** If possible, d/c diuretic 2-3 days prior to therapy. Initial: 10mg qd, 5mg qd with diuretic. Usual: 20-40mg qd. Resume diuretic if BP not controlled. Max: 80mg/day. **CrCl 10-30mL/min:** Initial: 5mg/day. Max: 40mg/day. CrCl <10mL/min: Initial: 2.5mg/day. Max: 40mg/day. **Heart Failure:** Initial: 5mg qd. Usual: 5-40mg qd. May increase by 10mg every 2 weeks. Max: 40mg/day. **Hyponatremia or CrCl ≤30mL/min:** Initial: 2.5mg qd. **AMI:** Initial: 5mg within 24 hrs, then 5mg after 24 hrs, then 10mg after 48 hrs, then 10mg qd. Use 2.5mg during first 3 days with low SBP. Maint: 10mg qd for 6 weeks, 2.5-5mg with hypotension. D/C with prolonged hypotension. **Elderly:** Caution with dose adjustment. *Pediatrics:* **≥6 yrs: HTN:** Initial: 0.07mg/kg qd up to 5mg total. Dose adjust according to response. Max: 0.61mg/kg or 40mg.	**BB:** ACE inhibitors can cause death/injury to developing fetus during 2nd and 3rd trimesters. D/C if pregnancy is detected. **W/P:** D/C if angioedema, jaundice, or marked LFT elevation occur. Risk of hyperkalemia, hypoglycemia with DM, renal dysfunction. Persistent nonproductive cough reported. Monitor WBCs in renal and collagen vascular disease. Anaphylactoid reactions during membrane exposure reported. Fetal/neonatal morbidity and death reported. Monitor for hypotension in high-risk patients (heart failure with SBP <100mmHg, surgery/anesthesia, hyponatremia, high-dose diuretic therapy, severe volume and/or salt depletion, etc). Caution with CHF, aortic stenosis/ hypertrophic cardiomyopathy, renal dysfunction, and renal artery stenosis. Less effective on BP in blacks and more reports of angioedema than nonblacks. **Contra:** History of ACE inhibitor-associated angioedema, hereditary or idiopathic angioedema. **P/N:** Category C (1st trimester) and D (2nd and 3rd trimesters), not for use in nursing.	Hypotension, diarrhea, headache, dizziness, hyperkalemia, chest pain, cough, cutaneous pseudolymphoma.

BB = black box warning; **W/P** = warnings/precautions; **Contra** = contraindications; **P/N** = pregnancy category rating and nursing considerations.

Table 13.2. Prescribing Information for Antihypertensive Agents

GENERIC (BRAND)	FORM/ STRENGTH	DOSAGE	WARNINGS/PRECAUTIONS & CONTRAINDICATIONS	ADVERSE REACTIONS
Moexipril HCl (Univasc)	**Tab:** 7.5mg*, 15mg* *scored	**Adults:** If possible, d/c diuretic 2-3 days prior to therapy. Take 1 hr before meals. Initial: 7.5mg qd, 3.75mg with concomitant diuretic therapy. Maint: 7.5-30mg/day given qd-bid. Resume diuretic if BP not controlled. Max: 60mg/day. **CrCl ≤40mL/min:** Initial: 3.75mg qd. Max: 15mg/day.	**BB:** ACE inhibitors can cause death/injury to developing fetus during 2nd and 3rd trimesters. Stop therapy if pregnancy detected. **W/P:** D/C if angioedema, jaundice, or if marked LFT elevation occurs. Intestinal angioedema reported. Risk of hyperkalemia with DM, renal dysfunction. Persistent nonproductive cough reported. Monitor WBCs in renal and collagen vascular disease. Anaphylactoid reactions reported. Fetal/ neonatal morbidity and death reported. Monitor for hypotension in high risk patients (heart failure, surgery/anesthesia, prolonged diuretic therapy, volume and/or salt depletion, etc.). Caution with CHF, renal dysfunction, and renal artery stenosis. Less effective on BP in blacks and more reports of angioedema than nonblacks. **Contra:** History of ACE inhibitor-associated angioedema. **P/N:** Category C (1st trimester) and D (2nd and 3rd trimesters), not for use in nursing.	Cough, dizziness, diarrhea, flu syndrome, fatigue, pharyngitis, flushing, rash, myalgia.
Perindopril erbumine (Aceon)	**Tab:** 2mg*, 4mg*, 8mg* *scored	**Adults: HTN:** If possible, d/c diuretic 2-3 days prior to therapy. Initial: 4mg qd; 2-4mg/day given qd-bid with concomitant diuretic. Maint: 4-8mg/day given qd-bid. Resume diuretic if BP not controlled. Max: 16mg/day. **Elderly (>65 yrs):** Initial: 4mg/ day given qd-bid. Max (usual): 8mg/ day. **Renal Impairment: CrCl >30mL/min:** Initial: 2mg/day. Max: 8mg/day. **CAD:** Initial: 4mg qd for 2 weeks. Maint: 8mg qd. **Elderly (>70 yrs):** Initial: 2mg qd for 1 week. Titrate: 4mg qd for Week 2. Maint: 8mg qd.	**BB:** ACE inhibitors can cause death/injury to developing fetus during 2nd and 3rd trimesters. Stop therapy if pregnancy detected. **W/P:** D/C if angioedema, jaundice, or if marked LFT elevation occurs. Risk of hyperkalemia with DM, renal dysfunction. Persistent nonproductive cough reported. Monitor WBCs in renal and collagen vascular disease. Anaphylactoid reactions reported. Fetal/neonatal morbidity and death reported. Monitor for hypotension in high-risk patients (heart failure, surgery/ anesthesia, hyponatremia, prolonged diuretic therapy, or volume and/or salt depletion). Caution with CHF, renal dysfunction, and renal artery stenosis. Less effective on BP in blacks and more reports of angioedema than nonblacks. Avoid if CrCl <30mL/min. **Contra:** History of ACE inhibitor-associated angioedema. **P/N:** Category C (1st trimester) and D (2nd and 3rd trimesters), caution in nursing.	Cough, headache, asthenia, dizziness, diarrhea, edema, respiratory infection, lower extremity pain.
Quinapril HCl (Accupril)	**Tab:** 5mg*, 10mg, 20mg, 40mg *scored	**Adults: HTN:** If possible, d/c diuretic 2-3 days prior to therapy. Initial: 10-20mg qd; 5mg qd with concomitant diuretic. Titrate at intervals of at least 2 weeks. Usual: 20-80mg/day given qd-bid. **CrCl >60mL/min:** Initial: 10mg/day. **CrCl 30-60mL/min:** Initial: 5mg/day. **CrCl 10-30mL/min:** Initial: 2.5mg/day. **Heart Failure:** Initial: 5mg bid. Titrate at weekly intervals. Usual: 10-20mg bid. **CrCl >30mL/min:** Initial: 5mg/day. **CrCl 10-30mL/min:** Initial: 2.5mg/day.	**BB:** ACE inhibitors can cause death/injury to developing fetus during 2nd and 3rd trimesters. Stop therapy if pregnancy detected. **W/P:** D/C if angioedema, jaundice, or if marked LFT elevation occurs. Risk of hyperkalemia with DM, renal dysfunction. Persistent nonproductive cough reported. Monitor WBCs in renal or collagen vascular disease. Anaphylactoid reactions reported. Fetal/neonatal morbidity and death reported. Monitor for hypotension in high risk patients (heart failure, surgery/anesthesia, hyponatremia, high-dose diuretic therapy, recent intensive diuresis, dialysis, or severe volume and/or salt depletion, etc). Caution with CHF, renal dysfunction, and renal artery stenosis. Less effective on BP in blacks and more reports of angioedema than nonblacks. **Contra:** History of ACE inhibitor-associated angioedema. **P/N:** Category C (1st trimester) and D (2nd and 3rd trimesters), not for use in nursing.	Fatigue, headache, dizziness, cough, nausea, vomiting, hypotension, chest pain.

BB = black box warning; **W/P** = warnings/precautions; **Contra** = contraindications; **P/N** = pregnancy category rating and nursing considerations.

Table 13.2. Prescribing Information for Antihypertensive Agents

GENERIC (BRAND)	FORM/ STRENGTH	DOSAGE	WARNINGS/PRECAUTIONS & CONTRAINDICATIONS	ADVERSE REACTIONS
ANGIOTENSIN CONVERTING ENZYME (ACE) INHIBITORS *(Cont.)*				
Ramipril (Altace)	**Cap:** 1.25mg, 2.5mg, 5mg, 10mg	***Adults:* HTN:** Initial: 2.5mg qd. Maint: 2.5-20mg/day given qd or bid. Add diuretic if BP not controlled. **CrCl <40mL/ min:** Initial: 1.25mg qd. Titrate/Max: 5mg/ day. **CHF Post-MI:** Initial: 2.5mg bid, 1.25mg bid if hypotensive. Titrate: Increase to 5mg bid. **CrCl <40mL/min:** Initial: 1.25mg qd. Titrate: May increase to 1.25mg bid. Max: 2.5mg bid. **Risk Reduction of MI, Stroke, Death (≥55 yrs):** Initial: 2.5mg qd for 1 week. Increase to 5mg qd for next 3 weeks. Maint: 10mg qd. Reduce or d/c diuretic if possible. **With Volume Depletion/Renal Artery Stenosis:** Initial: 1.25mg qd.	**BB:** ACE inhibitors can cause death/injury to developing fetus during 2nd and 3rd trimesters. Stop therapy if pregnancy detected. **W/P:** D/C if angioedema, jaundice, or if marked LFT elevation occurs. Risk of hyperkalemia with DM, renal dysfunction. Persistent nonproductive cough and anaphylactoid reactions reported. Monitor WBCs in renal and collagen vascular disease. Fetal/neonatal morbidity and death reported. Monitor for hypotension in high-risk patients (heart failure, surgery/anesthesia, hyponatremia, high dose diuretic therapy, recent intensive diuresis, dialysis, or severe volume and/or salt depletion, etc). Caution with CHF, renal dysfunction, severe liver cirrhosis and/or ascites, and renal artery stenosis. Less effective on BP in blacks and more reports of angioedema than nonblacks. May reduce RBCs, Hgb, WBCs or platelets. May cause agranulocytosis, pancytopenia, and bone marrow depression. **Contra:** History of ACE inhibitor-associated angioedema. **P/N:** Category C (1st trimester) and D (2nd and 3rd trimesters), not for use in nursing.	Hypotension, cough, dizziness, fatigue, angina, impotence, Stevens-Johnson syndrome.
Trandolapril (Mavik)	**Tab:** 1mg*, 2mg, 4mg *scored	***Adults:* HTN:** If possible, d/c diuretic 2-3 days before therapy. Initial: 1mg qd in nonblack patients; 2mg qd in black patients; 0.5mg with concomitant diuretic. Titrate: Adjust at 1-week intervals. Usual: 2-4mg qd. Resume diuretic if not controlled. Max: 8mg/day. **Post-MI:** Initial: 1mg qd. Titrate: Increase to target dose of 4mg qd as tolerated. **CrCl <30mL/min/Hepatic Cirrhosis for HTN or Post-MI:** Initial: 0.5mg qd.	**BB:** ACE inhibitors can cause death/injury to developing fetus during 2nd and 3rd trimesters. Stop therapy if pregnancy detected. **W/P:** D/C if angioedema or jaundice occurs. Risk of hyperkalemia with DM, renal dysfunction. Persistent nonproductive cough reported. Monitor WBCs in renal impairment and/or collagen vascular disease. Anaphylactoid reactions reported. Fetal/neonatal morbidity and death reported. Monitor for hypotension in high-risk patients (heart failure, surgery/anesthesia, prolonged diuretic therapy, volume and/or salt depletion, etc). Caution with CHF, renal dysfunction, and renal artery stenosis. More reports of angioedema in blacks than nonblacks. **Contra:** History of ACE inhibitor-associated angioedema. **P/N:** Category C (1st trimester) and D (2nd and 3rd trimesters), not for use in nursing.	Cough, dizziness, hypotension, elevated serum uric acid, elevated BUN, elevated creatinine, asthenia, syncope, myalgia, gastritis, hypocalcemia, hyperkalemia, dyspepsia.
ACE INHIBITOR COMBINATIONS				
Benazepril HCl/ Hydrochloro- thiazide (Lotensin HCT)	**Tab:** (Benazepril-HCTZ) 5mg-6.25mg*, 10mg-12.5mg*, 20mg-12.5mg*, 20mg-25mg* *scored	***Adults:*** Initial (if not controlled on benazepril monotherapy): 10mg-12.5mg or 20mg-12.5mg. Titrate: May increase after 2-3 weeks. **Initial (if controlled on 25mg HCTZ/day with hypokalemia):** 5mg-6.25mg. **Replacement Therapy:** Substitute combination for titrated components.	**BB:** When used in pregnancy, ACE inhibitors can cause injury and even death to the developing fetus. D/C therapy when pregnancy detected. **W/P:** Avoid if CrCl ≤30mL/min/1.73m². D/C if angioedema, jaundice, or marked LFT elevation occur. Risk of hyperkalemia with DM, renal dysfunction. May cause persistent nonproductive cough, hypokalemia, hyperuricemia, hypomagnesemia, hypercalcemia, hypophosphatemia. Monitor WBCs in renal and collagen vascular disease. Anaphylactoid reactions reported. Fetal/ neonatal morbidity and death reported. Monitor for hypotension in high risk patients (eg, surgery/anesthesia, prolonged diuretic therapy, heart failure, volume and/or salt depletion, etc). Caution with	Cough, dizziness/postural dizziness, headache, fatigue.

BB = black box warning; **W/P** = warnings/precautions; **Contra** = contraindications; **P/N** = pregnancy category rating and nursing considerations.

Table 13.2. Prescribing Information for Antihypertensive Agents

GENERIC (BRAND)	FORM/ STRENGTH	DOSAGE	WARNINGS/PRECAUTIONS & CONTRAINDICATIONS	ADVERSE REACTIONS
Benazepril HCl/ Hydrochlorothiazide (Lotensin HCT) *(Cont.)*			CHF, renal dysfunction, and renal artery stenosis. More reports of angioedema in blacks than nonblacks. Monitor for fluid/ electrolyte imbalance. May increase cholesterol and TG levels. May exacerbate/ activate SLE. **Contra:** Anuria, sulfonamide hypersensitivity. **P/N:** Category D, not for use in nursing.	
Captopril/ Hydrochlorothiazide (Capozide)	**Tab:** (Captopril-HCTZ) 25mg-15mg*, 25mg-25mg*, 50mg-15mg*, 50mg-25mg* *scored	***Adults:*** Initial: 25mg-15mg tab qd. Titrate: Adjust dose at 6-week intervals. Max: 150mg captopril/50mg HCTZ per day. **Replacement Therapy:** Substitute combination for titrated components. **Renal Impairment:** Decrease dose or increase interval. Take 1 hr before meals.	**BB:** ACE inhibitors can cause death/injury to developing fetus during 2nd and 3rd trimesters. Stop therapy if pregnancy detected. **W/P:** D/C if angioedema, jaundice, or if marked LFT elevation occurs. Risk of hyperkalemia with DM, renal dysfunction. Monitor WBCs in renal and collagen vascular disease. Fetal/neonatal morbidity and death reported. Monitor for hypotension in high-risk patients (eg, surgery/anesthesia, volume/salt depletion). Caution with renal or hepatic dysfunction. More reports of angioedema in blacks than nonblacks. May exacerbate or activate systemic lupus erythematosus. Monitor electrolytes. Hypercalcemia, hypomagnesemia, hyperuricemia may occur. With renal impairment, monitor WBCs and differential before therapy, every 2 weeks for 3 months, then periodically. Neutropenia with myeloid hypoplasia, persistent nonproductive cough, anaphylactoid reactions, proteinuria reported. **Contra:** History of ACE inhibitor-associated angioedema, anuria, sulfonamide hypersensitivity. **P/N:** Category C (1st trimester) and D (2nd and 3rd trimesters), not for use in nursing.	Cough, hypotension, rash, pruritus, fever, arthralgia, eosinophilia, dysgeusia, neutropenia/thrombocytopenia.
Enalapril maleate/ Hydrochlorothiazide (Vaseretic)	**Tab:** (Enalapril-HCTZ) 5mg-12.5mg, 10mg-25mg	***Adults:*** Initial (if not controlled with enalapril/HCTZ monotherapy): 5mg-12.5mg tab or 10mg-25mg tab qd. Titrate: May increase after 2-3 weeks. Max: 20mg enalapril/50mg HCTZ per day. **Replacement Therapy:** Substitute combination for titrated components.	**BB:** ACE inhibitors can cause death/injury to developing fetus during 2nd and 3rd trimesters. Stop therapy if pregnancy detected. **W/P:** D/C if angioedema, jaundice, or if marked LFT elevation occurs. Risk of hyperkalemia with DM, renal dysfunction. Persistent nonproductive cough reported. Monitor WBCs in renal and collagen vascular disease. Anaphylactoid reactions reported. Fetal/ neonatal morbidity and death reported. Monitor for hypotension in high-risk patients (surgery/anesthesia, hyponatremia, severe volume/salt depletion, etc). Caution with CHF, renal or hepatic dysfunction, obstruction to left ventricle outflow tract, elderly, renal artery stenosis. More reports of angioedema in blacks than nonblacks. May exacerbate or activate SLE. Monitor serum electrolytes. Avoid if CrCl ≤30mL/ min/1.73m^2. May increase cholesterol, TG, uric acid levels, and blood glucose. Intestinal angioedema reported. **Contra:** History of ACE inhibitor-associated angioedema and hereditary or idiopathic angioedema. Anuria, sulfonamide hypersensitivity. **P/N:** Category C (1st trimester) and D (2nd and 3rd trimesters), not for use in nursing.	Dizziness, cough, fatigue, orthostatic effects, diarrhea, nausea, muscle cramps, asthenia, impotence.

BB = black box warning; **W/P** = warnings/precautions; **Contra** = contraindications; **P/N** = pregnancy category rating and nursing considerations.

Table 13.2. Prescribing Information for Antihypertensive Agents

GENERIC (BRAND)	FORM/ STRENGTH	DOSAGE	WARNINGS/PRECAUTIONS & CONTRAINDICATIONS	ADVERSE REACTIONS
ACE INHIBITOR COMBINATIONS *(Cont.)*				
Fosinopril sodium/ Hydrochlorothiazide (Monopril HCT)	Tab: (Fosinopril-HCTZ) 10mg-12.5mg, 20mg-12.5mg	***Adults:* Initial (if not controlled with fosinopril/HCTZ monotherapy):** 12.5mg-10mg tab or 12.5mg-20mg tab qd.	**BB:** ACE inhibitors can cause death/injury to developing fetus during 2nd and 3rd trimesters. Stop therapy if pregnancy detected. **W/P:** D/C if angioedema, jaundice, or marked LFT elevation occurs. Risk of hyperkalemia with DM, renal dysfunction. Persistent nonproductive cough reported. Monitor WBCs in renal and collagen vascular disease. Anaphylactoid reactions reported. Fetal/neonatal morbidity and death reported. Monitor for hypotension in high-risk patients (eg, surgery/anesthesia, volume/salt depletion). Caution with CHF, renal or hepatic dysfunction. More reports of angioedema in blacks than nonblacks. May exacerbate or activate SLE. Monitor electrolytes. Avoid if CrCl ≤30mL/min/1.73m². May increase cholesterol, TG. Hypercalcemia, hypomagnesemia, hyperuricemia may occur. **Contra:** Anuria, sulfonamide hypersensitivity. **P/N:** Category C (1st trimester) and D (2nd and 3rd trimesters), not for use in nursing.	Headache, cough, fatigue, dizziness, upper respiratory infection, musculoskeletal pain.
Lisinopril/ Hydrochlorothiazide (Prinzide, Zestoretic)	Tab: (Lisinopril-HCTZ) 10mg-12.5mg, 20mg-12.5mg, 20mg-25mg	***Adults:* Initial (If Not Controlled with Lisinopril/HCTZ monotherapy):** 10mg-12.5mg tab or 20mg-12.5mg tab daily. Titrate: May increase after 2-3 weeks. **Initial (If Controlled on 25mg HCTZ/Day with Hypokalemia):** 10mg-12.5mg tab. Replacement Therapy: Substitute combination for titrated components.	**BB:** ACE inhibitors can cause death/injury to developing fetus during 2nd and 3rd trimesters. Stop therapy if pregnancy detected. **W/P:** D/C if angioedema, jaundice, or marked LFT elevation occur. Risk of hyperkalemia with DM, renal dysfunction. Persistent nonproductive cough reported. Monitor WBCs in renal and collagen vascular disease. Anaphylactoid reactions during membrane exposure reported. Fetal/neonatal morbidity and death reported. Monitor for hypotension in high-risk patients (eg, surgery/anesthesia, volume/salt depletion). Caution with CHF, renal or hepatic dysfunction. More reports of angioedema in blacks than nonblacks. May exacerbate or activate SLE. Monitor electrolytes. Avoid if CrCl ≤30mL/min/1.7m². May increase cholesterol, TG. Hypercalcemia, hypomagnesemia, hyperuricemia may occur. Caution with left ventricle outflow obstruction. **Contra:** History of ACE inhibitor-associated angioedema, hereditary or idiopathic angioedema, anuria, sulfonamide hypersensitivity. **P/N:** Category C (1st trimester) and D (2nd and 3rd trimesters), not for use in nursing.	Dizziness, headache, cough, fatigue, orthostatic effects, diarrhea, nausea, muscle cramps, angioedema, cutaneous pseudolymphoma.
Moexipril HCl/ Hydrochlorothiazide (Uniretic)	Tab: (Moexipril-HCTZ) 7.5mg-12.5mg*, 15mg-12.5mg*, 15mg-25mg* *scored	***Adults:* Initial (if not controlled on moexipril/HCTZ monotherapy):** Switch to 7.5mg-12.5mg tab, 15mg-12.5mg tab, or 15mg-25mg tab qd. Titrate: May increase after 2-3 weeks. **Initial (if controlled on 25mg HCTZ/day with hypokalemia):** 3.75mg-6.25mg (1/2 of 7.5mg-12.5mg tab). If excessive reduction with 7.5mg-12.5mg tab, may switch to 3.75mg-6.25mg. **Replacement Therapy:** Substitute combination for titrated components. Take 1 hr before meals.	**BB:** ACE inhibitors can cause death/injury to developing fetus during 2nd and 3rd trimesters. Stop therapy if pregnancy detected. **W/P:** D/C if angioedema, jaundice, or if marked LFT elevation occurs. Intestinal angioedema reported. Risk of hyperkalemia with DM, renal dysfunction. Persistent nonproductive cough reported. Monitor WBCs in renal and collagen vascular disease. Anaphylactoid reactions reported. Fetal/ neonatal morbidity and death reported. Monitor for hypotension in high-risk patients (eg, surgery/anesthesia, volume/ salt depletion). Caution in elderly, CHF, renal or hepatic dysfunction. More reports of angioedema in blacks than nonblacks. May exacerbate or activate SLE. Monitor	Cough, dizziness, fatigue.

BB = black box warning; **W/P** = warnings/precautions; **Contra** = contraindications; **P/N** = pregnancy category rating and nursing considerations.

Table 13.2. Prescribing Information for Antihypertensive Agents

GENERIC (BRAND)	FORM/ STRENGTH	DOSAGE	WARNINGS/PRECAUTIONS & CONTRAINDICATIONS	ADVERSE REACTIONS
Moexipril HCl/ Hydrochloro- thiazide (Uniretic) (Cont.)			electrolytes. Avoid if CrCl ≤40mL/min/ 1.73m². May increase cholesterol, TG. Hypercalcemia, hypomagnesemia, hyperuricemia may occur. **Contra:** History of ACE inhibitor-associated angioedema, anuria, sulfonamide hypersensitivity. **P/N:** Category C (1st trimester) and D (2nd and 3rd trimesters), not for use in nursing.	
Quinapril HCl/ Hydrochloro- thiazide (Accuretic)	**Tab:** (Quinapril-HCTZ) 10mg-12.5mg*, 20mg-12.5mg*, 20mg-25mg* *scored	**Adults: Initial (if not controlled on quinapril monotherapy):** 10mg-12.5mg or 20mg-12.5mg tab qd. Titrate: May increase after 2-3 weeks. **Initial (if controlled on HCTZ 25mg/day but significant K+ loss):** 10mg-12.5mg or 20mg-12.5mg tab qd. If previously treated with 20mg quinapril and 25mg HCTZ, may switch to 20mg-25mg tab qd.	**BB:** ACE inhibitors can cause death/injury to developing fetus during 2nd and 3rd trimesters. Stop therapy if pregnancy detected. **W/P:** D/C if angioedema, jaundice, or marked LFT elevation occurs. Risk of hyperkalemia with DM, renal dysfunction. Persistent nonproductive cough reported. Monitor WBCs in renal or collagen vascular disease. Anaphylactoid reactions reported. Fetal/neonatal morbidity and death reported. Monitor for hypotension in high-risk patients (heart failure, surgery/anesthesia, hyponatremia, severe volume/salt depletion, etc). Caution with CHF, renal or hepatic dysfunction, and renal artery stenosis. Less effective on BP in blacks and more reports of angioedema than nonblacks. May exacerbate or activate SLE. Monitor serum electrolytes. Avoid if CrCl ≤30mL/min/ 1.73m². May increase cholesterol, TG, and uric acid levels and decrease glucose tolerance. **Contra:** History of ACE inhibitor-associated angioedema, anuria, sulfonamide hypersensitivity. **P/N:** Category C (1st trimester) and D (2nd and 3rd trimesters), not for use in nursing.	Dizziness, headache, cough, myalgia.
ANGIOTENSIN RECEPTOR BLOCKERS (ARBs)				
Candesartan cilexetil (Atacand)	**Tab:** 4mg, 8mg, 16mg, 32mg	**Adults: HTN: Monotherapy Without Volume Depletion:** Initial: 16mg qd. Usual: 8-32mg/day given qd-bid. May add diuretic if BP not controlled. **Intravascular Volume Depletion/Moderate Hepatic Impairment:** Lower initial dose. Initial: 4mg qd. Usual: 32mg qd. Titrate: Double dose every 2 weeks, as tolerated.	**BB:** Can cause death/injury to developing fetus during 2nd and 3rd trimesters. Stop therapy if pregnancy is detected. **W/P:** Can cause fetal injury/death. Correct volume or salt depletion before therapy or monitor closely. Changes in renal function may occur; caution with renal artery stenosis, CHF. Risk of hypotension; caution in major surgery and anesthesia, or when initiating therapy in heart failure. May cause hyperkalemia in heart failure patients; monitor serum potassium. **P/N:** Category C (1st trimester) and D (2nd and 3rd trimesters), not for use in nursing.	Back pain, dizziness, upper respiratory infection.
Eprosartan mesylate (Teveten)	**Tab:** 400mg, 600mg	**Adults:** Initial: 600mg qd. Usual: 400-800mg/day, given qd-bid. **Moderate to Severe Renal Impairment:** Max: 600mg/day.	**BB:** Can cause death/injury to developing fetus during 2nd and 3rd trimesters. Stop therapy if pregnancy detected. **W/P:** Can cause fetal injury/death. Correct volume or salt depletion before therapy. Changes in renal function may occur; caution with renal artery stenosis, severe CHF. **P/N:** Category C (1st trimester) and D (2nd and 3rd trimesters), not for use in nursing.	Upper respiratory infection, rhinitis, pharyngitis, cough.
Irbesartan (Avapro)	**Tab:** 75mg, 150mg, 300mg	**Adults: HTN:** Initial: 150mg qd. Titrate: May increase to 300mg qd. **Intravascular Volume/Salt Depletion:** Initial: 75mg qd. **Nephropathy:** Maint: 300mg qd. **Pediatrics: HTN: ≥17 yrs:** Initial: 150mg qd. Titrate: May increase to 300mg qd. **Intravascular Volume/Salt Depletion:** Initial: 75mg qd.	**BB:** Can cause death/injury to developing fetus during 2nd and 3rd trimesters. Stop therapy if pregnancy detected. **W/P:** Can cause fetal injury/death. Correct volume or salt depletion before therapy. Changes in renal function may occur; caution with renal artery stenosis, severe CHF. Angioedema reported. **P/N:** Category C (1st trimester) and D (2nd and 3rd trimesters), not for use in nursing.	Diarrhea, dyspepsia/ heartburn, musculoskeletal trauma, fatigue, upper respiratory infection.

BB = black box warning; **W/P** = warnings/precautions; **Contra** = contraindications; **P/N** = pregnancy category rating and nursing considerations.

Table 13.2. Prescribing Information for Antihypertensive Agents

GENERIC (BRAND)	FORM/ STRENGTH	DOSAGE	WARNINGS/PRECAUTIONS & CONTRAINDICATIONS	ADVERSE REACTIONS
ANGIOTENSIN RECEPTOR BLOCKERS (ARBs) *(Cont.)*				
Losartan potassium (Cozaar)	**Tab:** 25mg, 50mg, 100mg	***Adults: HTN:*** Initial: 50mg qd. Usual: 25-100mg/day given qd-bid. **Intravascular Volume Depletion/Hepatic Impairment:** Initial: 25mg qd. **HTN with LVH:** Initial: 50mg qd. Add hydrochlorothiazide (HCTZ) 12.5mg qd and/or increase losartan to 100mg qd, followed by an increase in HCTZ to 25mg qd based on BP response. **Nephropathy:** Initial: 50 mg qd. Titrate: Increase to 100mg qd based on BP response. ***Pediatrics:*** **≥6 yrs: HTN:** Initial: 0.7mg/kg qd (up to 50mg/day). Max: 1.4mg/kg/day (100mg/day).	**BB:** Can cause death/injury to developing fetus during 2nd and 3rd trimesters. Stop therapy if pregnancy detected. **W/P:** Can cause fetal injury/death. Correct volume or salt depletion before therapy. Changes in renal function may occur; caution with renal artery stenosis, severe CHF. Angioedema reported. Consider dose adjustment with hepatic dysfunction. **P/N:** Category C (1st trimester) and D (2nd and 3rd trimesters), not for use in nursing.	Dizziness, cough, upper respiratory infection, diarrhea.
Olmesartan medoxomil (Benicar)	**Tab:** 5mg, 20mg, 40mg	***Adults:* Monotherapy Without Volume Depletion:** Initial: 20mg qd. Titrate: May increase to 40mg qd after 2 weeks if needed. May add diuretic if BP not controlled. **Intravascular Volume Depletion** (eg, with diuretics, impaired renal function): Lower initial dose; monitor closely.	**BB:** Can cause death/injury to developing fetus during 2nd and 3rd trimesters. Stop therapy if pregnancy detected. **W/P:** Can cause fetal injury/death. Symptomatic hypotension may occur in volume- and/or salt-depleted patients; monitor closely. Changes in renal function may occur; caution with severe CHF. Increases in serum creatinine or BUN reported with renal artery stenosis. **P/N:** Category C (1st trimester) and D (2nd and 3rd trimesters), not for use in nursing.	Dizziness, transient hypotension, hyperkalemia.
Telmisartan (Micardis)	**Tab:** 20mg, 40mg*, 80mg* *scored	***Adults:*** Initial: 40mg qd. Usual: 20-80mg/day. May add diuretic if need additional BP reduction after 80mg/day.	**BB:** Can cause death/injury to developing fetus during 2nd and 3rd trimesters. Stop therapy if pregnancy detected. **W/P:** Can cause fetal injury/death. Correct volume or salt depletion before therapy. Changes in renal function may occur; caution with renal artery stenosis, severe CHF. Closely monitor with biliary obstructive disorders or hepatic dysfunction. **P/N:** Category C (1st trimester) and D (2nd and 3rd trimesters), not for use in nursing.	Upper respiratory infection, back pain, sinusitis, diarrhea, bradycardia, eosinophilia, thrombocytopenia, increased uric acid, increased CPK, increased hepatic function/liver sweating, abnormal disorder, renal impairment failure, anemia, edema and cough.
Valsartan (Diovan)	**Tab:** 40mg*, 80mg, 160mg, 320mg *scored	***Adults: HTN:* Monotherapy Without Volume Depletion:** Initial: 80mg or 160mg qd. Titrate: May increase to 320mg qd or add diuretic (greater effect than increasing dose >80mg). **Hepatic/ Severe Renal Dysfunction:** Use with caution. **Heart Failure:** Initial: 40mg bid. Titrate: May increase to 80mg or 160mg bid (use highest dose tolerated). Max: 320mg/day in divided doses. **Post-MI:** Initial: 20mg bid. Titrate: May increase to 40mg bid within 7 days, with subsequent titrations up to 160mg bid. ***Pediatrics:*** **6-16 yrs: HTN:** Initial: 1.3mg/kg qd (up to 40mg total). Adjust dose according to BP response. Max: 2.7mg/kg (up to 160mg) qd. Use of a sus recommended for children who cannot swallow tabs, or children for whom calculated dosage (mg/kg) does not correspond to available tab strengths. Adjust dose accordingly when switching dosage forms. **Hepatic/ Severe Renal Impairment:** Use with caution. Avoid use in pediatrics with GFR <30mL/min/1.73m².	**BB:** When used in pregnancy, drugs that act directly on the renin-angiotensin system can cause injury and even death to the developing fetus. D/C therapy when pregnancy is detected. **W/P:** Changes in renal function may occur; caution with renal artery stenosis, severe CHF. Caution with hepatic dysfunction, renal dysfunction, and obstructive biliary disorder. Risk of hypotension; caution when initiating therapy in heart failure or post-MI. Correct volume or salt depletion before therapy. Avoid use in pediatric patients with GFR <30mL/min/1.73m². May cause fetal harm when administered to pregnant women. **P/N:** Category D, not for use in nursing.	(HTN) Headache, dizziness, viral infection, fatigue, abdominal pain. (Heart Failure) dizziness, hypotension, diarrhea, arthralgia, fatigue, back pain, hyperkalemia. (Post-MI) hypotension, cough, increased blood creatinine.

BB = black box warning; **W/P** = warnings/precautions; **P/N** = pregnancy category rating and nursing considerations.

Table 13.2. Prescribing Information for Antihypertensive Agents

GENERIC (BRAND)	FORM/ STRENGTH	DOSAGE	WARNINGS/PRECAUTIONS & CONTRAINDICATIONS	ADVERSE REACTIONS
ARBs COMBINATIONS				
Candesartan cilexetil/ Hydrochloro-thiazide (Atacand HCT)	**Tab:** (Candesartan-HCTZ) 16mg-12.5mg, 32mg-12.5mg	***Adults:*** Initial: If BP not controlled on HCTZ 25mg/day or controlled but serum K+ decreased: 16mg-12.5mg tab qd. If BP not controlled on 32mg candesartan/day, give 32mg-12.5mg qd; may increase to 32mg-25mg qd.	**BB:** Can cause death/injury to developing fetus during 2nd and 3rd trimesters. Stop therapy if pregnancy detected. **W/P:** Can cause fetal injury/death. Correct volume or salt depletion before therapy. Caution with hepatic or renal dysfunction, renal artery stenosis, severe CHF, history of allergies, and asthma. May exacerbate or activate SLE. Monitor serum electrolytes. Avoid if CrCl ≤30mL/min. Hyperuricemia, hyperglycemia, hypokalemia, hypomagnesemia, hypercalcemia may occur. Enhanced effects in post-sympathectomy patient. May increase cholesterol and triglyceride levels. Risk of hypotension; caution in major surgery or anesthesia. **Contra:** Anuria, sulfonamide hypersensitivity. **P/N:** Category C (1st trimester) and D (2nd and 3rd trimesters), not for use in nursing.	Upper respiratory infection, back pain, influenza-like symptoms, dizziness, headache.
Eprosartan mesylate/ Hydrochloro-thiazide (Teveten HCT)	**Tab:** (Eprosartan-HCTZ) 600mg-12.5mg, 600mg-25mg	***Adults:*** Usual (Not Volume Depleted): 600mg-12.5mg qd. Titrate: May increase to 600mg-25mg qd if needed. **Renal Impairment:** Max: 600mg/day (eprosartan).	**BB:** Can cause death/injury to developing fetus during 2nd and 3rd trimesters. Stop therapy if pregnancy detected. **W/P:** Hypersensitivity reactions reported. Fetal/neonatal morbidity and death reported. Monitor for hypotension in volume/salt depletion. Caution with CHF, renal or hepatic dysfunction. May exacerbate or activate SLE. Monitor electrolytes periodically. Hypercalcemia, hypomagnesemia, hyperuricemia, hyperglycemia may occur. Enhanced effects in post-sympathectomy patient. **Contra:** Anuria, sulfonamide hypersensitivity. **P/N:** Category C (1st trimester) and D (2nd and 3rd trimesters), not for use in nursing.	Dizziness, headache, back pain, fatigue, myalgia, upper respiratory tract infection, sinusitis, viral infection.
Irbesartan/ Hydrochloro-thiazide (Avalide)	**Tab:** (Irbesartan-HCTZ) 150mg-12.5mg, 300mg-12.5mg, 300mg-25mg	***Adults:*** **Not controlled on Monotherapy:** 150mg/12.5mg qd. Titrate: May increase to 300mg/12.5mg, then 300mg/25mg qd if needed. **Intial Therapy:** Initiate with 150mg/12.5mg qd for 1 to 2 weeks. Titrate: As needed to maximum 300mg/25mg qd. **Replacement Therapy:** May substitute for titrated components. **Elderly:** Start at low end of dosing range. Avoid with CrCl ≤30mL/min.	**BB:** Can cause death/injury to developing fetus during 2nd and 3rd trimesters. Stop therapy if pregnancy detected. **W/P:** Can cause fetal injury/death when administered to pregnant women. Correct volume or salt depletion before therapy. Caution with hepatic or renal dysfunction, renal artery stenosis, severe CHF, history of allergies, elderly, and asthma. May exacerbate or activate SLE. Monitor serum electrolytes. Avoid if CrCl ≤30mL/min. Hyperuricemia, hyperglycemia, hypokalemia, hypomagnes-emia, and hypercalcemia may occur. Enhanced effects in post-sympathectomy patient. May increase cholesterol and TG levels. Caution in elderly. **Contra:** Anuria, sulfonamide hypersensitivity. **P/N:** Category D, not for use in nursing.	Dizziness, fatigue, musculoskeletal pain, influenza, edema, nausea, vomiting, fever, chills, flushing, HTN, pruritus, sexual dysfunction, diarrhea, anxiety, vision disturbance, pancreatitis, aplastic anemia.
Losartan potassium/ Hydrochloro-thiazide (Hyzaar)	**Tab:** (Losartan-HCTZ) 50mg-12.5mg, 100mg-12.5mg, 100mg-25mg	***Adults:*** **HTN:** If BP uncontrolled on losartan monotherapy, HCTZ alone or controlled with HCTZ 25mg/day but hypokalemic: 50mg-12.5mg tab qd. Titrate/Max: If uncontrolled after 3 weeks, increase to 2 tabs of 50mg-12.5mg qd or 1 tab of 100mg-25mg qd. If uncontrolled on losartan 100mg monotherapy, may switch to 100mg-12.5mg qd. **Severe HTN:** Initial: 50mg-12.5mg qd. Titrate/Max: If inadequate response after 2-4 weeks, increase to 1 tab of 100mg-25mg qd.	**BB:** Can cause death/injury to developing fetus during 2nd and 3rd trimesters. D/C if pregnancy detected. **W/P:** Can cause fetal injury/death. Correct volume or salt depletion before therapy. Caution with hepatic or renal dysfunction, renal artery stenosis, severe CHF, history of allergies, asthma. May exacerbate or activate SLE. Monitor serum electrolytes. Avoid if CrCl ≤30mL/min. Observe for signs of fluid or electrolyte imbalance. May precipitate hyperuricemia or gout.	Dizziness, upper respiratory infection, back pain, cough.

BB = black box warning; **W/P** = warnings/precautions; **Contra** = contraindications; **P/N** = pregnancy category rating and nursing considerations.

Table 13.2. Prescribing Information for Antihypertensive Agents

GENERIC (BRAND)	FORM/ STRENGTH	DOSAGE	WARNINGS/PRECAUTIONS & CONTRAINDICATIONS	ADVERSE REACTIONS
ARBs COMBINATIONS *(Cont.)*				
Losartan potassium/ Hydrochloro-thiazide (Hyzaar) *(Cont.)*		**HTN With Left Ventricular Hypertrophy:** Initial: Losartan 50mg qd. If BP reduction inadequate, add HCTZ 12.5mg or substitute losartan/HCTZ 50-12.5. If additional BP reduction is needed, losartan 100mg and HCTZ 12.5mg or losartan/HCTZ 100-12.5 may be substituted, followed by losartan 100mg and HCTZ 25mg or losartan/HCTZ 100-25.	Enhanced effects in post-sympathectomy patient. May increase cholesterol, TG levels. Angioedema reported. Not recommended with hepatic dysfunction requiring losartan titration. **Contra:** Anuria, sulfonamide hypersensitivity. **P/N:** Category C (1st trimester) and D (2nd and 3rd trimesters), not for use in nursing.	
Olmesartan medoxomil/ Hydrochloro-thiazide (Benicar HCT)	**Tab:** (Olmesartan-HCTZ) 20mg-12.5mg, 40mg-12.5mg, 40mg-25mg	**Adults:** If BP not controlled with olmesartan alone: Add HCTZ 12.5mg qd. May titrate to 25mg qd if BP uncontrolled after 2-4 weeks. If BP not controlled with HCTZ alone: Add olmesartan 20mg qd. May titrate to 40mg qd if BP uncontrolled after 2-4 weeks. **Intravascular Volume Depletion** (eg, with diuretics, impaired renal function): Lower initial dose; monitor closely. **Elderly:** Start at lower end of dosing range.	**BB:** Can cause death/injury to developing fetus during 2nd and 3rd trimesters. Stop therapy if pregnancy detected. **W/P:** Can cause fetal injury/death. Correct volume or salt depletion before therapy or monitor closely. Caution with hepatic or severe renal dysfunction, progressive liver disease, history of allergies or asthma, renal artery stenosis, severe CHF. Avoid if CrCl ≤30mL/min. May exacerbate or activate SLE. Monitor serum electrolytes. Hyperuricemia, hyperglycemia, hypercalcemia, hypomagnesemia may occur. May increase cholesterol and triglyceride levels. **Contra:** Sulfonamide hypersensitivity. **P/N:** Category C (1st trimester) and D (2nd and 3rd trimesters), not for use in nursing.	Dizziness, upper respiratory tract infection, hyperuricemia, nausea, asthenia, angioedema, vomiting, hyperkalemia, rhabdomyolysis, ARF, alopecia, urticaria.
Telmisartan/ Hydrochloro-thiazide (Micardis HCT)	**Tab:** (HCTZ-Telmisartan) 12.5mg-40mg, 12.5mg-80mg, 25mg-80mg	**Adults:** If BP not controlled on 80mg telmisartan, or 25mg HCTZ/day, or controlled on 25mg HCTZ/day but serum K+ decreased, 80mg-12.5mg tab qd. Titrate/Max: If uncontrolled after 2-4 weeks, increase to 160mg-25mg. **Biliary Obstruction/Hepatic Dysfunction:** Initial: 40mg-12.5mg tab qd; monitor closely.	**BB:** Can cause death/injury to developing fetus during 2nd and 3rd trimesters. Stop therapy if pregnancy detected. **W/P:** Can cause fetal injury/death. Correct volume or salt depletion before therapy. Caution with hepatic or renal dysfunction, biliary obstructive disorders, renal artery stenosis, severe CHF, history of allergies, and asthma. May exacerbate or activate SLE. Monitor serum electrolytes. Avoid if CrCl ≤30mL/min. Hyperuricemia, hyperglycemia, hypokalemia, hypomagnesemia, hypercalcemia may occur. Enhanced effects in post-sympathectomy patient. May increase cholesterol and triglyceride levels. **Contra:** Anuria, sulfonamide hypersensitivity. **P/N:** Category C (1st trimester) and D (2nd and 3rd trimesters), not for use in nursing.	Dizziness, fatigue, sinusitis, upper respiratory infection, diarrhea, bradycardia, eosinophilia, thrombocytopenia, uric acid increased, abnormal hepatic function/liver disorder, renal impairment including acute renal failure, anemia, and increased CPK.
Valsartan/ Hydrochloro-thiazide (Diovan HCT)	**Tab:** (Valsartan-HCTZ) 80mg-12.5mg, 160mg-12.5mg, 160mg-25mg, 320mg-12.5mg, 320mg-25mg	**Adults:** Initial: **Uncontrolled on Valsartan Monotherapy:** Switch to 80mg-12.5mg, 160mg-12.5mg, or 320mg-12.5mg qd. May increase dose if uncontrolled after 3-4 weeks. Max: 320mg-25mg/day. **Uncontrolled on 25mg HCTZ/day or Controlled on 25mg HCTZ/day with Hypokalemia:** Switch to 80mg-12.5mg or 160mg-12.5mg qd. May titrate if uncontrolled after 3-4 weeks. Max: 320mg-25mg/day. **CrCl ≤30mL/min:** Use not recommended.	**BB:** When used in pregnancy, drugs that act directly on the renin-angiotensin system can cause injury and even death to the developing fetus. D/C therapy when pregnancy is detected. **W/P:** Correct volume or salt depletion before therapy. Caution with hepatic or renal dysfunction, biliary obstructive disorders, renal artery stenosis, severe CHF, history of allergies, and asthma. May exacerbate or activate SLE. Monitor serum electrolytes. Avoid if CrCl ≤30mL/min. Hyperuricemia, hyperglycemia, hypokalemia, hypomagnesemia, hypercalcemia may occur. Enhanced effects in post-sympathectomy patient. May increase cholesterol and triglyceride levels. May cause fetal and neonatal morbidity and death when given to pregnant women. **Contra:** Anuria, sulfonamide hypersensitivity. **P/N:** Category C (1st trimester) and D (2nd and 3rd trimesters), not for use in nursing.	Cough, headache, dizziness, fatigue, viral infection, pharyngitis, diarrhea.

BB = black box warning; **W/P** = warnings/precautions; **Contra** = contraindications; **P/N** = pregnancy category rating and nursing considerations.

Table 13.2. Prescribing Information for Antihypertensive Agents

GENERIC (BRAND)	FORM/ STRENGTH	DOSAGE	WARNINGS/PRECAUTIONS & CONTRAINDICATIONS	ADVERSE REACTIONS
BETA-BLOCKERS (Nonselective)				
Nadolol (Corgard)	**Tab:** 20mg*, 40mg*, 80mg*, 120mg*, 160mg* *scored	***Adults:* Angina Pectoris:** Initial: 40mg qd. Titrate: Increase by 40-80mg every 3-7 days. Usual: 40-80mg qd. Max: 240mg/day. **HTN:** Initial: 40mg qd. Titrate: Increase by 40-80mg. Max: 320mg/day. **CrCl 31-50mL/min:** Dose q24-36h. **CrCl 10-30mL/min:** Dose q24-48h. **CrCl <10mL/min:** Dose q40-60h.	**W/P:** Caution in well-compensated cardiac failure, nonallergic bronchospasm, renal dysfunction. Exacerbation of ischemic heart disease with abrupt withdrawal. Withdrawal before surgery is controversial. May mask hyperthyroidism or hypoglycemia symptoms. Can cause cardiac failure. **Contra:** Bronchial asthma, sinus bradycardia and >1st-degree conduction block, cardiogenic shock, overt cardiac failure. **P/N:** Category C, not for use in nursing.	Bradycardia, peripheral vascular insufficiency, dizziness, fatigue.
Penbutolol sulfate (Levatol)	**Tab:** 20mg* *scored	***Adults:*** 20mg qd.	**W/P:** Caution with well-compensated heart failure, elderly, nonallergic bronchospasm, renal impairment. Can cause cardiac failure. Avoid abrupt withdrawal. Withdrawal before surgery is controversial. May mask hypoglycemia or hyperthyroidism symptoms. **Contra:** Cardiogenic shock, sinus bradycardia, 2nd- and 3rd-degree AV block, bronchial asthma. **P/N:** Category C, caution in nursing.	Diarrhea, nausea, dyspepsia, dizziness, fatigue, headache, insomnia, cough.
Pindolol*	**Tab:** 5mg, 10mg	***Adults:*** Initial: 5mg bid. Titrate: May increase by 10mg/day after 3-4 weeks. Max: 60mg/day.	**W/P:** Caution with well-compensated heart failure, nonallergic bronchospasm, renal or hepatic impairment. Can cause cardiac failure. Avoid abrupt withdrawal. Withdrawal before surgery is controversial. May mask hypoglycemia or hyperthyroidism symptoms. **Contra:** Bronchial asthma, overt cardiac failure, cardiogenic shock, 2nd- and 3rd-degree heart block, severe bradycardia. **P/N:** Category B, not for use in nursing.	Dizziness, fatigue, insomnia, nervousness, dyspnea, edema, joint pain, muscle cramps/pain.
Propranolol HCl (Inderal)	**Inj:** 1mg/mL; **Tab:** 10mg*, 20mg*, 40mg*, 60mg*, 80mg* *scored	***Adults:* HTN: (Tab)** Initial: 40mg bid. Titrate: Increase gradually. Maint: 120-240mg/day. **Angina: (Tab)** 80-320mg/day, given bid-qid. **Arrhythmia: (Inj)** 1-3mg IV at 1 mg/min. **(Tab)** 10-30mg tid-qid ac and qhs. **MI: (Tab)** 180-240mg/day, given bid-tid. **Migraine: (Tab)** Initial: 80mg/day in divided doses. Usual: 160-240mg/day in divided doses. **Tremor: (Tab)** Initial: 40mg bid. Maint: 120mg/day. Max: 320mg/day. **Hypertrophic Subaortic Stenosis: (Tab)** 20-40mg tid-qid, ac and qhs. **Pheochromocytoma: (Tab)** 60mg/day in divided doses for 3 days before surgery with β-blocker. **Inoperable Tumor: (Tab)** 30mg/day in divided doses. ***Pediatrics:* HTN (Tab):** Initial: 1mg/kg/day PO. Usual: 1-2mg/kg bid. Max: 16mg/kg/day.	**W/P:** Caution with well-compensated cardiac failure, nonallergic bronchospasm, Wolff-Parkinson-White (WPW) syndrome, hepatic or renal dysfunction. Withdrawal before surgery is controversial. May mask hypoglycemia or hyperthyroidism symptoms. Avoid abrupt discontinuation. May reduce IOP. Can cause cardiac failure. Both digitalis glycosides and β-blockers slow atrioventricular conduction and decrease HR. Concomitant use can increase risk of bradycardia. **Contra:** Cardiogenic shock, sinus brady-cardia and >1st-degree block, bronchial asthma, CHF (unless failure is secondary to tachyarrhythmia treatable with propranolol). **P/N:** Category C, caution in nursing. Intrauterine growth retardation, small placenta, and congenital abnormalities have been reported in neonates whose mothers received propranolol during pregnancy. Neonates whose mothers received propranolol at parturition have exhibited bradycardia, hypoglycemia, and/or respiratory depression.	Bradycardia, CHF, hypotension, lightheaded ness, mental depression, nausea, vomiting, allergic reactions, agranulocytosis.
Propranolol HCl (Inderal LA)	**Cap, Extended-Release:** 60mg, 80mg, 120mg, 160mg	***Adults:* HTN:** Initial: 80mg qd. Maint: 120-160mg qd. **Angina:** Initial: 80mg qd. Titrate: Increase gradually every 3-7 days. Maint: 160mg qd. Max: 320mg/day. **Migraine:** Initial: 80mg qd. Maint: 160-240mg qd. Discontinue gradually if no response within 4-6 weeks. **Hypertrophic Subaortic Stenosis:** 80-160mg qd.	**W/P:** Caution with well-compensated cardiac failure, nonallergic bronchospasm, Wolff-Parkinson-White (WPW) syndrome, hepatic or renal dysfunction. Withdrawal before surgery is controversial. May mask hypoglycemia or hyperthyroidism symptoms. Avoid abrupt discontinuation. May reduce IOP. Can cause cardiac failure. Exacerbation of angina, in some cases	Bradycardia, CHF, hypotension, lightheadedness, mental depression, nausea, vomiting, allergic reactions, agranulocytosis, dry eyes, alopecia, SLE-like reactions, male impotence,

* Available only in generic form.
W/P = warnings/precautions; **Contra** = contraindications; **P/N** = pregnancy category rating and nursing considerations.

Table 13.2. Prescribing Information for Antihypertensive Agents

GENERIC (BRAND)	FORM/ STRENGTH	DOSAGE	WARNINGS/PRECAUTIONS & CONTRAINDICATIONS	ADVERSE REACTIONS
BETA-BLOCKERS (Nonselective) *(Cont.)*				
Propranolol HCl (Inderal LA) *(Cont.)*			myocardial reported. D/C if these occured. Stevens-Johnson Syndrome, toxic epidermal necrolysis, exfoliative dermatitis, erythema multiforme, and urticaria reported. Hypoglycemia and postural hypotension reported. **Contra:** Cardiogenic shock, sinus bradycardia and >1st-degree block, bronchial asthma, CHF (unless failure is secondary to tachyarrhythmia treatable with propranolol). **P/N:** Category C, caution in nursing.	Peyronie's disease.
Propranolol HCl (InnoPran XL)	Cap, **Extended-Release:** 80mg, 120mg	**Adults:** Initial: 80mg qhs (approximately 10 PM) consistently either on empty stomach or with food. Titrate: Based on response may titrate to dose of 120mg.	**W/P:** Caution with well-compensated cardiac failure, nonallergic bronchospasm (eg, chronic bronchitis, emphysema), Wolff-Parkinson-White syndrome, hepatic or renal dysfunction or with history of severe anaphylactic reactions. Withdrawal before surgery is controversial. May mask hypoglycemia or hyperthyroidism symptoms. Avoid abrupt discontinuation. May reduce IOP. Can cause cardiac failure. Caution in patients with impaired hepatic or renal function. Not for treatment of hypertensive emrgencies. **Contra:** Cardiogenic shock, sinus bradycardia and >1st-degree block, bronchial asthma. **P/N:** Category C; caution in nursing.	Fatigue, dizziness (except vertigo), constipation.
Timolol Maleate*	**Tab:** 5mg, 10mg*, 20mg* *scored	**Adults: HTN:** Initial: 10mg bid. Maint: 20-40mg/day. Wait at least 7 days between dose increases. Max: 60mg/day given bid. **MI:** 10mg bid. **Migraine:** Initial: 10mg bid. Maint: 20mg qd. Max: 30mg/day in divided doses. May decrease to 10mg qd. D/C if inadequate response after 6-8 weeks with max dose.	**W/P:** Caution with well-compensated cardiac failure, DM, mild to moderate COPD, bronchospastic disease, dialysis, hepatic/renal impairment, or cerebrovascular insufficiency. Exacerbation of ischemic heart disease with abrupt cessation. May mask hyperthyroidism or hypoglycemia symptoms. Withdrawal before surgery is controversial. May potentiate weakness with myasthenia gravis. Can cause cardiac failure. Caution and consider monitoring renal function in elderly. **Contra:** Active or history of bronchial asthma, severe COPD, sinus bradycardia, 2nd- and 3rd-degree AV block, overt cardiac failure, cardiogenic shock. **P/N:** Category C, not for use in nursing.	Fatigue, headache, nausea, arrhythmia, pruritus, dizziness, dyspnea, asthenia, bradycardia, dizziness.
BETA-BLOCKERS (Selective Beta1)				
Acebutolol HCl (Sectral)	**Cap:** 200mg, 400mg	**Adults: HTN:** Initial: 400mg/day, given qd-bid. Usual: 200-800mg/day. Max: 1200mg/day. **Ventricular Arrhythmia:** Initial: 200mg bid. Maint: Increase gradually to 600-1200mg/day. **Elderly:** Lower daily doses. Max: 800mg/day. **CrCl <50mL/min:** Decrease daily dose by 50%. **CrCl <25mL/min:** Decrease daily dose by 75%.	**W/P:** Withdrawal before surgery is controversial. Caution with bronchospastic disease, peripheral or mesenteric vascular disease, aortic or mitral valve disease, left ventricular dysfunction, heart failure controlled by digitalis and/or diuretics, hepatic or renal dysfunction. May mask hypoglycemia or hyperthyroidism symptoms. Avoid abrupt discontinuation. May develop antinuclear antibodies (ANA). **Contra:** Persistently severe bradycardia, 2nd- and 3rd-degree heart block, overt cardiac failure, cardiogenic shock. **P/N:** Category B, not for use in nursing.	Fatigue, dizziness, headache, constipation, diarrhea, dyspepsia, flatulence, nausea, dyspnea, urinary frequency, insomnia.
Atenolol (Tenormin)	**Tab:** 25mg, 50mg*, 100mg *scored	**Adults: HTN:** Initial: 50mg qd. Titrate: May increase after 1-2 weeks. Max: 100mg qd. **Angina:** Initial: 50mg qd. Titrate: May increase to 100mg after 1 week. Max: 200mg qd. **AMI:** Initial: 5mg IV over 5 min, repeat 10 min later. If tolerated, give 50mg PO 10 min after the last IV dose, followed by another 50mg PO	**BB:** Avoid abrupt discontinuation of therapy in coronary artery disease. Severe exacerbation of angina and occurrence of MI and ventricular arrhythmias reported in angina patients following abrupt discontinuation of therapy with β-blockers. **W/P:** Withdrawal before surgery is not recommended. Caution with bronchospastic	Bradycardia, hypotension, dizziness, fatigue, nausea, depression, dyspnea.

* Available only in generic form.
BB = black box warning; **W/P** = warnings/precautions; **Contra** = contraindications; **P/N** = pregnancy category rating and nursing considerations.

Table 13.2. Prescribing Information for Antihypertensive Agents

GENERIC (BRAND)	FORM/ STRENGTH	DOSAGE	WARNINGS/PRECAUTIONS & CONTRAINDICATIONS	ADVERSE REACTIONS
Atenolol (Tenormin) *(Cont.)*		12 hrs later. Maint: 100mg qd or 50mg bid for 6-9 days. **Renal Impairment/Elderly: HTN:** Initial: 25mg qd. **HTN/Angina/AMI:** Max: CrCl 15-35mL/min: 50mg/day. **CrCl <15mL/min:** 25mg/day. **Hemodialysis:** 25-50mg after each dialysis.	disease, conduction abnormalities, left ventricular dysfunction, heart failure controlled by digitalis and/or diuretics, renal or hepatic dysfunction. Can cause heart failure with prolonged use, hyperuricemia, hypercalcemia, hypokalemia, hypophosphatemia. May mask hypoglycemia or hyperthyroidism symptoms. Avoid abrupt discontinuation. Avoid with untreated pheochromocytoma. Possible fetal harm in pregnancy. May aggravate peripheral arterial circulatory disorders. May manifest latent DM. Monitor for fluid or electrolyte imbalance. May develop antinuclear antibodies (ANA). Neonates born to mothers receiving atenolol may be at risk of hypoglycemia and bradycardia. **Contra:** Sinus bradycardia, >1st-degree heart block, cardiogenic shock, overt cardiac failure. **P/N:** Category D, caution in nursing.	
Betaxolol HCl (Kerlone)	**Tab:** 10mg, 20mg	*Adults:* Initial: 10mg qd. Titrate: May increase to 20mg qd after 7-14 days. Max (usual): 20mg/day. **Severe Renal Impairment/Dialysis:** Initial: 5mg qd. Titrate: May increase by 5mg/day every 2 weeks. Max: 20mg/day. **Elderly:** Initial: 5mg qd.	**W/P:** Caution in CHF controlled by digitalis and diuretics, bronchospastic disease, renal or hepatic dysfunction. Can cause cardiac failure. Avoid abrupt withdrawal. Withdrawal before surgery is controversial. hyperthyroidism symptoms. May decrease IOP and interfere with glaucoma-screening test. Bradycardia may occur more often in elderly. May develop antinuclear antibodies (ANA). **Contra:** Sinus bradycardia, >1st degree heart block, cardiogenic shock, overt cardiac failure. **P/N:** Category C caution in nursing.	Bradycardia, fatigue, dyspnea, lethargy, impotence, dyspepsia, arthralgia, headache, dizziness, insomnia.
Bisoprolol fumarate (Zebeta)	**Tab:** 5mg*, 10mg *scored	*Adults:* Initial: 2.5-5mg qd. Max: 20mg/day. **Hepatic Dysfunction or CrCl <40mL/min:** Initial: 2.5mg qd; caution with dose titration.	**W/P:** Avoid abrupt withdrawal. May mask hypoglycemia or hyperthyroidism symptoms. Caution with compensated cardiac failure, DM, bronchospastic disease, hepatic/renal impairment, or peripheral vascular disease. May precipitate cardiac failure. Both digitalis glycosides and β-blockers slow atrioventricular conduction and decrease HR. Concomitant use can increase risk of bradycardia. **Contra:** Cardiogenic shock, overt cardiac failure, 2nd- or 3rd-degree AV block, marked sinus bradycardia. **P/N:** Category C, caution in nursing.	Diarrhea, upper respiratory infection, fatigue.
Metoprolol succinate (Toprol-XL)	**Tab, Extended-Release:** 25mg*, 50mg*, 100mg*, 200mg* *scored	*Adults:* **HTN:** Initial: 25-100mg qd. Titrate: May increase weekly. Max: 400mg/day. **Angina:** Initial: 100mg qd. Titrate: May increase weekly. Max: 400mg/day. **Heart Failure:** Initial: (NYHA Class II) 25mg qd for 2 weeks. **Severe Heart Failure:** 12.5mg qd for 2 weeks. Titrate: Double dose every 2 weeks as tolerated. Max: 200mg/day. *Pediatrics:* ≥6 yrs: **HTN:** 1mg/kg qd. Max: 50mg/day. Dose adjust according to BP response. Doses above 2mg/kg have not been studied.	**W/P:** Exacerbation of angina pectoris and MI reported following abrupt withdrawal; taper over 1-2 weeks. Caution with heart failure, bronchospastic disease, DM, hepatic dysfunction, hyperthyroidism, or peripheral vascular disease. May mask symptoms of hyperthyroidism and hypoglycemia. Withdrawal prior to surgery is controversial. **Contra:** Severe bradycardia, >1st degree heart block, cardiogenic shock, sick sinus syndrome (unless a pacemaker is present), decompensated cardiac failure. **P/N:** Category C, caution with nursing.	Bradycardia, shortness of breath, fatigue, dizziness, depression, diarrhea, pruritus, rash, hepatitis, arthralgia.
Metoprolol tartrate (Lopressor)	**Inj:** 1mg/mL; **Tab:** 50mg*, 100mg* *scored	*Adults:* **HTN:** Initial: 100mg/day in single or divided doses. Titrate: May increase at weekly (or longer) intervals. Usual: 100-450mg/day. Max: 450mg/day. **Angina:** Initial: 50mg bid. Titrate: May increase weekly. Usual: 100-400mg/day. Max: 400mg/day. **MI (Early Phase):** 5mg IV every 2 min for 3 doses (monitor BP,	**W/P:** Caution with ischemic heart disease, avoid abrupt withdrawal; taper over 1-2 weeks. Withdrawal before surgery is controversial. May mask hyperthyroidism and hypoglycemia symptoms. May exacerbate cardiac failure. Caution with hepatic dysfunction, CHF controlled by digitalis. Avoid in bronchospastic disease.	Bradycardia, shortness of breath, fatigue, dizziness, depression, diarrhea, pruritus, rash, heart block, hypotension.

W/P = warnings/precautions; **Contra** = contraindications; **P/N** = pregnancy category rating and nursing considerations.

Table 13.2. Prescribing Information for Antihypertensive Agents

GENERIC (BRAND)	FORM/ STRENGTH	DOSAGE	WARNINGS/PRECAUTIONS & CONTRAINDICATIONS	ADVERSE REACTIONS
BETA-BLOCKERS (Selective Beta₁) *(Cont.)*				
Metoprolol tartrate (Lopressor) *(Cont.)*		HR, and ECG). If tolerated, give 50mg PO q6h for 48 hrs. If not tolerated, give 25-50mg PO q6h. Initiate PO dose 15 min after last IV dose. **MI (Late Phase):** 100mg bid for at least 3 months. Take PO with or immediately following meals.	May decrease sinus HR and/or slow AV conduction. D/C if heart block or hypotension occurs. **Contra:** (HTN, Angina) Sinus bradycardia, >1st degree heart block, cardiogenic shock, overt cardiac failure, sick-sinus syndrome, severe peripheral arterial circulatory disorders, pheochromocytoma. (MI) HR <45 beats/min, 2nd- and 3rd-degree heart block, significant 1st-degree heart block, SBP <100mmHg, moderate to severe cardiac failure. **P/N:** Category C, caution in nursing.	
Nebivolol (Bystolic)	Tab: 2.5mg, 5mg, 10mg	*Adults:* **Monotherapy/Combination Therapy:** Initial: 5mg qd. Titrate: May increase dose if needed at 2-week intervals. Max: 40mg. **Hepatic Impairment/ CrCl <30mL/min:** 2.5mg qd; upward titration may be performed cautiously.	**W/P:** Exacerbation of angina, and occurrence of MI and ventricular arrhythmias reported in patients with CAD following abrupt withdrawal; taper over 1-2 weeks when possible. Avoid with bronchospastic disease. Caution with compensated CHF; consider d/c if heart failure worsens. Caution with PVD, severe renal/moderate hepatic impairment. May mask signs/symptoms of hypoglycemia or hyperthyroidism. Abrupt withdrawal may also exacerbate symptoms of hyperthyroidism or precipitate a thyroid storm. Caution with history of severe anaphylactic reactions. Patients with known/suspected pheochromocytoma should initially receive an α-blocker prior to use of any β-blocker. No studies done in patients with angina pectoris, recent MI, or severe hepatic impairment. **Contra:** Severe bradycardia, heart block >1st degree, cardiogenic shock, decompensated cardiac failure, sick sinus syndrome (unless permanent pacemaker in place), severe hepatic impairment (Child-Pugh >B). **P/N:** Category C, not for use in nursing.	Headache, fatigue, dizziness, diarrhea, nausea.
BETA-BLOCKER COMBINATIONS				
Atenolol/ Chlorthalidone (Tenoretic)	Tab: (Atenolol-Chlorthalidone) 50mg-25mg*, 100mg-25mg *scored	*Adults:* Initial: 50mg-25mg tab qd. May increase to 100mg-25mg tab qd. **CrCl 15-35mL/min:** Max: 50mg atenolol/ day. **CrCl <15mL/min:** Max: 25mg qd.	**W/P:** Withdrawal before surgery is not recommended. Caution with bronchospastic disease, conduction abnormalities, left ventricular dysfunction, heart failure controlled by digitalis and/or diuretics, renal dysfunction. Can cause heart failure with prolonged use. May mask hypoglycemia or hyperthyroidism symptoms. Avoid abrupt discontinuation. Avoid with untreated pheochromocytoma. Possible fetal harm in pregnancy. May aggravate peripheral arterial circulatory disorders. Enhanced effects in postsympathectomy patient. Neonates born to mothers receiving atenolol may be at risk of hypoglycemia and bradycardia. **Contra:** Sinus bradycardia, >1st degree heart block, cardiogenic shock, overt cardiac failure, anuria, sulfonamide hypersensitivity. **P/N:** Category D, caution in nursing.	Bradycardia, hypotension, dizziness, fatigue, nausea, depression, dyspnea, blood dyscrasias.
Bisoprolol fumarate/ Hydrochloro-thiazide (Ziac)	Tab: (Bisoprolol-HCTZ) 2.5mg-6.25mg, 5mg-6.25mg, 10mg-6.25mg	*Adults:* Initial: 2.5mg-6.25mg tab qd. Maint: May increase every 14 days. Max: 20mg bisoprolol-12.5mg HCTZ/day. **Renal/Hepatic Dysfunction:** Caution in dosing/titrating.	**W/P:** Caution with compensated cardiac failure, DM, bronchospastic disease, hepatic/renal impairment, or peripheral vascular disease. Avoid abrupt withdrawal. Photosensitivity reactions, hypokalemia, hypercalcemia, hypophosphatemia reported. May activate/exacerbate SLE. Enhanced effects in post-sympathectomy patients.	Cough, diarrhea, myalgia, headache, dizziness, fatigue, upper respiratory infection.

W/P = warnings/precautions; **Contra** = contraindications; **P/N** = pregnancy category rating and nursing considerations.

Table 13.2. Prescribing Information for Antihypertensive Agents

GENERIC (BRAND)	FORM/ STRENGTH	DOSAGE	WARNINGS/PRECAUTIONS & CONTRAINDICATIONS	ADVERSE REACTIONS
Bisoprolol fumarate/ Hydrochloro-thiazide (Ziac) *(Cont.)*			May mask hyperthyroidism or hypoglycemia symptoms. Monitor for fluid/electrolyte imbalance. May precipitate hyperuricemia, acute gout, cardiac failure. **Contra:** Cardiogenic shock, overt cardiac failure, 2nd- or 3rd-degree AV block, marked sinus bradycardia, anuria, sulfonamide hypersensitivity. **P/N:** Category C, not for use in nursing.	
Metoprolol tartrate/ Hydrochloro-thiazide (Lopressor HCT)	**Tab:** (Metoprolol-HCTZ) 50mg-25mg*, 100-25mg*, 100mg-50mg* *scored	***Adults:*** Usual: 100-450mg metoprolol/day and 12.5-50mg HCTZ/day. Max: 50mg HCTZ/day.	**W/P:** Avoid abrupt withdrawal; taper over 1-2 weeks. Withdrawal before surgery is controversial. May mask hyperthyroidism and hypoglycemia symptoms. May cause cardiac failure. Caution with hepatic dysfunction, CHF controlled by digitalis, severe renal disease, allergy or asthma history. Avoid in bronchospastic disease. Monitor for fluid/electrolyte imbalance. May manifest latent DM. Hypokalemia, hyperuricemia, hypercalcemia, hypophosphatemia, and hypomagnesemia may occur. May exacerbate SLE. Enhanced effects in post-sympathectomy patient. **Contra:** Sinus bradycardia, >1st degree heart block, cardiogenic shock, overt cardiac failure, sick-sinus syndrome, severe peripheral arterial circulatory disorders, pheochromocytoma, anuria, sulfonamide hypersensitivity. **P/N:** Category C, not for use in nursing.	Fatigue, dizziness, flu syndrome, drowsiness, hypokalemia, headache, bradycardia.
Nadolol/ Bendroflume-thiazide (Corzide)	**Tab:** (Nadolol-Bendroflumethiazide) 40mg-5mg*, 80mg-5mg* *scored	***Adults:*** Initial: 40mg-5mg tab qd. Max: 80mg-5mg tab qd. **CrCl >50mL/min:** Dose q24h. **CrCl 31-50mL/min:** Dose q24-36h. **CrCl 10-30mL/min:** Dose q24-48h. **CrCl <10mL/min:** Dose q40-60h.	**W/P:** Caution in well-compensated cardiac failure, nonallergic bronchospasm, progressive hepatic disease, and renal or hepatic dysfunction. Exacerbation of ischemic heart disease with abrupt withdrawal. Withdrawal before surgery is controversial. May mask hyperthyroidism or hypoglycemia symptoms. Can cause cardiac failure, sensitivity reactions, hypokalemia, hyperuricemia, hypomagnesemia, hypophosphatemia. May activate or exacerbate SLE. Monitor for fluid/electrolyte imbalance. Enhanced effects in postsympathectomy patient. May manifest latent DM. May decrease PBI levels. **Contra:** Bronchial asthma, sinus bradycardia and >1st degree conduction block, cardiogenic shock, overt cardiac failure, anuria, sulfonamide hypersensitivity. **P/N:** Category C, not for use in nursing.	Bradycardia, peripheral vascular insufficiency, dizziness, fatigue, nausea, vomiting, blood dyscrasias, hypersensitivity reactions.
Propranolol HCl/ Hydrochloro-thiazide (Inderide)	**Tab:** (Propranolol-HCTZ) 40mg-25mg*, 80mg-25mg* * scored	***Adults:*** Initial: 80-160mg propranolol/day; 25mg-50mg HCTZ/day. Max: (propranolol-HCTZ) 160mg-50mg/day. **Elderly:** Start at low end of dosing range. Do not substitute mg-for-mg of extended-release cap for immediate-release tab plus HCTZ. Dose tab bid and extended-release cap qd.	**W/P:** Caution with well-compensated cardiac failure, nonallergic bronchospasm, Wolff-Parkinson-White Syndrome, hepatic or renal dysfunction. Withdrawal before surgery is controversial. May mask hypoglycemia or hyperthyroidism symptoms. Avoid abrupt discontinuation. May reduce IOP. Can cause cardiac failure, hypokalemia, hyperuricemia, hypercalcemia, hypophosphatemia. May exacerbate or activate SLE. Monitor for fluid/electrolyte imbalance. May manifest latent DM. Enhanced effect in postsympathectomy patient. Concomitant use with alcohol may increase plasma levels of propranolol. **Contra:** Cardiogenic shock, sinus bradycardia and >1st degree block, bronchial asthma, CHF (unless failure is secondary to tachyarrhythmia treatable with propranolol), anuria, sulfonamide	Bradycardia, CHF, hypotension, lightheadedness, mental depression, nausea, vomiting, allergic reactions, blood dyscrasias, pancreatitis.

W/P = warnings/precautions; **Contra** = contraindications; **P/N** = pregnancy category rating and nursing considerations.

Table 13.2. Prescribing Information for Antihypertensive Agents

GENERIC (BRAND)	FORM/ STRENGTH	DOSAGE	WARNINGS/PRECAUTIONS & CONTRAINDICATIONS	ADVERSE REACTIONS
BETA-BLOCKER COMBINATIONS *(Cont.)*				
Propranolol HCl/ Hydrochloro-thiazide (Inderide) *(Cont.)*			hypersensitivity. **P/N:** Category C, not for use in nursing. Intrauterine growth retardation, small placenta, and congenital abnormalities have been reported in neonates whose mothers received propranolol during pregnancy. Neonates whose mothers received propranolol at parturition have exhibited bradycardia, hypoglycemia, and/or respiratory depression.	
CALCIUM CHANNEL BLOCKERS (Dihydropyridines)				
Amlodipine besylate (Norvasc)	Tab: 2.5mg, 5mg, 10mg	*Adults:* **HTN:** Initial: 5mg qd. Titrate over 7-14 days. Max: 10mg qd. **Small, Fragile, or Elderly/Hepatic Dysfunction/ ConcomitantAntihypertensive:** Initial: 2.5mg qd. **Angina:** 5-10mg qd. **Elderly/Hepatic Dysfunction:** 5mg qd. CAD: 5-10mg qd. *Pediatrics:* **6-17 yrs:** HTN: 2.5-5mg qd.	**W/P:** May increase angina or MI with severe obstructive CAD. Caution with severe aortic stenosis, CHF, severe hepatic impairment, and in elderly. **P/N:** Category C, not for use in nursing.	Edema, flushing, palpitation, dizziness, headache, fatigue.
Felodipine (Plendil)	Tab, Extended-Release: 2.5mg, 5mg, 10mg	*Adults:* Initial: 5mg qd. Titrate: Adjust at no less than 2 week intervals. Maint: 2.5-10mg qd. **Elderly/Hepatic Dysfunction:** Initial: 2.5mg qd. Take without food or with a light meal. Swallow tab whole.	**W/P:** May cause hypotension and lead to reflex tachycardia with precipitation of angina. Caution with heart failure or ventricular dysfunction, especially with concomitant β-blockers. Monitor dose adjustment with hepatic dysfunction or elderly. Peripheral edema reported. Maintain good dental hygiene; gingival hyperplasia reported. **P/N:** Category C, not for use in nursing.	Peripheral edema, headache, flushing, dizziness.
Isradipine (DynaCirc*)	Cap: 2.5mg, 5mg	*Adults:* Initial: 2.5mg bid alone or with a thiazide diuretic. Titrate: May adjust by 5mg/day at 2-4 week intervals. Max: 20mg/day.	**W/P:** May produce symptomatic hypotension. Caution in CHF, especially with concomitant β-blockers. Increased bioavailability in elderly, patients with hepatic functional impairment, and mild renal impairment. **P/N:** Category C, not for use in nursing.	Headache, edema, dizziness, palpitations, chest pain, constipation, fatigue, flushing, abdominal discomfort, tachycardia, rash, pollakiura, weakness, vomiting.
Isradipine (DynaCirc CR)	Tab, Controlled-Release: 5mg, 10mg	*Adults:* Initial: 5mg qd alone or with a thiazide diuretic. Titrate: May adjust by 5mg/day at 2-4 week intervals. Max: 20mg/day. Swallow whole.	**W/P:** May produce symptomatic hypotension. Caution in CHF, especially with concomitant β-blockers. Caution with pre-existing severe GI narrowing. Peripheral edema reported. Increased bioavailability in elderly. **P/N:** Category C, not for use in nursing.	Headache, edema, dizziness, constipation, fatigue, flushing, abdominal discomfort.
Nicardipine HCl (Cardene IV)	Inj: 2.5mg/mL	*Adults:* IV: Individualized dose; Administer by slow continuous infusion at a concentration of 0.1mg/mL. **Gradual Reduction:** Initial: 50mL/hr (5mg/hr). Titrate: May increase by 25mL/hr (2.5mg/hr) q15 min. Max: 150mL/hr (15mg/hr). **Rapid BP Reduction:** Initial 50mL/hr (5mg/hr). Titrate: 25mL/hr (2.5mg/hr) q5 min. Max 150mL/hr (15mg/hr). Decrease rate to 30mL/hr (3mg/hr) after BP reduction is achieved. **Equiv. PO/IV Dose:** 20mg q8h=0.5mg/hr, 30mg q8h=1.2mg/hr, 40mg q8h=2.2mg/hr.	**W/P:** May induce or exacerbate angina. Caution with CHF, significant left ventricular dysfunction, or pheochromocytoma. Change IV site every 12 hrs to minimize risk of peripheral venous irritation. Monitor BP during administration. Caution in hepatic/renal impairment or reduced hepatic blood flow. **Contra:** Advanced aortic stenosis. **P/N:** Category C, not for use in nursing.	Headache, hypotension, tachycardia, nausea/vomiting.
Nicardipine HCl (Cardene SR)	Cap, Extended-Release: 30mg, 45mg, 60mg	*Adults:* Initial: 30mg bid. Usual: 30-60mg bid.	**W/P:** Increased angina reported in patients with angina. Caution with CHF when titrating dose. Caution in hepatic/renal impairment, or reduced hepatic blood flow. May cause symptomatic hypotension. Measure BP 2-4 hrs after 1st dose or dose increase. **Contra:** Advanced aortic stenosis. **P/N:** Category C, not for use in nursing.	Headache, pedal edema, vasodilation, palpitations, nausea, dizziness, asthenia, flushing, increased angina.

* Available only in generic form (brand not available).
W/P = warnings/precautions; **Contra** = contraindications; **P/N** = pregnancy category rating and nursing considerations.

Table 13.2. Prescribing Information for Antihypertensive Agents

GENERIC (BRAND)	FORM/ STRENGTH	DOSAGE	WARNINGS/PRECAUTIONS & CONTRAINDICATIONS	ADVERSE REACTIONS
Nifedipine (Adalat CC, Afeditab CR)	**Tab, Extended-Release:** (Adalat CC, Afeditab CR) 30mg, 60mg, (Adalat CC) 90mg	**Adults:** Initial: 30mg qd. Titrate over 7-14 days. Usual: 30-60mg qd. Max: 90mg/day. Take on empty stomach. Swallow tab whole.	**W/P:** May cause hypotension; monitor BP initially or with titration. May exacerbate angina from β-blocker withdrawal. CHF risk, especially with aortic stenosis or β-blockers. Peripheral edema reported. May increase angina or MI with severe obstructive CAD. Caution in elderly. **P/N:** Category C, not for use in nursing.	Headache, flushing, heat sensation, dizziness, peripheral edema, fatigue, asthenia.
Nifedipine (Procardia)	**Cap:** 10mg, 20mg	**Adults:** Initial: 10mg tid. Titrate over 7-14 days. Usual: 10-20mg tid. Max: 180mg/day. **Elderly:** Start at low end of dosing range.	**W/P:** May cause hypotension; monitor BP initially or with titration. May exacerbate angina from β-blocker withdrawal. CHF risk, especially with aortic stenosis or β-blockers. Peripheral edema reported. Not for acute reduction of BP or essential HTN. May increase angina or MI with severe obstructive CAD. Avoid with acute coronary syndrome or within 1-2 weeks of MI. Caution in elderly. **P/N:** Category C, unknown use in nursing.	Dizziness, lightheadedness, giddiness, flushing, muscle cramps, headache, peripheral edema, nervousness/mood changes.
Nifedipine (Procardia XL)	**Tab, Extended-Release:** 30mg, 60mg, 90mg	**Adults: Angina/HTN:** Initial: 30-60mg qd. Titrate over 7-14 days. Max: 120mg/day. Caution if dose >90mg with angina.	**W/P:** May cause hypotension; monitor BP initially or with titration. May exacerbate angina from β-blocker withdrawal. CHF risk, especially with aortic stenosis or β-blockers. Peripheral edema reported. May increase angina or MI with severe obstructive CAD. Caution in pre-existing severe GI narrowing. **P/N:** Category C, unknown use in nursing.	Dizziness, lightheadedness, giddiness, flushing, muscle cramps, headache, weakness, nausea, peripheral edema, nervousness/mood changes.
Nimodipine (Nimotop)	**Cap:** 30mg	**Adults:** 60mg q 4 hrs for 21 days, 1 hr before or 2 hrs after meals. **Hepatic Cirrhosis:** 30mg q 4 hrs for 21 days. Start therapy within 96 hrs of SAH. If cannot swallow cap, extract contents into syringe and empty into NG tube, then flush with 30mL of 0.9% NaCl.	**BB:** Do not administer IV or by other parenteral routes. Deaths and serious, life-threatening adverse events have occurred when contents of capsules injected parenterally. **W/P:** Carefully monitor BP. Monitor BP and HR closely with hepatic dysfunction. Do not administer IV or by other parenteral routes. **P/N:** Category C, not for use in nursing.	Decreased BP, headache, rash, diarrhea, bradycardia, nausea, abnormal LFTs.
Nisoldipine (Sular)	**Tab, Extended-Release:** 10mg, 20mg, 30mg, 40mg	**Adults:** Initial: 20mg qd. Titrate: Increase by 10mg weekly or longer. Maint: 20-40mg qd. Max: 60mg/day. **Elderly >65 yrs/Hepatic Dysfunction:** Initial: Do not exceed 10mg/day. Do not chew, divide, or crush tabs.	**W/P:** May increase angina or MI with severe obstructive CAD. May cause hypotension; monitor BP initially or with titration. Caution with heart failure or compromised ventricular function, especially with concomitant β-blockers. Caution with severe hepatic dysfunction or in elderly. **P/N:** Category C, not for use in nursing.	Peripheral edema, headache, dizziness, pharyngitis, vasodilation, sinusitis, palpitations.
CALCIUM CHANNEL BLOCKERS (Nondihydropyridines)				
Diltiazem HCl (Cardizem)	**Tab:** 30mg, 60mg*, 90mg*, 120mg* *scored	**Adults:** Initial: 30mg qid (before meals and qhs). Adjust at 1-2 day intervals. Usual: 180-360mg/day.	**W/P:** Caution in renal, hepatic, or ventricular dysfunction. Monitor LFTs and renal function with prolonged use. D/C if persistent rash occurs. Symptomatic hypotension may occur. Acute hepatic injury reported. **Contra:** Sick sinus syndrome and 2nd- or 3rd-degree AV block (except with functioning pacemaker), hypotension (<90mmHg systolic), acute MI, pulmonary congestion. **P/N:** Category C, not for use in nursing.	Headache, dizziness, asthenia, flushing, 1st-degree AV block, edema, nausea, bradycardia, rash.

BB = black box warning; **W/P** = warnings/precautions; **Contra** = contraindications; **P/N** = pregnancy category rating and nursing considerations.

Table 13.2. Prescribing Information for Antihypertensive Agents

GENERIC (BRAND)	FORM/ STRENGTH	DOSAGE	WARNINGS/PRECAUTIONS & CONTRAINDICATIONS	ADVERSE REACTIONS
CALCIUM CHANNEL BLOCKERS (Nondihydropyridines) *(Cont.)*				
Diltiazem HCl (Cardizem CD, Cardizem LA, Cartia XT)	Cap, **Extended-Release:** (Cardizem CD, Cartia XT) 120mg, 180mg, 240mg, 300mg, (Cardizem CD) 360mg; **Tab, Extended-Release:** (Cardizem LA) 120mg, 180mg, 240mg, 300mg, 360mg, 420mg	**Adults: HTN:** (CD, Cartia XT) Initial (monotherapy): 180-240mg qd. Titrate: Adjust at 2-week intervals. Usual: 240-360mg qd. Max: 480mg qd. (LA) Initial: 180-240mg qd. Adjust at 2-week intervals. Max: 540mg qd. **Angina:** (CD, Cartia XT) Initial: 120-180mg qd. Adjust at 1-2 week intervals. Max: 480mg/day. (LA) Initial: 180mg qd. Adjust at 1-2 week intervals.	**W/P:** Caution in renal, hepatic, or ventricular dysfunction. Monitor LFTs and renal function with prolonged use. D/C if persistent rash occurs. Symptomatic hypotension may occur. Acute hepatic injury reported. **Contra:** Sick sinus syndrome and 2nd- or 3rd-degree AV block (except with functioning pacemaker), hypotension (<90mmHg systolic), acute MI, pulmonary congestion. **P/N:** Category C, not for use in nursing.	Headache, dizziness, asthenia, flushing, 1st-degree AV block, edema, nausea, bradycardia, rash.
Diltiazem HCl (Dilacor XR, Diltia XT)	Cap, **Extended-Release:** 120mg, 180mg, 240mg	**Adults: HTN:** Initial: 180-240mg qd. Usual: 180-480mg qd. Max: 540mg qd. **≥60 yrs:** Initial: 120mg qd. **Angina:** Initial: 120mg qd. Titrate: Adjust at 1-2 week intervals. Max: 480mg/day. Swallow whole on an empty stomach in the am.	**W/P:** Caution in renal, hepatic, or ventricular dysfunction. Monitor LFTs and renal function with prolonged use. D/C if persistent rash occurs. Symptomatic hypotension may occur. Acute hepatic injury reported. **Contra:** Sick sinus syndrome, 2nd- or 3rd-degree AV block (except with functioning pacemaker), hypotension (<90mmHg systolic), acute MI, pulmonary congestion. **P/N:** Category C, not for use in nursing.	Rhinitis, pharyngitis, cough, flu syndrome, peripheral edema, myalgia, vomiting, sinusitis, asthenia, nausea, vasodilation, headache, constipation, diarrhea.
Diltiazem HCl (Tiazac, Taztia XT)	Cap, Extended- **Release:** (Taztia XT, Tiazac) 120mg, 180mg, 240mg, 300mg, 360mg; (Tiazac) 420mg	**Adults: HTN:** Initial: 120-240mg qd. Titrate: Adjust at 2-week intervals. Usual: 120-540mg qd. Max: 540mg qd. **Angina:** Initial: 120-180mg qd Titrate: Increase over 7-14 days. Max: 540mg qd.	**W/P:** Caution in renal, hepatic, or ventricular dysfunction. Monitor LFTs and renal function with prolonged use. D/C if persistent rash occurs. Symptomatic hypotension may occur. Acute hepatic injury reported. **Contra:** Sick sinus syndrome and 2nd- or 3rd-degree AV block (except with functioning pacemaker), severe hypotension (<90mm Hg systolic), acute MI, pulmonary congestion. **P/N:** Category C, not for use in nursing.	Headache, peripheral edema, vasodilation, dizziness, rash, dyspepsia.
Verapamil HCl (Calan)	Tab: 40mg, 80mg*, 120mg* *scored	**Adults: HTN:** Initial: 80mg tid. Usual: 360-480mg/day. **Elderly/Small Stature:** Initial: 40mg tid. **Angina:** Usual: 80-120mg tid. **Elderly/Small Stature:** Initial: 40mg tid. Titrate: Increase daily or weekly. **A-Fib (Digitalized):** Usual: 240-320mg/day given tid-qid. **PSVT Prophylaxis (Non-Digitalized):** 240-480mg/day given tid-qid. Max: 480mg/day. **Severe Hepatic Dysfunction:** Give 30% of normal dose.	**W/P:** Avoid with moderate to severe cardiac failure, and ventricular dysfunction if taking a β-blocker. May cause hypotension, AV block, transient bradycardia, PR interval prolongation. Monitor LFTs periodically; hepatocellular injury reported. Caution with hypertrophic cardiomyopathy, renal or hepatic dysfunction. Decrease dose with decreased neuromuscular transmission. **Contra:** Severe ventricular dysfunction, hypotension, cardiogenic shock, sick sinus syndrome or 2nd- or 3rd-degree AV block (except with functioning ventricular pacemaker), A-Fib/Flutter with an accessory bypass tract. **P/N:** Category C, not for use in nursing.	Constipation, dizziness, nausea, hypotension, headache, edema, CHF, fatigue, elevated liver enzymes, dyspnea, bradycardia, AV block, rash, flushing.
Verapamil HCl (Calan SR)	Tab, **Extended-Release:** 120mg, 180mg*, 240mg* *scored	**Adults: ≥18 yrs:** Initial: 180mg qam. Titrate: If inadequate response, increase to 240mg qam, then 180mg bid; or 240mg qam plus 120mg qpm, then 240mg q12h. **Elderly/Small Stature:** Initial: 120mg qam. Take with food.	**W/P:** Avoid with moderate to severe cardiac failure, and ventricular dysfunction if taking a β-blocker. May cause hypotension, AV block, transient bradycardia, PR interval hepatocellular injury reported. Caution with hypertrophic cardiomyopathy, renal or hepatic dysfunction. Decrease dose with decreased neuromuscular transmission. **Contra:** Severe ventricular dysfunction, hypotension, cardiogenic shock, sick sinus syndrome or 2nd- or 3rd-degree AV block (except with functioning ventricular pacemaker), A-Fib/Flutter with an accessory bypass tract. **P/N:** Category C, not for use in nursing.	Constipation, dizziness, nausea, hypotension, headache, edema, CHF, fatigue, elevated liver enzymes, dyspnea, bradycardia, AV block, rash, flushing.

W/P = warnings/precautions; **Contra** = contraindications; **P/N** = pregnancy category rating and nursing considerations.

Table 13.2. Prescribing Information for Antihypertensive Agents

GENERIC (BRAND)	FORM/ STRENGTH	DOSAGE	WARNINGS/PRECAUTIONS & CONTRAINDICATIONS	ADVERSE REACTIONS
Verapamil HCl (Covera-HS)	Tab, Extended-Release: 180mg, 240mg	*Adults:* Initial: 180mg qhs. Titrate: May increase to 240mg qhs, then 360mg qhs, then 480mg qhs, if needed. Swallow tab whole. **Elderly:** Start at the low end of the dosing range.	**W/P:** Avoid with moderate to severe cardiac failure, and ventricular dysfunction if taking a β-blocker. May cause hypotension, AV block, transient bradycardia, PR interval prolongation. Monitor LFTs periodically; hepatocellular injury reported. Give 30% of normal dose with severe hepatic dysfunction. Caution with hypertrophic cardiomyopathy, renal or hepatic dysfunction. Decrease dose with decreased neuromuscular transmission. **Contra:** Severe ventricular dysfunction, hypotension, cardiogenic shock, sick sinus syndrome or 2nd- or 3rd-degree AV block (except with functioning ventricular pacemaker), A-Fib/Flutter with an accessory bypass tract. **P/N:** Category C, not for use in nursing.	Constipation, dizziness, nausea, hypotension, headache, edema, CHF, pulmonary edema, fatigue, dyspnea, bradycardia, AV block, rash, flushing.
Verapamil HCl (Isoptin SR)	Tab, Extended-Release: 120mg, 180mg*, 240mg* *scored	*Adults:* Initial: 180mg qam. Titrate: If inadequate response, increase to 240mg qam, then 180mg bid; or 240mg qam plus 120mg qpm, then 240mg q12h. **Elderly/Small Stature:** Initial: 120mg qam. Take with food.	**W/P:** Avoid with moderate to severe cardiac failure, and ventricular dysfunction if taking a β-blocker. May cause hypotension, AV block, transient bradycardia, PR interval prolongation. Monitor LFTs periodically; hepatocellular injury reported. Give 30% of normal dose with severe hepatic dysfunction. Caution with hypertrophic cardiomyopathy, renal or hepatic dysfunction. Decrease dose in those with decreased neuromuscular transmission. **Contra:** Severe ventricular dysfunction, hypotension, cardiogenic shock, sick sinus syndrome or 2nd- or 3rd-degree AV block (except with functioning ventricular pacemaker), A-Fib/Flutter with an accessory bypass tract. **P/N:** Category C, not for use in nursing.	Constipation, dizziness, nausea, hypotension, headache, edema, CHF, pulmonary edema, fatigue, dyspnea, bradycardia, AV block, rash, flushing.
Verapamil HCl (Verelan)	Cap, Extended-Release: 120mg, 180mg, 240mg, 360mg	*Adults:* Usual: 240mg qam. Titrate: May increase by 120mg qam. Max: 480mg qam. **Elderly/Small Stature:** Initial: 120mg qam. Titrate: May increase to 180mg qam, then 240mg qam, then 360mg qam, then 480mg qam. May sprinkle on applesauce; do not crush or chew.	**W/P:** Avoid with moderate to severe cardiac failure, and ventricular dysfunction if taking a β-blocker. May cause hypotension, AV block, transient bradycardia, PR interval prolongation. Monitor LFTs periodically; hepatocellular injury reported. Give 30% of normal dose with severe hepatic dysfunction. Caution with hypertrophic cardiomyopathy, renal or hepatic dysfunction. Decrease dose in those with decreased neuromuscular transmission **Contra:** Severe ventricular dysfunction, hypotension, cardiogenic shock, sick sinus syndrome or 2nd- or 3rd-degree AV block (except with functioning ventricular pacemaker), A-Fib/Flutter with an accessory bypass tract. **P/N:** Category C, not for use in nursing.	Constipation, dizziness, nausea, hypotension, headache, peripheral edema, infection, flu syndrome, fatigue, bradycardia, AV block.
Verapamil HCl (Verelan PM)	Cap, Extended-Release: 100mg, 200mg, 300mg	*Adults:* Usual: 200mg qhs. Titrate: May increase to 300mg qhs, then 400mg qhs. **Renal or Hepatic Dysfunction/Elderly/ Small Stature:** Initial: 100mg qhs. Max: 400mg qhs. May sprinkle on applesauce; do not crush or chew.	**W/P:** Avoid with moderate to severe cardiac failure, and ventricular dysfunction if taking a β-blocker. May cause hypotension, AV block, transient bradycardia, PR interval prolongation. Monitor LFTs periodically; hepatocellular injury reported. Give 30% of normal dose with severe hepatic dysfunction. Caution with hypertrophic cardiomyopathy, renal or hepatic dysfunction. Decrease dose in those with decreased neuromuscular transmission. **Contra:** Severe ventricular dysfunction, hypotension, cardiogenic shock, sick sinus syndrome or 2nd- or	Constipation, dizziness, nausea, hypotension, headache, peripheral edema, infection, flu syndrome, fatigue, bradycardia, AV block.

W/P = warnings/precautions; **Contra** = contraindications; **P/N** = pregnancy category rating and nursing considerations.

Table 13.2. Prescribing Information for Antihypertensive Agents

GENERIC (BRAND)	FORM/ STRENGTH	DOSAGE	WARNINGS/PRECAUTIONS & CONTRAINDICATIONS	ADVERSE REACTIONS
CALCIUM CHANNEL BLOCKERS (Nondihydropyridines) *(Cont.)*				
Verapamil HCl (Verelan PM) *(Cont.)*			3rd-degree AV block (except with functioning ventricular pacemaker), A-Fib/Flutter with an accessory bypass tract. **P/N:** Category C, not for use in nursing.	
CALCIUM CHANNEL BLOCKER COMBINATIONS				
Amlodipine besylate/ Atorvastatin calcium (Caduet)	**Tab:** (Amlodipine-Atorvastatin) 2.5mg-10mg, 2.5mg-20mg, 2.5mg-40mg, 5mg-10mg, 5mg-20mg, 5mg-40mg, 5mg-80mg, 10mg-10mg, 10mg-20mg, 10mg-40mg, 10mg-80mg	***Adults:*** Dosing should be individualized and based on the appropriate combination of recommendations for the monotherapies. (Amlodipine): **HTN:** Initial: 5mg qd. Titrate over 7-14 days. Max: 10mg qd. **Small, Fragile, or Elderly/ Hepatic Dysfunction/Concomitant Antihypertensive:** Initial: 2.5mg qd. **Angina:** 5-10mg qd. **Elderly/Hepatic Dysfunction:** 5mg qd. (Atorvastatin): **Hypercholesterolemia/Mixed Dyslipidemia:** Initial: 10-20mg qd (or 40mg qd for LDL-C reduction >45%). Titrate: Adjust dose if needed at 2-4 week intervals. Usual: 10-80mg qd. **Homozygous Familial Hypercholesterolemia:** 10-80mg qd. ***Pediatrics:*** **≥10 yrs (postmenarchal):** (Amlodipine): **HTN:** 2.5-5mg qd. **10-17 yrs (postmenarchal):** (Atorvastatin): **Heterozygous Familial Hypercholesterolemia:** Initial: 10mg/day. Titrate: Adjust dose if needed at intervals of ≥4 weeks. Max: 20mg/day.	**W/P:** May rarely increase angina or MI with severe obstructive CAD. Monitor LFTs prior to therapy, at 12 weeks after initiation, with dose elevation, and periodically thereafter. Reduce dose or withdraw if AST or ALT >3x ULN persist. Caution with heavy alcohol use and/or history of hepatic disease, severe aortic stenosis, CHF. D/C if markedly elevated CPK levels occur, if myopathy is diagnosed or suspected, or if predisposition to renal failure secondary to rhabdomyolysis. Increased risk of hemorrhagic stroke in patients with recent stroke or TIA. **Contra:** Active liver disease, unexplained persistent elevations of serum transaminases, pregnancy, nursing mothers. **P/N:** Category X, not for use in nursing	Headache, edema, palpitation, dizziness, fatigue, constipation, flatulence, dyspepsia, abdominal pain.
Amlodipine besylate/ Benazepril HCl (Lotrel)	**Cap:** (Amlodipine-Benazepril) 2.5mg-10mg, 5mg-10mg, 5mg-20mg, 5mg-40mg, 10mg-20mg, 10mg-40mg	***Adults:*** Usual: 2.5-10mg amlodipine and 10-80mg benazepril per day. **Small/Elderly/Frail/Hepatic Impairment:** Initial: 2.5mg amlodipine.	**BB:** When used in pregnancy, ACE inhibitors can cause injury and even death to the developing fetus. D/C therapy when pregnancy detected. **W/P:** D/C if angioedema, jaundice, or if marked LFT elevation occurs. Risk of hyperkalemia with DM, renal dysfunction. Persistent nonproductive cough reported. Monitor WBCs in collagen vascular disease. Anaphylactoid reactions reported. Fetal/neonatal morbidity and death reported. Monitor for hypotension in high-risk patients (heart failure, surgery/ anesthesia, volume and/or salt depletion, etc). Caution with CHF, severe hepatic or renal dysfunction, and renal artery stenosis. Avoid if CrCl ≤30mL/min. **P/N:** Category C (1st trimester) and D (2nd and 3rd trimesters), not for use in nursing.	Cough, headache, dizziness, edema.
Amlodipine besylate/ Olmesartan medoxomil (Azor)	**Tab:** (Amlodipine-Olmesartan) 5mg-20mg, 10mg-20mg, 5mg-40mg, 10mg-40mg	***Adults:* Replacement Therapy:** May substitute for individually titrated components for patients on amlodipine and olmesartan. When substituting for individual components, the dose of 1 or both components may be increased if needed. **Add-On Therapy:** May use as add-on therapy when not adequately controlled on amlodipine or olmesartan. May increase dose after 2 weeks to maximum dose of 10mg-40mg qd.	**BB:** When used in pregnancy during 2nd and 3rd trimesters, drugs that act directly on the renin-angiotensin system can cause injury and even death to developing fetus. When pregnancy is detected, d/c therapy asap. **W/P:** Hypotension, especially in volume- or salt-depleted patients, may occur with treatment initiation; monitor closely. Caution with severe aortic stenosis, heart failure, or severe hepatic impairment. Increased angina or MI with CCBs may occur with dosage initiation or increase. Changes in renal function, oliguria, progressive azotemia, or acute renal failure may occur. **P/N:** Category C (1st trimester) and D (2nd and 3rd trimester), not for use in nursing.	Edema.

BB = black box warning; **W/P** = warnings/precautions; **Contra** = contraindications; **P/N** = pregnancy category rating and nursing considerations.

Table 13.2. Prescribing Information for Antihypertensive Agents

GENERIC (BRAND)	FORM/ STRENGTH	DOSAGE	WARNINGS/PRECAUTIONS & CONTRAINDICATIONS	ADVERSE REACTIONS
Amlodipine besylate/ Valsartan (Exforge)	**Tab:** (Amlodipine-Valsartan) 5mg-160mg, 10mg-160mg, 5mg-320mg, 10mg-320mg	***Adults:* Combination Therapy from Monotherapy (amlodipine or valsartan):** Initial: 5mg-10mg amlodipine and 160mg-320mg valsartan qd. Titrate: If inadequate control, may increase after 3-4 weeks of therapy. Max: 10mg-320mg. If receiving amlodipine and valsartan separately, may give same component doses. **Elderly:** Lower initial dose may be required	**BB:** When used in pregnancy, drugs that act directly on the renin-angiotensin system can cause injury and even death to the developing fetus. D/C therapy when pregnancy is detected. **W/P:** May cause excessive hypotension. May increase risk of angina and MI in patients with severe obstructive CAD. Caution with CHF, severe hepatic impairment, renal dysfunction, or renal artery stenosis. **P/N:** Category C (1st trimester) and D (2nd and 3rd trimester), not for use in nursing.	Peripheral edema, vertigo, nasopharyngitis, upper respiratory tract infection, dizziness.
Verapamil HCl/ Trandolapril (Tarka)	**Tab:** (Trandolapril-Verapamil) 2mg-180mg, 1mg-240mg, 2mg-240mg, 4mg-240mg	***Adults:* Replacement Therapy:** 1 tab qd with food. **Severe Hepatic Dysfunction:** Give 30% of normal dose.	**BB:** ACE inhibitors can cause death/injury to developing fetus during 2nd and 3rd trimesters. Stop therapy if pregnancy detected. **W/P:** Monitor for hypotension with surgery or anesthesia. Risk of hyperkalemia with renal insufficiency, DM. D/C if jaundice develops. Avoid with moderate to severe cardiac failure and ventricular dysfunction if taking a β-blocker. May cause angioedema, cough, fetal/ neonatal morbidity, hypotension, AV block, anaphylactoid reactions, transient bradycardia, PR-interval prolongation. Monitor LFTs periodically. Give 30% of normal dose with severe hepatic dysfunction. Caution with CHF, hypertrophic cardiomyopathy, renal or hepatic dysfunction. Decrease dose in those with decreased neuromuscular transmission. Monitor WBC with collagen-vascular disease and/or renal disease. **Contra:** Severe ventricular dysfunction, hypotension, cardiogenic shock, sick sinus syndrome or 2nd- or 3rd-degree AV block (except with functioning ventricular pacemaker), A-Fib/Flutter with an accessory bypass tract, history of ACE inhibitor-associated angioedema. **P/N:** Category C (1st trimester) and D (2nd and 3rd trimesters), not for use in nursing.	AV block, constipation, cough, dizziness, fatigue, headache, increased hepatic enzymes, chest pain, upper respiratory tract infection/congestion.
DIRECT RENIN INHIBITOR & COMBINATION				
Aliskiren (Tekturna)	**Tab:** 150mg, 300mg	***Adults:*** Usual: 150mg qd. Titrate: May increase to 300mg/day if needed. High-fat meals decrease absorption.	**BB:** When used in pregnancy, drugs that act directly on the renin-angiotensin system can cause injury and even death to the developing fetus. D/C therapy when pregnancy is detected. **W/P:** Caution with greater than moderate renal dysfunction (SCr >1.7mg/dL (women) or >2mg/dL (men) and/or GFR <30mL/min), history of dialysis, nephrotic syndrome, or renovascular hypertension. May increase serum K+, especially when used in combination with especially when especially when in diabetics. Angioedema of face, extremities, lips, tongue, glottis, and/or larynx reported; d/c and monitor until complete resolution of signs and symptoms. Hypotension rarely seen. **P/N:** Category C (1st trimester) and D (2nd and 3rd trimesters); not for use in nursing.	Diarrhea, headache, nasopharyngitis, dizziness, fatigue, upper respiratory tract infection, back pain, cough.
Aliskiren/ Hydrochloro-thiazide (Tekturna HCT)	**Tab:** (Aliskiren-HCTZ) 150mg-12.5mg, 150mg-25mg, 300mg-12.5mg, 300mg-25mg	***Adults:*** Initial: Not Controlled on Monotherapy: 150mg/12.5mg qd. Titrate: May increase to 150mg/25mg, 300mg/12.5mg qd if uncontrolled after 2-4 weeks. Max: 300mg/25mg. Avoid with CrCl ≤30mL/min.	**BB:** Drugs that act directly on the renin-angiotensin system can cause injury and even death to the developing fetus. D/C therapy when pregnancy is detected. **W/P:** Angioedema of head and neck may occur; d/c therapy and monitor until	Dizziness, influenza, diarrhea, cough, vertigo, asthenia, arthralgia.

BB = black box warning; **W/P** = warnings/precautions; **Contra** = contraindications; **P/N** = pregnancy category rating and nursing considerations.

Table 13.2. Prescribing Information for Antihypertensive Agents

GENERIC (BRAND)	FORM/ STRENGTH	DOSAGE	WARNINGS/PRECAUTIONS & CONTRAINDICATIONS	ADVERSE REACTIONS
DIRECT RENIN INHIBITOR & COMBINATION *(Cont.)*				
Aliskiren/ Hydrochloro-thiazide (Tekturna HCT) *(Cont.)*			signs and symptoms resolve. May cause symptomatic hypotension in volume- and/or salt-depleted patients; correct condition prior to therapy. Avoid with CrCl <30mL/min. Caution with hepatic impairment, or history of allergy or bronchial asthma. May exacerbate or activate SLE. Monitor serum electrolytes periodically to detect possible electrolyte imbalance. **Contra:** Anuria, sulfonamide hypersensitivity. **P/N:** Category D, not for use in nursing.	
DIURETICS (Aldosterone Receptor Blockers)				
Eplerenone (Inspra)	Tab: 25mg, 50mg	***Adults:* CHF Post-MI:** Initial: 25mg qd. Titrate: To 50mg qd within 4 weeks. Maint: 50mg qd. Adjust dose based on K+ level: See PI. **HTN:** Initial: 50mg qd. May increase to 50mg bid if inadequate effect on BP. Max: 100mg/day. **With Weak CYP3A4 Inhibitors:** Initial: 25mg qd.	**W/P:** Risk of hyperkalemia (>5.5mEq/L); monitor periodically. With CHF post-MI use caution with SCr >2mg/dL (males) or >1.8mg/dL (females), CrCl ≤50mL/min, and in diabetics (also with proteinuria). **Contra:** All: Serum K+ >5.5mgEq/L at initiation, CrCl ≤30mL/min, with potent CYP3A4 inhibitors (eg, ketoconazole, itraconazole, nefazodone, troleandomycin, clarithromycin, ritonavir, nelfinavir). When treating HTN: Type 2 diabetes with microalbuminuria, SCr >2mg/dL (males) or >1.8mg/dL (females), CrCl >50mg/min, with K+ supplements or K+-sparing diuretics (eg, amiloride, spironolactone, triamterene). **P/N:** Category B, not for use in nursing.	Headache, dizziness, hyperkalemia, increased SCr/triglycerides/GGT, angina/MI.
Spironolactone (Aldactone)	Tab: 25mg, 50mg*, 100mg* *scored	***Adults:* Hyperaldosteronism:** (Diagnostic) 400mg/day for 3-4 weeks or 400mg/day for 4 days. (Preoperative) 100-400mg/day. Maint: Lowest effective dose. **Edema:** Initial: 100mg/day given qd or in divided doses for at least 5 days. Maint: 25-200mg/day given qd-bid. **HTN:** Initial: 50-100mg/day given qd or in divided doses. Titrate: Adjust at 2-week intervals. **Hypokalemia:** 25-100mg/day.	**BB:** Tumorigenic in chronic toxicity animal studies; avoid unnecessary use. **W/P:** Monitor for fluid/electrolyte imbalance. Caution with renal and hepatic dysfunction. Hyperchloremic metabolic acidosis reported with decompensated hepatic cirrhosis. Mild acidosis, gynecomastia, transient BUN elevation may occur. D/C and monitor ECG if hyperkalemia occurs. Risk of dilutional hyponatremia. **Contra:** Anuria, acute renal insufficiency, significantly impaired renal excretory function, hyperkalemia. **P/N:** Category C, not for use in nursing.	Gastric bleeding, ulceration, gynecomastia, impotence, agranulocytosis, fever, urticaria, confusion, ataxia, renal dysfunction, irregular menses, amenorrhea.
DIURETICS (Loop)				
Bumetanide (Bumex)	Inj: 0.25mg/mL; Tab: 0.5mg*, 1mg*, 2mg* *scored	***Adults:* ≥18 yrs: PO:** Usual: 0.5-2mg qd. Maint: May give every other day or every 3-4 days. Max: 10mg/day. **IV/IM:** Initial: 0.5-1mg over 1-2 min, may repeat every 2-3 hrs for 2-3 doses. Max: 10mg/day. **Elderly:** Start at low end of dosing range.	**BB:** Can lead to profound water and electrolyte depletion with excessive use. **W/P:** Monitor for volume/electrolyte depletion, hypokalemia, blood dyscrasias, hepatic damage. Elderly are prone to volume/electrolyte depletion. Caution in elderly, hepatic cirrhosis and ascites. Associated with ototoxicity, hypocalcemia, thrombocytopenia, hypomagnesemia, hypokalemia, and hyperuricemia. Hypersensitivity with sulfonamide allergy. D/C if marked increase in BUN or creatinine or if develop oliguria with progressive renal disease. **Contra:** Anuria, hepatic coma, severe electrolyte depletion. **P/N:** Category C, not for use in nursing.	Muscle cramps, dizziness, hypotension, headache, nausea, hyperuricemia, hypokalemia, hyponatremia, hyperglycemia, azotemia, increase serum creatinine.
Ethacrynic acid (Edecrin)	Tab: 25mg* *scored	***Adults:*** Initial: 50-100mg qd. Titrate: 25-50mg increments. Usual: 50-200mg/day. After diuresis achieved, give smallest effective dose continuously or intermittently. ***Pediatrics:*** Initial: 25mg. Titrate: Increase by 25mg increments.	**W/P:** Caution in advanced liver cirrhosis. Monitor serum electrolytes, CO_2, BUN early in therapy and periodically during active diuresis. Vigorous diuresis may induce acute hypotensive episode and in elderly cardiac patients, hemoconcentration	Anorexia, malaise, abdominal discomfort, gout, deafness, tinnitus, vertigo, headache, fatigue, rash, chills.

BB = black box warning; W/P = warnings/precautions; **Contra** = contraindications; **P/N** = pregnancy category rating and nursing considerations.

Table 13.2. Prescribing Information for Antihypertensive Agents

GENERIC (BRAND)	FORM/ STRENGTH	DOSAGE	WARNINGS/PRECAUTIONS & CONTRAINDICATIONS	ADVERSE REACTIONS
Ethacrynic acid (Edecrin) *(Cont.)*		Maint: Reduce dose and frequency once dry weight achieved; may give intermittently.	resulting in thromboembolic disorders. Ototoxicity reported with severe renal dysfunction. Hypomagnesemia and transient increase in serum urea nitrogen may occur. Reduce dose or withdraw if excessive electrolyte loss occurs. Initiate therapy in the hospital for cirrhotic patients with ascites. Liberalize salt intake and supplement with K⁺ if needed. Reduced responsiveness in renal edema with hypoproteinemia; use salt poor albumin. **Contra:** Anuria, infants. D/C if increasing electrolyte imbalance, azotemia, or oliguria develops during treatment of severe, progressive renal disease. D/C if severe, watery diarrhea occurs. **P/N:** Category B, not for use in nursing.	
Furosemide (Lasix)	**Inj:** 10mg/mL; **Sol:** 10mg/mL, 40mg/5mL; **Tab:** 20mg, 40mg*, 80mg *scored	***Adults:*** **(PO) HTN:** Initial: 40mg bid. **Edema:** Initial: 20-80mg PO. May repeat or increase by 20-40mg after 6-8 hrs. Max: 600mg/day. Alternative Regimen: Dose on 2-4 consecutive days each week. Closely monitor if on >80mg/day. **(Inj) Edema:** Initial: 20-40mg IV/IM. May repeat or increase by 20mg after 2 hrs. **Acute Pulmonary Edema:** Initial: 40mg IV. May increase to 80mg IV after 1 hr. ***Pediatrics:*** **Edema: (PO)** Initial: 2mg/kg single dose. May increase by 1mg/kg after 6-8 hrs. Max: 6mg/kg. **(Inj)** Initial: 1mg/kg IV/IM single dose. May increase by 1mg/kg IV/IM after 2 hrs. Max: 6mg/kg.	**BB:** Can lead to profound water and electrolyte depletion with excessive use. **W/P:** Monitor for fluid/electrolyte imbalance (eg, hypokalemia), renal or hepatic dysfunction. Initiate in hospital with hepatic cirrhosis and ascites. Tinnitus, hearing impairment, hyperglycemia, hyperuricemia reported. May activate SLE. Cross-sensitivity with sulfonamide allergy. Avoid excessive diuresis, especially in elderly. **Contra:** Anuria. **P/N:** Category C, caution in nursing.	Pancreatitis, jaundice, anorexia, paresthesias, ototoxicity, blood dyscrasias, dizziness, rash, urticaria, photosensitivity, fever, thrombophlebitis, restlessness.
Torsemide (Demadex)	**Inj:** 10mg/mL; **Tab:** 5mg*, 10mg*, 20mg*, 100mg* *scored	***Adults:*** **PO/IV** (bolus over 2 min or continuous): **CHF:** Initial: 10-20mg qd. Max: 200mg single dose. **Chronic Renal Failure:** Initial: 20mg qd. Max: 200mg single dose. **Hepatic Cirrhosis:** Initial: 5-10mg qd with aldosterone antagonist or K+-sparing diuretic. Titrate: Double dose. Max: 40mg single dose. **HTN:** Initial: 5mg qd. Titrate: May increase to 10mg qd in 4-6 weeks, then may add additional antihypertensive agent.	**W/P:** Caution with cirrhosis and ascites in hepatic disease. Tinnitus and hearing loss (usually reversible) reported. Avoid excessive diuresis, especially in elderly. Caution with brisk diuresis, inadequate oral intake of electrolytes, and cardiovascular disease, especially with digitalis glycosides. Monitor for electrolyte/volume depletion. Hyperglycemia, hypokalemia, hypermagnesemia, hypercalcemia, gout reported. May increase cholesterol and TG. **Contra:** Anuria, sulfonamide hypersensitivity. **P/N:** Category B, caution in nursing.	Headache, excessive urination, dizziness, cough, ECG abnormality, asthenia, rhinitis, diarrhea.
DIURETICS (Potassium-Sparing)				
Amiloride HCl*	**Tab:** 5mg	***Adults:*** Initial: 5mg qd. Titrate: Increase to 10mg/day. If hyperkalemia persists, may increase to 15mg/day then to 20mg/day with careful monitoring. Take with food.	**W/P:** Risk of hyperkalemia (≥5.5mEq/L) especially with renal impairment, elderly, DM; monitor levels frequently. D/C if hyperkalemia occurs. Caution in severely ill in whom respiratory or metabolic acidosis may occur; monitor acid-base balance frequently. Hepatic encephalopathy reported with severe hepatic disease. Increased BUN reported. D/C at least 3 days before glucose tolerance test. Monitor electrolytes and renal function in DM. **Contra:** Hyperkalemia, anuria, acute or chronic renal insufficiency, diabetic neuropathy, K⁺-sparing agents (eg, diuretics), and K⁺ supplements, K⁺ salt substitutes, K⁺-rich diet (except with severe hypokalemia). **P/N:** Category B, not for use in nursing.	Headache, nausea, anorexia, vomiting, elevated serum potassium, diarrhea, muscle cramps, impotence.

* Available only in generic form.
BB = black box warning; **W/P** = warnings/precautions; **Contra** = contraindications; **P/N** = pregnancy category rating and nursing considerations.

Table 13.2. Prescribing Information for Antihypertensive Agents

GENERIC (BRAND)	FORM/ STRENGTH	DOSAGE	WARNINGS/PRECAUTIONS & CONTRAINDICATIONS	ADVERSE REACTIONS
DIURETICS (Potassium-Sparing) *(Cont.)*				
Triamterene (Dyrenium)	Cap: 50mg, 100mg	**Adults:** Initial: 100mg bid pc. Max: 300mg/day.	**BB:** Abnormal elevation of serum K⁺ levels (≥5.5mEq/L) can occur with all K⁺-sparing agents, including triamterene. Hyperkalemia is more likely to occur with renal impairment and diabetes (even without evidence of renal impairment), and in the elderly, or severely ill. Monitor serum K⁺ at frequent intervals. **W/P:** Check ECG if hyperkalemia occurs. May cause decreased alkali reserve with possibility of metabolic acidosis, mild nitrogen retention. Monitor BUN periodically. May contribute to megaloblastosis in folic acid deficiency. Caution with gouty arthritis; may elevate uric acid levels. May aggravate or cause electrolyte imbalances in CHF, renal disease, or cirrhosis. Caution with history of renal stones. **Contra:** Anuria, severe or progressive kidney disease or dysfunction (except with nephrosis), severe hepatic disease, hyperkalemia, K⁺ supplements, K⁺ salt substitutes, K⁺-sparing agents (eg, diuretics). **P/N:** Category C, not for use in nursing.	Hypersensitivity reactions, hyper- or hypokalemia, azotemia, renal stones, jaundice, nausea, vomiting, diarrhea, weakness, dizziness.
DIURETICS (Thiazide)				
Chlorothiazide (Diuril)	Inj: 0.5g; Sus: 250mg/5mL [237mL]	**Adults: (PO/IV) Edema:** 0.5-1g qd-bid. May give every other day or 3-5 days/week. Substitute IV for oral using same dosage. **(PO) HTN:** 0.5-1g qd or in divided doses. Max: 2g/day. **Pediatrics: (PO) Diuresis/ HTN:** Usual: 10-20mg/kg/day given qd-bid. Max: **Infants up to 2 yrs:** 375mg/day. **2-12 yrs:** 1g/day. **<6 months:** Up to 15mg/kg bid may be required.	**W/P:** Caution in severe renal disease, liver dysfunction, electrolyte/fluid imbalance. Monitor electrolytes. Hyperuricemia, hyperglycemia, hypokalemia, hyponatremia, hypomagnesemia, hypercalcemia may occur. Increases in cholesterol and triglyceride levels reported. May exacerbate SLE. Sensitivity reactions reported. D/C prior to parathyroid test. Enhanced effects in post-sympathectomy patient. IV use not recommended in infants or children. **Contra:** Anuria, sulfonamide hypersensitivity. **P/N:** Category C, not for use in nursing.	Weakness, hypotension, pancreatitis, jaundice, diarrhea, vomiting, blood dyscrasias, rash, photosensitivity, electrolyte imbalance, impotence.
Chlorthalidone (Thalitone)	Tab: 15mg	**Adults: HTN:** Initial: 15mg qd. Titrate: May increase to 30mg qd, then to 45-50mg qd. **Edema:** Initial: 30-60mg/day or 60mg every other day, up to 90-120mg/day. Maint: May be lower than initial; adjust to patient. Take in the morning with food.	**W/P:** Caution in severe renal disease, liver dysfunction, allergy history, asthma. May exacerbate or activate SLE. Monitor for fluid and electrolyte imbalance. Hyperuricemia, hypomagnesemia, hypokalemia, hypercalcemia, hypophosphatemia, and hyperglycemia may occur. May manifest latent DM. **Contra:** Anuria, sulfonamide hypersensitivity. **P/N:** Category B, not for use in nursing.	Pancreatitis, jaundice, diarrhea, vomiting, constipation, nausea, blood dyscrasias, rash, photosensitivity, dizziness, headache, electrolyte disturbance, impotence.
Hydrochloro-thiazide*	Tab: 12.5mg, 25mg*, 50mg* *scored	**Adults: Edema:** 25-100mg qd or in divided doses. May give every other day or 3-5 days/week. **HTN:** Initial: 25mg qd. Titrate: May increase to 50mg/day. **Pediatrics: Diuresis/HTN:** 1-2mg/kg/day given qd-bid. Max: **Infants up to 2 yrs:** 37.5mg/day. **2-12 yrs:** 100mg/day. **<6 months:** Up to 1.5mg/kg bid may be required.	**W/P:** Caution in severe renal disease, liver dysfunction, electrolyte/fluid imbalance. Monitor electrolytes. Hyperuricemia, hyperglycemia, hypokalemia, hyponatremia, hypomagnesemia, hypercalcemia may occur. Increases in cholesterol and triglyceride levels reported. May exacerbate SLE. Sensitivity reactions reported. D/C prior to parathyroid test. Enhanced effects in post-sympathectomy patients. **Contra:** Anuria, sulfonamide hypersensitivity. **P/N:** Category B, not for use in nursing.	Weakness, hypotension, pancreatitis, jaundice, diarrhea, vomiting, blood dyscrasias, rash, photosensitivity, electrolyte imbalance, impotence.

* Available only in generic form.
BB = black box warning; **W/P** = warnings/precautions; **Contra** = contraindications; **P/N** = pregnancy category rating and nursing considerations.

Table 13.2. Prescribing Information for Antihypertensive Agents

GENERIC (BRAND)	FORM/ STRENGTH	DOSAGE	WARNINGS/PRECAUTIONS & CONTRAINDICATIONS	ADVERSE REACTIONS
Hydrochloro-thiazide (Microzide)	**Cap:** 12.5mg	**Adults:** Initial: 12.5mg qd. Max: 50mg/day.	**W/P:** Caution in severe renal disease, liver dysfunction, electrolyte/fluid imbalance. Monitor electrolytes. Hyperuricemia, hyperglycemia, hypokalemia, hyponatremia, hypomagnesemia, hypercalcemia may occur. Increases in cholesterol and triglyceride levels reported. May exacerbate SLE. Sensitivity reactions reported. D/C prior to parathyroid test. Enhanced effects in post-sympathectomy patient. **Contra:** Anuria, sulfonamide hypersensitivity. **P/N:** Category B, not for use in nursing.	Weakness, hypotension, pancreatitis, jaundice, diarrhea, vomiting, blood dyscrasias, rash, photosensitivity, electrolyte imbalance, impotence.
Indapamide (Lozol)	**Tab:** 1.25mg, 2.5mg	**Adults: HTN:** 1.25mg qam. Titrate: May increase to 2.5mg qd after 4 weeks, then to 5mg qd after another 4 weeks. Max: 5mg/day. **CHF:** 2.5mg qam. Titrate: May increase to 5mg qd after 1 week. Max: 5mg/day.	**W/P:** Caution in severe renal disease, liver dysfunction. May exacerbate or activate SLE. Monitor for fluid/electrolyte imbalance. Hyperuricemia, hypercalcemia, hypokalemia, hypophosphatemia, and hyperglycemia may occur. Monitor renal function, serum uric acid levels periodically. May precipitate gout. May manifest latent DM. Enhanced effects in post-sympathectomy patient. **Contra:** Anuria, sulfonamide hypersensitivity. **P/N:** Category B, not for use in nursing.	Headache, infection, pain, back pain, dizziness, rhinitis, fatigue, muscle cramps, nervousness, numbness of extremities, electrolyte imbalance, anxiety, agitation.
Methyclothiazide (Enduron)	**Tab:** 5mg* *scored	**Adults: Edema:** 2.5-10mg qd. Max: 10mg/dose. **HTN:** 2.5-5mg qd.	**W/P:** Caution in severe renal disease, liver dysfunction, electrolyte/fluid imbalance. Monitor electrolytes. Hyperuricemia, hyperglycemia, hypokalemia, hyponatremia, hypomagnesemia, hypercalcemia may occur. Increases in cholesterol and triglyceride levels reported. May exacerbate SLE. Sensitivity reactions reported. D/C prior to parathyroid test. Enhanced effects in post-sympathectomy patient. **Contra:** Anuria, sulfonamide hypersensitivity. **P/N:** Category B, not for use in nursing.	Headache, cramping, weakness, orthostatic hypotension, pancreatitis, hyperglycemia, hyperuricemia, electrolyte imbalance, blood dyscrasias, hypersensitivity reactions.
Metolazone (Zaroxolyn)	**Tab:** 2.5mg, 5mg, 10mg	**Adults: Edema:** 5-20mg qd. **HTN:** 2.5-5mg qd. **Elderly:** Start at low end of dosing range.	**BB:** Do not interchange rapid and complete bioavailability metolazone formulations for other slow and incomplete bioavailability metolazone formulations; they are not therapeutically equivalent. **W/P:** Risk of hypokalemia, orthostatic hypotension, hypercalcemia, hyperuricemia, azotemia and rapid onset hyponatremia. Cross-allergy with sulfonamide-derived drugs, thiazides, or quinethazone. Sensitivity reactions may occur with 1st dose. Monitor electrolytes. May cause hyperglycemia and glycosuria in diabetics. Caution in elderly or severe renal impairment. May exacerbate or activate SLE. **Contra:** Anuria, hepatic coma or precoma. **P/N:** Category B, not for use in nursing.	Chest pain/discomfort, orthostatic hypotension, syncope, neuropathy, necrotizing angiitis, hepatitis, jaundice, pancreatitis, blood dyscrasias, joint pain.
DIURETIC COMBINATIONS†				
Amiloride HCl/ Hydrochloro-thiazide*	**Tab:** (Amiloride-HCTZ) **Tab:** (Amiloride-HCTZ) 5mg-50mg* *scored	**Adults:** Initial: 1 tab qd. Titrate: May increase to 2 tabs qd or in divided doses. Max: 2 tabs/day. May give intermittently once diuresis is achieved. Take with food.	**W/P:** Risk of hyperkalemia (≥5.5mEq/L) especially with renal impairment or DM; d/c if hyperkalemia occurs. Monitor for fluid/electrolyte imbalance; hyponatremia and hypochloremia may occur. Caution in severely ill (risk of respiratory or metabolic acidosis). Increases BUN, cholesterol, and TG levels. D/C at least 3 days before glucose tolerance test. May precipitate gout or exacerbate SLE. May precipitate azotemia with renal disease. **Contra:** Hyperkalemia,	Nausea, anorexia, rash, headache, weakness, hyperkalemia, dizziness.

* Available only in generic form. † More combination products are on page 187 (α-Antagonist Combinations), page 192 (ACE Inhibitor Combinations), page 197 (ARBs Combinations), page 202 (Beta-Blocker Combinations), and page 209 (Direct Renin Inhibitor & Combination).
BB = black box warning; **W/P** = warnings/precautions; **Contra** = contraindications; **P/N** = pregnancy category rating and nursing considerations.

Table 13.2. Prescribing Information for Antihypertensive Agents

GENERIC (BRAND)	FORM/ STRENGTH	DOSAGE	WARNINGS/PRECAUTIONS & CONTRAINDICATIONS	ADVERSE REACTIONS
DIURETIC COMBINATIONS *(Cont.)*				
Amiloride HCl/ Hydrochlorothiazide* *(Cont.)*			anuria, sulfonamide hypersensitivity, acute or chronic renal insufficiency, diabetic neuropathy. Concomitant K⁺-sparing agents (eg, spironolactone, triamterene), K⁺ supplements, salt substitutes, K⁺-rich diet (except with severe hypokalemia). **P/N:** Category B, not for use in nursing.	
Chlorthalidone/ Clonidine HCl (Clorpres)	**Tab:** (Clonidine-Chlorthalidone) 0.1mg-15mg*, 0.2mg-15mg*, 0.3mg-15mg* *scored	**Adults:** Determine dose by individual titration. 0.1mg clonidine-15mg chlorthalidone tab qd-bid; Max: 0.6 mg clonidine-30mg chlorthalidone/day.	**W/P:** Caution with severe renal disease, hepatic dysfunction, asthma, severe coronary insufficiency, recent MI, cerebrovascular disease. May develop allergic reaction to oral clonidine if sensitive to clonidine patch. Avoid abrupt withdrawal. Continue therapy to within 4 hrs of surgery and resume after. Monitor for fluid/electrolyte imbalance. Hyperuricemia, hypokalemia, hyponatremia, hypochloremic alkalosis, and hyperglycemia may occur. **Contra:** Anuria, sulfonamide hypersensitivity. **P/N:** (Clonidine) Category C, caution in nursing. (Chlorthalidone) Category B, not for use in nursing.	Drowsiness, dizziness, constipation, sedation, nausea, vomiting, blood dyscrasias, hypersensitivity reactions, orthostatic symptoms, impotence.
Spironolactone/ Hydrochlorothiazide (Aldactazide)	**Tab:** (Spironolactone-HCTZ) 25mg-25mg, 50mg-50mg* *scored	**Adults: Edema:** 100mg/day per component qd or in divided doses. **Maint:** 25-200mg/day per component. **HTN:** 50-100mg/day per component qd or in divided doses.	**BB:** Tumorigenic in chronic toxicity animal studies; avoid unnecessary use. Not for initial therapy. **W/P:** Monitor for fluid/ electrolyte imbalance. Caution with renal and hepatic dysfunction. Hyperchloremic metabolic acidosis reported with decompensated hepatic cirrhosis. Mild acidosis, gynecomastia, transient BUN elevation, hypercalcemia, hyperglycemia, hyperuricemia, hypomagnesemia, and sensitivity reactions may occur. D/C if hyperkalemia occurs. Risk of dilutional hyponatremia. Enhanced effects in post-sympathectomy patient. May increase cholesterol and TG levels. May manifest latent DM. **Contra:** Acute renal impairment, significantly impaired renal excretory function, hyperkalemia, acute or severe hepatic dysfunction, anuria, sulfonamide hypersensitivity. **P/N:** Category C, not for use in nursing.	Gastric bleeding, ulceration, gynecomastia, impotence, agranulocytosis, fever, urticaria, confusion, ataxia, renal dysfunction, blood dyscrasias, electrolyte disturbances, weakness, irregular menses, amenorrhea.
Triamterene/ Hydrochlorothiazide (Dyazide)	**Cap:** (Triamterene-HCTZ) 37.5mg-25mg	**Adults:** 1-2 caps qd.	**W/P:** Risk of hyperkalemia (≥5.5mEq/L) especially with renal impairment, elderly, DM or severely ill; monitor levels frequently. Caution in severely ill in whom respiratory or metabolic acidosis may occur; monitor acid-base balance frequently. May manifest DM. Caution with hepatic dysfunction, history of renal stones. Increases uric acid levels, BUN, creatinine. May decrease PBI levels. D/C before parathyroid function tests. May potentiate electrolyte imbalance with heart failure, renal disease, cirrhosis. **Contra:** Hyperkalemia, anuria, acute or chronic renal insufficiency, sulfonamide hypersensitivity, diabetic neuropathy, K⁺-sparing agents (eg, diuretics), K⁺ supplements (except with severe hypokalemia), K⁺ salt substitutes, K⁺-rich diet. **P/N:** Category C, not for use in nursing.	Muscle cramps, GI effects, weakness, blood dyscrasias, arrhythmia, impotence, dry mouth, jaundice, paresthesia, renal stones, hypersensitivity reactions.

* Available only in generic form.
BB = black box warning; **W/P** = warnings/precautions; **Contra** = contraindications; **P/N** = pregnancy category rating and nursing considerations.

Table 13.2. Prescribing Information for Antihypertensive Agents

GENERIC (BRAND)	FORM/ STRENGTH	DOSAGE	WARNINGS/PRECAUTIONS & CONTRAINDICATIONS	ADVERSE REACTIONS
Triamterene/ hydrochloro-thiazide (Maxzide/ Maxzide-25)	(Triamterene-HCTZ) **Tab:** (Maxzide) 75mg-50mg*, (Maxzide-25) 37.5mg-25mg* *scored	***Adults:*** (37.5mg-25mg tab) 1-2 tabs qd. (75mg-50mg tab) 1 tab qd.	**W/P:** Risk of hyperkalemia (≥5.5mEq/L) especially with renal impairment, elderly, DM or severely ill; monitor levels frequently. Check ECG if hyperkalemia occurs. Caution with history of renal lithiasis, hepatic dysfunction. Monitor BUN and creatinine periodically. D/C if azotemia increases. May contribute to megaloblastosis in folic acid deficiency. Hyperuricemia, hypercalcemia, hypophosphatemia, hypokalemia may occur. May manifest latent DM. May decrease serum PBI levels. Monitor for fluid/electrolyte imbalance. **Contra:** Hyperkalemia, anuria, acute or chronic renal insufficiency, sulfonamide hypersensitivity, diabetic neuropathy, K⁺-sparing agents (eg, diuretics), K⁺ supplements, K⁺ salt substitutes, K⁺-rich diet. **P/N:** Category C, not for use **P/N:** Category C, not for use in nursing.	Jaundice, pancreatitis, nausea, vomiting, taste alteration, drowsiness, anxiety, tachycardia, dry mouth, depression, blood dyscrasias, electrolyte disturbances.
VASODILATORS				
Hydralazine HCl*	**Inj:** 20mg/mL; **Tab:** 10mg, 25mg, 50mg, 100mg	***Adults:*** Initial: 10mg qid for 2-4 days. Titrate: Increase to 25mg qid for the rest of the week, then increase to 50mg qid. Maint: Use lowest effective dose. **Resistant Patients:** 300mg/day or titrate to lower dose combined with thiazide diuretic and/or reserpine, or β-blocker. **Pediatrics:** Initial: 0.75mg/kg/day given qid. Titrate: Increase gradually over 3-4 weeks to a max of 7.5mg/kg/day or 200mg/day.	**W/P:** D/C if SLE symptoms occur. May cause angina and ECG changes of MI. Caution with suspected CAD, CVA, advanced renal impairment. May increase pulmonary artery pressure in mitral valvular disease. Postural hypotension reported. Add pyridoxine if peripheral neuritis develops. Monitor CBC and ANA titer before and periodically during therapy. **Contra:** CAD and mitral valvular rheumatic heart disease. **P/N:** Category C, safety in nursing not known.	Headache, anorexia, nausea, vomiting, diarrhea, tachycardia, angina.
Isosorbide dinitrate (Isordil, Isordil titradose)	**Tab:** 5mg*, 10mg*, 20mg*, 30mg*; **Tab, Extended-Release:** 40mg; **Tab, Sublingual:** 2.5mg *scored	***Adults:*** **Prevention:** Initial: 5-20mg bid-tid. Maint: 10-40mg bid-tid. Allow a dose-free interval of at least 14 hrs for both formulations. **Elderly:** Start at low end of dosing range.	**W/P:** Not for use with acute MI or CHF. Severe hypotension may occur. May aggravate angina caused by hypertrophic cardiomyopathy. Caution with volume depletion, hypotension, elderly. Monitor for tolerance. **P/N:** Category C, caution in nursing.	Headache, lightheadedness, hypotension, syncope, rebound HTN.
Isosorbide mononitrate (Imdur)	**Tab, Extended-Release:** 30mg*, 60mg*, 120mg *scored	***Adults:*** Initial: 30-60mg qd in am. Titrate: May increase after several days to 120mg/day. Swallow whole with fluids. **Elderly:** Start at lower end of dosing range.	**W/P:** Not for use with acute MI or CHF. Severe hypotension may occur; caution with volume depletion and hypotension. Hypotension may increase angina pectoris. May aggravate angina caused by hypertrophic cardiomyopathy. Monitor for tolerance. May interfere with cholesterol test. **P/N:** Category B, caution with nursing.	Headache, dizziness, hypotension.
Isosorbide mononitrate (Ismo)	**Tab:** 20mg* *scored	***Adults:*** 20mg bid; first dose on awakening, then 7 hrs later.	**W/P:** Not for use with acute MI or CHF. Severe hypotension may occur. May aggravate angina caused by hypertrophic cardiomyopathy. Caution with volume depletion and hypotension. Monitor for tolerance. **P/N:** Category C, caution in nursing.	Headache, dizziness, nausea, vomiting.
Minoxidil*	**Tab:** 2.5mg*, 10mg* *scored	***Adults:*** Initial: 5mg qd. Titrate: Increase by no less than 3 days; may increase every 6 hrs if closely monitored. Usual: 10-40mg/day. Max: 100mg/day. Frequency: Give qd if diastolic BP is reduced to <30mmHg and if reduced to >30mmHg give bid. Give with a diuretic (eg, HCTZ 50mg bid, furosemide 40mg bid) and a β-blocker (equivalent to propranolol 80-160mg/day) or methyldopa (250-750mg bid starting	**BB:** May cause pericardial effusion, occasionally progressing to tamponade, and angina pectoris may be exacerbated. Only for nonresponders to maximum therapeutic doses of two other antihypertensives and a diuretic. Administer under supervision with a β-blocker and diuretic. Monitor in hospital for a decrease in BP in those receiving guanethidine with malignant hypertension. **W/P:** Administer with a	Salt and water retention, pericarditis, pericardial effusion, tamponade, hypertrichosis, nausea, vomiting, rash, ECG changes, hemodilution effects.

* Available only in generic form.
BB = black box warning; **W/P** = warnings/precautions; **Contra** = contraindications; **P/N** = pregnancy category rating and nursing considerations.

Table 13.2. Prescribing Information for Antihypertensive Agents

GENERIC (BRAND)	FORM/ STRENGTH	DOSAGE	WARNINGS/PRECAUTIONS & CONTRAINDICATIONS	ADVERSE REACTIONS
VASODILATORS *(Cont.)*				
Minoxidil* *(Cont.)*		24 hrs before therapy). **Renal Failure/ Dialysis:** Reduce dose. *Pediatrics:* **>12 yrs:** Initial: 5mg qd. Titrate: Increase by no less than 3 days; may increase every 6 hrs if closely monitored. Usual: 10-40mg/day. Max: 100mg/day. Frequency: Give qd if diastolic BP is reduced to <30mmHg and if reduced to >30mmHg give bid. Give with a diuretic (eg, HCTZ 50mg bid, furosemide 40mg bid) and a β-blocker (equivalent to propranolol 80-160mg/day) or methyldopa (250-750mg bid starting 24 hrs before therapy). **<12 yrs:** 0.2mg/kg qd. Titrate: May increase by 50-100% increments. Usual: 0.25-1mg/kg/day. Max: 50mg/day. **Renal Failure/Dialysis:** Reduce dose.	diuretic and β-blocker. Pericarditis, pericardial effusion and tamponade reported. With renal failure or dialysis, reduce dose to prevent renal failure exacerbation and precipitation of cardiac failure. Avoid rapid control with severe HTN. Monitor body weight, fluid and electrolyte balance. Extreme caution with post-MI. Hypersensitivity reactions reported. **Contra:** Pheochromocytoma. **P/N:** Category C, not for use in nursing.	
VASODILATOR COMBINATION				
Hydralazine HCl/ Isosorbide dinitrate (BiDil)	**Tab:** (Hydralazine-Isosorbide) 37.5mg-20mg	*Adults:* Initial: 1 tab tid. Max: 2 tabs tid.	**W/P:** May produce a clinical picture simulating systemic lupus erythematosus including glomerulonephritis. May cause symptomatic hypotension, tachycardia, peripheral neuritis. Caution in patients with acute MI, hemodynamic and clinical monitoring recommended. May aggravate angina associated with hypertrophic cardiomyopathy. **Contra:** Allergies to organic nitrates. **P/N:** Category C, caution in nursing.	Headache, dizziness, chest pain, asthenia, nausea, bronchitis, hypotension, sinusitis, ventricular tachycardia, palpitations, hyperglycemia, rhinitis, paresthesia, vomiting, amblyopia, hyperlipidemia.
MISCELLANEOUS				
Clonidine** (Catapres, Catapres-TTS)	**Patch, Extended-Release** (TTS): 0.1mg/24 hr [4*], 0.2mg/24 hr [4*], 0.3mg/24 hr [4*]; **Tab:** 0.1mg*, 0.2mg*, 0.3mg* *scored	*Adults:* **(Patch)** Apply to hairless, intact area of upper arm or chest weekly. Taper withdrawal of previous antihypertensive. Initial: 0.1mg/24 hr patch weekly. Titrate: May increase after 1-2 weeks. Max: 0.6mg/24 hr. **(Tab)** Initial: 0.1mg bid. Titrate: May increase by 0.1mg weekly. Usual: 0.2-0.6mg/day in divided doses. Max: 2.4mg/day. **(Patch, Tab) Renal Impairment:** Adjust according to degree of impairment.	**W/P:** Avoid abrupt discontinuation. Tabs may cause rash if have allergic reaction to patch. Continue tabs to within 4 hrs of surgery resume and as soon as possible thereafter. Do not remove patch for surgery. Caution with severe coronary insufficiency, conduction disturbances, recent MI, cerebrovascular disease or chronic renal failure. Remove patch before defibrillation or cardioversion due to the potential risk of altered electrical conductivity or MRI due to the occurrence of burns. **P/N:** Category C, caution in nursing.	Dry mouth, drowsiness, dizziness, constipation, sedation, impotence/ sexual dysfunction, nausea, vomiting, alopecia, weakness, orthostatic symptoms, nervousness, localized skin reactions (patch).
Fenoldopam mesylate (Corlopam)	**Inj:** 10mg/mL	*Adults:* Range: Initial: 0.01-0.8 mcg/kg/min IV. Titrate: Increase/decrease by 0.05-0.1mcg/kg/min no more frequently than every 15 min. May use for up to 48 hrs. Refer to PI for detailed dosing info. *Pediatrics:* **<1 month-12 years:** Initial: 0.2mcg/kg/min. May increase dose every 20-30 min up to 0.3-0.5 mcg/kg/min. Refer to PI for detailed dosing info.	**W/P:** Contains sodium metabisulfite; may cause allergic-type reactions especially in asthmatics. Caution in glaucoma or intraocular HTN. Dose-related tachycardia reported. Symptomatic hypotension may occur; monitor BP. Avoid hypotension with acute cerebral infarction or hemorrhage. Hypokalemia reported; monitor serum electrolytes. **P/N:** Category B, caution in nursing.	Headache, nausea, flushing, extrasystoles, palpitations, bradycardia, heart failure, elevated BUN/glucose/ transaminase, chest pain, leukocytosis, bleeding, dyspnea.
Guanfacine HCl (Tenex)	**Tab:** 1mg, 2mg	*Adults:* 1mg qhs. Titrate: May increase to 2mg qhs after 3-4 weeks. Max: 3mg/day.	**W/P:** Caution with severe coronary insufficiency, recent MI, cerebrovascular disease, chronic renal or hepatic failure. Avoid abrupt discontinuation. Dose-related drowsiness and sedation. **P/N:** Category B, caution with nursing.	Dry mouth, somnolence, asthenia, dizziness, constipation, impotence, headache.

* Available only in generic form.
** Combination information for clonidine/chlorthalidone (Clorpres) is on page 214.
W/P = warnings/precautions; **Contra** = contraindications; **P/N** = pregnancy category rating and nursing considerations.

Table 13.2. Prescribing Information for Antihypertensive Agents

GENERIC (BRAND)	FORM/ STRENGTH	DOSAGE	WARNINGS/PRECAUTIONS & CONTRAINDICATIONS	ADVERSE REACTIONS
Mecamylamine HCl (Inversine)	Tab: 2.5mg	*Adults:* Initial: 2.5mg bid after meals. Titrate: Increase by 2.5mg/day at intervals of not less than 2 days. Usual: 25mg/day given tid. Give larger doses at noontime and evening. Reduce dose by 50% with thiazides.	W/P: Caution with renal, cerebral, or cardiovascular dysfunction, marked cerebral or coronary insufficiency, prostatic hypertrophy, bladder neck obstruction, urethral stricture. Large doses in cerebral or renal insufficiency may produce CNS effects. Withdraw gradually and add other antihypertensives. May be potentiated by excessive heat, fever, infection, hemorrhage, pregnancy, anesthesia, surgery, vigorous exercise, other antihypertensive drugs, alcohol, salt depletion. D/C if paralytic ileus occurs. Contra: Coronary insufficiency, recent MI, uremia, glaucoma, organic pyloric stenosis, uncooperative patients, mild to moderate or labile HTN, with antibiotics or sulfonamides. Administer with great discretion in renal insufficiency. P/N: Category C, not for use in nursing.	Ileus, constipation, vomiting, nausea, anorexia, dryness of mouth, syncope, postural hypotension, convulsions, tremor, interstitial pulmonary edema, urinary retention, impotence, blurred vision.
Methyldopa*	Tab: 125mg, 250mg, 500mg	*Adults:* Initial: 250mg bid-tid for 48 hrs. Adjust dose at intervals of not less than 2 days. Maint: 500mg-2g/day given bid-qid. Max: 3g/day. Concomitant **Antihypertensives (other than thiazides):** Initial: Limit to 500mg/day. **Renal Impairment:** May respond to lower doses. *Pediatrics:* Initial: 10mg/kg/day given bid-qid. Max: 65mg/kg/day or 3g/day, whichever is less.	W/P: Positive Coombs test, hemolytic anemia, and liver disorders may occur. Fever reported within the first 3 weeks of therapy. HTN has recurred after dialysis. Caution with liver disease or dysfunction. D/C if signs of heart failure, or involuntary choreoathetotic movements develop. Edema and weight gain reported. Blood count, Coombs test and LFTs prior to therapy and periodically thereafter. Contra: Active hepatic disease, history of methyldopa associated liver disorder, concomitant MAOIs. P/N: Category B, caution in nursing.	Sedation, headache, asthenia, edema/weight gain, hepatic disorders, vomiting, diarrhea, nausea, sore or black tongue, blood dyscrasias, BUN increase, gynecomastia, impotence.
Phenoxybenza-mine HCl (Dibenzyline)	Cap: 10mg	*Adults:* Initial: 10mg bid. Titrate: Increase every other day to 20-40mg bid-tid, until BP is controlled.	W/P: Caution with marked cerebral or coronary arteriosclerosis, or renal damage. May aggravate symptoms of respiratory infections. Contra: Conditions where fall in BP may be undesirable. P/N: Category C, not for use in nursing.	Postural hypotension, tachycardia, ejaculation nhibition, nasal congestion, miosis, GI irritation, drowsiness, fatigue.
Reserpine*	Tab: 0.1mg, 0.25mg	*Adults:* HTN: Initial: 0.5mg/day for 1-2 weeks. Maint: reduce to 0.1-0.25mg/day. **Psychotic Disorders:** Initial: 0.5mg/day. Range: 0.1-1mg/day.	W/P: Caution with renal insufficiency. May cause depression; d/c at 1st sign. Caution with history of peptic ulcer, ulcerative colitis, or gallstones. Contra: Active or history of mental depression, active peptic ulcer, ulcerative colitis, current electroconvulsive therapy. P/N: Category C, not for use in nursing.	GI effects, dry mouth, hypersecretion, arrhythmia, syncope, edema, dyspnea, muscle aches, dizziness, depression, nervousness, impotence, gynecomastia, rash.

* Available only in generic form.
BB = black box warning; **W/P** = warnings/precautions; **Contra** = contraindications; **P/N** = pregnancy category rating and nursing considerations.

Table 13.3. Drug Interactions for Antihypertensive Agents

ALPHA ANTAGONISTS

Prazosin HCl (Minipress)

Alcohol	Concomitant use may cause dizziness or syncope.
Antihypertensive agents	Concomitant use produces additive hypotensive effects.
Beta-blockers	Concomitant use produces additive hypotensive effects.
Diuretics	Concomitant use produces additive hypotensive effects.

Terazosin HCl (Hytrin)

Antihypertensive agents	Risk of significant hypotension with concomitant use; may require dosage adjustment or retitration of either agent.
Verapamil	Concomitant use may increase levels of terazosin.

ALPHA ANTAGONIST COMBINATION

Prazosin HCl-Polythiazide (Minizide)

ACTH	Increased risk of hypokalemia with concomitant use.
Alcohol	May potentiate orthostatic hypotension.
Antihypertensive drugs	May potentiate effects of antihypertensive drugs.
Barbiturates	May potentiate orthostatic hypotension.
Corticosteroids	Increased risk of hypokalemia with concomitant use.
Ganglionic or peripheral adrenergic blockers	Potentiation with ganglionic or peripheral adrenergic blockers.
Insulin	Concomitant use may alter insulin requirements.
Narcotics analgesics	May potentiate orthostatic hypotension.
Norepinephrine	May decrease arterial responsiveness to norepinephrine.
Tubocurarine	May increase responsiveness to tubocurarine.

ALPHA- AND BETA-BLOCKERS

Carvedilol (Coreg, Coreg CR)

Alcohol	May affect release properties of extended release caps; separate administration by >2 hrs.
Anesthetic agents (eg, ether, cyclopropane, trichloroethylene)	Caution with anesthetic agents that depress myocardium function.
Antidiabetic drugs (eg, insulins, oral hypoglycemic drugs)	May potentiate hypoglycemic effect of antidiabetic drugs; monitor blood glucose levels.
Calcium channel blockers (eg, verapamil, diltiazem)	Caution with calcium channel blockers that depress myocardial function; monitor ECG and blood pressure.
Catecholamine-depleting drugs (eg, reserpine, MAOIs)	Monitor for hypotension and bradycardia with concomitant use.

Table 13.3. Drug Interactions for Antihypertensive Agents

Cimetidine	May increase the AUC of carvedilol.
Clonidine	May potentiate blood pressure and heart rate lowering effects; carvedilol should be discontinued followed by discontinuation of clonidine gradually over several days.
Cyclosporine	Monitor cycloporine levels.
CYP2D6 inhibitors (eg, quinidine, fluoxetine, paroxetine, and propafenone)	May increase blood levels of carvedilol.
Digitalis glycosides	May increase the risk of bradycardia; monitor digoxin levels.
Rifampin	May reduce plasma levels of carvedilol.
Labetalol HCl (Trandate)	
Antidiabetic drugs (eg, insulins, oral hypoglycemic drugs)	Concomitant use may require dosage adjustment of antidiabetic drugs.
Beta-receptor agonist drugs (bronchodilators)	May blunt the bronchodilator effect in beta-receptor agonist drugs.
Calcium channel blockers (eg, verapamil)	Caution with concomitant use.
Cimetidine	Increases the bioavailability of cimetidine; may need to reduce dose of labetalol.
Halothane	Produces synergistic effects with concomitant use.
Nitroglycerin	Blunts the reflex tachycardia produced by nitroglycerin without preventing its hypotensive effect; may produce additional antihypertensive effects if angina pectoris is present.
Tricyclic antidepressants	May experience an increased amount of tremors with concomitant use.

ANGIOTENSIN CONVERTING ENZYME (ACE) INHIBITORS

Benazepril HCl (Lotensin)	
Diuretics	Risk of hypotension risk with concomitant use.
Lithium	May increase serum lithium levels.
Potassium-containing salt substitutes	May increase the risk of hyperkalemia; monitor serum potassium levels.
Potassium-sparing diuretics (eg, spironolactone, triamterene, amiloride)	May increase the risk of hyperkalemia; monitor serum potassium levels.
Potassium supplements	May increase the risk of hyperkalemia; monitor serum potassium levels.
Captopril (Capoten)	
Adrenergic blocking agents	Caution with concomitant use.
Antihypertensive drugs (eg, thiazides)	Augments the antihypertensive effect of captopril.
Ganglionic blocking agents	Caution with concomitant use.

Table 13.3. Drug Interactions for Antihypertensive Agents

Lithium	May increase serum lithium levels; monitor levels.
NSAIDs	May reduce the antihypertensive effects of captopril.
Potassium-containing salt substitutes	May increase the risk of hyperkalemia; monitor serum potassium levels.
Potassium-sparing diuretics (eg, spironolactone, triamterene, amiloride)	May increase the risk of hyperkalemia; monitor serum potassium levels.
Potassium supplements	May increase the risk of hyperkalemia; monitor serum potassium levels.
Vasodilator drugs (eg, nitroglycerin, other nitrates)	Caution with concomitant use.
Enalapril maleate (Vasotec)	
Antihypertensive drugs (eg, diuretics)	Augments the antihypertensive effect of enalapril.
Diuretics	Risk of hypotension with concominant use.
Lithium	May increase serum lithium levels; monitor levels.
NSAIDs	May diminish the antihypertensive effects of enalapril; may further decrease renal function in patients with compromised renal function.
Potassium-containing salt substitutes	May increase the risk of hyperkalemia; monitor serum potassium levels.
Potassium-sparing diuretics (eg, spironolactone, triamterene, amiloride)	May increase the risk of hyperkalemia; monitor serum potassium levels.
Potassium supplements	May increase the risk of hyperkalemia; monitor serum potassium levels.
Enalaprilat (Vasotec I.V.)	
Antihypertensive drugs (eg, diuretics)	Augments the antihypertensive effect of enalaprilat.
Diuretics	Risk of hypotension with concomitant use.
Lithium	May increase serum lithium levels; monitor levels.
NSAIDs	May diminish the antihypertensive effects enalaprilat; may further decrease renal function in patients with compromised renal function.
Potassium-containing salt substitutes	May increase the risk of hyperkalemia; monitor serum potassium levels.
Potassium-sparing diuretics (eg, spironolactone, triamterene, amiloride)	May increase the risk of hyperkalemia; monitor serum potassium levels.
Potassium supplements	May increase the risk of hyperkalemia; monitor serum potassium levels.
Fosinopril sodium (Monopril)	
Antacids	Decreases absorption of fosinopril; separate dosing by 2 hrs.
Diuretics	Risk of hypotension with concomitant use.

Table 13.3. Drug Interactions for Antihypertensive Agents

Lithium	May increase serum lithium levels.
Potassium-containing salt substitutes	May increase the risk of hyperkalemia; monitor serum potassium levels.
Potassium-sparing diuretics (eg, spironolactone, triamterene, amiloride)	May increase the risk of hyperkalemia; monitor serum potassium levels.
Potassium supplements	May increase the risk of hyperkalemia; monitor serum potassium levels.
Lisinopril (Prinivil, Zestril)	
COX-2 Inhibitors	May diminish the antihypertensive effects of lisinopril; may further decrease renal function in patients with compromised renal function.
Diuretics	Risk of hypotension with concomitant use.
Gold, injectable (sodium aurothiomalate)	Nitroid reactions have been reported rarely in patients on therapy with injectable gold and concomitant therapy with ACE inhibitors
Hypoglycemic drugs, oral	Concomitant use with antidiabetic medications may increase risk of hypoglycemia.
Indomethacin	May reduce antihypertensive effects of lisinopril.
Insulin	Concomitant use with insulin may increase risk of hypoglycemia.
Lithium	May increase serum lithium levels; monitor levels.
NSAIDs	May diminish the antihypertensive effects of lisinopril; may further decrease renal function in patients with compromised renal function.
Potassium-containing salt substitutes	May increase the risk of hyperkalemia; monitor serum potassium levels.
Potassium-sparing diuretics (eg, spironolactone, eplerenone, triamterene, amiloride)	May increase the risk of hyperkalemia; monitor serum potassium levels.
Potassium supplements	May increase the risk of hyperkalemia; monitor serum potassium levels.
Moexipril HCl (Univasc)	
Diuretics	Risk of hypotension with concomitant use.
Lithium	May increase serum lithium levels; monitor levels.
Potassium-containing salt substitutes	May increase the risk of hyperkalemia; monitor serum potassium levels.
Potassium-sparing diuretics (eg, spironolactone, triamterene, amiloride)	May increase the risk of hyperkalemia; monitor serum potassium levels.
Potassium supplements	May increase the risk of hyperkalemia; monitor serum potassium levels.
Perindopril erbumine (Aceon)	
Diuretics	Risk of hypotension with concomitant use.
Gentamicin	Caution with concomitant use.
Lithium	May increase serum lithium levels; monitor levels.
Potassium-containing salt substitutes	May increase the risk of hyperkalemia; monitor serum potassium levels.

Table 13.3. Drug Interactions for Antihypertensive Agents

Potassium-sparing diuretics (eg, spironolactone, triamterene, amiloride)	May increase the risk of hyperkalemia; monitor serum potassium levels.
Potassium supplements	May increase the risk of hyperkalemia; monitor serum potassium levels.
Quinapril HCl (Accupril)	
Diuretics	Risk of hypotension risk with concomitant use.
Lithium	May increase serum lithium levels; monitor levels.
Magnesium	Caution with use of drugs that interact with magnesium.
Potassium-containing salt substitutes	May increase the risk of hyperkalemia; monitor serum potassium levels.
Potassium-sparing diuretics (eg, spironolactone, triamterene, amiloride)	May increase the risk of hyperkalemia; monitor serum potassium levels.
Potassium supplements	May increase the risk of hyperkalemia; monitor serum potassium levels.
Tetracycline	Decreases the absorption of tetracycline, may be due to a reaction with magnesium that is contained within quinapril.
Ramipril (Altace)	
Diuretics	Risk of hypotension with concomitant use.
Lithium	May increase serum lithium levels; monitor levels.
NSAIDs	May worsen renal failure and increase serum potassium.
Potassium-containing salt substitutes	May increase the risk of hyperkalemia; monitor serum potassium levels.
Potassium-sparing diuretics (eg, spironolactone, triamterene, amiloride)	May increase the risk of hyperkalemia; monitor serum potassium levels.
Potassium supplements	May increase the risk of hyperkalemia; monitor serum potassium levels.
Trandolapril (Mavik)	
Diuretics	Risk of hypotension with concomitant use.
Lithium	May increase serum lithium levels; monitor levels.
Potassium-containing salt substitutes	May increase the risk of hyperkalemia; monitor serum potassium levels.
Potassium-sparing diuretics (eg, spironolactone, triamterene, amiloride)	May increase the risk of hyperkalemia; monitor serum potassium levels.
Potassium supplements	May increase the risk of hyperkalemia; monitor serum potassium levels.

ACE INHIBITOR COMBINATIONS

Benazepril HCl-Hydrochlorothiazide (Lotensin HCT)	
Cholestyramine	Reduces the absorption of hydrochlorothiazide.
Colestipol	Reduces the absorption of hydrochlorothiazide.
Insulin	May alter insulin requirements.

Table 13.3. Drug Interactions for Antihypertensive Agents

Lithium	Risk of lithium toxicity; monitor serum lithium levels.
Norephinephrine	May decrease arterial responsiveness to norepinephrine.
NSAIDs	May reduce the diuretic, natriuretic, and antihypertensive effects of hydrochlorothiazide.
Potassium-sparing diuretics (eg, spironolactone, triamterene, amiloride)	May increase the risk of hyperkalemia; monitor serum potassium levels.
Potassium supplements	May increase the risk of hyperkalemia; monitor serum potassium levels.
Tubocurarine	May increase responsiveness to tubocurarine.
Captopril-Hydrochlorothiazide (Capozide)	
ACTH	May intensify electrolyte imbalance, particularly hypokalemia; monitor potassium levels.
Adrenergic blocking agents	Caution with concomitant use.
Alcohol	May potentiate orthostatic hypotension with concomitant use.
Amphotercin B	May intensify electrolyte imbalance, particularly hypokalemia; monitor potassium levels.
Anesthetics	May potentiate effects of anesthetics.
Anticoagulant drugs	May require dosage adjustment; hydrochlorothiazide may decrease anticoagulant effect.
Antidiabetic drugs (eg, oral hypoglycemic drugs, insulin)	May require dosage adjustment of antidiabetic drugs; hydrochlorothiazide may elevate blood glucose levels.
Antigout drugs	May require dosage adjustment; hydrochlorothiazide may raise uric acid blood levels.
Antihypertensive drugs	May require dosage adjustment; hydrochlorothiazide may potentiate antihypertensive effect.
Barbiturates	May potentiate orthostatic hypotension with concomitant use.
Calcium salts	Concomitant use increases serum calcium levels; monitor levels.
Cardiac glycosides	May potentiate the possibility of digitalis toxicity; monitor serum potassium levels.
Cholestyramine	Reduces the absorption of hydrochlorothiazide.
Colestipol	Reduces the absorption of hydrochlorothiazide.
Corticosteroids	May intensify electrolyte imbalance, particularly hypokalemia; monitor potassium levels.
Diazoxide	Concomitant use potentiates hyperglycemic, hyperuricemic, and antihypertensive effects; monitor blood glucose and serum uric acid levels.
Ganglionic blocking agents	Caution with concomitant use.
Lithium	Risk of lithium toxicity; monitor serum lithium levels.
MAO inhibitors	Potentiates hypotensive effects with concomitant use.
Methenamine	May decrease effects of methenamine.

Table 13.3. Drug Interactions for Antihypertensive Agents

Muscle relaxants, nondepolarizing (eg, tubocurarine)	May potentiate effects of nondepolarizing muscle relaxants.
Narcotic analgesics	May potentiate orthostatic hypotension with concomitant use.
NSAIDs (eg, indomethacin)	May reduce the diuretic, natriuretic, and antihypertensive effects of hydrochlorothiazide.
Potassium-containing salt substitutes	May increase the risk of hyperkalemia; monitor serum potassium levels.
Potassium-sparing diuretics (eg, spironolactone, triamterene, amiloride)	May increase the risk of hyperkalemia; monitor serum potassium levels.
Potassium supplements	May increase the risk of hyperkalemia; monitor serum potassium levels.
Pressor amines (eg, norephinephrine)	May decrease response to pressor amines.
Probenecid	Hydrochlorothiazide may produce hyperuricemic effects; dosage adjustment of probenecid may be necessary.
Sulfinpyrazone	Hydrochlorothiazide may produce hyperuricemic effects; dosage adjustment of sulfinpyrazone may be necessary.
Vasodilators (eg, nigtroglycerin, other nitrates)	Discontinue use with vasodilators prior to initiation of therapy; caution should be used and vasodilator dose should be decreased if therapy is resumed.
Enalapril maleate-Hydrochlorothiazide (Vaseretic)	
ACTH	Intensifies electrolyte depletion, particularly hypokalemia.
Alcohol	May potentiate orthostatic hypotension.
Antidiabetic drugs (eg, oral hypoglycemic drugs, insulin)	May require dosage adjustment of antidiabetic drugs.
Antihypertensives	Potentiates antihypertensive effect.
Barbiturates	May potentiate orthostatic hypotension.
Cholestyramine	Reduces the absorption of hydrochlorothiazide.
Colestipol	Reduces the absorption of hydrochlorothiazide.
Corticosteroids	Intensifies electrolyte depletion, particularly hypokalemia.
Lithium	Risk of lithium toxicity; monitor serum lithium levels.
Muscle relaxants, nondepolarizing (eg, tubocurarine)	May increase responsiveness to skeletal muscle relaxants.
Narcotic analgesics	May potentiate orthostatic hypotension.
NSAIDs	May reduce the diuretic, natriuretic, and antihypertensive effects of hydrochlorothiazide; may worsen renal function in patients with renal impairment.
Potassium-containing salt substitutes	May increase the risk of hyperkalemia; monitor serum potassium levels.

Table 13.3. Drug Interactions for Antihypertensive Agents

Potassium-sparing diuretics (eg, spironolactone, triamterene, amiloride)	May increase the risk of hyperkalemia; monitor serum potassium levels.
Potassium supplements	May increase the risk of hyperkalemia; monitor serum potassium levels.
Pressor amines (eg, norepinephrine)	May decrease response to pressor amines.
Fosinopril sodium-Hydrochlorothiazide (Monopril HCT)	
Antacids	May impair absorbtion; separate doses by 2 hours.
Antihypertensives	Caution with concomitant use.
Cholestyramine	Reduces the absorption of hydrochlorothiazide
Colestipol	Reduces the absorption of hydrochlorothiazide
Insulin	May alter insulin requirements.
Lithium	Risk of lithium toxicity; monitor serum lithium levels.
Methenamine	May decrease the effectiveness of methenamine.
Norepinephrine	May decrease arterial responsiveness to norepinephrine.
NSAIDs	May reduce the diuretic, natriuretic, and antihypertensive effects of hydrochlorothiazide.
Potassium-containing salt substitutes	May increase the risk of hyperkalemia; monitor serum potassium levels.
Potassium-sparing diuretics (eg, spironolactone, triamterene, amiloride)	May increase the risk of hyperkalemia; monitor serum potassium levels.
Potassium supplements	May increase the risk of hyperkalemia; monitor serum potassium levels.
Tubocurarine	May increase responsiveness to tubocurarine.
Lisinopril-Hydrochlorothiazide (Prinzide, Zestoretic)	
ACTH	Intensifies electrolyte depletion, particularly hypokalemia.
Alcohol	May potentiate orthostatic hypotension.
Antidiabetic drugs (eg, oral hypoglycemic drugs, insulin)	May require dosage adjustment of antidiabetic drugs.
Antihypertensives	Potentiates antihypertensive effect.
Barbiturates	May potentiate orthostatic hypotension.
Cholestyramine	Reduces the absorption of hydrochlorothiazide.
Colestipol	Reduces the absorption of hydrochlorothiazide.
Corticosteroids	Intensifies electrolyte depletion, particularly hypokalemia.
Gold, injectable (sodium aurothiomalate)	Nitroid reactions have been reported rarely in patients on therapy with injectable gold and concomitant therapy with ACE inhibitors
Lithium	Risk of lithium toxicity; monitor serum lithium levels.
Muscle relaxants, nondepolarizing (eg, tubocurarine)	May increase responsiveness to skeletal muscle relaxants.

Table 13.3. Drug Interactions for Antihypertensive Agents

Narcotic analgesics	May potentiate orthostatic hypotension.
NSAIDs	May reduce the diuretic, natriuretic, and antihypertensive effects of hydrochlorothiazide; may worsen renal function in patients with renal impairment.
Potassium-containing salt substitutes	May increase the risk of hyperkalemia; monitor serum potassium levels.
Potassium-sparing diuretics (eg, spironolactone, triamterene, amiloride)	May increase the risk of hyperkalemia; monitor serum potassium levels.
Potassium supplements	May increase the risk of hyperkalemia; monitor serum potassium levels.
Pressor amines (eg, norepinephrine)	May decrease response to pressor amines.
Moxepril HCl-Hydrochlorothiazide (Uniretic)	
ACTH	May intensify electrolyte depletion, particularly hypokalemia.
Alcohol	May potentiate orthostatic hypotension.
Antidiabetic drugs (eg, oral hypoglycemic drugs, insulin)	May require dosage adjustment of antidiabetic drugs.
Antihypertensives	Potentiates antihypertensive effect.
Barbiturates	May potentiate orthostatic hypotension.
Cholestyramine	Reduces the absorption of hydrochlorothiazide.
Colestipol	Reduces the absorption of hydrochlorothiazide.
Corticosteroids	May intensify electrolyte depletion, particularly hypokalemia.
Guanabenz	Increases the absorption of hydrochlorothiazide with concomitant use.
Lithium	Risk of lithium toxicity; monitor serum lithium levels.
Muscle relaxants, nondepolarizing (eg, tubocurarine)	May increase responsiveness to skeletal muscle relaxants.
Narcotics analgesics	May potentiate orthostatic hypotension.
NSAIDs	May reduce the diuretic, natriuretic, and antihypertensive effects of hydrochlorothiazide.
Potassium-containing salt substitutes	May increase the risk of hyperkalemia; monitor serum potassium levels.
Potassium-sparing diuretics (eg, spironolactone, triamterene, amiloride)	May increase the risk of hyperkalemia; monitor serum potassium levels.
Potassium supplements	May increase the risk of hyperkalemia; monitor serum potassium levels.
Pressor amines (eg, norepinephrine)	May decrease response to pressor amines.
Propantheline	Increases the absorption of hydrochlorothiazide with concomitant use.

Table 13.3. Drug Interactions for Antihypertensive Agents

Quinapril HCI-Hydrochlorothiazide (Accuretic)

ACTH	May intensify electrolyte imbalance, particularly hypokalemia.
Alcohol	May potentiate orthostatic hypotension.
Antidiabetic drugs (eg, oral hypoglycemic drugs, insulin)	May interact with hydrochlorothiazide; may require dosage adjustment of the antidiabetic drug.
Antihypertensives	May potentiate antihypertensive effect.
Barbiturates	May potentiate orthostatic hypotension.
Cholestyramine	Reduces the absorption of hydrochlorothiazide
Colestipol	Reduces the absorption of hydrochlorothiazide
Corticosteroids	May intensify electrolyte imbalance, particularly hypokalemia.
Lithium	Risk of lithium toxicity; monitor serum lithium levels.
Magnesium	Caution with use of drugs that interact with magnesium.
Muscle relaxants, nondepolarizing (eg, tubocurarine)	May increase responsiveness to muscle relaxants.
Narcotic analgesics	May potentiate orthostatic hypotension.
NSAIDs	May reduce the diuretic, natriuretic, and antihypertensive effects of hydrochlorothiazide.
Potassium-containing salt substitutes	May increase the risk of hyperkalemia; monitor serum potassium levels.
Potassium-sparing diuretics (eg, spironolactone, triamterene, amiloride)	May increase the risk of hyperkalemia; monitor serum potassium levels.
Potassium supplements	May increase the risk of hyperkalemia; monitor serum potassium levels.
Pressor amines (eg, norepinephrine)	May decrease response to pressor amines.
Tetracycline	Decreases the absorption of tetracycline, may be due to a reaction with magnesium that is contained within quinapril.

ANGIOTENSIN RECEPTOR BLOCKERS (ARBs)

Candesartan cilextil (Atacand)

Lithium	Increases serum lithium levels; monitor levels.

Eprosartan mesylate (Teveten)

Diuretics	Risk of hypotension with concomitant use.

Losartan potassium (Cozaar)

COX-2 Inhibitors	May reduce antihypertensive effects; in patients with compromised renal function, may lead to further deterioration of renal function.
Lithium	May reduce lithium excretion; monitor serum lithium levels.
NSAIDs	May reduce antihypertensive effects; in patients with compromised renal function, may lead to further deterioration of renal function.

Table 13.3. Drug Interactions for Antihypertensive Agents

Potassium-containing salt substitutes	May lead to increases in serum potassium levels; avoid use.
Potassium-sparing diuretics (eg, spironolactone, triamterene, amiloride)	May lead to increases in serum potassium levels.
Potassium supplements	May lead to increases in serum potassium levels.
Olmesartan medoxomil (Benicar)	
Diuretics	Caution, risk of hypotension when concomitantly using high dose diuretics.
Telmisartan (Micardis)	
Digoxin	Increases digoxin plasma levels; monitor digoxin levels when initiating, adjusting, or discontinuing telmisartan.
Warfarin	May alter warfarin plasma levels.
Valsartan (Diovan)	
Potassium-containing salt substitutes	May lead to increases in serum potassium levels; may cause increases in serum creatine in heart failure patients.
Potassium-sparing diuretics (eg, spironolactone, triamterene, amiloride)	May lead to increases in serum potassium levels; may cause increases in serum creatine in heart failure patients.
Potassium supplements	May lead to increases in serum potassium levels; may cause increases in serum creatine in heart failure patients.

ARBs COMBINATIONS

Candesartan cilexetil-Hydrochlorothiazide (Atacand HCT)	
ACTH	Concomitant use intensifies electrolyte depletion, particularly hypokalemia.
Alcohol	May potentiate orthostatic hypotension.
Antihypertensive drugs	Potentiates antihypertensive effect.
Barbiturates	May potentiate orthostatic hypotension.
Cholestyramine	Impairs absorption of hydrochlorothiazide.
Colestipol	Impairs absorption of hydrochlorothiazide.
Corticosteroids	Concomitant use intensifies electrolyte depletion, particularly hypokalemia.
Hypoglycemic drugs, oral	May require dosage adjustment of oral hypoglycemic drugs.
Insulin	May require dosage adjustment of insulin.
Lithium	Reduces renal clearance of lithium and increases risk of lithium toxicity; avoid concomitant use.
Muscle relaxants, nondepolarizing (eg, tubocurarine)	May increase responsiveness to skeletal muscle relaxants.
Narcotic analgesics	May potentiate orthostatic hypotension.
NSAIDs	May reduce the diuretic, natriuretic, and antihypertensive effects of hydrochlorothiazide.

Table 13.3. Drug Interactions for Antihypertensive Agents

Pressor amines (eg, norepinephrine)	May decrease response to pressor amines.

Eprosartan mesylate-Hydrochlorothiazide (Teveten HCT)

ACTH	Concomitant use intensifies electrolyte depletion, particularly hypokalemia.
Alcohol	May potentiate orthostatic hypotension.
Antihypertensive drugs	Potentiates antihypertensive effect.
Barbiturates	May potentiate orthostatic hypotension.
Cholestyramine	Impairs absorption of hydrochlorothiazide.
Colestipol	Impairs absorption of hydrochlorothiazide.
Corticosteroids	Concomitant use intensifies electrolyte depletion, particularly hypokalemia.
Hypoglycemic drugs, oral	May require dosage adjustment of oral hypoglycemic drugs.
Insulin	May require dosage adjustment of insulin.
Lithium	Reduces renal clearance of lithium and increases risk of lithium toxicity; avoid concomitant use.
Muscle relaxants, nondepolarizing (eg, tubocurarine)	May increase responsiveness to skeletal muscle relaxants.
Narcotic analgesics	May potentiate orthostatic hypotension.
NSAIDs	May reduce the diuretic, natriuretic, and antihypertensive effects of hydrochlorothiazide.
Potassium-containing salt substitutes	May lead to increases in serum potassium levels; avoid use.
Potassium-sparing diuretics (eg, spironolactone, triamterene, amiloride)	May lead to increases in serum potassium levels.
Potassium supplements	May lead to increases in serum potassium levels.
Pressor amines (eg, norepinephrine)	May decrease response to pressor amines.

Irbesartan-Hydrochlorothiazide (Avalide)

ACTH	Concominant use intensifies electrolyte depletion, particularly hypokalemia.
Alcohol	May potentiate orthostatic hypotension.
Antihypertensive drugs	Potentiates antihypertensive effect.
Barbiturates	May potentiate orthostatic hypotension.
Cholestyramine	Impairs absorption of hydrochlorothiazide.
Colestipol	Impairs absorption of hydrochlorothiazide.
Corticosteroids	Concominant use intensifies electrolyte depletion, particularly hypokalemia.
Hypoglycemic drugs, oral	May require dosage adjustment of oral hypoglycemic drugs.
Insulin	May require dosage adjustment of insulin.
Lithium	Reduces renal clearance of lithium and increases risk of lithium toxicity; avoid concomitant use.

Table 13.3. Drug Interactions for Antihypertensive Agents

Muscle relaxants, nondepolarizing (eg, tubocurarine)	May increase responsiveness to skeletal muscle relaxants.
Narcotic analgesics	May potentiate orthostatic hypotension.
NSAIDs	May reduce the diuretic, natriuretic, and antihypertensive effects of hydrochlorothiazide.
Pressor amines (eg, norepinephrine)	May decrease response to pressor amines.
Losartan potassium-Hydrochlorothiazide (Hyzaar)	
ACTH	Concomitant use intensifies electrolyte depletion, particularly hypokalemia.
Alcohol	May potentiate orthostatic hypotension.
Antihypertensive drugs	Potentiates antihypertensive effect.
Barbiturates	May potentiate orthostatic hypotension.
Cholestyramine	Impairs absorption of hydrochlorothiazide.
Colestipol	Impairs absorption of hydrochlorothiazide.
Corticosteroids	Concomitant use intensifies electrolyte depletion, particularly hypokalemia.
COX-2 inhibitors	May reduce the diuretic, natriuretic, and antihypertensive effects of hydrochlorothiazide; may result in a further deterioration of renal function in the renally impaired.
Fluconazole	Increases levels of losartan.
Hypoglycemic drugs, oral	May require dose adjustment of oral hypoglycemic drugs.
Insulin	May require dose adjustment of insulin.
Lithium	Reduces renal clearance of lithium and increases risk of lithium toxicity; avoid concomitant use.
Muscle relaxants, nondepolarizing (eg, tubocurarine)	May increase responsiveness to skeletal muscle relaxants.
Narcotic analgesics	May potentiate orthostatic hypotension.
NSAIDs	May reduce the diuretic, natriuretic, and antihypertensive effects of hydrochlorothiazide; may result in a further deterioration of renal function in the renally impaired.
Potassium-containing salt substitutes	May lead to increases in serum potassium levels; avoid use.
Potassium-sparing diuretics (eg, spironolactone, triamterene, amiloride)	May lead to increases in serum potassium levels.
Potassium supplements	May lead to increases in serum potassium levels.
Pressor amines (eg, norepinephrine)	May decrease response to pressor amines.
Rifampin	Decreases drug levels of losartan.

Table 13.3. Drug Interactions for Antihypertensive Agents

Olmesartan medoxomil-Hydrochlorothiazide (Benicar HCT)

ACTH	Concomitant use intensifies electrolyte depletion, particularly hypokalemia.
Alcohol	May potentiate orthostatic hypotension.
Antihypertensive drugs	Potentiates antihypertensive effect.
Barbiturates	May potentiate orthostatic hypotension.
Cholestyramine	Impairs absorption of hydrochlorothiazide.
Colestipol	Impairs absorption of hydrochlorothiazide.
Corticosteroids	Concomitant use intensifies electrolyte depletion, particularly hypokalemia.
Hypoglycemic drugs, oral	May require dose adjustment of oral hypoglycemic drugs.
Insulin	May require dose adjustment of insulin.
Lithium	Reduces renal clearance of lithium and increases risk of lithium toxicity; avoid concomitant use.
Muscle relaxants, nondepolarizing (eg, tubocurarine)	May increase responsiveness to skeletal muscle relaxants.
Narcotic analgesics	May potentiate orthostatic hypotension.
NSAIDs	May reduce the diuretic, natriuretic, and antihypertensive effects of hydrochlorothiazide.
Pressor amines (eg, norepinephrine)	May decrease response to pressor amines.

Telmisartan-Hydrochlorothiazide (Micardis HCT)

ACTH	Concomitant use intensifies electrolyte depletion, particularly hypokalemia.
Alcohol	May potentiate orthostatic hypotension.
Antihypertensive drugs	Potentiates antihypertensive effect.
Barbiturates	May potentiate orthostatic hypotension.
Cholestyramine	Impairs absorption of hydrochlorothiazide.
Colestipol	Impairs absorption of hydrochlorothiazide.
Corticosteroids	Concomitant use intensifies electrolyte depletion, particularly hypokalemia.
Digoxin	Increases plasma levels of digoxin; monitor levels.
Hypoglycemic drugs, oral	May require dose adjustment of oral hypoglycemic drugs.
Insulin	May require dose adjustment of insulin.
Lithium	Reduces renal clearance of lithium and increases risk of lithium toxicity; avoid concomitant use.
Narcotic analgesics	May potentiate orthostatic hypotension.
NSAIDs	May reduce the diuretic, natriuretic, and antihypertensive effects of hydrochlorothiazide.
Pressor amines (eg, norepinephrine)	May decrease response to pressor amines.
Warfarin	May alter warfarin levels.

Table 13.3. Drug Interactions for Antihypertensive Agents

Valsartan-Hydrochlorothiazide (Diovan HCT)

ACTH	Concomitant use intensifies electrolyte depletion, particularly hypokalemia.
Alcohol	May potentiate orthostatic hypotension.
Antihypertensive drugs	Potentiates antihypertensive effect.
Barbiturates	May potentiate orthostatic hypotension.
Cholestyramine	Impairs absorption of hydrochlorothiazide.
Colestipol	Impairs absorption of hydrochlorothiazide.
Corticosteroids	Concomitant use intensifies electrolyte depletion, particularly hypokalemia.
Hypoglycemic drugs, oral	May require dose adjustment of oral hypoglycemic drugs.
Insulin	May require dosage adjustment of insulin.
Lithium	Reduces renal clearance of lithium and increases risk of lithium toxicity; avoid concomitant use.
Muscle relaxants, nondepolarizing (eg, tubocurarine)	May increase responsiveness to skeletal muscle relaxants.
Narcotic analgesics	May potentiate orthostatic hypotension.
NSAIDs	May reduce the diuretic, natriuretic, and antihypertensive effects of hydrochlorothiazide.
Pressor amines (eg, norepinephrine)	May decrease response to pressor amines.

BETA-BLOCKERS (NONSELECTIVE)

Nadolol (Corgard)

Anesthetics	May exaggerate hypotension.
Antidiabetic drugs (eg, insulins, oral hypoglycemic drugs)	May require dosage adjustment of antidiabetic drugs.
Catecholamine-depleting drugs (eg, reserpine)	Additive hypotension and/or bradycardia with catecholamine-depleting drugs.
Epinephrine	May block the effects of epinephrine.

Penbutolol sulfate (Levatol)

Alcohol	Caution with concomitant use.
Anesthetics	Caution with anesthetics that depress the myocardium (eg, ether, cyclopropane, trichloroethylene).
Calcium channel blockers	Produces synergistic hypotensive effects, bradycardia, and arrhythmias when used with oral calcium channel blockers.
Catecholamine-depleting drugs	Avoid concomitant use.
Epinephrine	May antagonize epinephrine.

Table 13.3. Drug Interactions for Antihypertensive Agents

Lidocaine	Increases volume of distribution of lidocaine; may require higher loading doses of lidocaine.
Pindolol*	
Catecholamine-depleting drugs	Additive hypotension and/or bradycardia with catecholamine-depleting drugs.
Thioridazine	Both thioridazine and pindolol levels may increase when used concomitantly.
Propranolol HCl (Inderal, Inderal LA)	
Aluminum hydroxide gel	Concomitant use may decrease propranolol plasma concentrations.
Cholestyramine	Decreases propranolol plasma concentrations.
Clorpromazine	Increases propranolol plasma concentrations with concomitant use.
Colestipol	Decreases propranolol plasma concentrations.
CYP1A2 inhibitors (eg, imipramine, cimetidine, ciprofloxacin, fluvoxamine, isoniazid, ritonavir, theophylline, zileuton, zolmitriptan, rizatriptan)	May increase blood levels and/or toxicity of propranolol with concomitant use.
CYP2C19 inhibitors (eg, fluconazole, cimetidine, fluoxetine, fluvoxamine, tenioposide, tolbutamide)	May increase blood levels and/or toxicity of propranolol with concomitant use.
CYP2D6 inhibitors (eg, amiodarone, cimetidine, fluoxetine, paroxetine, quinidine, ritonavir)	May increase blood levels and/or toxicity of propranolol with concomitant use.
Diazepam	Increases concentrations of diazepam and its metabolites with concomitant use.
Digitalis glycosides	Concominant use may increase the risk of bradycardia.
Hepatic enzyme inducers (eg, rifampin, ethanol, phenytoin, phenobarbital, cigarette smoking)	May decrease blood levels of propranolol with concomitant use.
Lidocaine	Lidocaine metabolism is inhibited with coadministration.
Nicardipine	Increases levels of propranolol.
Nisoldipine	Increases levels of propranolol.
Propafenone	Increases levels of propafenone with concomitant use.
Rizatriptan	Increases levels of rizatriptan with concomitant use.
Theophylline	Decreases theophylline clearance with concomitant use.
Thioridazine	Concomitant use with doses of propranolol >160 mg/day resulted in increased thioridazine plasma concentrations.
Warfarin	Concomitant use increases warfarin levels and prothrombin time.
Zolmitriptan	Increases levels of zolmitriptan with concomitant use.

*Available only in generic form.

Table 13.3. Drug Interactions for Antihypertensive Agents

Propranolol HCl (InnoPran XL)

ACE inhibitors	ACE inhibitors can cause hypotension and certain ACE inhibitors may increase bronchial hyperactivity.
Alpha-blockers (eg, prazosin, terazosin, doxazosin)	Potentiates effects of propranolol.
Aluminum hydroxide gel	Decreases levels of propranolol.
Anesthetics (eg, methoxyflurane, trichloroethylene)	May depress myocardial contractility with concomitant use.
Antiarrhythmics (eg, propafenone, quinidine, amiodarone)	Potentiates effects of propranolol.
AV conduction-slowing drugs (eg, digitalis, lidocaine, calcium channel blockers)	Caution with concomitant use.
Beta-agonists (eg, dobutamine, isoproterenol)	May reverse effects of propranolol.
Chlorpromazine	Increases levels of both propranolol and chlorpromazine.
Cholestyramine	Decreases levels of propranolol.
Cigarette smoke	Decreases levels of propranolol.
Clonidine	May antagonize clonidine effects; caution when withdrawing from clonidine.
Colestipol	Decreases levels of propranolol.
CYP1A2 substrates or inhibitors (eg, imipramine, cimetidine, ciprofloxacin, fluvoxamine, isoniazid, theophylline, zileuton, zolmitriptan, rizatriptan)	Potentiates effects of propranolol. Caution with concomitant use.
CYP2C19 substrates or inhibitors (eg, fluconazole, fluoxetine, fluvoxamine, teniposide, tolbutamide)	Potentiates effects of propranolol. Caution with concomitant use.
CYP2D6 substrates or inhibitors (eg, cimetidine, delavudin, fluoxetine, paroxetine, quinidine, ritonavir)	Potentiates effects of propranolol. Caution with concomitant use.
Diazepam	Increases levels of diazepam.
Disopyramide	Concomitant use associated with severe bradycardia, asystole, and heart failure.

Table 13.3. Drug Interactions for Antihypertensive Agents

Epinephrine	May develop uncontrolled hypertension with concomitant use.
Ethanol	Decreases levels of propranolol.
Haloperidol	Hypotension and cardiac arrest reported with concomitant use.
Lidocaine	Decreases clearance of lidocaine.
Lovastatin	Decreases levels of lovastatin.
MAO inhibitors	May exacerbate the hypotensive effects of MAO inhibitors.
NSAIDs	May decrease the antihypertensive effects of propranolol.
Pravastatin	Decreases levels of pravastatin.
Reserpine	Monitor for excessive reduction of resting sympathetic nervous activity (eg, hypotension, bradycardia, vertigo, orthostatic hypotension, syncope) with concomitant use; may also potentiate depression with concomitant use.
Rifampin	Decreases levels of propranolol.
Rizatriptan	Increases levels of rizatriptan.
Theophylline	Decreases oral clearance of theophylline.
Thioridazine	Increases levels of thioridazine.
Thyroxine	May result in lower than expected T_3 levels when used concomitantly.
Tricyclic antidepressants	May exacerbate the hypotensive effects of tricyclic antidepressants.
Warfarin	Increases the levels of warfarin; monitor prothrombin time.
Zolmitriptan	Increases levels of zolmitriptan.
Timolol maleate*	
Antidiabetic drugs (eg, insulins, oral hypoglycemic drugs)	Caution with concomitant use.
Calcium channel blockers	Concomitant use may cause AV conduction disturbances, left ventricular failure, or hypotension; avoid use if cardiac dysfunction present.
Catecholamine-depleting drugs (Reserpine)	Concomitant use may produce additive effects; may cause hypotension and/or marked bradycardia.
Clonidine	May exacerbate rebound hypertension following withdrawal from clonidine.
Digitalis	Concomitant use prolongs AV conduction time.
Epinephrine	May block effects of epinephrine.
NSAIDs	May reduce antihypertensive effects.
Quinidine	May potentiate systemic beta-blockade.

BETA-BLOCKERS (SELECTIVE BETA₁)

Acebutolol HCl (Sectral)	
Alpha adrenergic stimulants	May produce exaggerated hypertensive response when used concomitantly.
Catecholamine-depleting drugs (eg, reserpine)	May produce an additive effect; monitor for marked bradycardia or hypotension.
Epinephrine	May block the effects of epinephrine.

*Available only in generic form.

Table 13.3. Drug Interactions for Antihypertensive Agents

Insulin	May potentiate insulin-induced hypoglycemia.
NSAIDs	May reduce antihypertensive effects.
Atenolol (Tenormin)	
Anesthetic agents	Caution with anesthetic agents which depress myocardium function.
Calcium channel blockers	May produce an additive effect; bradycardia, heart block, and left ventricular end diastolic pressure can rise with verapamil or diltiazem.
Catecholamine-depleting drugs (eg, reserpine)	May produce an additive effect; monitor for marked bradycardia or hypotension.
Clonidine	Caution with clonidine withdrawal; may exacerbate rebound hypertension following withdrawal.
Epinephrine	May block epinephrine effects.
Prostaglandin synthase inhibitors (eg, indomethacin)	May decrease the hypotensive effects of atenolol.
Betaxolol HCl (Kerlone)	
Calcium channel blockers	Avoid concomitant use with oral calcium channel blockers in patients with cardiac dysfunction, may increase cardiac adverse effects.
Catecholamine-depleting drugs (eg, reserpine)	May produce an additive effect; monitor for marked bradycardia or hypotension.
Clonidine	Caution with clonidine withdrawal; betaxolol should be discontinued gradually over several days before clonidine withdrawal.
Epinephrine	May block epinephrine effects.
Bisoprolol fumarate (Zebeta)	
Anesthetic agents (eg, ether, cyclopropane, trichloroethylene)	Caution with anesthetic agents that depress myocardium function.
Antiarrhythmics (eg, disopyramide)	Caution with antiarrhymics that depress myocardial function.
Antidiabetic drugs (eg, insulins, oral hypoglycemic drugs)	Caution with concomitant use; may potentiate insulin induced hypoglycemia and delay recovery of serum glucose levels.
Beta-blockers	Avoid concomitant use with other beta-blockers.
Calcium channel blockers (eg, verapamil, diltiazem)	Caution with calcium channel blockers that depress myocardial function.
Catecholamine-depleting drugs (eg, reserpine, guanethidine)	May produce excessive reduction of sympathetic activity with concomitant use.
Clonidine	Caution with clonidine withdrawal; bisoprolol should be discontinued for several days before withdrawal from clonidine.
Epinephrine	May block epinephrine effects.
Rifampin	Increases the clearance of bisoprolol.

Table 13.3. Drug Interactions for Antihypertensive Agents

Metoprolol succinate (Toprol-XL); Metoprolol tartrate (Lopressor)

Calcium channel blockers (eg, verapamil, diltiazem)	Caution with calcium channel blockers that depress myocardial function.
Catecholamine-depleting drugs (eg, reserpine, MAOIs)	May produce additive effects; monitor for marked bradycardia or hypotension.
Clonidine	May exacerbate rebound hypertension following clonidine withdrawal; metoprolol should be withdrawn several days before gradual withdrawal from clonidine.
CYP2D6 inhibitors (eg, quinidine, fluoxetine, paroxetine, propafenone)	May increase levels of metoprolol.
Digitalis glycosides	May increase the risk of bradycardia. Both slow AV conduction.
Epinephrine	May block epinephrine effects.

Nebivolol (Bystolic)

Anesthetic agents (eg, ether, cyclopropane, trichloroethylene)	Caution with concomitant use; monitor closely.
Antiarrhythmic agents (eg, disopyramide)	Caution with concomitant use.
Antidiabetic drugs (eg, insulins, oral hypoglycemic drugs)	May potentiate hypoglycemic effect of antidiabetic drugs; caution with concomitant use.
Calcium channel blockers, non-dihydropyridine (eg, diltiazem, verapamil)	Caution with concomitant use; monitor closely.
Catecholamine-depleting drugs (eg, reserpine, guanethidine)	May produce excessive reduction of sympathetic activity; monitor closely.
Clonidine	Nebivolol should be discontinued for several days before gradually tapering clonidine.
CYP2D6 inhibitors (eg, fluoxetine, quinidine, propafenone, paroxetine)	May increase nebivolol levels; monitor and consider dosage adjustment.
Sildenafil	May decrease nebivolol levels.

BETA-BLOCKER COMBINATIONS

Atenolol-Chlorthalidone (Tenoretic)

ACTH	May develop hypokalemia with concomitant use.
Anesthetic agents	Caution with anesthetic agents that may depress the myocardium.
Calcium channel blockers	May produce additive effects.
Catecholamine-depleting drugs (eg, reserpine)	May produce additive effect; monitor for marked bradycardia and/or hypotension.

Table 13.3. Drug Interactions for Antihypertensive Agents

Clonidine	May exacerbate rebound hypertension with clonidine withdrawal.
Corticosteroids	May develop hypokalemia with concomitant use.
Digitalis	May produce additive effects.
Diltiazem	Bradycardia, heart block, and left ventricular end diastolic pressure can rise with concomitant use.
Epinephrine	May block the effects of epinephrine.
Insulin	May alter insulin requirements.
Lithium	Increases the risk of lithium toxicity.
Norepinephrine	May decrease arterial response to norepinephrine.
Prostaglandin synthase inhibitors (eg, indomethacin)	May decrease hypotensive effects of atenolol.
Verapamil	Bradycardia, heart block, and left ventricular end diastolic pressure can rise with concomitant use.
Bisoprolol fumarate-Hydrochlorothiazide (Ziac)	
ACTH	Intensifies electrolyte imbalance, particularly hypokalemia.
Alcohol	May potentiate orthostatic hypotension.
Anesthetic agents (eg, ether, cyclopropane, trichloroethylene)	Caution with anesthetic agents that depress myocardium function.
Antiarrhythmic drugs	Caution with concomitant use.
Antidiabetic drugs (insulin, oral hypoglycemic drugs)	May require dosage adjustment of the antidiabetic drug.
Antihypertensive drugs	Potentiates antihypertensive effect with concomitant use.
Barbiturates	May potentiate orthostatic hypotension.
Beta-blockers	Slows atrioventricular conduction and decreases heart rate; concomitant use can increase the risk of bradycardia. Avoid concomitant use with other beta-blockers.
Calcium channel blockers	Caution with concomitant use.
Catecholamine-depleting drugs (eg, reserpine, guanethidine)	Concomitant use may produce excessive reduction of sympathetic activity.
Cholestyramine	May impair the absorption of hydrochlorothiazide.
Clonidine	Caution with clonidine withdrawal.
Colestipol	May impair the absorption of hydrochlorothiazide.
Corticosteroids	Intensifies electrolyte imbalance, particularly hypokalemia.
Digitalis glycosides	Slows atrioventricular conduction and decreases heart rate; concomitant use can increase the risk of bradycardia.
Epinephrine	May block the effects of epinephrine.
Lithium	Increases the risk of lithium toxicity.

Table 13.3. Drug Interactions for Antihypertensive Agents

Muscle relaxants, nondepolarizing (eg, tubocurarine)	May potentiate to nondepolarizing muscle relaxants.
Myocardial depressant drugs	Caution with concomitant use.
Narcotic analgesics	May potentiate orthostatic hypotension.
NSAIDs	May reduce the diuretic, natriuretic, and antihypertensive effects of hydrochlorothiazide.
Pressor amines (eg, norepinephrine)	May decrease response to pressor amines.
Rifampin	Increases the clearance of bisoprolol.

Metoprolol tartrate-Hydrochlorothiazide (Lopressor HCT)

ACTH	May develop hypokalemia with concomitant use.
Alcohol	May potentiate orthostatic hypotension.
Antihypertensive drugs	Potentiates antihypertensive effect with concomitant use.
Barbiturates	May potentiate orthostatic hypotension.
Catecholamine-depleting drugs (eg, reserpine)	May produce additive effect; monitor for hypotension or marked bradycardia.
Cholestyramine	Impairs the absorption of hydrochlorothiazide.
Clonidine	Metoprolol-hydrochlorothiazide should be stopped several days before clonidine discontinuation.
Colestipol	Impairs the absorption of hydrochlorothiazide.
Corticosteroids	May develop hypokalemia with concomitant use.
CYP2D6 inhibitors	Concomitant use with strong CYP2D6 inhibitors may increase the plasma concentrations of metoprolol.
Digitalis glycosides	Caution with concomitant use, may increase the risk of bradycardia.
Epinephrine	May block the effects of epinephrine.
Insulin	May alter insulin requirements.
Lithium	Increases the risk of lithium toxicity.
Narcotic analgesics	May potentiate orthostatic hypotension.
Norepinephrine	May decrease arterial responsiveness to norepinephrine.
NSAIDs	May reduce the diuretic, natriuretic, and antihypertensive effects of hydrochlorothiazide.
Tubocurarine	May increase responsiveness to tubocurarine.

Nadolol-Bendroflumethazide (Corzide)

ACTH	May intensify electrolyte imbalance, particularly hypokalemia; monitor potassium levels.
Alcohol	May potentiate orthostatic hypotension.
Amphotericin B	May intensify electrolyte imbalance, particularly hypokalemia; monitor potassium levels.
Anesthetics	General anesthetics may exaggerate hypotension.
Anticoagulants, oral	May decrease effects of oral anticoagulants; dosage adjustment may be required.

Table 13.3. Drug Interactions for Antihypertensive Agents

Antidiabetic agents (insulins, oral hypoglycemic drugs)	May cause hypoglycemia or hyperglycemia; dosage adjustment may be required.
Antigout drugs	May raise blood uric acid levels; dosage adjustment may be required.
Antihypertensive drugs	May potentiate antihypertensive effects; dosage adjustment may be required.
Barbiturates	May potentiate orthostatic hypotension.
Calcium salts	Concomitant use increases serum calcium levels; monitor levels.
Catecholamine-depleting drugs (eg, reserpine)	May produce additive effect; monitor for hypotension and/or excessive bradycardia.
Cholestyramine	May delay or decrease absorption of bendroflumethazide.
Colestipol	May delay or decrease absorption of bendroflumethazide.
Corticosteroids	May intensify electrolyte imbalance, particularly hypokalemia; monitor potassium levels.
Diazoxide	Potentiates hyperglycemic, hyperuricemic, and antihypertensive effects; monitor blood glucose and serum uric acid levels.
Digoxin	Monitor digoxin levels with concomitant use.
Epinephrine	May block the effects of epinephrine.
Lithium	Increases the risk of lithium toxicity.
MAO inhibitors	Concomitant use potentiates hypotensive effects.
Methenamine	Possible decreased effectiveness with methenamine.
Muscle relaxants, nondepolarizing (eg, tubocurarine)	May potentiate effects of nondepolarizing muscle relaxants.
Narcotic analgesics	May potentiate orthostatic hypotension.
NSAIDs	May reduce the diuretic, natriuretic, and antihypertensive effects of bendroflumethazide.
Preanesthetic drugs	May potentiate effects of preanesthetic drugs.
Pressor amines (eg, norepinephrine)	Decreased arterial responsiveness with pressor amines.
Probenecid	Concomitant use may require a dosage increase of probenecid.
Sulfinpyrazone	Concomitant use may require a dosage increase of sulfinpyrazone.
Propranolol HCl-Hydrochlorothiazide (Inderide)	
ACTH	May develop hypokalemia with concomitant use.
Alcohol	Concomitant use may cause increases in plasma levels of propranolol; may potentiate orthostatic hypotension.
Aluminum hydroxide gel	Reduces the intestinal absorption of propranolol.
Antipyrine	Concomitant use reduces the clearance of antipyrine.
Barbiturates	May potentiate orthostatic hypotension.
Calcium channel blockers	May increase cardiac effects of calcium channel blockers.
Catecholamine-depleting drugs (eg, reserpine)	Concomitant use may produce excessive reduction of sympathetic activity which may produce marked bradycardia or hypotension.

Table 13.3. Drug Interactions for Antihypertensive Agents

Chlorpromazine	Increases plasma levels of chlorpromazine and propranolol.
Cimetidine	Increases blood levels of propranolol.
Corticosteroids	May develop hypokalemia with concomitant use.
Digoxin	Caution with concomitant use, may increase the risk of bradycardia.
Epinephrine	May block the effects of epinephrine.
Ganglionic or peripheral adrenergic-blockers	Concomitant use potentiates the effects of propranolol-hydrochlorothiazide.
Haloperidol	Concomitant use may cause hypotension and cardiac arrest.
Insulin	May alter insulin requirements.
Lidocaine	Concomitant use reduces the clearance of lidocaine.
Narcotic analgesics	May potentiate orthostatic hypotension.
Norepinephrine	May decrease arterial response to norepinephrine.
NSAIDs	Blunts the antihypertensive effects of propranolol.
Phenobarbital	Acclerates the clearance of propranolol.
Phenytoin	Acclerates the clearance of propranolol.
Rifampin	Acclerates the clearance of propranolol.
Theophylline	Concomitant use reduces the clearance of theophylline.
Thyroxine	May result in lower than expected T_3 levels when used concomitantly.
Tubocurarine	May increase responsiveness to tubocurarine.

CALCIUM CHANNEL BLOCKERS (DIHYDROPYRIDINES)

Felodipine (Plendil)

Anticonvulsant drugs	Decreases plasma levels of felodipine.
CYP3A4 inhibitors (eg, itraconazole, ketoconazole, erythromycin, grapefruit juice, cimetidine)	May increase plasma levels of felodipine.
Metoprolol	May increase metoprolol levels.

Isradipine (DynaCirc, DynaCirc CR)

Anesthesia	May produce severe hypotension.
Cimetidine	Increased mean peak plasma concentrations of isradipine.
Fentanyl	May produce severe hypotension.
Hydrochlorothiazide	Concomitant use produces additive hypertensive effects.
Propranolol	Increases AUC and C_{max} of propranolol.
Rifampicin	Decreases isradipine levels.

Nicardipine HCl (Cardene IV, Cardene SR)

Anesthesia	May produce severe hypotension.
Antihypertensive drugs	Caution with concomitant use; monitor blood pressure levels.
Beta-blockers	Caution with concomitant use in patients who have congestive heart failure.

Table 13.3. Drug Interactions for Antihypertensive Agents

Cimetidine	Increases plasma levels of nicardipine.
Cyclosporine	May increase cyclosporine levels.
Digoxin	Monitor digoxin levels.
Fentanyl	May produce severe hypotension.
Nifedipine (Adalat CC, Afeditab CR, Procardia, Procardia XL)	
Anesthesia	May produce severe hypotension.
Beta-blockers	Concomitant use in patients with patients with cardiovascular disease may increase risk of CHF, severe hypotension, or angina exacerbation.
Coumarin anticoagulants	May increase prothrombin time with concomitant use.
CYP3A4 inducers (eg, phenytoin, St. John's wort)	May decrease levels of nifedipine.
CYP3A4 inhibitors (eg, ketoconazole, erythromycin, protease inhibitors)	May increase levels of nifedipine.
Digoxin	May increase digoxin levels; monitor levels.
Fentanyl	May produce severe hypotension.
Grapefruit juice	Increases plasma levels of nifedipine; avoid concomitant use.
Quinidine	Monitor heart rate and dosage of nifedipine with concomitant use.
Nimodipine (Nimotop)	
Antihypertensive drugs	May intensify antihypertensive effect.
Calcium channel blockers	May enhance cardiovascular effects of other calcium channel blockers.
CYP3A4 Inhibitors (eg, ketoconazole, erythromycin, fluoxetine, protease inhibitors, cimetidine)	Increases plasma levels of nimodipine.
Nisoldipine (Sular)	
Cimetidine	Increases AUC and Cmax of nisoldipine.
CYP3A4 inducers	Avoid concomitant use.
Grapefruit juice	Increases the bioavailabilty of nisoldpine; avoid concomitant use.
High-fat meals	Increases peak concentrations of nisoldipine; avoid high-fat meals.
Phenytoin	Lowers nisoldipine plasma concentrations; avoid concomitant use.
Quinidine	Decreases bioavailability of nisoldipine.

CALCIUM CHANNEL BLOCKERS (NONDIHYDROPYRIDINES)

Diltiazem HCl (Cardizem, Cardizem CD, Cardizem LA, Cartia XT, Dilacor XR, Diltia XT, Tiazac, Taztia XT)	
Anesthetics	Concomitant use potentiates depression of cardiac contractility, conductivity, automaticity, and vascular dilation.
Beta-blockers	May produce additive cardiac conduction effects.

Table 13.3. Drug Interactions for Antihypertensive Agents

Buspirone	May potentiate the effects and increase the toxicity of buspirone.
Carbamazepine	Increases serum levels of carbamazepine.
Cimetidine	Increases levels of diltiazem.
Cyclosporine	Monitor cyclosporine levels with concomitant use.
CYP3A4 inducers (eg, rifampin)	Avoid concomitant use.
CYP3A4 substrates	May require dosage adjustment of diltiazem.
Digitalis	May increase plasma levels of digoxin; may produce additive cardiac conduction effects with concomitant use.
Lovastatin	Increases levels of lovastatin.
Midazolam	May increase levels of midazolam.
Propranolol	Increases levels of propranolol.
Quinidine	Increases levels of quinidine; monitor for adverse effects associated with quinidine.
Triazolam	May increase levels of triazolam.
Verapamil HCI (Calan, Calan SR, Covera HS, Isoptin SR, Verelan, Verelan PM)	
Alcohol	May increase blood alcohol levels and prolong its effects.
Anesthetics	Caution with concomitant use.
Antihypertensive drugs	May produce an additive antihypertensive effect.
Aspirin	May increase bleeding time with concomitant use.
Beta-blockers	May produce additive effects on heart rate, AV conduction, and/or cardiac contractility.
Carbamazepine	May increase levels of carbamazepine.
Cyclosporine	May increase serum levels of cyclosporine.
CYP3A4 inducers (eg, rifampin)	Decreases plasma levels of verapamil.
CYP3A4 inhibitors (eg, erythromycin, ritonavir)	Increases plasma levels of verapamil.
Cytotoxic agents	May reduce absorption of verapamil.
Digoxin	May increase serum digoxin levels.
Disopyramide	Avoid administration of disopyramide within 48 hrs before or 24 hrs after verapamil administration.
Doxorubicin	May increase the efficacy of doxorubicin; raises the levels of doxorubicin.
Flecainide	May produce additive negative inotropic effects and prolongation of AV conduction with concomitant use.
Grapefruit juice	Increases plasma levels of verapamil.
Lithium	Monitor lithium levels.
Neuromuscular blocking agents	May potentiate the effects of neuromuscular blockers; both verapamil and the neuromuscular blocker agent may require a dosage reduction.
Paclitaxel	May decrease clearance of paclitaxel.
Phenobarbital	May increased clearance of verapamil.

Table 13.3. Drug Interactions for Antihypertensive Agents

Quinidine	Avoid concomitant use with quinidine if hypertrophic cardiomyopathy is present.
Rifampin	May reduce the oral bioavailability of verapamil.
Theophylline	May increase plasma levels of theophylline.
VAC cytotoxic drug regimen	Mar reduce absorption of verapamil.

CALCIUM CHANNEL BLOCKER COMBINATIONS

Amlodipine besylate-Atorvastatin calcium (Caduet)

Azole antifungals	Concomitant use may increase the risk of myopathy.
Cimetidine	Caution with concomitant use.
Colestipol	Decreases plasma concentrations of atorvastatin, however greater reduction of LDL cholesterol levels were found when used concomitantly than when used alone.
Contraceptives, oral (norethindrone, ethinyl estradiol)	Increases concentrations of oral contraceptives.
Cyclosporine	Concomitant use may increase the risk of myopathy.
Digoxin	Increases plasma levels of digoxin.
Erythromycin	Increases plasma levels of atorvastin; concomitant use may increase the risk of myopathy.
Fibric acid derivatives	May increase the risk of myopathy; avoid concomitant use.
Ketoconazole	Caution with concomitant use.
Maalox TC Suspension	Decreases plasma concentrations of atorvastatin, however does not affect LDL cholesterol levels.
Niacin	Concomitant use may increase the risk of myopathy.
Spironolactone	Caution with concomitant use.

Amlodipine besylate-Benazepril HCl (Lotrel)

Diuretics	Caution, risk of hypotension with concomitant use.
Lithium	May increase serum lithium levels; monitor levels.
Peripheral vasodilators	Caution with concomitant use of other peripheral vasodilators.
Potassium-containing salt substitutes	May increase the risk of hyperkalemia.
Potassium-sparining diuretics (eg, spironolactone, triamterene, amiloride)	May increase the risk of hyperkalemia.
Potassium supplements	May increase the risk of hyperkalemia.

Amlodipine besylate-Valsartan (Exforge)

Potassium-containing salt substitutes	Concomitant use may lead to increases in serum potassium levels; may lead to increases in serum creatinine levels in heart failure patients.
Potassium-sparing diuretics (eg, spironolactone, triamterene, amiloride)	Concomitant use may lead to increases in serum potassium levels; may lead to increases in serum creatinine levels in heart failure patients.

Table 13.3. Drug Interactions for Antihypertensive Agents

Potassium supplements	Concomitant use may lead to increases in serum potassium levels; may lead to increases in serum creatinine levels in heart failure patients.

Verapamil HCl-Trandolapril (Tarka)

Alcohol	May increase alcohol blood levels and prolong effects.
Anesthetics	Caution with concomitant use.
Antihypertensive drugs	Concomitant use may potentiate antihypertensive effect.
Beta-blockers	May produce additive negative effects on heart rate, AV conduction, and/or cardiac contractility.
Carbamazepine	May increase levels of carbamazepine.
Cyclosporine	May increase serum levels of cyclosporine.
Digoxin	May increase plasma levels of digoxin.
Disopyramide	Avoid administration of disopyramide within 48 hrs before or 24 hrs after verapamil administration.
Flecainide	May produce additive negative inotropic effects and prolongation of AV conduction with concomitant use.
Lithium	May increase serum lithium levels; monitor levels.
Neuromuscular blocker agents	May potentiate the effects of neuromuscular blockers; both trandolapril-verapamil and the neuromuscular blocker agent may require a dosage reduction.
Phenobarbital	May increased clearance of verapamil.
Potassium-containing salt substitutes	May increase the risk of hyperkalemia.
Potassium-sparing diuretics (eg, spironolactone, triamterene, amiloride)	May increase the risk of hyperkalemia.
Potassium supplements	May increase the risk of hyperkalemia.
Quinidine	Avoid concomitant use with quinidine if hypertrophic cardiomyopathy is present.
Rifampin	May reduce the oral bioavailability of verapamil.
Theophylline	May increase plasma levels of theophylline.

DIRECT RENIN INHIBITOR & COMBINATION

Aliskiren (Tekturna)

Atorvastatin	May increase plasma levels of aliskiren.
Cyclosporine	Avoid concomitant use.
Furosemide	Coadministration may decrease levels of furosemide.
Irbesartan	May reduce levels of aliskiren.
Ketoconazole	May increase plasma levels of aliskiren.
Potassium-containing salt substitutes	Caution with concomitant use, may lead to increases in serum potassium levels.
Potassium-sparing diuretics	Caution with concomitant use, may lead to increases in serum potassium levels.
Potassium supplements	Caution with concomitant use, may lead to increases in serum potassium levels.

Table 13.3. Drug Interactions for Antihypertensive Agents

Aliskiren-Hydrochlorothiazide (Tekturna HCT)

ACTH	Intensifies electrolyte depletion, particularly hypokalemia.
Alcohol	May potentiate orthostatic hypotension.
Antidiabetic drugs (insulin, oral hypoglycemic drugs)	May cause changes in dosage requirements of antidiabetic drugs.
Atorvastatin	May increase plasma levels of aliskiren.
Barbiturates	May potentiate orthostatic hypotension.
Cholestyramine	Impairs absorption of hydrochlorothiazide.
Colestipol	Impairs absorption of hydrochlorothiazide.
Corticosteroids	Intensifies electrolyte depletion, particularly hypokalemia.
Cyclosporine	Avoid concomitant use.
Furosemide	Coadministration may decrease levels of furosemide.
Irbesartan	May reduce levels of aliskiren.
Ketoconazole	May increase plasma levels of aliskiren.
Lithium	Increases the risk of lithium toxicity.
Narcotic analgesics	May potentiate orthostatic hypotension.
NSAIDs	May reduce the diuretic, natriuretic, and antihypertensive effects of hydrochlorothiazide.
Potassium-containing salt substitutes	Caution with concomitant use, may lead to increases in serum potassium levels.
Potassium-sparing diuretics	Caution with concomitant use, may lead to increases in serum potassium levels.
Potassium supplements	Caution with concomitant use, may lead to increases in serum potassium levels.
Pressor amines (eg, norepinephrine)	May decrease response to pressor amines.

DIURETICS (ALDOSTERONE RECEPTOR BLOCKERS)

Eplerenone (Inspra)

ACE inhibitors	May increase risk of hyperkalemia.
Angiotensin II receptor antagonists	Caution with concomitant use, may increase risk of hyperkalemia.
CYP3A4 inhibitors	Increases levels of eplerenone; avoid concomitant use with potent CYP3A4 inhibitors (eg, ketoconazole, itraconazole, nefazodone, troleandomycin, clarithromycin, ritonavir, nelfinavir); caution with moderate inhibitors of CYP3A4.
Lithium	May increase risk of lithium toxicity; monitor lithium levels.
NSAIDs	Concomitant use may reduce the antihypertensive effects of eplerenone; monitor blood pressure levels.

Spironolactone (Aldactone)

ACE inhibitors	Caution, risk of hyperkalemia with concomitant use.
ACTH	Concomitant use may intensify electrolyte depletion, particularly hypokalemia.

Table 13.3. Drug Interactions for Antihypertensive Agents

Alcohol	May potentiate orthostatic hypotension.
Barbiturates	May potentiate orthostatic hypotension.
Corticosteroids	Concomitant use may intensify electrolyte depletion, particularly hypokalemia.
Digoxin	May increase serum digoxin levels; risk of digoxin toxicity.
Lithium	Increases the risk of lithium toxicity.
Narcotic analgesics	May potentiate orthostatic hypotension.
Norepinephrine	Reduces vascular responsiveness to norepinephrine.
NSAIDs (eg, indomethacin)	Caution, risk of hyperkalemia with concomitant use; may reduce the diuretic, natriuretic, and antihypertensive effects of spironolactone.
Potassium-sparing diuretics	Caution, risk of hyperkalemia with other potassium sparing diuretics.
Potassium supplements	Caution, risk of hyperkalemia with concomitant use.

DIURETICS (LOOP)

Bumetanide (Bumex)

Aminoglycosides	Avoid concomitant use.
Antihypertensive drugs	Concomitant use may potentiate antihypertensive effect.
Indomethacin	Avoid concomitant use.
Lithium	Increases the risk of lithium toxicity.
Nephrotoxic drugs	Avoid concomitant use.
Ototoxic drugs	Avoid concomitant use.
Probenecid	Reduces the effects of bumetanide.

Ethacrynic acid (Edecrin)

Aminoglycosides	May increase the ototoxic potential of aminoglycosides.
Antihypertensive drugs	Concomitant use may cause orthostatic hypotension.
Cephalosporins	May increase the ototoxic potential of some cephalosporins.
Corticosteroids	Concomitant use may increase the risk of gastric hemorrhage.
Digitalis glycosides	Excessive loss of potassium in patients receiving digitalis glycosides may precipitate digitalis toxicity.
Lithium	Increases the risk of lithium toxicity.
NSAIDs	May reduce the diuretic, natriuretic, and antihypertensive effects of ethacrynic acid.
Potassium-depleting steroids	Caution with concomitant use.
Warfarin	Displaces warfarin from plasma protein; may require dose reduction of warfarin.

Furosemide (Lasix)

ACTH	Concomitant use may cause hypokalemia.
Alcohol	May potentiate orthostatic hypotension.
Aminoglycosides	May increase ototoxic potential of aminoglycosides; avoid concomitant use.
Antihypertensive drugs	Concomitant use may potentiate antihypertensive effect.

Table 13.3. Drug Interactions for Antihypertensive Agents

Barbiturates	May potentiate orthostatic hypotension.
Corticosteroids	Concomitant use may cause hypokalemia.
Ethacrynic acid	Risk of ototoxiciy; avoid concomitant use.
Ganglionic or peripheral adrenergic blocking drugs	Potentiates the effects of ganglionic or peripheral adrenergic blocking drugs.
Indomethacin	May reduce the natriuretic and antihypertensive effects of furosemide.
Lithium	Risk of lithium toxicity.
Narcotic analgesics	May potentiate orthostatic hypotension.
Norepinephrine	May decrease arterial response to norepinephrine.
NSAIDs	Concomitant use may cause changes in renal function.
Salicylates	Caution with concomitant use of high dose salicylates, may lead to salicylate toxicity.
Succinylcholine	May potentiate the actions of succinylcholine.
Sucralfate	May reduce the natriuretic and antihypertensive effects of furosemide; separate sucralfate dose by 2 hrs.
Tubocurarine	Antagonizes the skeletal muscle relaxing effect of tubocurarine.
Torsemide (Demadex)	
ACTH	Risk of hypokalemia with concomitant use.
Aminoglycosides	Caution with concomitant use.
Cholestyramine	Avoid simultaneous administration.
Corticosteroids	Risk of hypokalemia with concomitant use.
Indomethacin	Partially inhibits the natriuretic effect of torsemide.
Lithium	May increase the risk of lithium toxicity.
NSAIDs	Concomitant use may cause renal dysfunction.
Probenecid	Decreases the diuretic effect of torsemide.
Salicylates	Caution with concomitant use of high dose salicylates, may lead to salicylate toxicity.
Spironolactone	Reduces renal clearance of spironolactone.

DIURETICS (POTASSIUM-SPARING)

Amiloride HCl*	
ACE inhibitors	May increase the risk of hyperkalemia.
Angiotensin II receptor antagonists	May increase the risk of hyperkalemia.
Cyclosporine	May increase the risk of hyperkalemia.
Diuretics	Risk of hyponatremia and hypochloremia when used concomitantly with other diuretics.
Indomethacin	May increase the risk of hyperkalemia.
Lithium	Increases the risk of lithium toxicity.
NSAIDs	May reduce the diuretic, natriuretic, and antihypertensive effects of amiloride.
Tacrolimus	May increase the risk of hyperkalemia.

*Available only in generic form.

Table 13.3. Drug Interactions for Antihypertensive Agents

Triamterene (Dyrenium)

ACE inhibitors	Increases the risk of hyperkalemia.
Anesthetic medications	May potentiate effects of anesthetic medications.
Antidiabetic drugs (insulin, oral hypoglycemic drugs)	May cause hyperglycemia; may require dosing adjustment of antidiabetic drugs.
Antihypertensives	May potentiate antihypertensive effects.
Blood from blood bank	Caution with concomitant use, may cause hyperkalemia.
Chlorpropamide	Concomitant use may increase risk of severe hyponatremia.
Diuretics	May potentiate diuretic effects.
Indomethacin	Concomitant use may cause renal failure.
Milk	Caution with concomitant use, may cause hyperkalemia.
Muscle relaxants, nondepolarizing	May potentiate effects of nondepolarizing skeletal muscle relaxants.
NSAIDs	Caution with concomitant use.
Potassium-containing salt substitutes	Caution with concomitant use, may cause hyperkalemia.
Potassium-containing medications (eg, parenteral penicillin G potassium)	Caution with concomitant use, may cause hyperkalemia.
Preanesthetic medications	May potentiate effects of preanesthetic medications.

DIURETICS (THIAZIDE)

Chlorothiazide (Diuril)

ACTH	Concomitant use intensifies electrolyte depletion, particularly hypokalemia.
Alcohol	May potentiate orthostatic hypotension.
Antidiabetic drugs (insulin, oral hypoglycemic drugs)	May cause changes in dosage requirements of the antidiabetic drug.
Antihypertensive drugs	May potentiate antihypertensive effect.
Barbiturates	May potentiate orthostatic hypotension.
Cholestyramine	May decrease absorption of chlorothiazide from the GI tract.
Colestipol	May decrease absorption of chlorothiazide from the GI tract.
Corticosteroids	Concomitant use intensifies electrolyte depletion, particularly hypokalemia.
COX-2 Inhibitors	May reduce the diuretic, natriuretic, and antihypertensive effects of chlorthiazide.
Lithium	Increases the risk of lithium toxicity.
Muscle relaxants, nondepolarizing (eg, tubocurarine)	May increase responsiveness to skeletal muscle relaxants.
Narcotic analgesics	May potentiate orthostatic hypotension.

Table 13.3. Drug Interactions for Antihypertensive Agents

NSAIDs	May reduce the diuretic, natriuretic, and antihypertensive effects of chlorothiazide.
Pressor amines (eg, norepinephrine)	May decrease response to pressor amines.
Chlorthalidone (Thalitone)	
Alcohol	May potentiate orthostatic hypotension.
Antidiabetic drugs (insulin, oral hypoglycemic drugs)	May cause changes in dosage requirements of the antidiabetic drug.
Antihypertensive drugs	May potentiate antihypertensive effect.
Barbiturates	May potentiate orthostatic hypotension.
Lithium	Increases the risk of lithium toxicity.
Narcotic analgesics	May potentiate orthostatic hypotension.
Norepinephrine	May decrease response to norepinephrine.
Tubocurarine	May increase responsiveness to tubocurarine.
Hydrochlorothiazide (Microzide)	
ACTH	Concomitant use intensifies electrolyte depletion, particularly hypokalemia.
Alcohol	May potentiate orthostatic hypotension.
Antidiabetic drugs (insulin, oral hypoglycemic drugs)	May cause changes in dosage requirements of the antidiabetic drug.
Antihypertensive drugs	Concomitant use may potentiate antihypertensive effect.
Barbiturates	May potentiate orthostatic hypotension.
Cholestyramine	May decrease absorption of hydrochlorothiazide from the GI tract.
Colestipol	May decrease absorption of hydrochlorothiazide from the GI tract.
Corticosteroids	Concomitant use intensifies electrolyte depletion, particularly hypokalemia.
Lithium	Increases the risk of lithium toxicity.
Muscle relaxants, nondepolarizing (eg, tubocurarine)	May increase responsiveness to skeletal muscle relaxants.
Narcotic analgesics	May potentiate orthostatic hypotension.
NSAIDs	May reduce the diuretic, natriuretic, and antihypertensive effects of hydrochlorothiazide.
Pressor amines (eg, norepinephrine)	May decrease response to pressor amines.
Indapamide (Lozol)	
ACTH	May increase the risk of hypokalemia.
Antidiabetic drugs (insulin, oral hypoglycemic drugs)	May cause changes in dosage requirements of the antidiabetic drug.
Antihypertensive drugs	Concomitant use may potentiate antihypertensive effect.
Corticosteroids	May increase the risk of hypokalemia.
Lithium	Increases the risk of lithium toxicity.

Table 13.3. Drug Interactions for Antihypertensive Agents

Norepinephrine	May decrease arterial response to norepinephrine.

Methyclothiazide (Enduron)

ACTH	May increase the risk of hypokalemia.
Antihypertensive drugs	Concomitant use may potentiate antihypertensive effect.
Corticosteroids	May increase the risk of hypokalemia.
Insulin	May alter insulin requirements.
Lithium	Increases the risk of lithium toxicity.
Norepinephrine	May decrease arterial response to norepinephrine.
Tubocurarine	May increase responsiveness to tubocurarine.

Metolazone (Zaroxolyn)

ACTH	May increase risk of hypokalemia and increase salt and water retention.
Alcohol	May potentiate orthostatic hypotension.
Anticoagulants	May require dosage adjustment of anticoagulants.
Antidiabetic drugs (insulin, oral hypoglycemic drugs)	May cause changes in dosage requirements of the antidiabetic drug.
Antihypertensive drugs	Concomitant use may require dose adjustment of other antihypertensive drugs.
Barbiturates	May potentiate orthostatic hypotension.
Corticosteroids	May increase risk of hypokalemia and increase salt and water retention.
Curariform drugs (eg, tubocurarine)	May increase neuromuscular blocking effects of curariform drugs.
Digitalis	Diuretic induced hypokalemia can increase sensitivity of the myocardium to digitalis which may cause serious arrthymias.
Furosemide	Concomitant use with furosemide or other loop diuretics may cause unusually large or prolonged losses of fluid and electrolytes.
Lithium	May increase the risk of lithium toxicity.
Methenamine	May decrease efficacy of methenamine.
Narcotic analgesics	May potentiate orthostatic hypotension.
Norepinephrine	May decrease arterial response to norepinephrine.
NSAIDs	May decrease antihypertensive effects of metolazone.
Salicylates	May decrease antihypertensive effects of metolazone.

DIURETIC COMBINATIONS†

Amiloride HCl-Hydrochlorothiazide*

ACE Inhibitors	May increase the risk of hyperkalemia.
ACTH	Intensifies electrolyte depletion, particularly hypokalemia.
Alcohol	May potentiate orthostatic hypotension.

*Available only in generic form.

† More combination interaction information is on page 219 (α-Antagonist Combinations), page 223 (ACE Inhibitor Combinations), page 229 (ARBs Combinations), page 238 (Beta-Blocker Combinations), and page 247 (Direct Renin Inhibitor & Combination).

Table 13.3. Drug Interactions for Antihypertensive Agents

Angiotensin II receptor antagonists	May increase the risk of hyperkalemia.
Antidiabetic drugs (insulin, oral hypoglycemic drugs)	May cause changes in dosage requirements of antidiabetic drugs.
Antihypertensives	May potentiate antihypertensive effects.
Barbiturates	May potentiate orthostatic hypotension.
Cholestyramine	Impairs absorption of hydrochlorothiazide.
Colestipol	Impairs absorption of hydrochlorothiazide.
Corticosteroids	Intensifies electrolyte depletion, particularly hypokalemia.
Cyclosporine	May increase the risk of hyperkalemia.
Indomethacin	May increase the risk of hyperkalemia.
Lithium	Increases the risk of lithium toxicity.
Muscle relaxants, nondepolarizing (eg, tubocurarine)	May increase responsiveness to skeletal muscle relaxants.
Narcotic analgesics	May potentiate orthostatic hypotension.
NSAIDs	May reduce the diuretic, natriuretic, and antihypertensive effects of amiloride-hydrochlorothiazide.
Pressor amines (eg, norepinephrine)	May decrease response to pressor amines.
Tacrolimus	May increase the risk of hyperkalemia.
Chlorthalidone-Clonidine HCl (Clorpres)	
Alcohol	May potentiate CNS-depressive effects and/or orthostatic hypotension.
Antidiabetic drugs (insulin, oral hypoglycemic drugs)	May cause changes in dosage requirements of the antidiabetic drug.
Antihypertensive drugs	Concomitant use may potentiate antihypertensive effect.
Barbiturates	May potentiate CNS-depressive effects and/or orthostatic hypotension.
Lithium	Increases the risk of lithium toxicity.
Narcotic analgesics	May potentiate orthostatic hypotension.
Norepinephrine	May decrease arterial response to norepinephrine.
Sedatives	May potentiate CNS-depressive effects.
Tricyclic antidepressants	May reduce the effect of clonidine; amitriptyline may enhance ocular toxicity.
Tubocurarine	May increase responsiveness to tubocurarine.
Spironolactone-Hydrochlorothiazide (Aldactazide)	
ACE inhibitors	Caution, risk of hyperkalemia with concomitant use.
ACTH	Concomitant use may intensify electrolyte depletion.
Alcohol	May potentiate orthostatic hypotension.

Table 13.3. Drug Interactions for Antihypertensive Agents

Antidiabetic drugs (insulin, oral hypoglycemic drugs)	May cause changes in dosage requirements of antidiabetic drugs.
Barbiturates	May potentiate orthostatic hypotension.
Corticosteroids	Concomitant use may intensify electrolyte depletion.
Digoxin	May increase serum digoxin levels and lead to digoxin toxicity.
Lithium	Increases the risk of lithium toxicity.
Muscle relaxants, nondepolarizing (eg, tubocurarine)	May increase responsiveness to skeletal muscle relaxants.
Narcotic analgesics	May potentiate orthostatic hypotension.
Norepinephrine	Reduces vascular responsiveness to norepinephrine.
NSAIDs	Caution, risk of hyperkalemia with concomitant use; may reduce the diuretic, natriuretic, and antihypertensive effects of hydrochlorothiazide-spironolactone.
Potassium supplements	Risk of hyperkalemia with concomitant use.
Potassium-sparing diuretics	Risk of hyperkalemia with concomitant use of other potassium sparing diuretics.
Triamterene-Hydrochlorothiazide (Dyazide, Maxzide, Maxzide-25)	
ACE inhibitors	Increases the risk of hyperkalemia.
ACTH	Concomitant use may intensify electrolyte depletion.
Alcohol	May potentiate orthostatic hypotension.
Amphotericin B	Concomitant use may intensify electrolyte depletion.
Anticoagulants, oral	Concomitant use may decrease effects of oral anticoagulants; dose of oral anticoagulant may need to be adjusted.
Antidiabetic drugs (insulin, oral hypoglycemic drugs)	May cause changes in dosage requirements of antidiabetic drugs.
Antigout medications	Hydrochlorothiazide may increase blood uric acid levels; may require dose adjustment of antigout medications.
Antihypertensives	May potentiate antihypertensive effects.
Barbiturates	May potentiate orthostatic hypotension.
Blood from blood bank	Caution with concomitant use, may cause hyperkalemia.
Chlorpropamide	Concomitant use may increase risk of severe hyponatremia.
Corticosteroids	Concomitant use may intensify electrolyte depletion.
Indomethacin	Concomitant use may cause renal failure.
Insulin	Concomitant use may alter insulin requirements.
Laxatives	Chronic or overuse of laxatives may reduce serum potassium levels.
Lithium	Increases the risk of lithium toxicity.
Methenamine	May decrease the effectiveness of methenamine.
Milk, low-salt	Caution with concomitant use, may cause hyperkalemia.

Table 13.3. Drug Interactions for Antihypertensive Agents

Muscle relaxants, nondepolarizing (eg, tubocurarine)	May increase effects of nondepolarizing skeletal muscle relaxants.
Narcotic analgesics	May potentiate orthostatic hypotension.
Norepinephrine	Decreases arterial response to norepinephrine.
NSAIDs	Caution with concomitant use.
Potassium-containing salt substitutes	Caution with concomitant use, may cause hyperkalemia.
Potassium-containing medications (eg, parenteral penicillin G potassium)	Caution with concomitant use, may cause hyperkalemia.
Sodium polystyrene sulfonate	Reduces serum potassium levels.
Tubocurarine	May increase responsiveness to tubocurarine.

VASODILATORS

Hydralazine HCl*

Antihypertensive drugs, parenteral (eg, diazoxide)	Concomitant use with potent parenteral antihypertensive drugs may cause profound hypotension.
Epinephrine	May reduce pressor response to epinephrine.
MAO inhibitors	Caution with concomitant use.

Isosorbide dinitrate (Isordil, Isordil titradose)

Alcohol	May produce additive vasodilating effects.
Sildenafil	Concomitant use may cause severe hypotension.
Vasodilators	May produce additive vasodilating effects.

Isosorbide mononitrate (Imdur, Ismo)

Alcohol	May produce additive vasodilating effects.
Calcium channel blockers	May cause orthostatic hypotension.
Sildenafil	Concomitant use may cause severe hypotension.
Vasodilators	May produce additive vasodilating effects.

Minoxidil*

Guanethidine	Risk of severe orthostatic hypotension with concomitant use.

VASODILATOR COMBINATION

Hydralazine HCl-Isosorbide dinitrate (BiDil)

Alcohol	May produce additive vasodilating effects.
Antihypertensive drugs, parenteral	Concomitant use with potent parenteral antihypertensive drugs may cause profound hypotension.
MAO inhibitors	Caution with concomitant use.

*Available only in generic form.

Table 13.3. Drug Interactions for Antihypertensive Agents

Phosphodiesterase inhibitors (eg, sildenafil, vardenafil, tadalafil)	Concomitant use may cause severe hypotension.
Vasodilators	May produce additive vasodilating effects.

MISCELLANEOUS

Clonidine (Catapres, Catapres-TTS)

Alcohol	Concomitant use may potentiate CNS depression.
Barbiturates	Concomitant use may potentiate CNS depression.
Beta-blockers	Concomitant use may produce additive bradycardia and AV block.
Calcium channel blockers	Concomitant use may produce additive bradycardia and AV block.
Digitalis	Concomitant use may produce additive bradycardia and AV block.
Sedatives	Concomitant use may potentiate CNS depression.
Tricyclic antidepressants	May reduce the hypotensive effect of clonidine.

Fenoldopam mesylate (Corlopam)

Beta-blockers	Avoid concomitant use, may cause unexpected hypotension.

Guanfacine HCl (Tenex)

CNS depressants	Concomitant use may produce additive sedative effects.
CYP450 inducers (eg, phenobarbital, phenytoin)	Caution with concomitant use in patients who have renal dysfunction.

Mecamylamine HCl (Inversine)

Alcohol	May potentiate effects of mecamylamine.
Anesthesia	May potentiate effects of mecamylamine.
Antibiotics	Avoid concomitant use.
Antihypertensive drugs	May potentiate effects of mecamylamine.
Sulfonamides	Avoid concomitant use.

Methyldopa*

Anesthetics	Concomitant use may require dose reductions of anesthetics.
Antihypertensive drugs	Concomitant use may potentiate antihypertensive effects.
Ferrous gluconate	May decrease bioavailability of methyldopa; avoid concomitant use.
Ferrous sulfate	May decrease bioavailability of methyldopa; avoid concomitant use.
Lithium	Monitor for signs of lithium toxicity.
MAO inhibitors	Warning, concomitant use is contraindicated.

Phenoxybenzamine HCl (Dibenzyline)

Alpha-adrenergic agonist	Concomitant use may produce an exaggerated hypotensive response and tachycardia.

*Available only in generic form.
**Combination information for clonidine/chlorthalidone (Clorpres) is on page 253.

Table 13.3. Drug Interactions for Antihypertensive Agents

Beta-adrenergic agonist	Concomitant use may produce an exaggerated hypotensive response and tachycardia.
Epinephrine	Concomitant use may produce an exaggerated hypotensive response and tachycardia.
Levarterenol	Blocks hyperthermia production by levarterenol
Reserpine	Blocks hypothermia production by reserpine.
Reserpine*	
Antihypertensive agents	Caution with concomitant use.
Digoxin	Risk of cardiac arrhythmias with concomitant use.
MAO inhibitors	Avoid or use with extreme caution.
Quinidine	Risk of cardiac arrhythmias with concomitant use.
Sympathomimetics, direct-acting (eg, epinephrine, isoproterenol, phenylephrine)	Concomitant use may prolong the actions of direct-acting sympathomimetics.
Sympathomimetics, indirect-acting (eg, ephedrine, tyramine)	Concomitant use may inhibit the effects of indirect-acting sympathomimetics.
Tricyclic antidepressants	Concomitant use may decrease the antihypertensive effect of reserpine.

*Available only in generic form.

Hypertension Management in Adults with Diabetes

American Diabetes Association

INTRODUCTION

Hypertension (defined as a blood pressure ≥140/90 mmHg) is an extremely common comorbid condition in diabetes, affecting ~20–60% of patients with diabetes, depending on obesity, ethnicity, and age. In type 2 diabetes, hypertension is often present as part of the metabolic syndrome of insulin resistance also including central obesity and dyslipidemia. In type 1 diabetes, hypertension may reflect the onset of diabetic nephropathy. Hypertension substantially increases the risk of both macrovascular and microvascular complications, including stroke, coronary artery disease, and peripheral vascular disease, retinopathy, nephropathy, and possibly neuropathy. In recent years, adequate data from well-designed randomized clinical trials have demonstrated the effectiveness of aggressive treatment of hypertension in reducing both types of diabetes complications.

Scope

These recommendations are intended to apply to nonpregnant adults with type 1 or type 2 diabetes.

Target Audience

These recommendations are intended for the use of health care professionals who care for patients with diabetes and hypertension, including specialist and primary care physicians, nurses and nurse practitioners, physicians' assistants, educators, dietitians, and others.

Method

These recommendations are based on the American Diabetes Association Technical Review "Treatment of Diabetes in Adult Patients with Hypertension." A technical review is a systematic review of the medical literature that has been peer-reviewed by the American Diabetes Association's Professional Practice Committee.

Abbreviations: ACE: angiotensin-converting enzyme; ALLHAT: Antihypertensive and Lipid-Lowering Treatment to Prevent Heart Attack Trial; ARB: angiotensin receptor blocker; DCCB: dihydropyridine calcium channel blocker; HOT: Hypertension Optimal Treatment; JNC VI: Sixth Report of the Joint National Committee on Prevention, Detection, Evaluation, and Treatment of High Blood Pressure; UKPDS: U.K. Prospective Diabetes Study

EVIDENCE REVIEW: HYPERTENSION AS A RISK FACTOR FOR COMPLICATIONS OF DIABETES

Diabetes increases the risk of coronary events twofold in men and fourfold in women. Part of this increase is due to the frequency of associated cardiovascular risk factors such as hypertension, dyslipidemia, and clotting abnormalities. In observational studies, people with both diabetes and hypertension have approximately twice the risk of cardiovascular disease as nondiabetic people with hypertension. Hypertensive diabetic patients are also at increased risk for diabetes-specific complications including retinopathy and nephropathy. In the U.K. Prospective Diabetes Study (UKPDS) epidemiological study, each 10-mmHg decrease in mean systolic blood pressure was associated with reductions in risk of 12% for any complication related to diabetes, 15% for deaths related to diabetes, 11% for myocardial infarction, and 13% for microvascular complications. No threshold of risk was observed for any end point.

EVIDENCE FOR TARGET LEVELS OF BLOOD PRESSURE IN PATIENTS WITH DIABETES

The UKPDS and the Hypertension Optimal Treatment (HOT) trial both demonstrated improved outcomes, especially in preventing stroke, in patients assigned to lower blood pressure targets. Optimal outcomes in the HOT study were achieved in the group with a target diastolic blood pressure of 80 mmHg (achieved 82.6 mmHg). Randomized clinical trials demonstrate the benefit of targeting a diastolic blood pressure of ≤80 mmHg. Epidemiological analyses show that blood pressures ≥120/70 mmHg are associated with increased cardiovascular event

rates and mortality in persons with diabetes. Therefore, a target blood pressure goal of <130/80 mmHg is reasonable if it can be safely achieved. There is no threshold value for blood pressure, and risk continues to decrease well into the normal range. Achieving lower levels, however, would increase the cost of care as well as drug side effects and is often difficult in practice. Whether even more aggressive treatment would further reduce the risk is an unanswered question, but may be answered by clinical trials now in progress.

EVIDENCE FOR NONDRUG MANAGEMENT OF HYPERTENSION

Dietary management with moderate sodium restriction has been effective in reducing blood pressure in individuals with essential hypertension. Several controlled studies have looked at the relationship between weight loss and blood pressure reduction. Weight reduction can reduce blood pressure independent of sodium intake and also can improve blood glucose and lipid levels. The loss of one kilogram in body weight has resulted in decreases in mean arterial blood pressure of ~1 mmHg. The role of very low calorie diets and pharmacologic agents that induce weight loss in the management of hypertension in diabetic patients has not been adequately studied. Some appetite suppressants may induce increases in blood pressure levels, so these must be used with care. Given the present evidence, weight reduction should be considered an effective measure in the initial management of mild-to-moderate hypertension, and these results could probably be extrapolated to the diabetic hypertensive population.

Sodium restriction has not been tested in the diabetic population in controlled clinical trials. However, results from controlled trials in essential hypertension have shown a reduction in systolic blood pressure of ~5 mmHg and diastolic blood pressure of 2–3 mmHg with moderate sodium restriction (from a daily intake of 200 mmol [4,600 mg] to 100 mmol [2,300 mg] of sodium per day). A dose response effect has been observed with sodium restriction. Even when pharmacologic agents are used, there is often a better response when there is concomitant salt restriction due to the aforementioned volume component of the hypertension that is almost always present. The efficacy of these measures in diabetic individuals is not known.

Moderately intense physical activity, such as 30–45 min of brisk walking most days of the week, has been shown to lower blood pressure and is recommended in the Sixth Report of the Joint National Committee on Prevention, Detection, Evaluation and Treatment of High Blood Pressure (JNC VI). The American Diabetes Association Consensus Development Conference on the Diagnosis of Coronary Heart Disease in People with Diabetes has recommended that diabetic patients who are 35 years of age or older and are planning to begin a vigorous exercise program should have exercise stress testing or other appropriate noninvasive testing. Stress testing is not generally necessary for asymptomatic patients beginning moderate exercise such as walking. Smoking cessation and moderation of alcohol intake are also recommended by JNC VI and are clearly appropriate for all patients with diabetes.

EVIDENCE FOR DRUG THERAPY OF HYPERTENSION

There are a number of trials demonstrating the superiority of drug therapy versus placebo in reducing outcomes including cardiovascular events and microvascular complications of retinopathy and progression of nephropathy. These studies used different drug classes, including angiotensin-converting enzyme (ACE) inhibitors, angiotensin receptor blockers (ARBs), diuretics, and ß-blockers, as the initial step in therapy. All of these agents were superior to placebo; however, it must be noted that many patients required three or more drugs to achieve the specified target levels of blood pressure control. Overall there is strong evidence that pharmacologic therapy of hypertension in patients with diabetes is effective in producing substantial decreases in cardiovascular and microvascular diseases.

There are limited data from trials comparing different classes of drugs in patients with diabetes and hypertension. The UKPDS-Hypertension in Diabetes Study showed no significant difference in outcomes for treatment based on an ACE inhibitor compared with a ß-blocker. There were slightly more withdrawals due to side effects and there was more weight gain in the ß-blocker group. In postmyocardial infarction patients, ß-blockers have been shown to reduce mortality.

There are numerous studies documenting the effectiveness of ACE inhibitors and ARBs in retarding the development and progression of diabetic nephropathy. ACE inhibitors have a favorable effect on cardiovascular outcomes, as demonstrated in the MICRO-HOPE study. This cardiovascular effect may be mediated by mechanisms other than blood pressure reduction. It is possible that other drug classes may behave similarly.

Some studies have shown an excess of selected cardiac events in patients treated with dihydropyridine calcium channel blockers (DCCBs) compared with ACE inhibitors. Ongoing trials including the Antihypertensive and Lipid-Lowering Treatment to Prevent Heart Attack Trial (ALLHAT) study should help to resolve this issue. DCCBs in combination with ACE inhibitors, ß-blockers, and diuretics, as in the HOT study and the Systolic Hypertension in Europe (Syst-Eur) Trial, did not appear to be associated with increased cardiovascular morbidity. However, ACE inhibitors and ß-blockers appear to be superior to DCCBs in reducing myocardial infarction and heart failure. Therefore, DCCBs appear to be appropriate agents in addition to, but not instead of, ACE inhibitors and ß-blockers. Non-DCCBs (ie, verapamil and diltiazem) may reduce coronary events. In short-term studies, non-DCCBs have reduced albumin excretion.

There are no long-term studies of the effect of β-blockers, loop diuretics, or centrally acting adrenergic blockers on long-term complications of diabetes. The α-blocker arm of the ALLHAT study was stopped by the data and safety monitoring committee because of an increase in cases of new-onset heart failure in patients assigned to the α-blocker. While this could merely represent unmasking of heart failure in patients previously treated with an ACE inhibitor or a diuretic, it seems reasonable to use these as second-line agents when preferred classes have been ineffective or when other specific indications, such as benign prostatic hypertrophy (BPH), are present.

SUMMARY

There is a strong epidemiological connection between hypertension in diabetes and adverse outcomes of diabetes. Clinical trials demonstrate the efficacy of drug therapy versus placebo in reducing these outcomes and in setting an aggressive blood pressure–lowering target of <130/80 mmHg. It is very clear that many people will require three or more drugs to achieve the recommended target. Achievement of the target blood pressure goal with a regimen that does not produce burdensome side effects and is at reasonable cost to the patient is probably more important than the specific drug strategy.

Because many studies demonstrate the benefits of ACE inhibitors on multiple adverse outcomes in patients with diabetes, including both macrovascular and microvascular complications, in patients with either mild or more severe hypertension and in both type 1 and type 2 diabetes, the established practice of choosing an ACE inhibitor as the first-line agent in most patients with diabetes is reasonable. In patients with microalbuminemia or clinical nephropathy, both ACE inhibitors (type 1 and type 2 patients) and ARBs (type 2 patients) are considered first-line therapy for the prevention of and progression of nephropathy. However, other strategies including diuretic and ß-blocker–based therapy are also supported by evidence. Because of lingering concerns about the lower effectiveness of DCCBs (compared with ACE inhibitors, ARBs, ß-blockers, or diuretics) in decreasing coronary events and heart failure and in reducing progression of renal disease in diabetes, these agents should be used as second-line drugs for patients who cannot tolerate the other preferred classes or who require additional agents to achieve the target blood pressure. Other classes, including α-blockers, may be used under specific indications (such as symptoms of BPH for α-blockers) or other agents have failed to control the blood pressure or have unacceptable side effects. Blood pressure, orthostatic changes, renal function, and serum potassium should be monitored at appropriate intervals.

Treatment decisions should be individualized based on the clinical characteristics of the patient, including comorbidities as well as tolerability, personal preferences, and cost.

Table 1— Indications for initial treatment and goals for adult hypertensive diabetic patients		
	Systolic	Diastolic
Goal (mmHg)	<130	<80
Behavioral therapy alone (maximum 3 months) then add pharmacologic treatment	130–139	80–89
Behavioral therapy + pharmacologic treatment	≥140	≥90

RECOMMENDATIONS

Refer to **Table 1** for recommendations on initial treatment and goals for adult hypertensive diabetic patients.

SCREENING AND DIAGNOSIS

- Blood pressure should be measured at every routine diabetes visit. Patients found to have systolic blood pressure ≥130 mmHg or diastolic blood pressure ≥80 mmHg should have blood pressure confirmed on a separate day. (C)
- Orthostatic measurement of blood pressure should be performed when clinically indicated to assess for the presence of autonomic neuropathy. (E)

GOALS

- Patients with diabetes should be treated to a systolic blood pressure <130mm Hg. (B)
- Patients with diabetes should be treated to a diastolic blood pressure <80 mmHg. (B)

TREATMENT

- Patients with a systolic blood pressure of 130–139 mmHg or a diastolic blood pressure of 80–89 mmHg should be given lifestyle/behavioral therapy alone for a maximum of 3 months and then, if targets are not achieved, should also be treated pharmacologically with agents that block the renin-angiotensin system. (E)
- Patients with hypertension (systolic blood pressure ≥140 mmHg or diastolic blood pressure ≥90 mmHg) should receive drug therapy in addition to lifestyle/behavioral therapy. (A)
- Multiple drug therapy (two or more agents at proper doses) is generally required to achieve blood pressure targets. (B)
- Initial drug therapy for those with a blood pressure >140/90 should be with a drug class demonstrated to reduce CVD events in patients with diabetes (ACE inhibitors, ARBs, ß-blockers, diuretics, calcium channel blockers). (A)
- All patients with diabetes and hypertension should be treated with a regimen that includes either an ACE inhibitor or ARB. If one class is not tolerated, the other should be substituted. If needed to achieve blood pressure targets, a thiazide diuretic should be added. (E)
- If ACE inhibitors or ARBs are used, monitor renal function and serum potassium levels. (E)
- While there are no adequate head-to-head comparisons of ACE inhibitors and ARBs, there is clinical trial support for each of the following statements:

  o In patients with type 1 diabetes with hypertension and any degree of albuminuria, ACE inhibitors have been shown to delay the progression of nephropathy. (A)
  o In patients with type 2 diabetes, hypertension, and microalbuminuria, ACE inhibitors and ARBs have been shown to delay the progression to macroalbuminuria. (A)

o In those with type 2 diabetes, hypertension, macroalbuminuria (>300 mg/day), and renal insufficiency, an ARB should be strongly considered. (A)
- In elderly hypertensive patients, blood pressure should be lowered gradually to avoid complications. (E)
- Patients not achieving target blood pressure on three drugs, including a diuretic, and patients with a significant renal disease should be referred to a physician experienced in the care of patients with hypertension. (E)

FOOTNOTES

The recommendations in this paper are based on the evidence reviewed in the following publication: The treatment of hypertension in adult patients with diabetes (Technical Review). *Diabetes Care* 25:134–147, 2002.

The initial draft of this position statement was prepared by Carlos Arauz-Pacheco, MD, Marian A. Parrott, MD, MPH, and Phillip Raskin, MD. The paper was peer-reviewed, modified, and approved by the Professional Practice Committee and the Executive Committee, October 2001.

BIBLIOGRAPHY

1. Arauz-Pacheco C, Parrott MA, Raskin P. The treatment of hypertension in adult patients with diabetes (Technical Review). *Diabetes Care* 25:134–147, 2002.
2. Bakris GL, Williams M, Dworkin L, Elliott WJ, Epstein M, Toto R, Tuttle K, Douglas J, Hsueh W, Sowers J. Preserving renal function in adults with hypertension and diabetes: a consensus approach. *Am J Kid Dis* 36:646–661, 2000.

Chapter 14

Management of Hyperlipidemia

Joshua J. Neumiller, PharmD, CGP, FASCP

INTRODUCTION

Macrovascular complications are the leading cause of morbidity and mortality in the United States. People with type 2 diabetes are estimated to be two to four times as likely to suffer from coronary artery disease (CAD). Hyperlipidemia is one of the major risk factors associated with the increased overall mortality by cardiovascular disease in people with diabetes, indicating that lipid management in this at-risk population is a critical component of patient care. The most common lipid abnormalities present in people with type 2 diabetes are elevated triglyceride levels, increased very-low-density lipoprotein (VLDL) levels, and decreased high-density lipoprotein (HDL) concentrations. Patients with type 1 diabetes under good glycemic control exhibit little overall differences in lipid profiles compared to nondiabetic patients. In those with poor control, however, elevations in triglyceride, VLDL, and LDL concentrations can occur as well as reductions in HDL concentrations. Various studies have demonstrated that abnormal LDL, HDL, and triglyceride concentrations are independent predictors of cardiovascular disease. All patients with type 1 and type 2 diabetes should be assessed periodically for hyperlipidemia and appropriate treatment strategies initiated, if needed.

A number of clinical trials have demonstrated benefits in lipid-lowering therapies in the prevention of cardiovascular events in patients with diabetes. The Heart Protection Study conducted in patients with type 2 diabetes over 40 years of age demonstrated a 22% risk reduction in the event rate for major cardiovascular events in those patients treated with simvastatin. The Veterans Affairs High-Density Lipoprotein Cholesterol Intervention Trial (VA-HIT) associated the use of gemfibrozil with a 24% decrease in cardiovascular events in patients with diabetes with preexisting cardiovascular disease, low HDL (<40mg/dL), and modestly elevated triglyceride levels.

The predominant causes of elevated triglycerides in both type 1 and type 2 diabetes include increased VLDL synthesis, impaired VLDL clearance, and reduced lipoprotein lipase (LPL) activity. The predominance of small, dense LDL particles in subjects with diabetes has also been identified. These LDL particles contain more triglycerides and may be more atherogenic than the larger, less dense LDL cholesterol particles found in those without diabetes. Oxidation and glycosylation of LDL and other lipoproteins may increase their uptake into atherosclerotic lesions in people with diabetes, thus placing this population at increased risk of cardiovascular events. Elevations in the triglyceride content of HDL

Table 14.1. Treatment Recommendations and Goals for the Management of Hyperlipidemia in Patients with Diabetes

- Lifestyle modification focusing on the reduction of saturated fat and cholesterol intake, weight loss, increased physical activity, and smoking cessation has been shown to improve the lipid profile in patients with diabetes.
- Patients who do not achieve lipid goals with lifestyle modifications require pharmacological therapy.
- Lower LDL cholesterol to <100mg/dL as the primary goal of therapy for adults.
- Lowering LDL cholesterol with a statin is associated with a reduction in cardiovascular events.
- In people with diabetes over the age of 40 years with a total cholesterol ≥135mg/dL, statin therapy to achieve an LDL reduction of ~30% regardless of baseline LDL levels may be appropriate.
- In children and adolescents with diabetes, LDL cholesterol should be lowered to <100mg/dL using medical nutrition therapy and medications, based on LDL level and other cardiovascular risk factors in addition to diabetes.
- Lower triglycerides to <150mg/dL, and raise HDL cholesterol to >40mg/dL. In women, an HDL goal 10mg/dL higher may be appropriate.
- Lowering triglycerides and increasing HDL cholesterol with a fibrate is associated with a reduction in cardiovascular events in patients with clinical cardiovascular disease, low HDL, and near-normal levels of LDL.
- Combination therapy using statins and fibrates or niacin may be necessary to achieve lipid targets, but has not been evaluated in outcomes studies for either event reduction or safety.

Source: Dyslipidemia Management in Adults with Diabetes. *Diabetes Care.* 2004;27 (S1):S68-71.

particles have also been reported. Obesity, smoking, and insulin resistance are contributing factors to lipoprotein alterations. Other factors theorized to play a role in lipid abnormalities in this population include nephropathy, renal disease, and uremia.

Table 14.1 outlines treatment recommendations and goals for patients with diabetes regarding the management of hyperlipidemia to prevent cardiovascular events.

NONPHARMACOLOGICAL MANAGEMENT OF HYPERLIPIDEMIA

Dietary and lifestyle modifications are the mainstay of therapy concerning the management of hyperlipidemia in patients with diabetes. Lipid abnormalities in people with diabetes are often secondary to inadequate control of blood glucose. Aggressive glycemic control should be a primary goal for all patients with diabetes, and effective management of blood glucose will convey beneficial effects to cholesterol concentrations.

Improved eating habits and increased physical activity can facilitate important metabolic benefits in patients with diabetes. Consultation with a dietitian can provide valuable assistance to patients with diabetes to optimize dietary habits. Physical activity (exercise) can result in favorable changes in body weight and body composition. Increased physical activity has been associated with improvements in triglyceride levels, total cholesterol, and LDL levels while increasing HDL cholesterol levels. Individualized exercise programs should be tailored to the patient's diabetic complications, history and medical status to avoid injury and optimize results. Physical limitations, including vascular complications and/or neuropathy associated with diabetes, may limit the extent or type of physical activity that can be implemented. Even modest weight loss (<10 pounds) has been shown to improve cholesterol profiles. Weight reduction is associated with improvements in triglycerides, insulin sensitivity, glucose control, reductions in total and LDL cholesterol, and increases in HDL cholesterol.

Table 14.2. Order of Priorities for Treatment of Dyslipidemia in Adults with Diabetes
1. **LDL lowering** Lifestyle interventions Preferred: HMG CoA reductase inhibitor (statin) Others: Bile acid binding resin, ezetimibe, fenofibrate or niacin
2. **HDL cholesterol raising** Lifestyle interventions Nicotinic acid or fibrates
3. **Triglyceride lowering** Lifestyle interventions Glycemic control Fibric acid derivative (gemfibrozil, fenofibrate) Niacin High-dose statins in those who also have elevated LDL cholesterol
4. **Combined hyperlipidemia** First choice: Improved glycemic control plus high-dose statin Second choice: Improved glycemic control plus statin plus fibric acid derivative Third choice: Improved glycemic control plus statin plus nicotinic acid
Source: Dyslipidemia management in adults with diabetes. *Diabetes Care.* 2004;27 (S1):S68-71.

PHARMACOLOGICAL MANAGEMENT OF HYPERLIPIDEMIA

When dietary modifications, lifestyle changes, and strict glycemic control fail to adequately control dyslipidemia in patients with diabetes, pharmacological intervention is warranted. **Table 14.2** outlines the order of priorities for the treatment of dyslipidemia in adults with diabetes and preferred treatment strategies.

Many therapies used in patients with diabetes exert effects upon lipoprotien concentrations. Insulin, metformin, thiazolidinediones, and sulfonylureas are all associated with improvents in glucose control, insulin sensitivity, and lipoprotien abnormalities. Metformin has been shown to decrease triglyceride levels via reductions in VLDL cholesterol. Positive effects of metformin therapy have also been documented on LDL and HDL cholesterol, albeit with less frequency and consistency than

with triglycerides. Likewise, sulfonylureas can reduce total cholesterol and triglyceride concentrations in patients with type 2 diabetes. Reductions in LDL and elevations in HDL cholesterol concentrations have also been observed in some studies. Intensification of insulin therapy can correct lipoprotien abnormalities in both type 1 and type 2 patients. Pioglitazone has been shown to decrease triglyceride levels and increase HDL concentrations with no changes in LDL or total cholesterol levels. Rosiglitazone therapy results in a reduction in free fatty acids and an increase in LDL and HDL.

HMG-CoA Reductase Inhibitors (Statins)

HMG-CoA reductase inhibitors, or statins, are useful agents in the treatment of hypercholesterolemia. Statins are widely utilized and are considered the gold standard of lipid lowering therapies. **Statins are particularly** useful pharmacological agents in the treatment of hyperlipidemia, particularly those with elevated LDL cholesterol, and are considered first-line agents by the ADA. Patients with diabetes and hyperlipidemia should be considered as candidates for statin therapy unless a contraindication exists.

Pharmacology

Mechanism of Action
HMG-CoA reductase inhibitors (statins) inhibit the rate-limiting hepatic enzyme responsible for converting HMG-CoA to mevalonate, a precursor of cholesterol. This inhibition in turn results in LDL receptor up-regulation and increased hepatic uptake of LDL cholesterol from the systemic circulation. Statins exhibit favorable effects on LDL, HDL, and triglyceride levels.

Pharmacokinetics
Specific pharmacokinetic characteristics vary depending on the statin agent being used. For specific pharmacokinetic parameters, refer to the full prescribing information for the drug in question.

Treatment Advantages and Disadvantages
HMG-CoA reductase inhibitors are especially valuable for diabetes patients with elevated LDL cholesterol, and are considered first-line agents by the ADA. Statins are associated with 18%-55% reductions in LDL, 7%-30% reductions in triglycerides, and increases of 5%-15% in HDL concentrations. Patients with diabetes with elevated LDL cholesterol and mild hypertriglyceridemia are prime candidates for statin therapy. Patients with autonomic neuropathy may obtain additional benefits from statin therapy due to reduced lithogenicity of bile, thus aiding in the prevention of cholelithiasis. Altered glycemic control has not been reported in patients with diabetes. The risk of myopathy due to statin therapy is of concern in patients with diabetic nephropathy and/or moderate to severe renal impairment. Given the potential for hepatic and muscular toxicity with these agents, careful consideration of individual patient characteristics is important prior to initiation of therapy.

Statins are effective in lowering apolipoprotein B (Apo B), the primary apolipoprotein of LDL cholesterol, which carries LDL to tissues. Each LDL, VLDL, and intermediate-density lipoprotein particle contains a single Apo B molecule. Because of the effects of statins on Apo B and LDL cholesterol, together with the direct relationship between Apo B concentrations and LDL/VLDL/intermediate-density lipoprotein concentrations, recent evidence suggests that Apo B serum concentrations are the optimal indicator of statin efficacy.

Therapeutic Considerations

Warnings and Precautions
Statins are contraindicated in patients with active hepatic disease or those with persistent elevations in hepatic enzymes such as ALT, and should be avoided in patients with alcoholic liver disease. Statins also should be used cautiously in patients with a history of rhabdomyolysis.

Special Populations
Statins are pregnancy category X medications because cholesterol biosynthesis pathways are crucial for fetal development, and statins can inhibit fetal synthesis of steroids and cell membranes. Additionally, statins are contraindicated during breastfeeding. Elderly patients may have an increased susceptibility to adverse effects as well as an increased cholesterol-lowering response to statin therapy, thus lower doses are often required in the aging population.

Adverse Effects and Monitoring

Common adverse events associated with statin therapy include arthralgia, dyspepsia, constipation, and abdominal pain. Serious myopathies and rhabdomyolysis can occur with statin therapy, and patients should report any abnormal muscle pain or discomfort to health care providers. While rare, severe hepatotoxicity can occur with statin therapy, including hepatitis, cholestasis with jaundice, cirrhosis, hepatic failure, and pancreatitis. Statin therapy can also induce elevations in hepatic enzymes, and thus periodic liver function tests (LFTs) are warranted in patients taking these medications.

Drug Interactions

Many of the statins are substrates of the cytochrome P450 system, and thus drug interactions are possible regarding the metabolism of the agents. Any patient under consideration for statin therapy should receive a thorough review of their medication regimen to assess the possibility of drug interactions prior to drug initiation. Rosuvastatin, unlike other statins, undergoes minimal hepatic metabolism and thus has less of a potential for drug interactions. For additional information regarding potential drug interactions with these agents, see **Table 14.4**, or refer to the full prescribing information for the drug in question.

Dosage and Administration

Statins are dosed once daily, excluding atorvastatin, which has a long, active half-life of 20-30 hours and thus can be dosed at any time of the day. Statins are typically dosed at bedtime since cholesterol production is at its highest during sleep. Dosing parameters vary depending on specific agent used. Doses should typically be titrated at four-week intervals. Refer to **Table 14.3**, or refer to the full prescribing information for specific dosing and administration information.

Fibric Acid Derivatives

Fibric acid derivatives, or fibrates for short, can be used with success in the treatment of hypertriglyceridemia, and have demonstrated efficacy in patients with diabetes. **Fenofibrate is considered a viable alternative for the treatment of elevated LDL cholesterol in patients with diabetes who cannot take statins or require multidrug therapy to meet goals set by the ADA, and may be synergistic when used in combination with statin therapy. Fibric acid derivatives are associated with reductions of 5%-20% in LDL cholesterol, decreases of 20%-50% in triglyceride levels, and increases of 10%-20% in HDL concentrations.**

Pharmacology

Mechanism of Action

While the exact mechanisms involved in the lipid-lowering effects of the fibrates are not fully understood, these agents have been shown to inhibit peripheral lipolysis and decrease hepatic extraction of free fatty acids, thus decreasing triglyceride production by the liver. Fibrates, such as gemfibrozil, also inhibit the synthesis and increase the clearance of apolipoprotein B, which is a carrier molecule for VLDL cholesterol. Fibrates may also increase lipoprotein lipase activity and stimulate the production of apoprotein A-I, which is thought to aid in maintaining the integrity of HDL cholesterol particles. These agents also appear to accelerate the removal of cholesterol from the liver, and increase the excretion of cholesterol via the feces.

Pharmacokinetics

Specific pharmacokinetic characteristics vary depending on the fibric acid derivative used. For specific pharmacokinetic parameters, refer to the full prescribing information for the drug in question.

Treatment Advantages and Disadvantages

Beneficial effects of fibric acid derivatives include reduction in triglycerides, reduction in VLDL cholesterol, and increases in HDL concentrations. Gemfibrozil has been demonstrated to be highly beneficial in patients with diabetes. Patients with severe mixed hyperlipidemia associated with elevated LDL cholesterol can benefit from fibrate therapy in combination with a statin. Patients taking this combination, however, should be monitored closely for creatinine phosphokinase (CPK) elevations and the development of myopathy. In the Helsinki Heart Study, gemfibrozil was associated with a reduction in overall cardiovascular events, thus gemfibrozil is the agent of choice in patients with diabetes in whom hypertriglyceridemia is the predominant lipid abnormality. Additionally, studies have indicated that fibric acid derivatives are beneficial in decreasing angiographic progression of coronary artery disease (CAD). Fibric acid derivatives require three to six months of therapy in most patients to reach maximal therapeutic effects. Fibrates can also increase the risk of cholelithiasis, and thus should be avoided in patients with diabetes with impaired gall bladder motility due to progressive autonomic neuropathy.

Therapeutic Considerations

Warnings and Precautions

Fibric acid derivatives are primarily eliminated renally, thus extreme caution is warranted in patients with severe diabetic nephropathy or chronic renal insufficiency, due to an increased risk of myopathy. Additionally, use is cautioned in elderly patients with suspected renal impairment. Caution is also warranted in patients with a history of cholecystitis and cholelithiasis due to a potential exacerbation of these conditions with fibrate therapy. For specific contraindications and warnings for individual agents, refer to the full prescribing information.

Special Populations

Fibrates have not been specifically studied in pregnant or nursing women, so use in this population should be avoided unless potential benefits justify potential risk to the fetus or breastfed infant. Use of fibric acid derivatives is also cautioned in patients with suspected renal impairment.

Adverse Effects and Monitoring

Gastrointestinal side effects are the most common adverse reactions to fibrate therapy and include dyspepsia, nausea, vomiting, constipation or diarrhea, abdominal pain, and flatulence. Fenofibrate is associated with rash in 2%-3% of patients. Cholelithiasis and cholecystitis can result in patients on fibrate therapy due to increased biliary excretion of cholesterol. Fibric acid derivatives are also associated with myopathies, and cautious use is particularly warranted when used in combination with statins. Gemfibrozil has also been associated with a variety of nervous system effects including dizziness, drowsiness, blurred vision, peripheral neuropathy, mental depression, and adverse effects on libido and erectile function.

Drug Interactions

In general, fibrates should be used cautiously in combination with statins due to an increased risk of myopathies and rhabdomyolysis. Clofibrate has been associated with prolonging the half-life and enhancing the hypoglycemic actions of oral sulfonylureas. Patients on concomitant fibrate and sulfonylurea regimens should be counseled regarding the increased risk of hypoglycemia upon drug initiation or upward dose titrations of these agents. For drug interaction information for specific agents, see **Table 14.4**, or refer to the full prescribing information for the drug in question.

Dosage and Administration

For specific product dosing information, see **Table 14.3**, or refer to the full prescribing information for individual product dosing and administration guidelines.

Bile Acid Sequestrants

Bile acid sequestrants, also known as bile acid binding resins (BARs), are associated with reductions in LDL cholesterol of 15%-30% and minor elevations in HDL concentrations can occur. BARs have the potential to increase triglyceride levels. **The ADA recognizes bile acid sequestrants as viable options for the treatment of dyslipidemia in patients with diabetes, and their LDL-lowering effects appear to synergistic when co-administered with HMG-CoA reductase inhibitors (statins). Colesevelam has also demonstrated efficacy in decreasing HbA_{1c} (A_{1c}) levels by 0.5% when compared with placebo as add-on therapy to existing diabetes therapies in patients with type 2 diabetes. This drug received FDA approval in January of 2008 as adjunct therapy to diet, exercise, and other antidiabetic agents to improve glycemic control in patients with type 2 diabetes.**

Pharmacology

Mechanism of Action

BARs bind with bile acids in the intestine to impede their absorption. Depletion of bile acid concentrations results in up-regulation of the hepatic enzyme cholesterol 7-α-hydroxylase, which is responsible for the conversion of cholesterol to bile acids. The increased conversion of cholesterol to bile acid results in up-regulation of LDL receptors and increased clearance of LDL from the blood. Overall, BARs reduce total cholesterol, LDL cholesterol, apoliproprotein B levels, and increase HDL cholesterol concentrations. The mechanisms resulting in reduced fasting plasma glucose and improvements in HBA_{1c} are unknown at this time.

Pharmacokinetics

For drug specific pharmacokinetic parameters, refer to individual drug information. In general, BARs are minimally absorbed and exert their effects within the gastrointestinal tract. Therapeutic effects regarding cholesterol reduction are typically seen within several weeks of initiation.

Treatment Advantages and Disadvantages

BARs are useful for the treatment of hypercholesterolemia, however, since these agents may induce or exacerbate hypertriglyceridemia, monitor triglyceride levels. BARs should be avoided in patients with preexisting elevated triglyceride levels. The high incidence of constipation with BAR therapy can be problematic in patients with diabetes. Colesevelam use can result in modest decreases in fasting blood glucose and HbA_{1c} levels, thus lending to the utility of this agent in people with diabetes. Dosing of BARs can be inconvenient for many patients, however, as these agents can adversely affect the bioavailability of other medications, including sulfonylureas, thus necessitating the administration of medications affected by BARs either one hour prior to or four to six hours after BAR administration.

Therapeutic Considerations

Warnings and Precautions

BARs are generally contraindicated in patients with cholelithiasis, complete biliary obstruction, or gastrointestinal obstruction. Use is cautioned in patients with significant hypertriglyceridemia due to the potential exacerbation of this condition with BAR therapy.

Special Populations

Because BARs undergo negligible absorption, specific caution in elderly patients with limited hepatic or renal function is of less concern as with agents that are systemically absorbed. Additionally, BARs have not been formally evaluated in pregnant or nursing women, however, effects of BAR therapy on vitamin absorption in this population is a theoretical concern.

Adverse Effects and Monitoring
The primary side effects of BARs involve gastrointestinal complaints including constipation and dyspepsia. Additional adverse effects reported in clinical trials include myalgia, fecal impaction, pancreatitis, hemorrhoid exacerbation, abdominal distension, and elevated hepatic enzymes.

Drug Interactions
The absorption and bioavailability of many drugs can be inhibited by BAR therapy. General drug classes reported as being adversely affected include sulfonylureas, anticonvulsants, antiarrhythmics, and oral contraceptives. Any medication considered to have a "narrow therapeutic range" with the potential for loss of efficacy should be administered four hours prior to or following BAR administration. For specific drug interactions, see **Table 14.4** or refer to the full prescribing information for the drug in question.

Dosage and Administration
Careful consideration is warranted in patients taking other medications that may bind to BARs. Such medications should not be administered either one hour prior to or four to six hours after BAR administration. For specific administration and dosing information, see **Table 14.3** or refer to the full prescribing information for the drug in question.

Ezetimibe
Ezetimibe is an oral antilipidemic agent approved for use as monotherapy or in combination with a statin or fenofibrate for the treatment of hypercholesterolemia. Ezetimibe is the first agent in the class of medications known as cholesterol absorption inhibitors, and is an effective inhibitor of cholesterol absorption from the gastrointestinal tract. Monotherapy with ezetimibe is associated with reductions in total cholesterol of approximately 13%, 18% reductions in LDL, and 18% reductions in triglyceride concentrations. Ezetimibe is also available in combination with simvastatin for the treatment of hyperlipidemia. **While recent data indicate that ezetimibe therapy may not be associated with decreases in cardiovascular risk despite decreases in LDL cholesterol levels, ezetimibe can be used in patients with diabetes in combination with statins for synergistic lowering of LDL and triglyceride levels for patients not reaching treatment goals on statin therapy alone.**

Pharmacology
Mechanism of Action
Ezetimibe selectively inhibits absorption of cholesterol and related compounds via sterol transporters in the small intestine. The mechanism of action of ezetimibe is very different from that of other antilipidemic agents, and is thought to compliment the effects of HMG-CoA reductase inhibitors (statins) in cholesterol reduction.

Pharmacokinetics
Following oral administration and absorption, ezetimibe is extensively conjugated to a pharmacologically active compound (ezetimibe-glucuronide). Mean peak plasma concentrations are reached within four to 12 hours following administration. Administration with food has no effect on the extent of ezetimibe absorption; however, administration with high-fat meals increases peak concentrations by approximately 38%. Ezetimibe and ezetimibe-glucuronide are slowly eliminated with a half-life of ~22 hours. Ezetimibe undergoes enterohepatic recirculation, and is mainly excreted via the feces.

Treatment Advantages and Disadvantages

Ezetimibe in combination with statins results in synergistic lipid-lowering effects, with improvements in total cholesterol, LDL cholesterol, triglyceride concentrations, and HDL levels when compared to either treatment approach when administered as monotherapy. Recent results from the Effect of Combination Ezetimibe and High-Dose Simvastatin vs. Simvastatin Alone on the Atherosclerotic Process in Patients with Heterozygous Familial Hypercholesterolemia (ENHANCE) trial, however, sheds doubt upon the utility of ezetimibe-statin combination therapy on the prevention of cardiovascular events and associated mortality. The ENHANCE trial evaluated the progression of atherosclerotic plaques in carotid arteries via carotid ultrasound monitoring. Early reports from the study indicate that no significant differences were identified between ezetimibe-simvastatin combination therapy and simvastatin monotherapy on the progression of carotid plaques despite favorable changes in LDL cholesterol. While the ENHANCE study was not a clinical outcomes study, these findings raise questions regarding the benefit of ezetimibe-statin combination therapy on morbidity and mortality associated with macrovascular disease.

Therapeutic Considerations

Warnings and Precautions

Ezetimibe is not recommended in patients with moderate or severe hepatic disease due to increased drug concentrations in this population.

Special Populations

While pharmacokinetic variations have been documented in the elderly, women, patients with mild hepatic impairment, and patients with severe renal impairment, dosage adjustments for ezetimibe are not indicated in these populations. Ezetimibe is not, however, recommended for use in patients with moderate to severe hepatic impairment. Ezetimibe should be used with caution in pregnant or nursing women as it has not been formally evaluated in this population. If given as a combination with simvastatin (marketed as Vytorin), use is contraindicated during pregnancy and breastfeeding.

Adverse Effects and Monitoring

Common adverse effects associated with ezetimibe monotherapy include fatigue, abdominal pain, diarrhea, increased risk of viral infection, and arthralgia. During post-marketing surveillance, reports of hypersensitivity reactions, angioedema, urticaria, arthralgia, and rash have been documented. When given in combination with simvastatin as the combination product Vytorin, side effects associated with statin therapy were also noted.

Drug Interactions

The oral absorption of ezetimibe can be decreased if given in combination with BAR therapy. Cyclosporine has been associated with increasing ezetimibe serum concentrations. The combination of ezetimibe with statins can result in increased risk or exacerbation of hepatic disease or elevation of serum transaminase levels. For specific drug interactions, see **Table 14.4** or refer to the full prescribing information for the drug in question.

Dosage and Administration

As monotherapy or in combination with statins, ezetimibe is orally dosed 10 mg once daily. Dose adjustments are not recommended in patients with renal impairment or mild hepatic disease. Use is not recommended, however, in patients with moderate to severe hepatic impairment. For specific administration and dosing information, see **Table 14.3** or refer to the full prescribing information for the drug in question.

Nicotinic Acid Derivative

Niacin is a water-soluble B vitamin used in the treatment of hyperlipidemia. Doses of niacin exceeding the recommended daily allowance are required for cholesterol reduction. Clinical trial data show that niacin is effective in lowering LDL by 5%-25%, triglycerides by 20%-50%, and can increase HDL by 15%-35%. Nicotinic acid was the first hypolipidemic agent shown to decrease the incidence of secondary myocardial infarction and reduce total mortality in myocardial infarction patients. **While niacin has demonstrated efficacy in the treatment of hyperlipidemia with significant effects on LDL, triglyceride, and HDL levels, it should be used with caution in patients with diabetes.**

Pharmacology

Mechanism of Action

The mechanism of action of niacin in terms of its favorable effects on lipids is not fully understood, but appears to be independent of its physiological role as a vitamin. Primarily, nicotinic acid decreases hepatic VLDL synthesis. A variety of mechanisms have been proposed as to how this occurs, including inhibition of free fatty acid release from adipose tissue, increased lipoprotein lipase activity, decreased triglyceride synthesis, decreased VLDL-triglyceride transport, and inhibition of lipolysis. Niacin is effective in elevating HDL cholesterol levels even in patients without other lipid abnormalities.

Pharmacokinetics

Following administration of immediate-release niacin, absorption is rapid, with peak plasma levels reached in approximately 45 minutes. Extended-release products reach peak concentrations in four to five hours following administration. Peripheral vasodilation occurs within 20 minutes with immediate release products, and can last for up to an hour. Niacin undergoes extensive first-pass metabolism. Roughly 12% of nicotinic acid is excreted unchanged in the urine, however, greater proportions of niacin are renally excreted unchanged as doses reach and exceed 1,000 mg/day and metabolic pathways become saturated. Niacin is widely distributed through the body and tends to concentrate in the liver, spleen, and fat tissue.

Treatment Advantages and Disadvantages

Although niacin is effective for treating hyperlipidemia, it should be used with caution in patients with diabetes. Niacin is associated with a number of bothersome side effects that hinder patient compliance, and more importantly, use is associated with a number of metabolic side effects including hyperglycemia, hyperuricemia, insulin resistance, and abnormalities in hepatic transaminase levels.

Therapeutic Considerations

Warnings and Precautions

Niacin is contraindicated in patients with significant or unexplained hepatic dysfunction, active peptic ulcer disease, or arterial bleeding. As mentioned previously, niacin can exacerbate glycemic control due to increased insulin resistance, thus niacin should be used judiciously in patients with diabetes. Recent findings suggest that extended-release forms of niacin, while beneficial in attenuating the flushing associated with niacin products, are associated with a greater incidence of hepatotoxicity when compared with immediate-release products. Due to this finding, many practitioners prefer the use of crystalline niacin products.

Special Populations

Niacin administration is considered safe at recommended daily allowance levels. When used at lipid-lowering doses, however, niacin is a pregnancy category C agent. Niacin accumulation within breast milk can have negative impacts on infants, thus nursing mothers should consider niacin discontinuation or the discontinuation of nursing when using niacin for lipid management. The safety of niacin at high doses for the treatment of hyperlipidemia has not been evaluated in children under the age of 16 years. Caution is warranted in patients with impaired renal function because metabolites of niacin are excreted renally.

Adverse Effects and Monitoring
Adverse effects associated with niacin administration can be quite bothersome and may limit adherence to therapy. Common side effects include flushing, pruritus, dry skin, headaches, nausea, epigastric pain, and exacerbation of gout.

Drug Interactions
Rare cases of rhabdomyolysis have been documented in patients taking niacin in combination with statins. Patients on combination therapy should be carefully monitored for worsening muscle pain, particularly upon upward dose titration of either drug. Bile acid sequestrants have been demonstrated to bind niacin and prevent absorption, with roughly 98% of a given niacin dose bound to colestipol and 10%-30% bound to cholestyramine in drug-interaction studies. Patients using niacin in combination with a bile acid sequestrant should separate the administration of these agents by a minimum of four to six hours. Additionally, due to the vasodilatory effects of niacin, niacin can augment the hypotensive effects of medications used in the treatment of hypertension, particularly agents that induce peripheral vasodilation such as nitrates and calcium channel blockers. For specific drug interactions, see **Table 14.4** or refer to the full prescribing information for the drug in question.

Dosage and Administration
Considering niacin is associated with a variety of side effects, niacin is often better tolerated if initiated at a low dose and titrated slowly. Niacin may be instituted at a dose of 100 mg twice daily, with dose escalations occurring weekly by 100-mg twice-daily increments as tolerated until a dose of 500 mg twice daily is achieved. The dose can then be titrated by 500-mg increments to the desired target dose and the desired therapeutic effect. Doses can be titrated up to 4 g/day if necessary, however, doses above 1,500 mg are rarely needed for the treatment of hypertriglyceridemia. For patients experiencing significant flushing, administration of 325 mg of aspirin approximately 30 minutes to 1 hour prior to niacin administration may decrease the incidence and severity. For specific administration and dosing information, see **Table 14.3** or refer to the full prescribing information for the drug in question.

Fatty Acid Derivatives

Omega-3 fatty acids have demonstrated efficacy in reduction of triglyceride levels in normal subjects. Clinically, fatty acid derivatives are promoted for a variety of health conditions; however, data regarding the efficacy of these products are largely limited and preliminary in nature. **Omega-3 fatty acids are a viable option for the treatment of diabetic patients with resistant hypertriglyceridemia, and are being widely utilized as add-on therapy to statin drugs due to potential benefits in triglyceride levels and decreased insulin resistance in patients with type 2 diabetes.**

Pharmacology
Mechanism of Action
For the treatment of hyperlipidemia, omega-3 essential fatty acids are thought to inhibit VLDL and triglyceride synthesis in the liver. Beneficial effects on triglyceride levels are the most consistent, with reductions ranging

from 25%-50% with doses of 3-6 g/day. Similar to gemfibrozil, omega-3 products can increase LDL and total cholesterol levels by roughly 10%, particularly in people with mixed dyslipidemia. No effects on HDL concentrations have been documented.

Pharmacokinetics
Omega-3 fatty acids are well absorbed upon oral administration, and distribute widely throughout the body. Fatty acids are eliminated primarily by oxidative catabolism to carbon dioxide and water with small quantities lost when skin and digestive cell sloughing. It is unknown if the metabolism of these products are altered in patients with renal or hepatic impairment.

Treatment Advantages and Disadvantages
Omega-3 fatty acids have demonstrated efficacy in lowering triglyceride levels in normal subjects, and have been used in patients with diabetes for the treatment of hypertriglyceridemia. Additionally, omega-3 fatty acids have demonstrated positive effects on platelet aggregation in some studies, and small dose-dependent reductions in systolic blood pressure have been reported in patients with untreated hypertension. When used in patients with type 2 diabetes, however, some adverse effects have been noted, namely modest elevations in LDL and total cholesterol concentrations. For type 2 diabetic patients with resistant hypertriglyceridemia, omega-3 fatty acids are being used as add-on therapy to statins due to potential benefits in triglyceride levels and decreased insulin resistance.

Therapeutic Considerations
Warnings and Precautions
Omega-3 fatty acid products should not be used in any patients with a known fish hypersensitivity. Additionally, due to the antiplatelet effects of these agents, caution is

advised in patients undergoing surgery or other invasive procedures that may increase bleeding risk. Use of these products in patients with mixed dyslipidemia is also cautioned due to potential increases in LDL and total cholesterol levels.

Special Populations
Omega-3 fatty acid therapy has not been formally studied during pregnancy, and it is unknown if these products are excreted in breast milk. Use during pregnancy is not recommended without the supervision of a qualified health care provider. Use in children under the age of 18 years is not recommended. It is unknown if the metabolism or elimination of omega-3 fatty acids are affected by renal or hepatic disease.

Adverse Effects and Monitoring
Common adverse effects associated with omega-3 fatty acid therapy include halitosis, altered taste (dyspepsia), and gastrointestinal discomfort. In studies evaluating the use of omega-3 products for hypertriglyceridemia, back pain, flulike symptoms, increased risk of infection, and angina pectoris were witnessed at rates higher than placebo controls. Alanine aminotransferase (ALT) and aspartate aminotransferase (AST) elevations have been observed in patients using omega-3 fatty acids, thus periodic liver function tests should be performed in patients using these products. Prolonged bleeding time has also been observed due to inhibition of platelet aggregation. Of particular concern in patients with type 2 diabetes, fish oil products have been associated with substantial weight gain in some patients.

Drug Interactions
Due to inhibition of platelet aggregation, caution is advised in patients on concurrent anticoagulants, platelet inhibitors, or thrombolytic agents. The clinical relevance of this

potential interaction is not known. For specific drug interactions, see **Table 14.4** or refer to the full prescribing information for the drug in question.

Dosage and Administration
The FDA-approved dosage for Lovaza (originally called Omacor) is 4 g/day by mouth either as a single 4-g dose once daily or as 2 g twice daily. Recommendations state that the drug should be withdrawn in patients that do not adequately respond to therapy after two months. Nonprescription omega-3 fatty acid products are often taken in dosages ranging from 3-6 g/day in divided doses. Optimal supplemental dosage for the adjunctive treatment of hypertriglyceridemia is unknown. See **Table 14.3** or refer to the full prescribing information for more dosing guidance.

Combination Therapies

Management of hyperlipidemia in patients with type 2 diabetes often requires the use of multiple medications to meet treatment goals for patients unresponsive to mono-therapy. It is important to consider that combinations involving statins and niacin are associated with an increased risk of myopathy, thus patients receiving this combination should be monitored closely.

Combination therapy with a fibrate and a statin can be considered for patients who have met LDL goals but in whom triglycerides remain greater than 200 mg/dL in the presence of vascular disease. Side effects such as myopathy and hepatitis must be monitored with this combination. Given that many patients will require multiple agents to meet lipid goals, some medications are available as combination pills to ease pill burden and aid in medication adherence. Products are available containing niacin in combination with statin drugs and ezetimibe in combination with simvastatin (Vytorin). Additionally, a product containing atorvastatin in combination with amlodipine is also available (Caduet). For additional information regarding combination products, see **Table 14.3** or refer to the full prescribing information.

SUGGESTED READING

Aguilar-Salinas CA, Mehta R, Gomez-Perez FJ et al. Management of the metabolic syndrome as a strategy for preventing the macro vascular complications of type 2 diabetes: controversial issues. *Curr Diabetes Rev.* 2005;1:145-158.

Dyslipidemia Management in Adults with Diabetes. *Diabetes Care.* 2004;27 (S1):S68-71.

Executive Summary of the Third Report of the National Cholesterol Education Program (NCEP) Expert Panel on Detection, Evaluation, and Treatment of High Blood Cholesterol in Adults (Adult Treatment Panel III). *JAMA.* 2001;285(19):2486-2497.

Haffner SM. Management of dyslipidemia in adults with diabetes (Technical Review). *Diabetes Care.* 1998;21:160-178.

O'Brien T, Nguyen TT, Zimmerman BR. Hyperlipidemia and diabetes mellitus. *Mayo Clin Proc.* 1998;73:969-976.

Table 14.3. Prescribing Information for Antilipidemic Agents

GENERIC (BRAND)	FORM/ STRENGTH	DOSAGE	WARNINGS/PRECAUTIONS & CONTRAINDICATIONS	ADVERSE REACTIONS
BILE ACID SEQUESTRANTS				
Cholestyramine (Questran, Questran Light)	**Powder:** 4g/pkt [60^s, 378g], **(Light)** 4g/scoopful [60^s, 268g]	***Adults:*** Initial: 1 pkt or scoopful qd or bid. Maint: 2-4 pkts or scoopfuls/day, given bid. Titrate: Adjust at no less than 4 week intervals. Max: 6 pkts/day or 6 scoopfuls/day. May also give as 1-6 doses/day. Mix with fluid or highly fluid food. ***Pediatrics:*** Usual: 240mg/kg/day of anhydrous cholestyramine resin in 2-3 divided doses. Max: 8g/day.	**W/P:** May produce hyperchloremic acidosis with prolonged use. Caution in renal insufficiency, volume depletion, and with concomitant spironolactone. Chronic use may produce or worsen constipation. Avoid constipation with symptomatic CAD. May increase bleeding tendency due to vitamin K deficiency. Serum or red cell folate reduced with chronic use. Constipation may aggravate hemorrhoids. Light formulation contains phenylalanine. Measure cholesterol during 1st few months; periodically thereafter. Measure TG periodically. **Contra:** Complete biliary obstruction. **P/N:** Category C, caution in nursing.	Constipation, heartburn, nausea, vomiting, abdominal pain, flatulence, diarrhea, anorexia, osteoporosis, rash, hyperchloremic acidosis (children), vitamin A and D deficiency, steatorrhea, hypoprothrombinemia (vitamin K deficiency).
Colesevelam HCl (Welchol)	**Tab:** 625mg	***Adults:* Hyperlipidemia/Type 2 DM:** 3 tabs bid or 6 tabs qd. Take with liquids and a meal.	**W/P:** Monitor lipids, including TG and non-HDL-cholesterol levels prior to initiation of treatment and periodically thereafter. Caution in TG levels >300mg/dL, dysphagia or swallowing disorders, gastroparesis, GI motility disorders, major GI tract surgery, bowel obstruction, and those susceptible to vitamin K or fat soluble vitamin deficiencies. Coadministered drugs should be given at least 4 hrs prior to treatment; monitor drug levels. Not for use in treatment of type 1 DM or for diabetic ketoacidosis. **Contra:** Bowel obstruction, hypertriglyceridemia-induced pancreatitis, serum TG concentrations >500mg/dL. **P/N:** Category B, caution in nursing.	Asthenia, constipation, dyspepsia, pharyngitis, myalgia, nausea, hypoglycemia, bowel obstruction, dysphagia, esophageal obstruction, fecal impaction, hypertriglyceridemia, pancreatitis, increased transaminases.
Colestipol HCl (Colestid)	**Granules:** 5g/pkt [30^s 90^s], 5g/ scoopful [300g, 500g]; **Tab:** 1g	***Adults:*** Initial: 2g, 1 pkt or 1 scoopful qd-bid. Titrate: Increase by 2g qd or bid at 1-2 month intervals. Usual: 2-16g/day (tab) or 1-6 pkts or scoopfuls qd or in divided doses. Always mix granules with liquid. Swallow tabs whole with plenty of liquid.	**W/P:** Exclude secondary causes of hypercholesterolemia and perform a lipid profile. May produce hyperchloremic acidosis with prolonged use. Monitor cholesterol and TG based on NCEP guidelines. May cause hypothyroidism. May interfere with normal fat absorption. Chronic use may produce or worsen constipation. Avoid constipation with symptomatic CAD. May increase bleeding tendency due to vitamin K deficiency. **P/N:** Safety in pregnancy not known, caution in nursing.	Constipation, musculoskeletal pain, headache, migraine headache, sinus headache.
CHOLESTEROL ABSORPTION INHIBITOR				
Ezetimibe (Zetia)	**Tab:** 10mg	***Adults:*** 10mg qd. May give with HMG-CoA reductase inhibitor (with primary hypercholesterolemia) or fenofibrate (with mixed hyperlipidemia) for incremental effect. **Concomitant Bile Acid Sequestrant:** Give either ≥2 hrs before or ≥4 hrs after bile acid sequestrant.	**W/P:** Monitor LFTs with concurrent statin therapy. Not recommended with moderate or severe hepatic insufficiency. **Contra:** When used with a statin, refer to the HMG-CoA reductase inhibitor prescribing information. **P/N:** Category C, contraindicated in nursing.	Back pain, arthralgia, diarrhea, sinusitis, abdominal pain, myalgia.
FATTY ACID DERIVATIVE				
Omega-3-acid ethyl esters (Lovaza)	**Cap:** 1g	***Adults:*** 4g qd. Given as single 4-g dose (4 caps) or as two 2-g doses (2 caps bid).	**W/P:** Caution in patients with diabetes, hypothyroidism, hepatic and pancreas problems, known sensitivity or allergy to fish. Lower alcohol use. Lose weight if overweight. Possible increases in alanine aminotransferase levels without a concurrent increase in aspartate aminotransferase levels. Possible increased LDL cholesterol levels. **P/N:** Category C, caution in nursing.	Eructation, infection, flu-syndrome, dyspepsia.

W/P = warnings/precautions; **Contra** = contraindications; **P/N** = pregnancy category rating and nursing considerations.

Table 14.3. Prescribing Information for Antilipidemic Agents

GENERIC (BRAND)	FORM/ STRENGTH	DOSAGE	WARNINGS/PRECAUTIONS & CONTRAINDICATIONS	ADVERSE REACTIONS
FIBRATES				
Fenofibrate (Antara)	Cap: 43mg, 130mg	*Adults:* **Hypercholesterolemia/Mixed Dyslipidemia:** Initial: 130mg qd. **Hypertriglyceridemia:** Initial: 43-130mg/day. Titrate: Adjust if needed after repeat lipid levels at 4-8 week intervals. Max: 130mg/day. **Renal Dysfunction/Elderly:** Initial: 43mg/day. Take with meals.	**W/P:** Monitor LFTs regularly; d/c if >3x ULN. May cause cholelithiasis; d/c if gallstones found. D/C if myopathy or marked CPK elevation occurs. Decreased Hgb, Hct, WBCs, thrombocytopenia, and agranulocytosis reported; monitor CBCs during first 12 months of therapy. Acute hypersensitivity reactions (rare) and pancreatitis reported. Rare cases of rhabdomyolysis. Evaluate for myopathy. Monitor lipids periodically initially, d/c if inadequate response after 2 months on 130mg/day. Minimize dose in severe renal impairment. Caution in elderly. **Contra:** Hepatic or severe renal dysfunction (including primary cirrhosis), unexplained persistent hepatic function abnormality, pre-existing gallbladder disease. **P/N:** Category C, not for use in nursing.	Abdominal pain, back pain, headache, abnormal LFTs, respiratory disorder, increased CPK, increased SGPT/SGOT.
Fenofibrate (Lofibra)	Cap: 67mg, 134mg, 200mg; Tab: 54mg, 160mg	*Adults:* **Hypercholesterolemia/Mixed Dyslipidemia:** Initial: **Cap:** 200mg qd. **Hypercholesterolemia/Mixed Hyperlipidemia: Tab:** 160mg qd. **Hypertriglyceridemia:** Initial: **Cap:** 67-200mg/day. **Tab:** 54-160mg qd. Titrate: Adjust if needed after repeat lipid levels at 4-8 week intervals. Max: **Cap:** 200mg/day. **Tab:** 160mg/day. **Renal Dysfunction/Elderly:** Initial: **Cap:** 67mg/day. **Tab:** 54mg/day. Take with meals.	**W/P:** Monitor LFTs regularly; d/c if >3x ULN. May cause cholelithiasis; d/c if gallstones found. D/C if myopathy or marked CPK elevation occurs. Decreased Hgb, Hct, WBCs, thrombocytopenia, and agranulocytosis reported; monitor CBCs during first 12 months of therapy. Acute hypersensitivity reactions (rare) and pancreatitis reported. Monitor lipids periodically initially, d/c if inadequate response after 2 months on 200mg/day. Minimize dose in severe renal impairment. Caution in elderly. **Contra:** Pre-existing gallbladder disease, unexplained persistent hepatic function abnormality, hepatic or severe renal dysfunction (including primary biliary cirrhosis). **P/N:** Category C, not for use in nursing.	Abdominal pain, back pain, headache, abnormal LFTs, increased CPK, respiratory disorder.
Fenofibrate (Tricor)	Tab: 48mg, 145mg	*Adults:* **Hypercholesterolemia/Mixed Dyslipidemia:** Initial: 145mg qd. **Hypertriglyceridemia:** Initial: 48-145mg/day. Titrate: Adjust if needed after repeat lipid levels at 4-8 week intervals. Max: 145mg/day. **Renal Dysfunction/Elderly:** Initial: 48mg/day. Take without regards to meals.	**W/P:** Monitor LFTs regularly; d/c if >3x ULN. May cause cholelithiasis; d/c if gallstones found. D/C if myopathy or marked CPK elevation occurs. Decreased Hgb, Hct, WBCs, thrombocytopenia, and agranulocytosis reported; monitor CBC during first 12 months of therapy. Acute hypersensitivity reactions (rare) and pancreatitis reported. Monitor lipids periodically initially, d/c if inadequate response after 2 months on 145mg/day. Minimize dose in severe renal impairment. Caution in elderly. **Contra:** Preexisting gallbladder disease, unexplained persistent hepatic function abnormality, hepatic or severe renal dysfunction (including primary biliary cirrhosis). **P/N:** Category C, not for use in nursing.	Abdominal pain, back pain, headache, abnormal LFTs, respiratory disorder, increased CPK.
Fenofibrate (Triglide)	Tab: 50mg, 160mg	*Adults:* **Hypercholesterolemia/Mixed Hyperlipidemia:** 160mg qd. **Hypertriglyceridemia:** Initial: 50-160mg/day. Titrate: Adjust if needed after repeat lipid levels at 4-8 week intervals. Max: 160mg/day. **Renal Dysfunction/Elderly:** Initial: 50mg/day. Take without regards to meals.	**W/P:** Monitor LFTs regularly; d/c if >3x ULN. May cause cholelithiasis; d/c if gallstones found. D/C if myopathy or marked CPK elevation occurs. Decreased Hgb, Hct, WBCs, thrombocytopenia, and agranulocytosis reported; monitor CBCs during first 12 months of therapy. Acute hypersensitivity reactions (rare) and pancreatitis reported. Monitor lipids periodically initially; d/c if inadequate response after 2 months on 160mg/day. Minimize dose in severe renal impairment. Caution in elderly. **Contra:** Severe renal	Abdominal pain, back pain, headache, abnormal LFTs, respiratory disorder, increased CPK, increased SGPT/SGOT.

W/P = warnings/precautions; **Contra** = contraindications; **P/N** = pregnancy category rating and nursing considerations.

Table 14.3. Prescribing Information for Antilipidemic Agents

GENERIC (BRAND)	FORM/ STRENGTH	DOSAGE	WARNINGS/PRECAUTIONS & CONTRAINDICATIONS	ADVERSE REACTIONS
Fenofibrate (Triglide) *(Cont.)*			dysfunction, hepatic dysfunction (including primary biliary cirrhosis and unexplained persistent liver function abnormality), pre-existing gallbladder disease. **P/N:** Category C, not for use in nursing.	
Gemfibrozil (Lopid)	Tab: 600mg* *scored	*Adults:* 600mg bid. Give 30 min before morning and evening meals.	**W/P:** Abnormal LFTs reported; monitor periodically. Only use if indicated and d/c if significant lipid response not obtained. Associated with myositis. D/C if suspect or diagnose myositis, if abnormal LFTs persist, or gallstones develop. Cholelithiasis reported. Monitor CBC periodically during first 12 months. May worsen renal insufficiency. **Contra:** Hepatic or severe renal dysfunction, including primary biliary cirrhosis; pre-existing gallbladder disease, concomitant cerivastatin. **P/N:** Category C, not for use in nursing.	Dyspepsia, abdominal pain, diarrhea, fatigue, bacterial and viral infections, musculoskeletal symptoms, abnormal LFTs, hematologic changes, hypoesthesia, paresthesia, taste perversion.
HMG-CoA REDUCTASE INHIBITORS (STATINS)				
Atorvastatin calcium (Lipitor)	Tab: 10mg, 20mg, 40mg, 80mg	*Adults:* **Hypercholesterolemia/Mixed Dyslipidemia:** Initial: 10-20mg qd (or 40mg qd for LDL-C reduction >45%). Titrate: Adjust dose if needed at 2-4 week intervals. Usual: 10-80mg qd. **Homozygous Familial Hypercholesterolemia:** 10-80mg qd. *Pediatrics:* **Heterozygous Familial Hypercholesterolemia: 10-17 yrs** (postmenarchal): Initial: 10mg/day. Titrate: Adjust dose if needed at intervals of ≥4 weeks. Max: 20mg/day.	**W/P:** Monitor LFTs prior to therapy, at 12 weeks or with dose elevation, and periodically thereafter. Reduce dose or withdraw if AST or ALT ≥3x ULN persist. Caution with heavy alcohol use and/or history of hepatic disease. D/C if markedly elevated CPK levels occur, if myopathy is diagnosed or suspected, or if predisposition to renal failure secondary to rhabdomyolysis. Caution in patients with recent stroke or TIA. Rare cases of rhabdomyolysis reported. **Contra:** Active liver disease, unexplained persistent elevations of serum transaminases, pregnancy, nursing mothers. **P/N:** Category X, not for use in nursing.	Constipation, flatulence, dyspepsia, abdominal pain, transaminase and CK elevation in higher doses.
Fluvastatin sodium (Lescol, Lescol XL)	Cap: (Lescol) 20mg, 40mg; Tab, Extended-Release: (Lescol XL) 80mg	*Adults:* ≥18 yrs: (For LDL-C reduction of ≥25%) Initial: 40mg cap qpm or 80mg XL tab at any time of day or 40mg cap bid. (For LDL-C reduction of <25%) Initial: 20mg cap qpm. Range: 20-80mg/day. **Severe Renal Impairment:** Caution with dose >40mg/day. Take 2 hrs after bile-acid resins qhs. *Pediatrics:* **Heterozygous Familial Hypercholesterolemia: 10-16 yrs (≥1 yr postmenarche):** Individualize dose: Initial: One 20mg cap. Titrate: Adjust dose at 6-week intervals. Max: 40mg cap bid or 80mg XL tab qd.	**W/P:** Monitor LFTs prior to therapy, at 12 weeks, or with dose elevation. D/C if AST or ALT ≥3x ULN on 2 consecutive occasions. Risk of myopathy and/or rhabdomyolysis reported. D/C if markedly elevated CPK levels occur, if myopathy is diagnosed or suspected, or if predisposition to renal failure secondary to rhabdomyolysis. Less effective with homozygous familial hypercholesterolemia. Caution with heavy alcohol use and/or history of hepatic disease. Evaluate if endocrine dysfunction develops. **Contra:** Active liver disease or unexplained, persistent elevations of serum transaminases, pregnancy, nursing mothers. **P/N:** Category X, not for use in nursing.	Dyspepsia, abdominal pain, headache, nausea, diarrhea, abnormal LFTs, myalgia, flu-like symptoms.
Lovastatin (Altoprev)	Tab: Extended-Release: 20mg, 40mg, 60mg	*Adults:* Initial: 20, 40, or 60mg qhs. Consider immediate-release lovastatin in patients requiring smaller reductions. May adjust at intervals of ≥4 weeks. **Concomitant Fibrates/Niacin** (≥1g/day): Try to avoid. Max: 20mg/day. **Concomitant Amiodarone/Verapamil:** Max: 20mg/day. **CrCl <30mL/min:** Consider dose increase of >20mg/day carefully and implement cautiously. Swallow whole; do not chew or crush.	**W/P:** May increase serum transaminases and CPK levels; consider in differential diagnosis of chest pain. D/C if AST or ALT ≥3x ULN persist, if myopathy diagnosed or suspected, and a few days before major surgery. Monitor LFTs prior to therapy, at 6 weeks, 12 weeks, then periodically or with dose elevation. Caution with heavy alcohol use and/or history of hepatic disease. Caution with dose escalation in renal insufficiency. Lovastatin immediate-release found to be less effective with homozygous familial hypercholesterolemia.	Nausea, abdominal pain, insomnia, dyspepsia, headache, asthenia, myalgia.

W/P = warnings/precautions; **Contra** = contraindications; **P/N** = pregnancy category rating and nursing considerations.

Table 14.3. Prescribing Information for Antilipidemic Agents

GENERIC (BRAND)	FORM/ STRENGTH	DOSAGE	WARNINGS/PRECAUTIONS & CONTRAINDICATIONS	ADVERSE REACTIONS
Lovastatin (Altoprev) *(Cont.)*			Rhabdomyolysis (rare), myopathy reported. **Contra:** Active liver disease, unexplained persistent elevations of serum transaminases, pregnancy, nursing mothers. **P/N:** Category X, not for use in nursing.	
Lovastatin (Mevacor)	**Tab:** 20mg, 40mg	***Adults:*** Initial: 20mg qd at dinner (10mg/day if need LDL-C reduction <20%). Usual: 10-80mg/day given qd or bid. May adjust every 4 weeks. Max: 80mg/day. **Concomitant Cyclosporine:** Initial: 10mg/day. Max: 20mg/day. **Fibrates/ Niacin (≥1g/day):** Max: 20mg/day. **Concomitant Amiodarone/Verapamil:** Max: 40mg/day. **CrCl <30mL/min:** Consider dose increase of >20mg/day carefully and implement cautiously. ***Pediatrics:* Heterozygous Familial Hypercholesterolemia: 10-17 yrs (at least 1-yr postmenarchal):** Initial: If <20% LDL-C Reduction Needed: 10mg qd. If ≥20% LDL-C Reduction Needed: 20mg qd. May adjust every 4 weeks. Max: 40mg/day. **Concomitant Cyclosporine:** Initial: 10mg/day. Max: 20mg/day. **Fibrates/Niacin (≥1g/day):** Max: 20mg/day. **Concomitant Amiodarone/Verapamil:** Max: 40mg/day. **CrCl <30mL/min:** Consider dose increase of >20mg/day carefully and implement cautiously.	**W/P:** May increase serum transaminases and CPK levels; consider in differential diagnosis of chest pain. D/C if AST or ALT 3x ULN persist, or if myopathy diagnosed or suspected. Monitor LFTs prior to therapy, at 6 weeks, 12 weeks, then periodically or with dose elevation. Caution with heavy alcohol use and/or history of hepatic disease. Caution with dose escalation in renal insufficiency. Less effective with homozygous familial hypercholesterolemia. Rhabdomyolysis (rare), myopathy reported. D/C a few days before elective major surgery and when any major acute medical or surgical condition supervenes. **Contra:** Active liver disease, unexplained persistent elevations of serum transaminases, pregnancy, nursing mothers. **P/N:** Category X, not for use in nursing.	Headache, constipation, flatulence, dizziness, rash, elevated transaminases or CK levels, GI upset, blurred vision.
Pravastatin sodium (Pravachol)	**Tab:** 10mg, 20mg, 40mg, 80mg	***Adults:* ≥18 yrs:** Initial: 40mg qd. Perform lipid tests within 4 weeks and adjust according to response and guidelines. Titrate: May increase to 80mg qd if needed. **Significant Renal/Hepatic Dysfunction:** Initial: 10mg qd. **Concomitant Immunosuppressives** (eg, cyclosporine): Initial:10mg qhs. Max: 20mg/day. ***Pediatrics:* Heterozygous Familial Hypercholesterolemia: 14-18 yrs:** Initial: 40mg qd. **8-13 yrs:** 20mg qd. **Concomitant Immunosuppressives** (eg, cyclosporine): Initial: 10mg qhs. Max: 20mg/day.	**W/P:** Perform LFTs before therapy, before dose increases, and if clinically indicated. Risk of myopathy, myalgia, and rhabdomyolysis. D/C if AST or ALT ≥3x ULN persists, if elevated CPK levels occur, or if myopathy diagnosed or suspected. Less effective with homozygous familial hypercholesterolemia. Monitor for endocrine dysfunction. Closely monitor with heavy alcohol use, recent history or signs of hepatic disease, or renal dysfunction. **Contra:** Active liver disease, unexplained persistent elevations of LFTs, pregnancy, nursing mothers. **P/N:** Category X, not for use in nursing.	Rash, nausea, vomiting, diarrhea, headache, chest pain, influenza, abdominal pain, dizziness, increases ALT, AST, CPK levels.
Rosuvastatin calcium (Crestor)	**Tab:** 5mg, 10mg, 20mg, 40mg	***Adults:* Hypercholesterolemia/Mixed Dyslipidemia/Hypertriglyceridemia/ Slowing Progression of Atherosclerosis:** Initial: 10mg qd. (20mg qd with LDL-C >190mg/dL). Titrate: Adjust dose if needed at 2-4 week intervals. Range: 5-40mg qd. **Homozygous Familial Hypercholesterolemia:** 20mg qd. Max: 40mg qd. **Asian Patients:** 5mg qd. **Concomitant Cyclosporine:** Max: 5mg qd. **Concomitant Lopinavir/Ritonavir:** Max 10mg qd. **Concomitant Gemfibrozil:** Max: 10mg qd. **Severe Renal Impairment: CrCl <30mL/min (not on hemodialysis):** Initial: 5mg qd. Max: 10mg qd.	**W/P:** Increased risk of myopathy with other lipid-lowering therapies, cyclosporine, or lopinavir/ritonavir. Rare cases of rhabdomyolysis with acute renal failure secondary to myoglobinuria reported. Monitor LFTs prior to therapy, at 12 weeks or with dose elevation, and periodically thereafter. Reduce dose or d/c if AST/ALT ≥3x ULN persist. Caution with heavy alcohol use, history of hepatic disease, renal impairment, hypothyroidism, elderly. D/C if markedly elevated CPK levels occur, if myopathy is diagnosed or failure secondary to rhabdomyolysis. Approximately 2-fold elevation in median exposure in Asian subjects. Persistent elevations in hepatic transaminase occurred. Monitor liver enzymes. **Contra:** Rash, pruritus, urticaria, angioedema, active liver disease, unexplained persistent elevations of serum transaminases, pregnancy, nursing mothers. **P/N:** Category X, not for use in nursing.	Headache, myalgia, abdominal pain, asthenia, diarrhea, dyspepsia, nausea, rhabdomyolysis with myoglobinuria and ARF and myopathy, liver enzyme abnormalities.

W/P = warnings/precautions; **Contra** = contraindications; **P/N** = pregnancy category rating and nursing considerations.

Table 14.3. Prescribing Information for Antilipidemic Agents

GENERIC (BRAND)	FORM/ STRENGTH	DOSAGE	WARNINGS/PRECAUTIONS & CONTRAINDICATIONS	ADVERSE REACTIONS
Simvastatin (Zocor)	**Tab:** 5mg, 10mg, 20mg, 40mg, 80mg	**Adults:** Initial: 20-40mg qpm. Usual: 5-80mg/day. Titrate: Adjust at ≥4-week intervals. **High Risk for CHD Events:** Initial: 40mg/day. **Homozygous Familial Hypercholesterolemia:** 40mg qpm or 80mg/day given as 20mg bid plus 40mg qpm. **Concomitant Cyclosporine:** Initial: 5mg/day. Max: 10mg/day. **Concomitant Gemfibrozil** (try to avoid): Max: 10mg/day. **Concomitant Amiodarone/Verapamil:** Max: 20mg/day. **Severe Renal Insufficiency:** 5mg/day; monitor closely. **Pediatrics: Heterozygous Familial Hypercholesterolemia: 10-17 yrs (at least 1 yr postmenarchal):** Initial: 10mg qpm. Usual: 10-40mg/day. Titrate: Adjust at ≥4-week intervals. Max: 40mg/day.	**W/P:** Caution with heavy alcohol use, severe renal insufficiency or history of hepatic disease. Monitor LFTs prior to therapy, periodically thereafter for 12 months, or until 12 months after last dose elevation (additional test at 3 months for 80mg dose). D/C if AST or ALT ≥3x ULN persist, if myopathy is suspected or diagnosed, a few days prior to major surgery. Rhabdomyolysis (rare), myopathy reported. **Contra:** Active liver disease, unexplained persistent elevations of serum transaminases, pregnancy, nursing mothers. **P/N:** Category X, not for use in nursing.	Abdominal pain, headache, CK and transaminase elevations, constipation, upper respiratory infection, hepatic failure.
NICOTINIC ACID DERIVATIVE				
Niacin (Niaspan)	**Tab, Extended-Release:** 500mg, 750mg, 1000mg	**Adults:** Take qhs after low-fat snack. Initial: 500mg qhs. Titrate: Increase by 500mg every 4 weeks. Maint: 1-2g qhs. Max: 2g/day. Take ASA or NSAIDs 30 min before to reduce flushing. Do not chew, crush, or break; swallow whole. Women may respond to lower doses than men.	**W/P:** Do not substitute with equivalent doses of immediate-release niacin (severe hepatic toxicity may occur). Associated with abnormal LFTs; monitor LFTs before therapy, every 6-12 weeks during 12 months, then periodically thereafter. D/C if LFTs ≥3x ULN persists or develop signs of hepatotoxicity. Monitor for rhabdomyolysis. Observe closely with history of jaundice, hepatobiliary disease, and peptic ulcer; monitor LFTs and blood glucose frequently. Dose-related rise in glucose tolerance in diabetics. Caution with history of hepatic disease, heavy alcohol use, renal dysfunction, unstable angina, and acute phase of MI. Elevated uric acid levels reported. May reduce platelet and phosphorous levels. **Contra:** Unexplained or significant hepatic dysfunction, active peptic ulcer disease, arterial bleeding. **P/N:** Category C, not for use in nursing.	Flushing episodes (eg, tachycardia, shortness of warmth, redness, itching, tingling), dizziness, breath, sweating, chills, edema, headache, diarrhea.
COMBINATIONS				
Amlodipine/ Atorvastatin (Caduet)	**Tab:** (Amlodipine-Atorvastatin) 2.5mg-10mg, 2.5mg-20mg, 2.5mg-40mg, 5mg-10mg, 5mg-20mg, 5mg-40mg, 5mg-80mg, 10mg-10mg, 10mg-20mg, 10mg-40mg, 10mg-80mg	**Adults:** Dosing should be individualized and based on the appropriate combination of recommendations for the monotherapies. **(Amlodipine): HTN:** Initial: 5mg qd. Titrate over 7-14 days. Max: 10mg qd. **Small, Fragile, or Elderly/ Hepatic Dysfunction/Concomitant Antihypertensive:** Initial: 2.5mg qd. Angina: 5-10mg qd. **Elderly/Hepatic Dysfunction:** 5mg qd. **(Atorvastatin): Hypercholesterolemia/Mixed Dyslipidemia:** Initial: 10-20mg qd (or 40mg qd for LDL-C reduction >45%). Titrate: Adjust dose if needed at 2-4 week intervals. Usual: 10-80mg qd. **Homozygous Familial Hypercholesterolemia:** 10-80mg qd. **Pediatrics: ≥10 yrs (postmenarchal): (Amlodipine): HTN:** 2.5-5mg qd. **10-17 yrs (postmenarchal): (Atorvastatin): Heterozygous Familial Hypercholesterolemia:** Initial: 10mg/day. Titrate: Adjust dose if needed at intervals of ≥4 weeks. Max: 20mg/day.	**W/P:** May rarely increase angina or MI with severe obstructive CAD. Monitor LFTs prior to therapy, at 12 weeks after initiation, with dose elevation, and periodically thereafter. Reduce dose or withdraw if AST or ALT >3x ULN persist. Caution with heavy alcohol use and/or history of hepatic disease, severe aortic stenosis, CHF. D/C if markedly elevated CPK levels occur, if myopathy is diagnosed or suspected, or if predisposition to renal failure secondary to rhabdomyolysis. Increased risk of hemorrhagic stroke in patients with recent stroke or TIA. **Contra:** Active liver disease, unexplained persistent elevations of serum transaminases, pregnancy, nursing mothers. **P/N:** Category X, not for use in nursing	Headache, edema, palpitation, dizziness, fatigue, constipation, flatulence, dyspepsia, abdominal pain.

W/P = warnings/precautions; **Contra** = contraindications; **P/N** = pregnancy category rating and nursing considerations.

Table 14.3. Prescribing Information for Antilipidemic Agents

GENERIC (BRAND)	FORM/ STRENGTH	DOSAGE	WARNINGS/PRECAUTIONS & CONTRAINDICATIONS	ADVERSE REACTIONS
Ezetimibe/ Simvastatin (Vytorin)	**Tab:** (ezetimibe-simvastatin) 10mg/ 10mg, 10mg/20mg, 10mg/40mg, 10mg/ 80mg	**Adults:** Take once daily in the evening. Initial: 10mg/20mg qd. **Less Aggressive LDL-C Reductions:** Initial: 10mg/10mg qd. **LDL-C Reduction >55%:** Initial: 10mg/ 40mg qd. Titrate: Adjust at ≥2 weeks. **Homozygous Familial Hypercholesterolemia:** 10mg/40mg or 10mg/80mg qd. **Severe Renal Insufficiency:** Avoid unless tolerant of ≥5mg of simvastatin; monitor closely. **Concomitant Bile Acid Sequestrant:** Take either ≥2 hrs before or ≥4 hrs after bile acid sequestrant. **Concomitant Cyclosporine:** Avoid unless tolerant of ≥5mg of simvastatin. Max: 10mg/10mg/ day. **Concomitant Amiodarone/Verapamil:** Max: 10mg/20mg/day.	**W/P:** Rhabdomyolysis (rare), myopathy reported. D/C therapy if myopathy is suspected or diagnosed, if AST or ALT ≥3x ULN persist, a few days prior to major surgery or when any major medical or surgical condition supervenes. Monitor LFTs prior to therapy and thereafter when clinically indicated. With 10mg/80mg dose, monitor LFTs prior to titration, 3 months after titration and periodically thereafter for 12 months. Caution with heavy alcohol use, severe renal insufficiency, or history of hepatic disease. Avoid use in moderate or severe hepatic insufficiency. **Contra:** Active liver disease, unexplained persistent elevations in serum transaminases, pregnancy, lactation. **P/N:** Category X, not for use in nursing.	Headache, upper respiratory tract infection, myalgia, CK and transaminase elevations, urticaria, arthralgia.
Niacin ER/ Lovastatin (Advicor)	**Tab: Extended-Release** (Niacin-Lovastatin) 500mg-20mg, 750mg-20mg, 1000mg-20mg, 1000mg-40mg	**Adults:** ≥18 yrs: Initial: 500mg-20mg qhs. Titrate: Increase by no more than 500mg of niacin every 4 weeks. Max: 2000mg-40mg. **Concomitant Cyclosporine/Danazol:** Max Lovastatin: 20mg/day. **Concomitant Amiodarone/Verapamil:** Max Lovastatin: 40mg/day. Swallow tab whole. Take with low-fat snack. Pretreat 30 min prior with ASA to reduce flushing.	**W/P:** Do not substitute for equivalent dose of immediate-release niacin. Myopathy, rhabdomyolysis, severe hepatotoxicity reported. Caution with history of liver disease or jaundice, heavy alcohol use, hepatobilliary disease, peptic ulcer, diabetes, unstable angina, acute phase of MI, gout, renal dysfunction. Monitor LFTs prior to therapy, every 6-12 weeks for 1st 6 months, and periodically thereafter. May elevate PT, uric acid levels. D/C if AST or ALT ≥3x ULN persist, if myopathy diagnosed or suspected, and a few days before surgery. May reduce phosphorous levels. May disrupt therapy during a course of treatment with systemic antifungal azole, a macrolide antibiotic or ketolide antibiotic. **Contra:** Active liver disease, unexplained persistent elevations in serum transaminases, active PUD, arterial bleeding, pregnancy, nursing mothers. **P/N:** Category X, not for use in nursing.	Flushing, asthenia, flu syndrome, headache, infection, pain, GI effects, hyperglycemia, myalgia, pruritus, rash.
Niacin ER/ Simvastatin (Simcor)	**Tab, Extended-Release:** (Niacin-Simvastatin) 500mg/ 20mg, 750mg/20mg, 1000mg/20mg	**Adults:** Patients not currently on niacin extended-release or switching from immediate-release niacin: Initial: 500mg/ 20mg qd hs, with a low fat snack. Titrate: Adjust dose at ≥4 weeks. After week 8, titrate to patient response and tolerance. Maint: 1000mg/20mg-2000mg/40mg qd. Max: 2000mg/40mg qd. Doses >2000mg/ 40mg qd are not recommended. Do not break, crush or chew before swallowing.	**W/P:** Do not substitute for equivalent dose of immediate-release niacin. Myopathy and rhabdomyolysis reported; monitor serum creatine kinase (CK) periodically. D/c therapy if myopathy is suspected or diagnosed, if transaminase levels increase ≥3 ULN persist, or a few days prior to major surgery or when any major medical or surgical condition supervenes. Increased risk with higher doses, advanced age (≥65), hypothyroidism, renal impairment. Caution with heavy alcohol use, or history of liver disease; monitor LFTs prior to therapy, every 12 weeks for the first 6 months and periodically thereafter. Severe hepatic toxicity may occur in patients substituting sustained-release niacin for immediate-release niacin at equivalent doses. May increase serum glucose levels in diabetic or potentially diabetic patients, particularly the first few months of therapy; adjust diet and/or hypoglycemic therapy or d/c if necessary. May reduce platelet count. Caution with those predisposed to gout. **Contra:** Active liver disease, unexplained persistent elevations of serum transaminases, active peptic ulcer disease, arterial bleeding, pregnancy, nursing mothers. **P/N:** Category X, not for use in nursing.	Flushing, headache, backpain, diarrhea, nausea, pruritus.

W/P = warnings/precautions; **Contra** = contraindications; **P/N** = pregnancy category rating and nursing considerations.

Table 14.4. Drug Interactions for Antilipidemic Agents

BILE ACID SEQUESTRANTS

Cholestyramine (Questran, Questran Light)

Digitalis	Cholestyramine may reduce or delay absorption.
Drugs that undergo enterohepatic circulation	Interferes with absorption. Take concomitant drugs 1 hr before or 4-6 hrs after.
Estrogens	Cholestyramine may reduce or delay absorption.
Fat-soluble vitamins (A, D, E, K)	Interferes with absorption. Take concomitant drugs 1 hr before or 4-6 hrs after.
HMG-CoA reductase inhibitors	Additive effects.
Nicotinic acid	Additive effects.
Penicillin G	Cholestyramine may reduce or delay absorption.
Phenobarbital	Cholestyramine may reduce or delay absorption.
Phenylbutazone	Cholestyramine may reduce or delay absorption.
Phosphate supplements (oral)	Interferes with absorption. Take concomitant drugs 1 hr before or 4-6 hrs after.
Progestins	Cholestyramine may reduce or delay absorption.
Propranolol	Cholestyramine may reduce or delay absorption.
Spironolactone	Exercise caution.
Tetracycline	Cholestyramine may reduce or delay absorption.
Thiazide diuretics	Cholestyramine may reduce or delay absorption.
Thyroid	Cholestyramine may reduce or delay absorption.
Warfarin	Cholestyramine may reduce or delay absorption.

Colesevelam HCl (Welchol)

Contraceptives, oral	Decreases levels of ethinyl estradiol and norethindrone.
Glyburide	Decreases levels of glyburide.
Insulin	Increases TG levels.
Levothyroxine	Decreases levels of levothyroxine.
Phenytoin	Decreases levels of phenytoin.
Sulfonylureas	Increases TG levels.
Thyroid hormone replacement therapy	Elevates TSH.
Warfarin	Concomitant use decreases International Normalized Ratio (INR); monitor INR levels.

Colestipol HCl (Colestid)

Chlorothiazide	Reduces absorption of chlorothiazide.
Digitalis agents	Exercise caution.
Fat-soluble vitamins (A, D, E, K)	Interferes with absorption.

Table 14.4. Drug Interactions for Antilipidemic Agents

Folic acid	Interferes with absorption.
Furosemide	Reduces absorption of furosemide.
Gemfibrozil	Reduces absorption of gemfibrozil.
Hydrochlorothiazide	Reduces absorption of hydrochlorothiazide.
Hydrocortisone	Interferes with absorption.
Oral medications	Take other drugs 1 hr before or 4 hrs after colestipol.
Penicillin G	Reduces absorption of penicillin G.
Phosphate supplements (oral)	Interferes with absorption.
Propranolol	Exercise caution.
Tetracycline	Reduces absorption of tetracycline.

CHOLESTEROL ABSORPTION INHIBITOR
Ezetimibe (Zetia)

Cholestyramine	Incremental LDL-C reduction may be reduced with concomitant cholestyramine.
Cyclosporine	Monitor cyclosporine levels with concomitant use.
Fenofibrate	Increased levels of ezetimibe.
Fibrates	May increase cholesterol excretion into the bile; concurrent use not recommended.
Gemfibrozil	Increased levels of ezetimibe.
Warfarin	Monitor INR levels.

FATTY ACID DERIVATIVE
Omega-3-acid ethyl esters (Lovaza)

Aspirin	May cause prolongation of bleeding time.
Clopidogrel	May cause prolongation of bleeding time.
Coumarin	May cause prolongation of bleeding time.
Warfarin	May cause prolongation of bleeding time.

FIBRATES
Fenofibrate (Antara, Lofibra, Tricor, Triglide)

Bile acid sequestrants	May impede absorption; take at least 1 hr before or 4-6 hrs after the resin.
Coumarin anticoagulants	Potentiates coumarin anticoagulants. Monitor PT/INR levels.
HMG-CoA reductase inhibitors	To be avoided.
Immunosuppressants (eg, cyclosporine)	Concomitant use may cause nephrotoxicity.

Gemfibrozil (Lopid)

HMG-CoA reductase inhibitors	Increases risk of myopathy and rhabdomyolysis. To be avoided.

Table 14.4. Drug Interactions for Antilipidemic Agents

Immunosuppressants (eg, cyclosporine)	Concomitant use may cause nephrotoxicity.
Itraconazole	Avoid in patients on itraconazole and gemfibrozil.
Repaglinide	Increases levels of repaglinide. Monitor levels.

HMG-CoA REDUCTASE INHIBITORS (STATINS)

Atorvastatin calcium (Lipitor)

Azole antifungals (eg, ketoconazole)	Increases risk of myopathy. Decreases levels of endogenous steroids, caution with concomitant use.
Cimetidine	Decreases levels of endogenous steroids, caution with concomitant use.
Colestipol	Decreases atorvastatin levels. LDL-C reduction greater on concomitant administration.
Contraceptives, oral	Increases levels of ethinyl estradiol and norethindrone.
Cyclosporine	Increases risk of myopathy.
Digoxin	Increases levels of digoxin. Monitor levels.
Erythromycin	Increases atorvastatin levels with concomitant use. Increases risk of myopathy.
Fibric acid derivatives	Increases risk of myopathy.
Maalox	Decreases atorvastatin levels.
Niacin	Increases risk of myopathy.
Spironolactone	Decreases levels of endogenous steroids, caution with concomitant use.

Fluvastatin sodium (Lescol, Lescol XL)

Anticoagulants	Monitor PT/INR levels.
Cholestyramine	Decreases fluvastatin levels when given within 4 hrs. Has an additive effect when given after 4 hrs.
Cimetidine	Increases fluvastain levels. Decreases levels of endogenous steroids; caution with concomitant use.
Colchicine	Increases risk of myopathy and rhabdomyolysis.
Cyclosporine	Increases risk of myopathy and rhabdomyolysis.
Diclofenac	Increases levels of diclofenac.
Digoxin	Monitor levels.
Erythromycin	Increases risk of myopathy and rhabdomyolysis.
Fibrates	To be avoided.
Gemfibrozil	Increases risk of myopathy and rhabdomyolysis.
Glyburide	Levels of both glyburide and fluvastatin is increased.
Ketoconazole	Decreases levels of endogenous steroids, caution with concomitant use.
Niacin	Increases risk of myopathy.
Omeprazole	Increases fluvastain levels.
Phenytoin	Levels of both phenytoin and fluvastatin is increased. Monitor phenytoin levels.
Ranitidine	Increases fluvastatin levels.

Table 14.4. Drug Interactions for Antilipidemic Agents

Rifampicin	Decreases fluvastatin levels.
Spironolactone	Decreases levels of endogenous steroids; caution with concomitant use.
Lovastatin (Altoprev, Mevacor)	
Amiodarone	Increases risk of myopathy.
Anticoagulants	Monitor PT/INR levels.
Cimetidine	Decreases levels of endogenous steroids; caution with concomitant use.
Clarithromycin	Increases risk of myopathy.
Cyclosporine	Increases risk of myopathy.
Danazol	Increases risk of myopathy.
Erythromycin	Increases risk of myopathy.
Grapefruit juice	Increases risk of myopathy.
Itraconazole	Increases risk of myopathy.
Ketoconazole	Increases risk of myopathy. Decreases levels of endogenous steroids; caution with concomitant use.
Nefazodone	Increases risk of myopathy.
Niacin	Increases risk of myopathy.
Protease inhibitors	Increases risk of myopathy.
Spironolactone	Decreases levels of endogenous steroids; caution with concomitant use.
Telithromycin	Increases risk of myopathy.
Verapamil	Increases risk of myopathy.
Pravastatin sodium (Pravachol)	
Cholestyramine	Decreases pravastatin levels.
Cimetidine	Decreases levels of endogenous steroids, caution with concomitant use.
Colestipol	Decreases pravastatin levels.
Cyclosporine	Increases risk of myopathy.
Erythromycin	Increases risk of myopathy.
Fibrates	Increases risk of myopathy. To be avoided.
Gemfibrozil	Increases pravastatin levels.
Itraconazole	Increases pravastatin levels.
Ketoconazole	Decreases levels of endogenous steroids, caution with concomitant use.
Niacin	Increases risk of myopathy.
Resins	Take 1 hr before or 4 hrs after resins.
Spironolactone	Decreases levels of endogenous steroids; caution with concomitant use.
Rosuvastatin calcium (Crestor)	
Antacids	Space antacid dosing by 2 hrs.
Cimetidine	Decreases levels of endogenous steroids; caution with concomitant use.
Contraceptives, oral	Increases levels of ethinyl estradiol and norethindrone.

Table 14.4. Drug Interactions for Antilipidemic Agents

Cyclosporine	Increases rosuvastatin levels and risk of myopathy.
Fibrates	Increases risk of myopathy.
Gemfibrozil	To be avoided.
Ketoconazole	Decreases levels of endogenous steroids; caution with concomitant use.
Lopinavir	Increases rosuvastatin levels and risk of myopathy.
Niacin	Increases rosuvastatin levels and risk of myopathy.
Ritonavir	Increases rosuvastatin levels and risk of myopathy.
Spironolactone	Decreases levels of endogenous steroids; caution with concomitant use.
Warfarin	Concomitant use increases International Normalized Ratio (INR); monitor INR levels.
Simvastatin (Zocor)	
Amiodarone	Do not exceed 20mg of simvastatin daily.
Clarithromycin	Increases risk of myopathy.
Cyclosporine	Do not exceed 10mg of simvastatin daily.
Danazol	Do not exceed 10mg of simvastatin daily.
Digoxin	Monitor digoxin levels.
Erythromycin	Increases risk of myopathy.
Fibrates	Exercise caution.
Gemfibrozil	Do not exceed 10mg of simvastatin daily.
Grapefruit juice	Increases risk of myopathy.
Itraconazole	Increases risk of myopathy.
Ketoconazole	Increases risk of myopathy.
Nefazodone	Increases risk of myopathy.
Niacin	Exercise caution with concomitant administration of 1g/day of niacin.
Protease inhibitors	Increases risk of myopathy.
Verapamil	Do not exceed 20mg of simvastatin daily.
Warfarin	Monitor warfarin levels.

NICOTINIC ACID DERIVATIVE

Niacin (Niaspan)	
Alcohol	Avoid concomitant alcohol. May cause flushing and pruritus.
Anticoagulants	Exercise caution.
Antidiabetic agents	May need adjustment.
Bile acid resins	Separate dosing from bile acid resins by at least 4-6 hrs.
Ganglionic blockers	May potentiate antihypertensives.
HMG-CoA reductase inhibitors	Rhabdomyolysis may occur.

Table 14.4. Drug Interactions for Antilipidemic Agents

Nicotinamide	High doses may potentiate adverse effects.
Vasoactive drugs	May potentiate antihypertensives.

COMBINATIONS

Amlodipine/Atorvastatin (Caduet)

Azole antifungals	Increases risk of myopathy.
Cimetidine	Decreases levels of endogenous steroids; caution with concomitant use.
Colestipol	Decreases atorvastatin levels. LDL-C reduction greater on concomitant administration.
Contraceptives, oral	Increases levels of ethinyl estradiol and norethindrone.
Cyclosporine	Increases risk of myopathy.
Digoxin	Increases levels of digoxin.
Erythromycin	Increases levels of Caduet and risk of myopathy.
Fibrates	To be avoided.
Fibric acid derivatives	Increases risk of myopathy.
Ketoconazole	Decreases levels of endogenous steroids; caution with concomitant use.
Maalox	Decreases atorvastatin levels.
Niacin	Increases risk of myopathy.
Spironolactone	Decreases levels of endogenous steroids; caution with concomitant use.

Ezetimibe/Simvastatin (Vytorin)

Amiodarone	Do not exceed 20mg of simvastatin.
Cholestyramine	Incremental LDL-C reduction may be reduced with concomitant cholestyramine.
Clarithromycin	Increases risk of myopathy.
Cyclosporine	Do not exceed 10mg of simvastatin.
Danazol	Do not exceed 10mg of simvastatin.
Digoxin	Monitor digoxin levels.
Erythromycin	Increases risk of myopathy.
Fibrates	Exercise caution.
Gemfibrozil	Do not exceed 10mg of Vytorin.
Grapefruit juice	Increases risk of myopathy.
Itraconazole	Increases risk of myopathy.
Ketoconazole	Increases risk of myopathy.
Nefazodone	Increases risk of myopathy.
Niacin	Exercise caution with concomitant administration of 1g/day of niacin.
Protease inhibitors	Increases risk of myopathy.
Verapamil	Do not exceed 20mg of simvastatin daily.
Warfarin	Monitor warfarin levels.

Table 14.4. Drug Interactions for Antilipidemic Agents

Lovastatin/Niacin ER (Advicor)

Adrenergic blockers	Exercise caution.
Alcohol	Avoid concomitant alcohol. May cause flushing and pruritis.
Amiodarone	Increases risk of myopathy.
Anticoagulants	Exercise caution; monitor levels.
Antidiabetic agents	May need adjustment.
ASA	Decreased niacin clearance.
Bile acid resins	Separate dosing from bile acid resins by at least 4-6 hrs.
Calcium channel blockers	Exercise caution.
Cimetidine	Decreases levels of endogenous steroids, caution with concomitant use.
Clarithromycin	Increases risk of myopathy.
Cyclosporine	Increases risk of myopathy.
Danazol	Increases risk of myopathy.
Erythromycin	Increases risk of myopathy.
Ganglionic blockers	May potentiate antihypertensives.
Grapefruit juice	Increases risk of myopathy.
HMG-CoA reductase inhibitors	Rhabdomyolysis may occur.
Itraconazole	Increases risk of myopathy.
Ketoconazole	Increases risk of myopathy. Decreases levels of endogenous steroids; caution with concomitant use.
Nefazodone	Increases risk of myopathy.
Niacin supplements	Exercise caution.
Nicotinamide	High doses may potentiate adverse effects.
Nitrates	Exercise caution.
Protease inhibitors	Increases risk of myopathy.
Spironolactone	Decreases levels of endogenous steroids; caution with concomitant use.
Telithromycin	Increases risk of myopathy.
Vasoactive drugs	May potentiate antihypertensives.
Verapamil	Increases risk of myopathy.

Niacin/Simvastatin (Simcor)

Amiodarone	Do not exceed 20mg of simvastatin daily.
Aspirin	Concomitant use decreases niacin levels.
Cholestyramine	Increase niacin-binding capacity.
Clarithromycin	Increases risk of myopathy.
Colestipol	Increases niacin-binding capacity.

Table 14.4. Drug Interactions for Antilipidemic Agents

Coumarin anticoagulants	Potentiates coumarin anticoagulants. Monitor PT/INR levels.
Cyclosporine	Do not exceed 10mg of simvastatin daily.
Danazol	Do not exceed 10mg of simvastatin daily.
Digoxin	Monitor digoxin levels.
Erythromycin	Increases risk of myopathy.
Fibrates	Exercise caution.
Grapefruit juice	Increases risk of myopathy.
Itraconazole	Increases risk of myopathy.
Ketoconazole	Increases risk of myopathy.
Nefazodone	Increases risk of myopathy.
Niacin supplements	Potentiates adverse effects.
Propranolol	Decreases simvastatin levels.
Protease inhibitors	Increases risk of myopathy.
Verapamil	Do not exceed 20mg of simvastatin daily.

Dyslipidemia Management in Adults with Diabetes

RATIONALE FOR TREATMENT OF DYSLIPIDEMIA

The rationale for the treatment of diabetic dyslipidemia is discussed in detail in the American Diabetes Association (ADA) technical review "Management of Dyslipidemia in Adults with Diabetes" (1). Type 2 diabetes is associated with a two- to fourfold excess risk of cardiovascular disease (CVD).

PREVALENCE OF DYSLIPIDEMIA IN TYPE 2 DIABETES

The most common pattern of dyslipidemia in patients with type 2 diabetes patients is elevated triglyceride levels and decreased HDL cholesterol levels. The mean concentration of LDL cholesterol in those with type 2 diabetes is not significantly different from that in those individuals who do not have diabetes. However, qualitative changes in LDL cholesterol may be present. In particular, patients with diabetes tend to have a higher proportion of smaller and denser LDL particles, which are more susceptible to oxidation and may thereby increase the risk of cardiovascular events. Insufficient data are available to make recommendations on the measurement of particle size in clinical practice.

As in those who do not have diabetes, lipid levels may be affected by factors unrelated to glycemia or insulin resistance, such as renal disease, hypothyroidism, and frequent occurrence of genetically determined lipoprotein disorders (e.g., familial combined hyperlipidemia and familial hypertriglyceridemia). These genetic disorders may contribute to the severe hypertriglyceridemia seen in some patients with diabetes. Furthermore, use of alcohol or estrogen may also contribute to hypertriglyceridemia.

LIPOPROTEIN RISK FACTORS FOR CVD

Available prospective cohort studies suggest that lipid abnormalities are associated with increased risk of cardiovascular events in patients both with and without diabetes. Various studies have demonstrated that LDL, HDL, and triglycerides are independent predictors of CVD (2).

Abbreviations: ADA, American Diabetes Association; CHD, coronary heart disease: CVD, cardiovascular disease; MNT, medical nutrition therapy; NCEP, National Cholesterol Education Program

CLINICAL TRIALS OF LIPID LOWERING IN DIABETIC SUBJECTS

The recently completed Heart Protection Study has been the largest study to date, enrolling and randomizing 5,963 patients age >40 years with diabetes and total cholesterol >135 mg/dL. In this trial, patients with diabetes assigned to simvastatin had a 22% reduction (95% CI 13–30) in the event rate for major CVD events. This risk reduction was similar across all LDL subcategories examined, including patients with lower pretreatment LDL cholesterol levels (<116 mg/dL) and those without identified vascular disease (3). Numerous other statin trials have included much smaller numbers of patients with diabetes but have demonstrated similar reductions in CVD events.

Two outcomes studies have been conducted with the fibric acid derivative gemfibrozil. In the Veterans Affairs High-Density Lipoprotein Cholesterol Intervention Trial (VA-HIT), gemfibrozil was associated with a 24% decrease in cardiovascular events in diabetic subjects with prior cardiovascular disease, low HDL (<40 mg/dL), and modestly elevated triglycerides (4).

MODIFICATION OF LIPOPROTEINS BY MEDICAL NUTRITION THERAPY AND PHYSICAL ACTIVITY

There is little evidence from clinical trials to determine the effect of different dietary interventions on the incidence of cardiovascular events. Observational studies suggest that patients who report healthier diets and greater physical activity have fewer cardiovascular events (5,6). The ADA has made recommendations for both medical nutrition therapy (MNT) (5) and physical activity (6).

Weight loss and increased physical activity will lead to decreased triglycerides and increased HDL cholesterol levels and also to modest lowering of LDL cholesterol levels. Patients with diabetes who are overweight should be given a prescription for MNT and for increased physical activity. The proportion of saturated fat in the meal plan should be reduced. The ADA suggests an increase in either carbohydrate or monounsaturated fat to compensate for the reduction in saturated fat. Some (but not all) studies suggest that a high–monounsaturated fat diet may have better metabolic effects than a high-carbohydrate diet, although other experts have suggested that such a dietary modification may make weight loss more difficult in obese patients with diabetes.

Recommendations of the American Heart Association for patients with CVD (7) have suggested that the maximal MNT typically reduces LDL cholesterol 15–25 mg/dL (0.40–0.65 mmol/L). Lifestyle intervention may be evaluated at regular intervals, with consideration of pharmacological therapy between 3 and 6 months.

MODIFICATION OF LIPOPROTEINS BY GLUCOSE-LOWERING AGENTS

Interventions to improve glycemia usually lower triglyceride levels modestly. In general, glucose-lowering agents do not change or have only a minimal effect on HDL levels. Thiazolidinediones may increase HDL and LDL levels, but the long-term effect of such changes is not known.

TREATMENT GOALS FOR LIPOPROTEIN THERAPY

No completed clinical trials have examined the effect of implementing different lipid treatment goals, including the question of what LDL cholesterol goal should be used and whether the use of multi-drug therapy is more effective than monotherapy for patients with complex lipid abnormalities. Current trials are examining these questions.

Because of frequent changes in glycemic control in patients with diabetes and the effects on levels of LDL, HDL, total cholesterol, and triglyceride, levels should be measured every year in adult patients. If values are at low-risk levels (LDL <100 mg/dL, triglycerides <150 mg/dL, and HDL >50 mg/dL), assessment may be repeated every 2 years.

Lipid-associated risk for CVD events is graded and continuous. Target LDL cholesterol levels for adults with diabetes are <100 mg/dL (2.60 mmol/L); HDL cholesterol levels are >40 mg/dL (1.02 mmol/L); and triglyceride levels are <150 mg/dL (1.7 mmol/L). In women, who tend to have higher HDL cholesterol levels than men, an HDL goal 10 mg/dL higher may be appropriate.

The recommendations for treatment of elevated LDL cholesterol generally follow the guidelines of both the NCEP (8) and an ADA consensus development conference (9),

with the following caveats. Pharmacological therapy should be initiated after lifestyle intervention has been implemented. However, in patients with clinical cardiovascular disease and LDL >100 mg/dL, pharmacological therapy should be initiated at the same time that lifestyle intervention is started.

For patients with diabetes without preexisting CVD, the current ADA recommendations for starting pharmacological therapy are 1) an LDL cholesterol level of 130 mg/dL (3.35 mmol/L) and 2) a goal of <100 mg/dL (2.60 mmol/L) for LDL cholesterol. These recommendations are based not only on the high incidence of CVD in patients with diabetes (10), but also on the higher case fatality rate of these patients once they have CVD. Since a large proportion of diabetic patients die before they reach the hospital, a preventive strategy based solely on secondary prevention would not be able to "save" large numbers of these diabetic patients. In patients with LDL between 100 mg/dL (2.60 mmol/L) and 129 mg/dl (3.30 mmol/L), a variety of treatment strategies are available, including more aggressive MNT and pharmacological treatment with a statin.

Table 1. Order of Priorities for Treatment of Diabetic Dyslipidemia in Adults

I. LDL cholesterol lowering	II. HDL cholesterol raising	IV. Combined hyperlipidemia
Lifestyle interventions	Lifestyle interventions	First choice
Preferred	Nicotinic acid or fibrates	Improved glycemic control plus high-dose statin
HMG CoA reductase inhibitor (statin)	III. Triglyceride lowering	Second choice
Others	Lifestyle interventions	Improved glycemic control plus statin plus fibric acid derivative
Bile acid binding resin (resin), cholesterol absorption inhibitor, fenofibrate or niacin	Glycemic control	Third choice
	Fibric acid derivative (gemfibrozil, fenofibrate)	Improved glycemic control plus statin plus nicotinic acid
	Niacin	
	High-dose statins (in those who also have high LDL cholesterol)	

Decision for treatment of high LDL before elevated triglyceride is based on clinical trial data indicating safety as well as efficacy of the available agents. The combination of statins with nicotinic acid, fenofibrate, and especially gemfibrozil may carry an increased risk of myositis. See text for recommendations for patients with triglyceride levels >400 mg/dL.

Recent findings from the Heart Protection Study (3), in people with diabetes over the age of 40 years with a total cholesterol ≥135 mg/dL, suggest that statin therapy to achieve an LDL reduction of ~30% regardless of baseline LDL levels may be appropriate.

Table 1 shows the order of priorities for treatment of dyslipidemia. Treatment of LDL cholesterol is considered the first priority for pharmacological therapy of dyslipidemia for a number of reasons (1).

Hypertriglyceridemia may be a risk factor for CVD in people with diabetes. The initial therapy for hypertriglyceridemia is lifestyle intervention with weight loss, increased physical activity, restricted intake of saturated fats, incorporation of monounsaturated fats, reduction of carbohydrate intake, and reduction of alcohol consumption. In the case of severe hypertriglyceridemia (1,000 mg/dL [11.3 mmol/L]), severe dietary fat restriction (<10% of calories) in addition to pharmacological therapy is necessary to reduce the risk of pancreatitis.

Improved glycemic control can be very effective for reducing triglyceride levels and should be aggressively pursued. Insulin therapy (alone or with insulin sensitizers) may also be particularly effective in lowering triglyceride levels. After the achievement of optimal glycemic control (or at least after the achievement of as much improvement as likely to be possible), the physician should consider adding a fibric acid and/or niacin.

The decision to start pharmacological therapy is dependent on the clinician's judgment between triglyceride levels of 200 mg/dL (2.30 mmol/L) and 400 mg/dL (4.50 mmol/L). Above 400 mg/dL (4.50 mmol/L), strong consideration should be given to pharmacological treatment of triglyceridemia to minimize the risk of pancreatitis. In some studies, higher-dose statins are moderately effective in reducing triglyceride levels in markedly hypertriglyceridemic subjects (triglyceride 300 mg/dL [3.40 mmol/L]).

Gemfibrozil should not be initiated alone in diabetic patients who have undesirable levels of both triglyceride and LDL cholesterol. Fenofibrate has greater LDL-lowering effects, is arguably safer in combination with statin therapy, and may be useful in those patients with diabetes with combined hyperlipidemia.

Although HDL cholesterol is a powerful predictor of CVD in patients with diabetes, it is difficult to raise HDL cholesterol levels without pharmacological intervention. Nicotinic acid, which should be used with caution in patients with diabetes, and fibrates can effectively increase HDL cholesterol levels. Low doses of nicotinic acid (2 g nicotinic acid/day) may not have much of a detrimental effect on glycemic control, and any deterioration may be easily remediable by adjustment of hypoglycemic medications. Behavioral interventions (weight loss, smoking cessation, increased physical activity) may increase HDL cholesterol.

In some cases, combined lipid therapy may be initiated. Several options are shown in Table 1. The combination of statins with nicotinic acid, fenofibrate, and especially gemfibrozil has been associated with increased risk of myositis, although the risk of clinical myositis (as opposed to elevated creatinine phosphokinase levels) appears to be low. However, the risk of myositis may be increased with the combination of gemfibrozil and a statin or in patients with renal disease. Combinations of statins with nicotinic acid and fibrates are extremely effective in modifying diabetic dyslipidemia.

LIPID-LOWERING AGENTS

The choice of statin should depend principally on the LDL reduction needed to achieve the target (<100 mg/dL [2.60 mmol/L]) and on the judgment of the treating physician.

It should also be noted that the higher doses of statins may be moderately effective at reducing triglyceride levels (though not necessarily at raising HDL levels) and thus may reduce the need for combination therapy. With the use of statins, LDL levels may be reduced to 50 mg/dL (1.30 mmol/L). There is no safety data at such low LDL levels. The use of very high-dose statin therapy (e.g., simvastatin 80 mg or atorvastatin 40 or 80 mg) to treat hypertriglyceridemia should be restricted to patients with both high LDL cholesterol levels and high triglyceride levels.

Changes in therapy should be based on laboratory follow-up between 4 and 12 weeks after initiating therapy. Once goals have been achieved, laboratory follow-up every 6–12 months is suggested.

CONSIDERATIONS IN THE TREATMENT OF ADULTS WITH TYPE ONE DIABETES

Patients with type 1 diabetes who are in good glycemic control tend to have normal levels of lipoproteins, unless they are overweight or obese, in which case they may get a lipid profile very similar to that seen in type 2 diabetes. Their composition of lipoproteins may be abnormal, but the effects of these compositional abnormalities in relation to CVD are unknown. There is relatively little observational data on lipoproteins and CVD, and there are no clinical trials relating lipoproteins to CVD. It seems reasonable that if patients with type 1 diabetes have LDL cholesterol levels that are above the goals recommended for those with type 2 diabetes (<100 mg/dL), they should be aggressively treated. Improved glycemic control may be even more important in those with type 1 diabetes than in those with type 2 diabetes for reduction of CVD (e.g., Wisconsin Epidemiologic Study of Diabetic Retinopathy [WESDR]).

CONCLUSIONS

Aggressive therapy of diabetic dyslipidemia will reduce the risk of CVD in patients with diabetes. Primary therapy should be directed first at lowering LDL levels. The goal is to reduce LDL concentrations to ≤100 mg/dL [2.60 mmol/L]. The initiation level for behavioral interventions is also an LDL cholesterol of ≥100 mg/dL (2.60 mmol/L). The initial pharmacological therapy should be to use statins. A cholesterol absorption inhibitor, a resin, niacin, or fenofibrate may be added if necessary to reach the LDL goal or in the case of statin intolerance. There are no outcome studies of combination lipid-lowering therapies.

In addition, if the HDL is <40 mg/dL, a fibric acid, such as fenofibrate, or niacin might be used in patients with LDL cholesterol between 100 and 129 mg/dL.

The initial therapy for hypertriglyceridemia is improved glycemic control and lifestyle intervention. Additional triglyceride lowering can be achieved with fibric acid derivatives (gemfibrozil or fenofibrate) or niacin. For subjects with both high LDL and triglyceride levels, high dose statins may be used.

RECOMMENDATIONS

Screening
- In adult patients, test for lipid disorders at least annually and more often if needed to achieve goals. In adults with low-risk lipid values (LDL <100 mg/dL, HDL >50 mg/dL, and triglycerides <150 mg/dL), repeat lipid assessments every 2 years. (E)

Treatment recommendations and goals
- Lifestyle modification focusing on the reduction of saturated fat and cholesterol intake, weight loss, increased physical

activity, and smoking cessation has been shown to improve the lipid profile in patients with diabetes. (A)

- Patients who do not achieve lipid goals with lifestyle modifications require pharmacological therapy. (A)
- Lower LDL cholesterol to <100 mg/dL (2.6 mmol/L) as the primary goal of therapy for adults. (B)
- Lowering LDL cholesterol with a statin is associated with a reduction in cardiovascular events. (A)
- In people with diabetes over the age of 40 years with a total cholesterol 135 mg/dL, statin therapy to achieve an LDL reduction of 30% regardless of baseline LDL levels may be appropriate. (A)
- In children and adolescents with diabetes, LDL cholesterol should be lowered to <100 mg/dL (2.60 mmol/L) using MNT and medications, based on LDL level and other cardiovascular risk factors in addition to diabetes. (E)
- Lower triglycerides to <150 mg/dL (1.7 mmol/L), and raise HDL cholesterol to >40 mg/dL (1.15 mmol/L). In women, an HDL goal 10 mg/dL higher may be appropriate. (C)
- Lowering triglycerides and increasing HDL cholesterol with a fibrate is associated with a reduction in cardiovascular events in patients with clinical CVD, low HDL, and near-normal levels of LDL. (A)
- Combination therapy using statins and fibrates or niacin may be necessary to achieve lipid targets, but has not been evaluated in outcomes studies for either event reduction or safety. (E)

FOOTNOTES

The recommendations in this paper are based on the evidence reviewed in the following publication: Management of dyslipidemia in adults with diabetes (Technical Review). *Diabetes Care* 21:160–178, 1998.

The initial draft of this paper was prepared by Steven M. Haffner, MD. This paper was peer-reviewed, modified, and approved by the Professional Practice Committee and the Executive Committee, November 1997. Most recent review/revision, 2003.

REFERENCES

1. Haffner SM: Management of dyslipidemia in adults with diabetes (Technical Review). *Diabetes Care* 21:160–178, 1998
2. Turner RC, Millns H, Neil HA, Stratton IM, Manley SE, Matthews DR, Holman RR: Risk factors for coronary artery disease in non-insulin dependent diabetes mellitus (UKPDS 23). *BMJ* 316:823–828, 1998.
3. Heart Protection Study Collaborative Group: MRC/BHF Heart Protection Study of cholesterol-lowering with simvastatin in 5963 people with diabetes: a randomised placebo-controlled trial. *Lancet* 361:2005–2016, 2003.
4. Rubins HB, Robins SJ, Collins D, Fye CL, Anderson JW, Elam MB, Faas FH, Linares E, Schaefer EJ, Schectman G, Wilt TJ, Wittes J: Gemfibrozil for the secondary prevention of coronary heart disease in men with low levels of high-density lipoprotein cholesterol: Veterans Affairs High-Density Lipoprotein Cholesterol Intervention Trial Study Group. *N Engl J Med* 341:410–418, 1999.
5. American Diabetes Association: Nutrition principles and recommendations in diabetes (Position Statement). *Diabetes Care* 27 (Suppl. 1):S36–S46, 2004.
6. American Diabetes Association: Physical activity/exercise and diabetes (Position Statement). *Diabetes Care* 27:S58–S62, 2004.
7. Grundy SM, Balady GJ, Criqui MH, Fletcher G, Greenland P, Hiratzka LF, Houston-Miller N, Kris-Etherton P, Krumholz HM, LaRosa J, Ockene IS, Pearson TA, Reed J, Smith SC, Washington R: When to start cholesterol-lowering therapy in patients with coronary heart disease: a statement for healthcare professionals from the American Heart Association task force on risk reduction. *Circulation* 95:1683–1685, 1997.
8. NCEP Expert Panel on Detection, Evaluation and Treatment of High Blood Cholesterol in Adults: Executive Summary of the Third Report of the National Cholesterol Education Program (NCEP) Expert Panel on Detection, Evaluation and Treatment of High Blood Cholesterol in Adults (Adult Treatment Panel III). *JAMA* 285:2486–2497, 2001.
9. American Diabetes Association: Detection and management of lipid disorders in diabetes (Consensus Statement). *Diabetes Care* 16:828–834, 1993.
10. Haffner SM, Lehto S, Rönnemaa T, Pyörälä K, Laakso M: Mortality from coronary heart disease in subjects with type 2 diabetes and in nondiabetic subjects with and without prior myocardial infarction. *N Engl J Med* 339:229–234, 1998.

Chapter 15

Antiplatelet Agents

Linda Garrelts MacLean, BPharm, CDE

INTRODUCTION

Patients with diabetes have an increased risk for cardiovascular events. The National Cholesterol Education Program (NCEP) recognizes diabetes as a cardiovascular disease (CVD) equivalent. Incorporating agents that will decrease this risk into the treatment regime for a patient with diabetes is an important part of the total care plan. Antiplatelet agents are used as a strategy for primary and secondary prevention of these cardiovascular events.

ASPIRIN

In 2004, the American Diabetes Association (ADA) issued a formal recommendation that persons with diabetes, who had no contraindications to aspirin (acetylsalicylic acid or ASA), should take a low-dose aspirin daily. However, it is estimated that fewer than half of eligible persons with diabetes are actually using aspirin routinely. There is some current debate surrounding the effectiveness of aspirin in persons with diabetes when compared with those without diabetes; this will be discussed under "Therapeutic Advantages and Disadvantages" later in this chapter. But until evidence indicates differently, the ADA position statement offers a challenge and opportunity for health care providers to improve the utilization of

aspirin. These professionals can communicate the value of incorporating a low-dose aspirin into the treatment regimen, ultimately resulting in a higher percentage of patients being treated appropriately.

Pharmacology

Mechanism of Action

The anti-inflammatory and anticoagulant properties of aspirin are believed to be responsible for its positive effects on the atherosclerosis and hypercoaguability associated with the insulin resistance of type 2 diabetes. Prostaglandins are associated with inflammation. It is aspirin's interference with prostaglandin production that is responsible for its anti-inflammatory action. The anticoagulation effects of aspirin are related to aspirin's ability to interfere with the production of thromboxane A_2 in the platelet. Since platelet aggregation is associated with thromboxane A_2, anticoagulation is associated with decreased levels of this compound.

Although the full mechanism of action regarding the cardioprotective effects of aspirin is not completely understood, the potential mechanisms by which these actions occur are well described by Nobles-James, et al in *Prevention of Cardiovascular Complications of Diabetes Mellitus by Aspirin*, which is referenced in the suggested reading at the end of the chapter.

Other positive effects on diabetes and its complications have been associated with aspirin. It may influence carbohydrate metabolism, improving glucose control. Additionally, the findings of a recent study in Spain indicate that low-dose aspirin given at night reduced daytime blood pressure in persons with prehypertension with a mean age of 43 years. These subjects did not have diabetes, therefore further study is needed in this population to determine if the body's circadian rhythm influences the effect of aspirin on blood pressure.

Pharmacokinetics

The low-dose aspirin therapy recommended for patients with diabetes is administered orally and is rapidly absorbed as unchanged drug (70%) and hydrolyzed salicylic acid (30%). Absorption occurs primarily from the small intestine, though to some extent via the stomach. The rate of absorption is affected by the tablet formulation (eg, uncoated, film coated, or enteric coated), stomach-emptying time, gastric and small intestine pH, and the presence of food. Most germane to this discussion would be the recommendation that a patient take the aspirin dose with a full glass of water or food to minimize gastric irritation; this will not decrease the extent of absorption. After absorption, the salicylate is widely distributed throughout body fluids and tissues. It crosses the placental barrier and is present in breast milk.

The liver is the primary site for salicylate metabolism with other tissues secondarily involved. The principal excretion route for salicylates is via the kidneys. The half-life of aspirin is approximately 15 to 20 minutes, because it is very quickly hydrolyzed to salicylic acid. Salicylic acid has a half-life that ranges between 3.5 and 4.5 hours, although this elimination half-life varies with dosage.

Treatment Advantages and Disadvantages

Unless a major contraindication is identified, the use of aspirin therapy in patients with diabetes is highly recommended. In light of the fact that diabetes increases the risk of developing cardiovascular disease by four-fold, the advantages of using aspirin as a primary and secondary preventive measure are well documented. The favorable results associated with low-dose aspirin therapy are also very cost-effective, adding to the body of evidence that supports this treatment modality for diabetes.

There has been recent discussion regarding the existence of a phenomenon resembling aspirin resistance in patients with diabetes. Aspirin may be less effective in preventing death in patients with diabetes. This conclusion was supported when a retrospective analysis on the data from the Evaluation of Methods and Management of Acute Coronary Events (EMMACE)-2 Study was performed. The researchers believe this indicates that more effective antiplatelet therapies must be developed for patients with diabetes and unstable coronary disease.

Therapeutic Considerations

Warnings/Precautions

Patients using aspirin should be warned that the risk for gastrointestinal bleeding is increased. A history of peptic ulcer disease or of a previous upper gastrointestinal bleed would indicate that aspirin should be used cautiously if at all. In this scenario, *H.pylori*, if present, should be eliminated; then aspirin therapy would be initiated along with a proton pump inhibitor. In general, the benefits of aspirin therapy outweigh the risk of serious bleeding in adults, although each person must be assessed individually. The age of the patient must be taken into consideration; patients >70 years of age experience a higher incidence of upper gastrointestinal bleeding, highlighting the need to carefully evaluate risks versus expected benefits.

Aspirin should be administered cautiously in the presence of other conditions, including:
• Asthma
• Other allergic conditions, including a hypersensitivity to other nonsteroidal anti-inflammatory drugs (NSAIDs)
• Gastrointestinal ulcerations
• Hypoprothrombinemia
• Significant anemia

Additionally, warn patients of the increased chance that a GI bleed may occur when alcohol is consumed concomitantly with aspirin.

Aspirin should also be administered cautiously in the presence of certain medications, including:
• Sulfonylureas (reduced dose of the hypoglycemic drug may be necessary)
• Insulin (dosing may need to be changed)
• Anticoagulants (salicylates can decrease the concentration of prothrombin in the plasma)
• Methotrexate (salicylates can decrease the elimination of methotrexate)

The ADA position statement on *Aspirin Therapy in Diabetes* lists the following as contraindications to aspirin therapy:
• Allergy
• Bleeding tendency
• Anticoagulant therapy
• Recent gastrointestinal bleeding
• Clinically active hepatic disease

Adverse Effects and Monitoring

Gastric mucosal injury and GI bleeding have been associated with aspirin therapy. Even at low doses, the risk for a GI bleed is increased and using an enteric-coated dosage form does not decrease this risk. Hence, counsel patients to watch for signs and symptoms of bleeding, which include but are not limited to the following: hematemesis, hematochezia, melena, lethargy, and pallor.

Other potential GI adverse reactions can include nausea, vomiting, diarrhea, dyspepsia, and heartburn. Patients should be advised to take their aspirin dose with a full glass of water to minimize stomach irritation.

Drug Interactions

A list of drug interactions associated with aspirin may be found in **Table 15.2** at the end of this chapter. When aspirin is combined with other anticoagulant agents, including many natural products, the risk of bleeding is increased. Chronic NSAID use with aspirin increases the potential for nephrotoxicity. Other agents that cause nephrotoxicity should not be taken concurrently with aspirin because of the prostaglandin inhibition by salicylates. Medications that cause GI toxicity should be used with caution with aspirin. Because salicylic acid is highly protein bound, other drugs that are highly protein bound may be displaced causing an increased effect of the displaced drug.

Dosage and Administration

The ADA recommends low-dose aspirin therapy (75-162 mg/day) for people with diabetes.
• This dosage is advised for individuals with a history of CVD (myocardial infarction, stroke, transient ischemic attacks, peripheral vascular disease, claudication, angina pectoris) for secondary prevention.
• Additionally, low-dose aspirin therapy is advised as a primary prevention strategy for eligible individuals with type 1 or type 2 diabetes. Eligible individuals would include:
  – Persons > 40 years of age
  – Persons who have an increased risk for CVD: high blood pressure, family history of CVD, smoking, albuminuria, dyslipidemia.
• Because of its association with Reye's syndrome when given to children with a viral infection, aspirin should NOT be

given to children. The ADA recommends that aspirin not be used in patients with diabetes under the age of 21 years.

For more dosing information, see **Table 15.1** at the end of this chapter.

Clopidogrel

The ADA position *Aspirin Therapy in Diabetes* makes a limited reference to the possible use of clopidogrel in patients with diabetes. Although limited data is available in this population, the recommendation is that clopidogrel may be considered as an alternative antiplatelet therapy in patients with an aspirin allergy. One study was noted (Clopidogrel Versus Aspirin in Patients at Risk of Ischemic Events: CAPRIE), where 75 mg of clopidogrel was found to be marginally more effective than a 325-mg dose of aspirin in reducing the combined risk of ischemic stroke, myocardial infarction, or vascular death in persons with and without diabetes. However, the clopidogrel dose was not found to be effective in reducing the rate of recurrent stroke or vascular death.

A current topic of interest concerns the possible rebound effect that may occur once clopidogrel is discontinued. The results of an observational study published in the February 6, 2008 issue of *JAMA* support the possibility of this effect. Increased adverse events were observed in the initial 90 days after the discontinuation of clopidogrel, indicating the aforementioned rebound effect. The current recommendation is that a patient be treated with clopidogrel for 1 year after acute coronary syndrome. It is urged that patients and physicians carefully evaluate the strategy for drug discontinuation once the acute coronary syndrome patient has been on clopidogrel for the recommended time. Until this rebound effect is confirmed and the mechanism by which it occurs is known, the following approaches may be considered:

• If the clopidogrel is well tolerated and affordable, consider continuing the clopidogrel therapy.
• If the decision to discontinue the clopidogrel is made, discontinuation should be gradual and tapered over at least three weeks.

SUGGESTED READING

Cubbon RM, Gale CP, Rajwani A, Abbas A, Morrell C, Das R, et al. Aspirin and mortality in patients with diabetes sustaining acute coronary syndrome. *Diabetes Care.* 2008;31:363-5.

Nobles-James C, James EA, Sowers JR. Prevention of cardiovascular complications of diabetes mellitus by aspirin. *Cardiovascular Drug Rev.* 2004;22:215-226.

Cohen HW, Crandall JP, Hailpern SM, Billett HH. Aspirin resistance associated with HbA1c and obesity in diabetic patients. *J Diabetes and Its Complications.* 2008; 22: 224-228.

Ho PM, Peterson ED, Wang L, et al. Incidence of death and acute myocardial infarction associated with stopping clopidogrel after acute coronary syndrome. *JAMA.* 2008;299(5):532-539.

Table 15.1. Prescribing Information for Antiplatelet Agents

GENERIC (BRAND)	FORM/ STRENGTH	DOSAGE	WARNINGS/PRECAUTIONS & CONTRAINDICATIONS	ADVERSE REACTIONS
Anagrelide HCl (Agrylin)	Cap: 0.5mg, 1mg	**Adults:** Initial: 0.5mg qid or 1mg bid for at least 1 week. **Moderate Hepatic Impairment:** Initial: 0.5mg qd for at least 1 week. Titrate: Increase by no more than 0.5mg/day per week. Max: 10mg/day or 2.5mg/dose. Adjust lowest effective dose to reduce and maintain platelets <600,000/mcL. Monitor platelets every 2 days during first week, then weekly thereafter until reach maintenance dose. **Pediatrics:** Initial: 0.5mg qd. Titrate: Increase by no more than 0.5mg/day per week. Max: 10mg/day or 2.5mg/dose. Adjust to lowest effective dose to reduce and maintain platelets <600,000/mcL. Monitor platelets every 2 days during first week, then weekly thereafter until reach maintenance dose.	**W/P:** Caution with heart disease, renal or hepatic dysfunction. Perform pre-treatment cardiovascular exam and monitor during treatment; may cause cardiovascular effects (eg, vasodilation, tachycardia, palpitations, CHF). Monitor closely for renal toxicity if creatinine ≥2mg/dL or hepatic toxicity if bilirubin, SGOT, or LFTs >1.5x ULN. Monitor blood counts, renal and hepatic function while platelets are lowered. Increase in platelets after therapy interruption. Reduce dose in moderate hepatic impairment. **Contra:** Severe hepatic impairment. **P/N:** Category C, not for use in nursing.	Headache, palpitations, asthenia, edema, GI effects, dizziness, pain, dyspnea, fever, chest pain, rash, tachycardia, malaise, pharyngitis, cough, paresthesia.
Aspirin (Bayer Aspirin)	Tab: (Genuine Bayer Aspirin) 325mg; Tab: (Bayer Aspirin Regimen with Calcium) 81mg; Tab, Chewable: (Bayer Aspirin Children's) 81mg; Tab, Delayed-Release: (Bayer Aspirin Regimen) 81mg, 325mg	**Adults: Ischemic Stroke/TIA:** 50-325mg qd. **Suspected Acute MI:** Initial: 160-162.5mg qd as soon as suspect MI. Maint: 160-162.5mg qd for 30 days post-infarction, consider further therapy for prevention/recurrent MI. **Prevention or Recurrent MI/Unstable Angina/Chronic Stable Angina:** 75-325mg qd. **CABG:** 325mg qd, start 6 hrs post-surgery. Continue for 1 yr. **PTCA:** Initial: 325mg, 2 hrs pre-surgery. Maint: 160-325mg qd. **Carotid Endarterectomy:** 80mg qd to 650mg bid, start pre-surgery. **RA:** Initial: 3g qd in divided doses. Increase for anti-inflammatory efficacy to 150-300mcg/mL plasma salicylate level. **Spondyloarthropathies:** Up to 4g/day in divided doses. **OA:** Up to 3g/day in divided doses. **Arthritis/SLE Pleurisy:** Initial: 3g/day in divided doses. Increase for anti-inflammatory efficacy to 150-300mcg/mL plasma salicylate level. **Pain:** 325-650mg q4-6h. Max: 4g/day. **Pediatrics: JRA:** Initial: 90-130mg/kg/day in divided doses. Increase for anti-inflammatory efficacy to 150-300mcg/mL plasma salicylate level. **Pain: ≥12 yrs:** 325-650mg q4-6h. Max: 4g/day.	**W/P:** Increased risk of bleeding with heavy alcohol use (≥3 drinks/day). May inhibit platelet function; can adversely affect inherited (hemophilia) or acquired (hepatic disease, vitamin K deficiency) bleeding disorders. Monitor for bleeding and ulceration. Avoid in history of active peptic ulcer, severe renal failure, severe hepatic insufficiency, and sodium restricted diets. Associated with elevated LFTs, BUN, and serum creatinine; hyperkalemia; proteinuria; and prolonged bleeding time. Avoid 1 week before and during labor. **Contra:** NSAID allergy, viral infections in children or teenagers, syndrome of asthma, rhinitis, and nasal polyps. **P/N:** Avoid in 3rd trimester of pregnancy and nursing.	Fever, hypothermia, dysrhythmias, hypotension, agitation, cerebral edema, dehydration, hyperkalemia, dyspepsia, GI bleed, hearing loss, tinnitus, problems in pregnancy.
Aspirin (Bayer Aspirin Extra Strength)	Tab: 500mg	**Adults:** 500-1000mg q4-6h prn. Max: 4g/24hrs. **Pediatrics: ≥12 yrs:** 500-1000mg q4-6h prn. Max: 4g/24hrs.	**W/P:** Avoid in children or teenagers for chickenpox or flu symptoms; Reye's syndrome may occur. Do not take >10 days for pain or >3 days for fever. Avoid in asthma, stomach problems that persist or recur, gastric ulcers, or bleeding problems. Stop therapy if ringing in the ears or loss of hearing occurs. **P/N:** Avoid in 3rd trimester of pregnancy; safety in nursing not known.	
Aspirin (Ecotrin)	Tab, Delayed-Release: 81mg, 325mg, 500mg	**Adults: Ischemic Stroke/TIA:** 50-325mg qd. **Suspected Acute MI:** Initial: 160-162.5mg qd as soon as suspect MI. Maint: 160-162.5mg for 30 days post-infarction, consider further therapy for prevention/recurrent MI. **Prevention or Recurrent MI/Unstable Angina/Chronic Stable Angina:** 75-325mg qd. **CABG:** 325mg qd, start 6 hrs post-surgery. Continue for 1 yr. **PTCA:** Initial: 325mg, 2 hrs pre-surgery. Maint: 160-325mg qd. **Carotid Endarterectomy:** 80mg qd to	**W/P:** Increased risk of bleeding with heavy alcohol use (≥3 drinks/day). May inhibit platelet function; can adversely affect inherited (hemophilia) or acquired (hepatic disease, vitamin K deficiency) bleeding disorders. Monitor for bleeding and ulceration. Avoid in history of active peptic ulcer, severe renal failure, severe hepatic insufficiency, and sodium restricted diets. Associated with elevated LFTs, BUN, and serum creatinine; hyperkalemia; proteinuria; and prolonged bleeding time.	Fever, hypothermia, dysrhythmias, hypotension, agitation, cerebral edema, dehydration, hyperkalemia, dyspepsia, GI bleed, hearing loss, tinnitus, problems in pregnancy.

BB = black box warning; **W/P** = warnings/precautions; **Contra** = contraindications; **P/N** = pregnancy category rating and nursing considerations.

Table 15.1. Prescribing Information for Antiplatelet Agents

GENERIC (BRAND)	FORM/ STRENGTH	DOSAGE	WARNINGS/PRECAUTIONS & CONTRAINDICATIONS	ADVERSE REACTIONS
Aspirin (Ecotrin) *(Cont.)*		650mg bid, start pre-surgery. **RA/Arthritis/SLE Pleurisy:** Initial: 3g qd in divided doses. Increase for anti-inflammatory efficacy to 150-300mcg/mL plasma salicylate level. **Spondyloarthropathies:** Up to 4g/day in divided doses. **OA:** Up to 3g/day in divided doses. ***Pediatrics:* JRA:** Initial: 90-130mg/kg/day in divided doses. Increase for anti-inflammatory efficacy to 150-300mcg/mL plasma salicylate level.	Avoid 1 week before and during labor. **Contra:** NSAID allergy, children or teenagers for viral infections with or without fever, syndrome of asthma, rhinitis, and nasal polyps. **P/N:** Avoid in 3rd trimester of pregnancy and nursing.	
Aspirin (Halfprin)	**Tab, Delayed-Release:** 81mg, 162mg	***Adults:*** 162mg as soon as MI suspected; continue qd for 30 days. May need to continue as prophylaxis for recurrent MI. Crush, chew, or suck the 1st dose.	**W/P:** Caution with marked HTN or renal dysfunction; monitor renal function with long-term therapy. **P/N:** Safety in pregnancy and nursing is not known.	Stomach pain, heartburn, nausea, vomiting, GI bleeding, small increases in BP.
Aspirin/ Dipyridamole ER (Aggrenox)	**Cap:** (ASA/ Dipyridamole Extended-Release) 25mg-200mg	***Adults:*** 1 cap bid (am and pm).	**W/P:** Increased risk of bleeding with chronic, heavy alcohol use. Caution with inherited or acquired bleeding disorders, severe CAD, and hypotension. Monitor for signs of GI ulcers and bleeding. Avoid with history of peptic ulcer disease, severe renal failure (CrCl <10mL/min). Risk of hepatic dysfunction. Not interchangeable with individual components of ASA and Persantine tabs. Avoid in 3rd trimester of pregnancy. **Contra:** NSAID allergy, children or teenagers with viral infections, syndrome of asthma, rhinitis, nasal polyps. **P/N:** Category D, caution in nursing.	Headache, dyspepsia, abdominal pain, nausea, diarrhea, vomiting, fatigue, arthralgia, pain, hemorrhage.
Cilostazol (Pletal)	**Tab:** 50mg, 100mg	***Adults:*** 100mg bid, 1/2 hr before or 2 hrs after breakfast and dinner. **Concomitant CYP3A4 and CYP2C19 Inhibitors:** Consider 50mg bid.	**BB:** Contraindicated with CHF of any severity due to possible decrease in survival. **W/P:** Risks not known in patients with severe underlying heart disease, moderate or severe hepatic impairment, or with long-term use. Rare cases of thrombocytopenia or leukopenia reported. **Contra:** CHF of any severity. Hemostatic disorders or active pathologic bleeding (eg, peptic ulcer, intracranial bleeding). **P/N:** Category C, not for use in nursing.	Headache, palpitations, tachycardia, abnormal stool, diarrhea, peripheral edema, dizziness, infection, rhinitis, blood pressure increase, aplastic anemia.
Clopidogrel bisulfate (Plavix)	**Tab:** 75mg, 300mg	***Adults:* MI/Stroke/PAD:** 75mg qd. **Acute Coronary Syndrome:** Take with 75-325mg ASA qd. LD: 300mg. Maint: 75mg qd. **STEMI:** 75mg, with 75-325mg ASA, qd with or without LD.	**W/P:** Caution with risk of increased bleeding, ulcers or lesions with a propensity to bleed, severe hepatic or renal impairment. D/C 5 days before surgery if antiplatelet effect is not desired. Monitor blood cell count and other appropriate tests if symptoms of bleeding or undesirable hematological effects arise. Thrombotic thrombocytopenic purpura (TTP) reported (rare). **Contra:** Active pathological bleeding (eg, peptic ulcer, intracranial hemorrhage). **P/N:** Category B, not for use in nursing.	Chest pain, influenza-like symptoms, pain, edema, HTN, headache, dizziness, abdominal pain, dyspepsia, diarrhea, arthralgia, purpura, upper respiratory tract infection, back pain, dyspnea.
Dipyridamole (Persantine)	**Tab:** 25mg, 50mg, 75mg	***Adults:*** 75-100mg qid.	**W/P:** Caution with hypotension or severe CAD (eg, unstable angina or recent MI); may aggravate chest pain. Elevated hepatic enzymes and hepatic failure reported. **P/N:** Category B, caution in nursing.	Dizziness, abdominal distress.
Ticlopidine HCl (Ticlid)	**Tab:** 250mg	***Adults:*** Take with food. **Stroke:** 250mg bid. **Coronary Artery Stenting:** 250mg bid with ASA up to 30 days after stent implant.	**BB:** Can cause life-threatening hematological adverse reactions, including neutropenia/agranulocytosis, thrombotic thrombocytopenic purpura (TTP), and aplastic anemia. Monitor for evidence of neutropenia or TTP during first 3 months;	Diarrhea, rash, nausea, GI pain, rash, dyspepsia, neutropenia.

BB = black box warning; **W/P** = warnings/precautions; **Contra** = contraindications; **P/N** = pregnancy category rating and nursing considerations.

Table 15.1. Prescribing Information for Antiplatelet Agents

GENERIC (BRAND)	FORM/ STRENGTH	DOSAGE	WARNINGS/PRECAUTIONS & CONTRAINDICATIONS	ADVERSE REACTIONS
Ticlopidine HCl (Ticlid) (Cont.)			d/c if any seen. **W/P:** Monitor for hematologic toxicity before treatment, then every 2 weeks for 1st 3 months, and 2 weeks after discontinuation. Monitor more frequently if signs of hematological adverse reactions; d/c if neutrophils <1200/mm^3, aplastic anemia or TTP occurs. D/C 10-14 days before surgery. Caution in trauma, surgery, bleeding disorders. May need dose adjustment with renal or hepatic impairment. May elevate LFTs, TG, and cholesterol. **Contra:** Hematopoietic disorders (eg, neutropenia, thrombocytopenia), history of TTP or aplastic anemia, hemostatic disorders, active pathological bleeding, severe liver impairment. **P/N:** Category B, not for use in nursing.	
Warfarin sodium (Coumadin, Jantoven)	**Inj:** (Coumadin) 5mg; **Tab:** (Coumadin, Jantoven) 1mg*, 2mg*, 2.5mg*, 3mg*, 4mg*, 5mg*, 6mg*, 7.5mg*, 10mg* *scored	***Adults:*** **≥18 yrs:** Adjust dose based on PT/INR. Give IV as alternate to PO. Initial: 2-5mg qd. Usual: 2-10mg qd. **Venous Thromboembolism** (including pulmonary embolism): INR 2-3. **Atrial Fibrillation:** INR 2-3. **Post-MI:** Initiate 2-4 weeks post-infarct and maintain INR 2.5-3.5. **Mechanical/Bioprosthetic Heart Valve:** INR 2-3 for 12 weeks after valve insertion, then INR 2.5-3.5 long term.	**BB:** May cause major or fatal bleeding; monitor INR regularly. **W/P:** Monitor PT/INR; many endogenous and exogenous factors may affect PT/INR. Weigh benefits/risks with severe-moderate hepatic or renal insufficiency, infectious disease, intestinal flora disturbance, lactation, surgery, trauma, severe-moderate HTN, protein C deficiency, polycythemia vera, vasculitis, severe DM, indwelling catheters. D/C if tissue necrosis, systemic cholesterol microembolization (purple toe syndrome) occurs. Caution with HIT, DVT, elderly. Warfarin resistance, allergic reactions reported. **Contra:** Hemorrhagic tendencies, blood dyscrasias, CNS surgery, ophthalmic or traumatic surgery, inadequate lab facility, threatened abortion, eclampsia, preeclampsia, major regional lumbar block anesthesia, malignant HTN, pregnancy and unsupervised senile, alcoholic or psychotic patients. Bleeding of GI, GU or respiratory tract, aneurysms, pericarditis and pericardial effusion, bacterial endocarditis, cerebrovascular hemorrhage, spinal puncture, procedures with potential for uncontrollable bleeding. **P/N:** Category X, weigh benefits/risks with nursing.	Tissue or organ hemorrhage/necrosis, paresthesia, vasculitis, fever, rash, abdominal pain, hepatic disorders, fatigue, headache, alopecia.

BB = black box warning; **W/P** = warnings/precautions; **Contra** = contraindications; **P/N** = pregnancy category rating and nursing considerations.

Table 15.2. Drug Interactions for Antiplatelet Agents

Anagrelide HCl (Agrylin)

Amrinone	Exacerbates the effects of amrinone.
Cilostazol	Exacerbates the effects of cilostazol.
Enoximone	Exacerbates the effects of enoximone.
Milrinone	Exacerbates the effects of milrinone.
Olparinone	Exacerbates the effects of olparinone.
Sucralfate	May interfere with absorption.

Aspirin (Bayer Aspirin, Ecotrin, Halfprin)

ACE inhibitors	Diminished hypotensive and hyponatremic effects of ACE inhibitors.
Acetazolamide	May increase levels of acetazolamide.
Beta-blockers	Decreased hypotensive effects of beta-blockers.
Diuretics	Decreased diuretic effects with renal or cardiovascular disease.
Heparin	Increased risk of bleeds.
Hypoglycemic agents	Increased effects of hypoglycemic agents.
Methotrexate	Decreased methotrexate clearance; increased risk of bone marrow toxicity.
NSAIDs	Avoid NSAIDs.
Phenytoin	Decreased levels of phenytoin.
Uricosuric agents	Antagonizes uricosuric agents
Valproic acid	May increase levels of valproic acid.
Warfarin	Increased risk of bleeds.

Aspirin/Dipyridamole (Aggrenox)

ACE inhibitors	Reduces effect.
Acetazolamide	Potentiates effect.
Adenosine	Potentiates effect.
Anticoagulants	May increase risk of bleeding.
Beta-blockers	Reduces effect.
Cholinesterase inhibitors	Reduces effect.
Diuretics	Decreased effects of diuretics in renal or cardiovascular disease.
Hypoglycemics, Oral	Potentiates effect.
Methotrexate	Potentiates effect.
NSAIDs	May increase risk of bleeding and decrease renal function.
Phenytoin	Reduces effect.
Uricosuric agents	May antagonize uricosuric agents.
Valproic acid	Potentiates effect.

Cilostazol (Pletal)

CYP2C19 inhibitors (eg, omeprazole)	May increase cilostazol levels.
CYP3A4 inhibitors	Exercise caution with use.

Table 15.2. Drug Interactions for Antiplatelet Agents

Diltiazem	Exercise caution with use.
Erythromycin	Exercise caution with use.
Grapefruit juice	Avoid grapefruit juice.
Ketoconazole	Exercise caution with use.
Clopidogrel bisulfate (Plavix)	
ASA	Potentiates effect of ASA on collagen-induced platelet aggregation.
Drugs that may induce GI lesions	Exercise caution with use.
Fluvastatin	Exercise caution with use.
NSAID	Increased occult GI loss with NSAIDs.
Phenytoin	Exercise caution with use.
Tamoxifen	Exercise caution with use.
Tolbutamide	Exercise caution with use.
Torsemide	Exercise caution with use.
Warfarin	Caution with warfarin.
Dipyridamole (Persantine)	
Adenosine	Increases levels of adenosine.
Cholinesterase inhibitors	May counteract effects of cholinesterase inhibitors.
Ticlopidine HCl (Ticlid)	
Antacids	Reduces plasma levels of ticlopidine.
Anticoagulants	D/C while on ticlopidine.
ASA	Potentiates effect of ASA on platelet aggregation.
Cimetidine	Reduces clearance of ticlopidine.
Digoxin	Reduces plasma digoxin. Monitor digoxin levels.
Fibrinolytics	D/C while on ticlopidine.
NSAIDs	Potentiates effect of ASA on platelet aggregation.
Phenytoin	Exercise caution with use.
Propranolol	Exercise caution with use.
Theophylline	Decrease of theophylline plasma clearance.
Warfarin sodium (Coumadin, Jantoven)	
Anticonvulsants	Potentiates the action of anticonvulsants.
Antihyperlipidemic drugs (eg, ezetimibe)	Potentiates the action of antihyperlipidemic drugs.
ASA	Exercise caution with use.
Hepatic enzyme inducers	May increase or decrease the effect of warfarin.
Hepatic enzyme inhibitors	May increase or decrease the effect of warfarin.
Hypoglycemic agents	Potentiates the action of hypoglycemics.
NSAIDs	Exercise caution with use.

Table 15.2. Drug Interactions for Antiplatelet Agents

Protein-bound drugs	May increase or decrease the effect of warfarin.
Streptokinase	To be avoided.
Urokinase	To be avoided.

Aspirin Therapy in Diabetes

American Diabetes Association

INTRODUCTION

People with diabetes have a two- to fourfold increase in the risk of dying from the complications of cardiovascular disease. Both men and women are at increased risk. Atherosclerosis and vascular thrombosis are major contributors, and it is generally accepted that platelets are contributory. Platelets from men and women with diabetes are often hypersensitive in vitro to platelet aggregating agents. A major mechanism is increased production of thromboxane, a potent vasoconstrictor and platelet aggregant. Investigators have found evidence in vivo of excess thromboxane release in type 2 diabetic patients with cardiovascular disease. Aspirin blocks thromboxane synthesis by acetylating platelet cyclo-oxygenase and has been used as a primary and secondary strategy to prevent cardiovascular events in nondiabetic and diabetic individuals. Meta-analyses of these studies and large-scale collaborative trials in men and women with diabetes support the view that low-dose aspirin therapy should be prescribed as a secondary prevention strategy, if no contraindications exist. Substantial evidence suggests that low-dose aspirin therapy should also be used as a primary prevention strategy in men and women with diabetes who are at high risk (over age 40 or with other CVD risk factors) for cardiovascular events (1–3). Despite its proven efficacy, aspirin therapy is underutilized in patients with diabetes. Available data suggest that less than half of eligible patients are being treated with aspirin.

EFFICACY

Secondary prevention trials

A meta-analysis of 145 prospective controlled trials of antiplatelet therapy in men and women after myocardial infarction, stroke or transient ischemic attack, or positive cardiovascular history (vascular surgery, angioplasty, angina, etc.) has been reported by the Anti-Platelet Trialists (APT) (4). Reductions in vascular events were about one-quarter in each of these categories, and diabetic subjects had risk reductions that were comparable to nondiabetic individuals. There was a trend toward increased risk reductions with doses of aspirin between 75 and 162 mg/day. It was estimated that 38 ± 12 vascular events per 1,000 diabetic patients would be prevented if they were treated with aspirin as a secondary prevention strategy. Comparable results were seen in males and females.

Abbreviations: APT, Anti-Platelet Trialists; ETDRS, Early Treatment Diabetic Retinopathy Study

Primary prevention trials

Two studies have examined the effect of aspirin in primary prevention and have included patients with diabetes. The U.S. Physicians' Health Study (5) was a primary prevention trial in which a low-dose aspirin regimen (325 mg every other day) was compared with placebo in male physicians. There was a 44% risk reduction in the treated group, and subgroup analyses in the diabetic physicians revealed a reduction in myocardial infarction from 10.1% (placebo) to 4.0% (aspirin), yielding a relative risk of 0.39 for the diabetic men on aspirin therapy.

These results are supported by the Early Treatment Diabetic Retinopathy Study (ETDRS), a mixed primary and secondary prevention trial (6). This population consisted of type 1 and type 2 diabetic men and women, about 48% of whom had a history of cardiovascular disease. The study, therefore, may be viewed as a mixed primary and secondary prevention trial. The relative risk for myocardial infarction in the first 5 years in those randomized to aspirin therapy was lowered significantly to 0.72 (CI 0.55–0.95).

The Hypertension Optimal Treatment (HOT) Trial examined the effects of 75 mg/day of aspirin vs. placebo in 18,790 hypertensive patients who were randomized to achieve diastolic blood pressure goals of 90, 85, or 80 mmHg (7). Aspirin significantly reduced cardiovascular events by 15% and myocardial infarction by 36%. This study provides further evidence for the efficacy and safety of aspirin therapy in diabetic patients with systolic blood pressure less than 160 mmHg.

SAFETY

A major risk of aspirin therapy is gastric mucosal injury and gastrointestinal hemorrhage. Aspirin increases the relative risk of major gastrointestinal bleeding (relative risk 1.6), even with relatively low doses. Enteric coating does not appear to reduce such risk. Minor bleeding episodes (epistaxis, bruising, etc.) are also increased. A well-conducted meta-analysis of primary and secondary prevention trials found a moderately increased relative risk of hemorrhagic stroke in aspirin users. Absolute risk was approximately 1 event per 1,000 users over 3–5 years. Risk did not appear to differ significantly by dosage, but power to detect such differences was limited. Contraindications to aspirin therapy include allergy, bleeding tendency, anticoagulant therapy, recent gastrointestinal bleeding, and clinically active hepatic disease.

The ETDRS (6) established that aspirin therapy was not associated with an increased risk for retinal or vitreous hemorrhage. Since the primary endpoint in this trial was retinopathy and maculopathy, these serial observations by ophthalmologists, using retinal photography in a group of diabetic subjects with retinopathy, established conclusively that aspirin therapy conveyed no increase in benefit or in risk regarding progression of diabetic retinopathy and maculopathy.

Regular use of nonsteroidal anti-inflammatory drugs may increase the risk for chronic renal disease and may impair blood pressure control in hypertensive patients. However, a low dose of aspirin is a very weak inhibitor of renal prostaglandin synthesis and has no clinically significant effect on renal function or on blood pressure control.

DOSAGE

The platelet release reaction is exquisitely sensitive to inhibition by aspirin. In this regard, it has been shown that a dose as low as 75 mg of enteric-coated aspirin is just as effective as higher doses of either plain or enteric-coated aspirin in inhibiting thromboxane synthesis. When platelet turnover is rapid, as may be the case with diabetic vascular disease, the steady plasma aspirin concentration from enteric preparations theoretically allows for constant suppression of thromboxane synthesis.

The APT meta-analysis (4) explored the results achieved with various doses of aspirin, alone or in combination with other antiplatelet agents, including dipyridamole and sulfinpyrazone. Whereas risk reductions of 21 ± 4% were seen in cardiovascular events in 30 trials in which doses of 500–1,500 mg/day were used, a trend for greater risk reductions of 29 ± 7% was seen in 5,000 patients in whom doses of 75 mg/day were used. Comparable risk reductions of 28 ± 3% were seen in 12 trials in which doses of 160–325 mg/day were used. No evidence was found that combinations of aspirin with other antiplatelet drugs were any more effective than aspirin alone. Because low-dose aspirin (75–162 mg/day) appears to be equally or more effective, and possibly to have lower risk than higher doses, low-dose aspirin should be recommended routinely.

SPECIAL CONSIDERATIONS

The meta-analysis of the secondary prevention trials provided sample sizes that were adequate to determine aspirin's efficacy in a wide variety of patients. Separate analyses were done in males and females, patients with or without diastolic hypertension, those over or under age 65 years, and in diabetic and nondiabetic subjects. Proportional benefits of aspirin therapy were seen in all subgroups studied. Absolute benefit was greater among those at high risk (over age 65 years, diastolic hypertension, diabetes). Intervention trials in women are underway. Case-control studies have shown that the use of one to six aspirins a week is associated with a reduced risk for myocardial infarction in women. Further, the APT meta-analysis of

secondary prevention trials showed no difference in responses in men and women, and the ETDRS included men and women in the trial. Diabetes appears to place women at high risk for myocardial infarction. For these reasons, recommendations in this article apply to men and women with diabetes.

Although data are limited in diabetic subjects, agents such as clopidogrel may be considered as a substitute in the case of aspirin allergy. In one large study (CAPRIE), clopidogrel (75 mg) was slightly more effective than aspirin (325 mg) in reducing the combined risk of stroke, myocardial infarction, or vascular death in diabetic and nondiabetic subjects (8). Other approaches, such as blocking a key platelet receptor (GPIIb/IIIa), are under study.

RECOMMENDATIONS

1. Use aspirin therapy (75–162 mg/day) as a secondary prevention strategy in diabetic men and women with a history of myocardial infarction, vascular bypass procedure, stroke or transient ischemic attack, peripheral vascular disease, claudication, and/or angina. (A)
2. Use aspirin therapy (75–162 mg/day) as a primary prevention strategy in men and women with type 2 diabetes at increased cardiovascular risk, including those over 40 years of age or who have additional risk factors (family history of CVD, hypertension, smoking, dyslipidemia, albuminuria). (A)
3. Use aspirin therapy as a primary prevention strategy in men and women with type 1 diabetes at increased cardiovascular risk, including those over 40 years of age or who have additional risk factors (family history of CVD, hypertension, smoking, dyslipidemia, albuminuria). (C)
4. People with aspirin allergy, bleeding tendency, anticoagulant therapy, recent

gastrointestinal bleeding, and clinically active hepatic disease are not candidates for aspirin therapy. Other antiplatelet agents may be a reasonable alternative for patients with high risk. (E)

5. Aspirin therapy should not be recommended for patients under the age of 21 years because of the increased risk of Reye's syndrome associated with aspirin use in this population. People under the age of 30 have generally not been studied. (E)

FOOTNOTES

The recommendations in this paper are based on the evidence reviewed in the following publication: Aspirin therapy in diabetes (Technical Review). *Diabetes Care* 20:1767–1771, 1997.

The initial draft of this paper was prepared by John A. Colwell, MD, PhD. This paper was peer-reviewed, modified, and approved by the Professional Practice Committee in May 1997 and by the Executive Committee in June 1997. Most recent review/revision, 2000.

REFERENCES

1. Colwell JA: Aspirin therapy in diabetes (Technical Review). *Diabetes Care* 20:1767–1771, 1997.
2. Hayden M, Pignone M, hillips C: Aspirin for the primary prevention of cardiovascular events: a summary of the evidence for the U.S. Preventive Services Task Force. *Ann Intern Med* 136:161–171, 2002.
3. US Preventive Services Task Force: Aspirin for the primary prevention of cardiovascular events: recommendation and rationale. *Ann Intern Med* 136:157–160, 2002.
4. Collaborative overview of randomised trials of antiplatelet therapy-I: prevention of death, myocardial infarction, and stroke by prolonged antiplatelet therapy in various categories of patients. Antipatelet Trialists' Collaboration. *BMJ* 308:81–106, 1994.
5. Final report on the aspirin component of the ongoing Physicians' Health Study Research Group. *N Engl J Med* 321:129–135, 1989.
6. The ETDRS Investigators: Aspirin effects on mortality and morbidity in patients with diabetes mellitus: Early Treatment Diabetic Retinopathy Study report 14, *JAMA* 268:1292–1300, 1992.
7. Hansson L, Zanchetti A, Carruthers SG, Dahlof B, Elmfeldt D, Julius S, Menard J, Rahn KH, Wedel H, Westerling S: Effects of intensive blood-pressure lowering and low dose aspirin on patients with hypertension: principal results of the Hypertension Optimal Treatment (HOT) randomized trial. *Lancet* 351:1755–1762, 1998.
8. CAPRIE Steering Committee: A randomised, blinded trial of clopidogrel versus aspirin in patients at risk of ischaemic events (CAPRIE). *Lancet* 348:1329–1339, 1996.

Chapter 16

Smoking Cessation

Joshua J. Neumiller, PharmD, CGP, FASCP

INTRODUCTION

Cigarette smoking accounts for approximately 400,000 deaths each year in the United States, and is considered the leading avoidable cause of death in the country. It is well known and documented that people with diabetes mellitus are at increased risk of experiencing morbidity and mortality related to circulatory and cardiovascular (CV) disease when compared to those without diabetes. Likewise, cigarette smoking is associated with significant morbidity and mortality primarily due to cardiovascular events. According to the U.S. Surgeon General's report in 2004, current evidence suggests a causal relationship between cigarette smoking and subclinical atherosclerosis, abdominal aneurysm, stroke and coronary artery disease (CAD). Studies have indicated that cessation of smoking leads to a 36% reduction in the relative risk of all-cause mortality for patients with CAD regardless of age or gender compared with those that continue to smoke. Given that people with diabetes are predisposed to CV disease, smoking can greatly increase the propensity of CV events in this population.

Studies performed in patients with diabetes that also smoke tobacco indicate a strong correlation with smoking on the progression of CV disease and death. The Multiple Risk Factor Intervention Trial (MRFIT), the Finnish Prospective Study, and the Paris Prospective Study have all identified cigarette smoking as a significant risk factor for death via heart disease in people with type 2 diabetes. In addition to increasing the risk of CV morbidity and mortality, evidence exists suggesting that smoking also increases the risk of microvascular complications of diabetes, including nephropathy, neuropathy, and retinopathy, and may even play a role in the pathogenesis of type 2 diabetes.

According to the American Diabetes Association (ADA) position statement on smoking and diabetes from 2004, smoking cessation is one of few interventions that can safely and cost-effectively be recommended for all patients who smoke. Additionally, smoking cessation interventions have been demonstrated to be effective in reducing tobacco use in patients with diabetes as a means to reduce CV event risk. Despite these findings, studies indicate that only about half of smokers with diabetes have been advised or counseled regarding smoking cessation by their health care providers. **Table 16.1** on the following page outlines smoking cessation and prevention recommendations from the ADA for health care practitioners.

The "5 A's" approach to counseling and treating tobacco use and dependence is widely utilized, and is recommended for

---

Table 16.1. Recommendations Regarding Diabetes and Smoking

Assessment of smoking status and history
- Systematic documentation of a history of tobacco use must be obtained from all adolescent and adult individuals with diabetes.

Counseling on smoking prevention and cessation
- All health care providers should advise individuals with diabetes not to initiate smoking. This advice should be consistently repeated to prevent smoking and other tobacco use among children and adolescents with diabetes under age 21 years.
- Among smokers, cessation counseling must be completed as a routine component of diabetes care.
- Every smoker should be urged to quit in a clear, strong, and personalized manner that describes the added risks of smoking and diabetes.
- Every diabetic smoker should be asked if he or she is willing to quit at this time.
   – If no, initiate brief and motivational discussion regarding need to stop using tobacco, risks of continued use, and encouragement to quit as well as support when ready.
   – If yes, assess preference for and initiate either minimal, brief, or intensive cessation counseling and offer pharmacological supplements as appropriate.

Effective systems for delivery of smoking cessation
- Training of all diabetes health care providers in the Public Health Service guidelines regarding smoking should be implemented.
- Follow-up procedures designed to assess and promote quitting status must be arranged for all diabetic smokers.

Source: Smoking and Diabetes. *Diabetes Care.* 2004;27(suppl1):S74-75.

---

clinician use by the U.S. Department of Health and Human Services (**see Table 16.2**).

While the core of smoking cessation intervention is patient counseling and lifestyle modification, pharmacological interventions are available for use when deemed appropriate. These pharmacological interventions may help prevent the symptoms of nicotine withdrawal that can include symptoms of irritability, difficulty with concentration, feelings of depression, difficulty sleeping, increased appetite, and headaches. FDA-approved pharmacological options include nicotine replacement therapy (NRT), the nicotine receptor agonist varenicline, and the antidepressant medication bupropion (marketed as Zyban for this use). Additionally, clonidine and nortriptyline are non-FDA-approved medications that may be used as second-line therapies. While a variety of other medications (such as other classes of antidepressants) have been studied as potential therapeutic interventions for smoking

cessation, the medications covered below represent those that are most often used in clinical practice and are supported by clinical data. The following section will provide discussion related to the use of these medications as a component of a smoking cessation strategy in conjunction with adequate counseling and lifestyle modification strategies.

PHARMACOLOGICAL MANAGEMENT OF SMOKING CESSATION

Nicotine Replacement Therapy

Nicotine replacement therapy (NRT) is the most widely utilized pharmacological intervention for smoking cessation. NRT provides nicotine that helps minimize the adverse symptoms associated with nicotine withdrawal. NRT products vary greatly and include nicotine gum, patches, lozenges, nasal sprays, and inhalers. Nicotine patches,

Table 16.2. Principles of the "5 A's" Approach

Ask about tobacco use	Identify and document tobacco use status for every patient at every visit.
Advise to quit	In a clear, strong, and personalized manner, urge every tobacco user to quit.
Assess willingness to make a quit attempt	Is the tobacco user willing to make a quit attempt at this time?
Assist in quit attempt	For the patient willing to make a quit attempt, offer medication and provide or refer for counseling or additional treatment to help the patient quit. For patients unwilling to quit at the time, provide interventions designed to increase future quite attempts.
Arrange follow-up	For the patient willing to make a quit attempt, arrange for follow-up contacts, beginning within the first week after the quit date. For patients willing to make a quit attempt at the time, address tobacco dependence and willingness to quit at next clinic visit.

Source: Treating tobacco use and dependence: 2008 update. U.S. Department of Health and Human Services.

gum, and lozenges are available as over-the-counter products that are available for purchase and use without a prescription. The consistent use of NRT products has been shown to double a person's chances of successfully quitting smoking. However, it is important to consider that these products are generally not successful unless used in combination with behavioral modification and support systems. **NRT therapy is appropriate as a first-line intervention for management of withdrawal symptoms associated with smoking cessation.**

Pharmacology
Mechanism of Action
The pharmacological actions of nicotine are complex and include effects on both the central and peripheral nervous systems. NRT products work by stimulating nicotine receptors in the absence of nicotine intake from cigarettes or other forms of tobacco. This "nicotine replacement" allows for continued nicotine receptor stimulation to alleviate the adverse withdrawal symptoms associated with smoking cessation.

Pharmacokinetics
As NRT is administered through a variety of dosage forms, the onset of action can vary among products. Following administration of gum or lozenges, absorption of nicotine readily occurs through the buccal mucosa, but the systemic absorption is slower when compared to that of cigarette smoke or with inhaled or nasal NRT products. Some studies indicate that nicotine lozenges deliver between 25% and 75% more nicotine than gum products. Peak plasma nicotine concentrations are achieved within 15-30 minutes after starting to chew nicotine gum, 15 minutes following inhalation, 4-15 minutes after nasal administration, and 4-12 hours following application of the patch.

Treatment Advantages and Disadvantages
NRT can be very beneficial for people desiring to quit smoking who find the withdrawal symptoms unbearable. While NRT has been demonstrated to approximately double a person's chances of quitting, it is important to explain to patients that these

products will not "make" them quit smoking. These products are useful when used in conjunction with behavioral modification strategies and/or support groups. The fact that some NRT products are available without a prescription can be very beneficial to some patients, however, this can be a downside if by not seeking a prescription, the individual is not receiving supportive care and counseling.

Therapeutic Considerations
Warnings and Precautions
NRT should be avoided in patients with serious cardiac arrhythmias, immediately following a myocardial infarction (MI), or in patients with severe or worsening angina pectoris. NRT therapy should also be used with caution in patients with uncontrolled hypertension, pheochromocytoma, vasospastic angina, or hyperthyroidism due to associated increases in blood pressure and heart rate following nicotine-induced catecholamine release. Increases in plasma glucose can also result following nicotine administration.

Special Populations
NRT therapy has not been evaluated during pregnancy, and pregnant smokers should be encouraged to quit smoking without the use of medications. NRT has not been studied in children who smoke, and doses currently available could result in toxicity if taken by children, thus their use is not recommended in this population. While NRT has not been formally studied in the elderly, clinical findings have not demonstrated a difference between geriatric and younger patients utilizing NRT. Elderly patients using NRT should be initiated at the lowest possible dose and titrate upward slowly to desired effect.

Adverse Effects and Monitoring
Many of the side effects associated with NRT therapy depend upon the route of administration. For example, inhaled nicotine is associated with local irritation of the mouth and throat, while nicotine patches can cause local skin irritation. Of note with NRT therapy, however, patients may experience acute increases in blood pressure and heart rate following administration. Refer to full prescribing information for a more complete list of product-specific adverse effects.

Drug Interactions
Hydrocarbons present in tobacco smoke are known to induce hepatic cytochrome P450 enzymes, and thus smoking cessation can lead to decreased metabolic clearance of drugs such as theophylline, warfarin, tricyclic antidepressants (TCAs) as well as others. Of note for patients with diabetes on insulin, nicotine is known to activate neuroendocrine pathways that can lead to elevations in blood glucose. Whenever smoking status or nicotine use is altered, people using insulin should monitor blood glucose more frequently and assess for the need of insulin dosage adjustments. Regarding nicotine gum products, ingestion of acidic foods or beverages immediately before or during gum use can impair nicotine absorption. See **Table 16.4** for more drug interaction information.

Dosage and Administration
NRT dosage and administration varies greatly depending upon the product used. See **Table 16.3**, or refer to the full prescribing information for specific guidelines.

Varenicline
Varenicline (Chantix) is classified as a nicotine receptor agonist, which actually possesses partial agonist properties at the nicotine receptor. **Varenicline is FDA-approved as a first-line therapy for treating tobacco use. The use of this product is being questioned due to some patients becoming depressed and considering suicide. Patients thus need to be screened carefully prior to receiving a prescription for varenicline.**

Pharmacology

Mechanism of Action

Varenicline is a partial agonist at α4-β2 neuronal nicotinic acetylcholine receptors, which are the receptors responsible for the physical effects of nicotine. Varenicline acts as a competitive inhibitor of nicotine at these receptor sites, thus blocking the effects of nicotine intake. Nicotine increases dopamine release in the prefrontal cortex of the brain, and nicotine cravings are mediated by low levels of dopamine release in the mesolimbic region of the brain. The efficacy of varenicline is attributed to its partial stimulation of α4-β2 neuronal nicotinic acetylcholine receptors to produce a small amount of mesolimbic dopamine release (smaller of that produced by nicotine), thus minimizing nicotine cravings and withdrawal symptoms.

Pharmacokinetics

Following oral administration, varenicline is nearly completely absorbed, with maximum plasma concentrations reached within three to four hours. Steady-state concentrations are reached in approximately four days of therapy, and the bioavailability of varenicline appears unaffected by time of administration or food intake. Less than 20% of a given dose of varenicline is protein bound, and varenicline is minimally metabolized. Approximately 92% is excreted unchanged in the urine, and varenicline is effectively removed via hemodialysis. The elimination half-life of varenicline is approximately 24 hours. No clinically meaningful pharmacokinetic differences have been observed due to age, race, gender, smoking status, or use of concomitant medications.

Treatment Advantages and Disadvantages

Clinical experience with varenicline is limited considering it received FDA approval in May 2006. Over the past few years, however, varenicline has become a popular smoking cessation agent, and many patients have very good success when using the drug. Another benefit of varenicline is that it has few if any clinically significant drug interactions identified to date. Due to its effects in the brain, varenicline has been associated with a variety of neuropsychiatric adverse events, and has been associated with attempted and completed suicide attempts.

Therapeutic Considerations

Warnings and Precautions

Extreme caution is warranted in any patient with a history or current symptoms of depression, agitation, or suicidal ideation. The FDA recommends that patients inform their health care providers of any history of psychiatric illness prior to initiation of varenicline therapy. Any patient using varenicline should receive periodic assessment for changes in mood or behavior.

Special Populations

Varenicline is an FDA pregnancy class C agent, and has not been studied in pregnant women or women who are breastfeeding. Use has not been evaluated in children under the age of 18 years, therefore its use in this population is not recommended. No differences in efficacy or safety parameters have been observed in elderly patients using varenicline. Cautious use is warranted in patients with kidney disease. Dose reduction is recommended in patients on hemodialysis or with a creatinine clearance <30mL/min.

Adverse Effects and Monitoring

All patients using varenicline should receive periodic assessment regarding changes in mood and behavior due to the association between varenicline use and neuropsychiatric effects. Common adverse effects include nausea and vomiting, insomnia, abnormal and vivid dreams, altered taste perception (dyspepsia), and fatigue.

Drug Interactions

Because varenicline is renally excreted by glomerular filtration and active tubular secretion, drugs that inhibit active tubular secretion, such as cimetidine, can increase concentrations of varenicline. These potential interactions are not expected to be clinically significant, however. See **Table 16.4** for more drug interaction information.

Dosage and Administration

Varenicline is initiated one week prior to the quit date at 0.5 mg once daily for three days, followed by 0.5 mg twice daily for four days, followed by 1 mg twice daily for three months. Patients should be instructed to quit smoking on Day 8 of therapy once the dosage is increased to 1 mg twice daily. For patients with a creatinine clearance ≤50 mL/min, recommendations state patients should be titrated to a maximum dose of 0.5 mg twice daily. Varenicline is approved for maintenance of smoking cessation for up to six months. To reduce the nausea associated with varenicline, this medication should be taken with food. Additionally, for those patients experiencing insomnia, the second pill of the day may be taken with the evening meal rather than at bedtime. See **Table 16.3,** or refer to the full prescribing information for more details.

Bupropion

While NRT has traditionally been the pharmacological treatment of choice for smoking cessation, bupropion has become increasingly popular in recent years. Bupropion was developed and marketed as an antidepressant medication in the United States, and was noted to reduce the desire to smoke cigarettes. **Clinical trials have demonstrated efficacy in smoking cessation with bupropion therapy, and bupropion (marketed as Zyban) is considered a first-line therapy for smoking cessation in patients with diabetes.**

Pharmacology

Mechanism of Action

Bupropion is an atypical antidepressant, and while the exact mechanism of action is not fully understood, bupropion inhibits the synaptic reuptake of dopamine, norepinephrine, and serotonin in the central nervous system. Additionally, bupropion has been shown to be a noncompetitive nicotine receptor antagonist, thus lending to its utility in smoking cessation. Inhibition of the typical reductions in dopamine and norepinephrine levels that occurs during nicotine withdrawal is likely important in the antismoking effects of bupropion. The antidepressant effects of bupropion appear to be unrelated to its antismoking effects as it appears to be equally effective in smoking cessation in those with and without depression.

Pharmacokinetics

Based on animal data, the bioavailability of oral bupropion is estimated to be 5%-20% with peak plasma concentrations achieved at approximately three hours following administration. Bupropion is approximately 85% protein bound, and readily crosses the blood-brain barrier. Steady-state concentrations are achieved within approximately five to eight days of therapy, with an onset of effect within approximately one to three weeks. Metabolism occurs in the liver producing several metabolites, some of which are active. The terminal elimination half-life of the sustained release (SR) form is roughly 21 hours. Over 60% of bupropion is excreted as metabolites in the urine within 24 hours of administration.

Treatment Advantages and Disadvantages

Bupropion presents a viable option for pharmacotherapy in patients wanting to quit smoking. For patients with concurrent depression, bupropion may present a viable option for therapy due to its demonstrated efficacy in both treatment of depression and smoking cessation. Another advantage to bupropion therapy is that in clinical studies, it was shown to reduce the weight gain associated with smoking cessation. Potential disadvantages of bupropion include possible drug interactions and bothersome side effects. Fortunately bupropion SR is available in generic form and thus may be more affordable for patients without insurance or on a fixed income when compared with varenicline or some NRT products.

Therapeutic Considerations

Warnings and Precautions

Bupropion is contraindicated for use in patients with a history of epilepsy, and should be used with extreme caution in patients with a predisposition to a low threshold for seizure (eg, history of head trauma or those taking concomitant medications that lower the seizure threshold). Contraindications also exist for those with a history of anorexia nervosa and/or bulimia, severe hepatic necrosis, and those on monoamine oxidase inhibitor (MAOI) therapy. Cautious use is warranted in those with bipolar disorder.

Special Populations

Bupropion is a pregnancy category C agent, and pregnant women who wish to stop smoking should be encouraged to do so without medication. The use of bupropion in children for smoking cessation has not been studied. Data in patients >65 years with the immediate-release bupropion do not indicate any significant differences in pharmacokinetic variables of the drug. The elderly should, however, be initiated at low doses and titrated upward slowly to therapeutic effect. For patients with hepatic cirrhosis, the dose of bupropion SR should not exceed 150 mg every other day. Dosage reduction should also be considered for patients with mild to moderate hepatic impairment. Dosage reduction may be necessary for those with renal impairment, however no specific recommendations are available.

Adverse Effects and Monitoring

Common adverse effects associated with bupropion therapy include dry mouth, insomnia, skin rashes, and pruritus. Bupropion use has been associated with inducing seizures in approximately one out of 1,000 patients, and can rarely induce a reaction resembling serum sickness.

Drug Interactions

Concomitant use with MAOIs is contraindicated. Bupropion should only be initiated after a minimum of 14 days following discontinuation of an MAOI. Bupropion is an inhibitor of the CYP2D6 enzyme, thus drug interactions exist between bupropion and drugs metabolized via this enzyme system. All patients under consideration for bupropion therapy should be checked for potential drug interactions between bupropion and their current drug regimen.

Of note in patients utilizing both bupropion and NRT, clinically significant elevations in blood pressure have been noted. Close monitoring of blood pressure is recommended in patients utilizing this combination. See **Table 16.4** for more drug interaction information.

Dosage and Administration

Patients should begin bupropion SR one to two weeks prior to their quit date. Therapy should be initiated at 150 mg every morning for three days, followed by a dose escalation to 150 mg twice daily. The bupropion dose for smoking cessation generally should not exceed a total daily dose of 300 mg. Once titrated to 150 mg twice daily, therapy should continue for seven to 12 weeks, however, treatment can be up to six months in duration. For patients with hepatic cirrhosis, the dose of bupropion SR should not exceed 150 mg every other day. Dosage reduction should also be considered for patients with mild to moderate hepatic impairment. Dosage reduction may be necessary for those with renal impairment, however no specific recommendations are available. For patients experiencing significant insomnia, the second dose of the day may be taken in the afternoon (at least eight hours after the first dose) to minimize this effect. See **Table 16.3**, or refer to the the the full prescribing information for further guidelines.

Clonidine

Clonidine is a centrally acting α-2 receptor agonist that is used as a second-line agent for smoking cessation. **Second-line agents such as clonidine can be considered for patients unable to use first-line medications due to contraindications, or for those who have unsuccessfully quit with use of first-line therapies.** In clinical trials with both oral and transdermal clonidine efficacy has been demonstrated in eight of nine trials as measured by rate of smoking cessation. The following discussion outlines the properties of clonidine, as well as considerations for the use of this drug in the diabetic population for smoking cessation.

Pharmacology
Mechanism of Action
Clonidine is a centrally acting alpha noradrenergic agonist. Clonidine has been used in the treatment of hypertension and to reduce withdrawal symptoms associated with alcohol and opioid use. The physiological mechanisms involved in the central nervous system associated with clonidine use are complex, and clonidine is used off-label for a variety of conditions. Clonidine use as second-line therapy for smoking cessation is theorized to decrease symptoms associated with nicotine withdrawal via inhibition of sympathetic outflow from the central nervous system.

Pharmacokinetics
Clonidine is rapidly absorbed following oral administration with bioavailability nearing 100%. Clonidine is highly lipid soluble and readily distributes into the central nervous system, with a CSF elimination half-life of ~1.3 hours and a serum half-life of ~12 hours. Clonidine undergoes hepatic metabolism with approximately 50% of a given dose processed by the liver to inactive metabolites, and is ~45% renally excreted. Transdermal clonidine preparations release the drug at a constant rate for seven days, with a therapeutic plasma concentration reached within two to three days of patch therapy.

Treatment Advantages and Disadvantages
While clonidine is not FDA-approved for treatment of withdrawal symptoms associated with smoking cessation, it is utilized as second-line therapy. While the administration of clonidine can be very convenient for patients who utilize the transdermal patch, clonidine use is associated with a variety of side effects that limit the utility of its use.

Therapeutic Considerations
Warnings and Precautions
Abrupt discontinuation of clonidine is not recommended due to the risk of severe rebound hypertension. Clonidine is also associated with sedation and drowsiness, so patients should be cautioned when performing potentially dangerous activities such as driving or operating machinery. For patients with a history of major depressive disorder, clonidine should be used cautiously due to the potential of this agent to induce depressive episodes. While clonidine has been used successfully in patients with diabetes, transient increases in blood

sugar have been noted. Clonidine should be used cautiously in patients with renal or hepatic dysfunction.

Special Populations
Clonidine is an FDA pregnancy class C agent, and should be avoided in pregnant women wishing to stop smoking. Clonidine should also be avoided in breastfeeding women as clonidine concentrations reach levels in breast milk approximately twice that achieved in maternal plasma. Elderly patients should be treated with caution because they are more likely to have decreased renal function and are more susceptible to the hypotensive and sedative effects of clonidine. If used in an elderly patient, initiate clonidine at a low dose and titrate slowly to desired therapeutic effect.

Adverse Effects and Monitoring
Clonidine is associated with a variety of anticholinergic side effects, and the most frequently reported side effects associated with clonidine use include dry mouth, drowsiness, dizziness, sedation, and constipation. Transdermal clonidine may decrease the severity of systemic anticholinergic side effects when compared to the oral formulation. Symptoms of fatigue and lethargy can be particularly bothersome in elderly patients, and symptomatic hypotension can occur and is a huge concern in the elderly population. Oral clonidine therapy can result in sodium and fluid retention during the first few days of therapy, which is typically responsive to diuretic therapy, and can cause adverse cardiovascular events including palpitations, sinus tachycardia, and sinus bradycardia. Of particular concern in patients with diabetes, clonidine use can result in transient increases in blood glucose as well as symptoms of sexual dysfunction including impotence, decreased libido, and ejaculatory dysfunction.

Drug Interactions
Prior to initiation of clonidine, patients should receive a thorough drug interaction screen to avoid harmful drug interactions with this medication. Clonidine can potentiate the effects of concomitant CNS depressants, and can lead to symptomatic hypotension when coadministered with other antihypertensive agents. Clonidine should also be used cautiously with other medications that slow the heart rate such as amiodarone, β-blockers, and cardiac glycosides. This drug interaction overview is not comprehensive, as clonidine interacts with a variety of medications. See **Table 16.4**, or refer to the full prescribing information for clonidine for additional drug interaction information.

Dosage and Administration
Doses of clonidine used in various clinical trials vary significantly from 0.15-0.75 mg/day orally and from 0.10-0.20 mg/day transdermally. Unfortunately, a clear dose-response relationship has not been identified in terms of efficacy in preventing withdrawal symptoms associated with smoking cessation. Treatment should be initiated up to three days prior or on the quit date, with a recommended initial dose of 0.10 mg twice daily by mouth, or 0.10 mg/day transdermally. The dose can be titrated by 0.10 mg/day per week if needed for therapeutic effect as tolerated. The duration of clonidine use also varied in clinical trials with a range of three to 10 weeks. Do not discontinue clonidine therapy abruptly, and titrate patients off of the drug due to the risk of rebound hypertension. See **Table 16.3**, or refer to the full prescribing information for more dosing guidance.

Nortriptyline
Nortriptyline, a tricyclic antidepressant (TCA), is a non-FDA-approved medication used as second-line therapy as a pharmacological intervention for smoking cessation.

Second-line agents such as nortriptyline can be considered for patients unable to use first-line medications due to contraindications, or for those who have failed with use of first-line therapies. Nortriptyline use may also be beneficial for patients with diabetes with peripheral neuropathy. When studied, nortriptyline led to an increased short-term cessation rate when compared to placebo, and appeared to exhibit efficacy in lessening withdrawal symptoms. The following discussion outlines the properties of nortriptyline, as well as considerations for the use of this drug in the diabetic population for smoking cessation.

Pharmacology

Mechanism of Action
Nortriptyline is a TCA. While the mechanism of action of nortriptyline is not fully understood, its actions are thought to be attributable to norepinephrine and serotonin reuptake inhibition. While nortriptyline enhances the actions of both norepinephrine and serotonin, its effects on serotonin are more pronounced. The mechanisms responsible for the beneficial effects seen with nortriptyline in terms of smoking cessation are unknown. Theories include an antidepressant effect that diminishes the need for smoking to improve patients affect or "mood," an antianxiety effect, inhibition of withdrawal symptoms via modulation of central noradrenergic receptor systems, or a diminished craving for tobacco and nicotine via the anticholinergic effects of nortriptyline such as dry mouth and altered taste perception.

Pharmacokinetics
Nortriptyline is well absorbed from the gastrointestinal tract following oral administration, however variation in individual responses to the medication can occur. In general, lower doses are required for adolescents or in the elderly. It can take several weeks to reach peak antidepressant effects with nortriptyline, and in studies utilizing nortriptyline for treatment of withdrawal symptoms associated with smoking cessation, improvements were seen within several weeks of medication initiation.

TCAs are highly protein bound, and the plasma half-life of nortriptyline can range from 16-90 hours. Nortriptyline is metabolized in the liver, and approximately one-third of a single dose is excreted in the urine as metabolites with a small amount excreted in the feces. Nortriptyline is metabolized to an active metabolite, 10-hydroxynortriptyline, which has been reported to accumulate in elderly patients with hepatic impairment.

Treatment Advantages and Disadvantages
Nortriptyline may be a viable treatment option for those who have failed first-line therapies or are unable to use first-line therapies due to contraindications. Nortriptyline use and effectiveness may be limited, however, due to its side effect profile. Nortriptyline use is associated with pronounced sedation and anticholinergic effects in many patients, and must be used cautiously with concomitant medications that can alter nortriptyline metabolism. Additionally, nortriptyline can accumulate in elderly patients or those with hepatic impairment.

Nortriptyline use may be beneficial in patients with comorbid depression or peripheral diabetic neuropathy, as nortriptyline has demonstrated efficacy in both conditions. Caution is warranted, however, in people with diabetes because nortriptyline has been associated with alterations in blood glucose (both low and high blood sugars). Patients with diabetes starting nortriptyline should be aware of the signs and symptoms of hyper- and hypoglycemia and consider increasing the frequency of blood glucose checks upon nortriptyline initiation.

Therapeutic Considerations

Warnings and Precautions

Nortriptyline use is associated with pronounced sedation in some people. Nortriptyline may impair the mental or physical abilities required to perform hazardous tasks such as driving or operating machinery. Nortriptyline has also been associated with an increased risk of arrhythmia (QT interval prolongation) and impairment of myocardial contractility, thus caution should be practiced in patients with a history of cardiovascular disease. Nortriptyline should also not be coadministered with MAOIs.

Special Populations

Nortriptyline is metabolized to an active metabolite, 10-hydroxynortriptyline, which has been reported to accumulate in elderly patients with hepatic impairment. Caution should be used in elderly patients due to the sedating and anticholinergic properties of nortriptyline. Pregnant smokers should be encouraged to quit without pharmacologic intervention. Nortriptyline is a pregnancy class D agent, and has not been evaluated in women who are breastfeeding.

Adverse Effects and Monitoring

Adverse effects associated with nortriptyline use are numerous. Anticholinergic side effects such as dry mouth, constipation, urinary retention, blurred vision, and confusion are common. Nortriptyline is also associated with sedation, particularly in the elderly population.

Therapeutic drug levels for smoking cessation have not been established. However, clinicians may consider plasma drug monitoring to assess nortriptyline levels as needed to monitor and prevent toxicity.

Drug Interactions

The TCAs, including nortriptyline, have a high propensity toward drug interactions. All patients under consideration for nortriptyline should undergo a thorough drug interaction screen prior to therapy. Refer to **Table 16.4** or the full prescribing information for nortriptyline for specific drug interaction information.

Dosage and Administration

Nortriptyline is available by prescription only. Doses used in smoking cessation trials have been initiated at 25 mg/day. The dose was escalated gradually to a target dose of 75-100 mg/day. The duration of treatment studied in trials was approximately 12 weeks in duration, although it has been used for up to six months. Therapy is initiated 10-28 days prior to the quit date to achieve steady state concentrations of nortriptyline upon smoking cessation. Abrupt discontinuation of nortriptyline is discouraged due to the potential of withdrawal effects. See **Table 16.3**, or refer to the full prescribing information for more dosing guidance.

SUGGESTED READING

Berlin I. Smoking-induced metabolic disorders: a review. *Diabetes Metab.* 2008; In Press.

Haire-Joshu D, Glasgow RE, Tibbs TL. Smoking and diabetes. *Diabetes Care.* 1999;22(11): 1887-1898.

Smoking and Diabetes. *Diabetes Care.* 2004;27(S1):S74-75.

Treating tobacco use and dependence: 2008 update. U.S. Department of Health and Human Services. 2008. Available at: http://www.surgeongeneral.gov/tobacco/treating_tobacco_use08.pdf

Table 16.3. Prescribing Information for Smoking Cessation Agents

GENERIC (BRAND)	INGREDIENT/ STRENGTH	DOSAGE
Bupropion HCl† (Zyban)	Tab, Extended-Release: 150mg	*Adults:* ≥18 yrs: **Initial:** 150mg qd for 3 days. **Usual:** 150mg bid; separate dose intervals by at least 8 hrs. **Max:** 300mg/day. Initiate treatment while patient is still smoking. Patient should set a target quit date within the first 2 weeks. Treat for 7-12 weeks; d/c at 7 weeks if no progress is seen. **Renal/Hepatic Dysfunction:** Reduce dose. **Severe Hepatic Cirrhosis:** 150mg every other day.
Clonidine†* (Catapres, Catapres-TTS)	Patch, Extended Release(TTS): 0.1mg/24 hr [4ˢ], 0.2mg/24 hr [4ˢ], 0.3mg/24 hr [4ˢ]; Tab: 0.1mg*, 0.2mg*, 0.3mg* *scored	*Adults:* **(Patch)** Apply to hairless, intact area of upper arm or chest weekly. Taper withdrawal of previous antihypertensive. **Initial:** 0.1mg/24 hr patch weekly. **Titrate:** May increase after 1-2 weeks. **Max:** 0.6mg/24 hr. **(Tab) Initial:** 0.1mg bid. **Titrate:** May increase by 0.1mg weekly. **Usual:** 0.2-0.6mg/day in divided doses. **Max:** 2.4mg/day. **(Patch, Tab) Renal Impairment:** Adjust according to degree of impairment.
Commit Stop Smoking 2mg Lozenges	Nicotine Polacrilex 2mg	*Adults:* If smoking first cigarettte >30 minutes after waking up use 2mg lozenge. **Weeks 1 to 6:** 1 lozenge q1-2h. **Weeks 7 to 9:** 1 lozenge q2-4h. **Weeks 10 to 12:** 1 lozenge q4-8h. **Max:** 5 lozenges/6 hours; 20 lozenges/day. Stop using at the end of 12 weeks.
Commit Stop Smoking 4mg Lozenges	Nicotine Polacrilex 4mg	*Adults:* If smoking first cigarettte within 30 minutes after waking up use 4mg lozenge. **Weeks 1 to 6:** 1 lozenge q1-2h. **Weeks 7 to 9:** 1 lozenge q2-4h. **Weeks 10 to 12:** 1 lozenge q4-8h. **Max:** 5 lozenges/6 hours; 20 lozenges/day. Stop using at the end of 12 weeks.
NicoDerm CQ Step 1 Clear Patch	Nicotine 21mg	*Adults:* If smoking >10 cigarettes/day. **Weeks 1 to 6:** Apply one 21mg patch/day. **Weeks 7 to 8:** Apply one 14mg patch/day. **Weeks 9 to 10:** Apply one 7mg patch/day.
NicoDerm CQ Step 2 Clear Patch	Nicotine 14mg	*Adults:* If smoking <10 cigarettes/day. **Weeks 1 to 6:** Apply one 14mg patch/day. **Weeks 7 to 8:** Apply one 7mg patch/day.
NicoDerm CQ Step 3 Clear Patch	Nicotine 7mg	*Adults:* Apply 1 patch qd Weeks 9 to 10 if smoking >10 cigarettes/day or **Weeks 7 to 8** if smoking ≤10 cigarettes/day.
Nicorette 2mg Original/Mint/Orange Gum	Nicotine Polacrilex 2mg	*Adults:* If smoking <25 cigarettes/day use 2mg gum. **Weeks 1 to 6:** 1 piece q1-2h. **Weeks 7 to 9:** 1 piece q2-4h. **Weeks 10 to 12:** 1 piece q4-8h. **Max:** 24 pieces/day.
Nicorette 4mg Original/Mint/Orange Gum	Nicotine Polacrilex 4mg	*Adults:* If smoking ≥25 cigarettes/day use 4mg gum. **Weeks 1 to 6:** 1 piece q1-2h. **Weeks 7 to 9:** 1 piece q2-4h. **Weeks 10 to 12:** 1 piece q4-8h. **Max:** 24 pieces/day.
Habitrol Nicotine Transdermal System Patch Step 1	Nicotine 21mg/24 hr	*Adults:* If smoking >10 cigarettes/day. **Weeks 1 to 4:** Apply one 21mg patch/day. **Weeks 5 to 6:** Apply one 14mg patch/day. **Weeks 7 to 8:** Apply one 7mg patch/day.
Habitrol Nicotine Transdermal System Patch Step 2	Nicotine 14mg/24 hr	*Adults:* If smoking >10 cigarettes/day. **Weeks 1 to 4:** Apply one 21mg patch/day. **Weeks 5 to 6:** Apply one 14mg patch/day. **Weeks 7 to 8:** Apply one 7mg patch/day. If smoking <10 cigarettes/day. **Weeks 1 to 6:** Apply one 14 mg patch/day. **Weeks 7 to 8:** Apply one 7mg patch/day.
Habitrol Nicotine Transdermal System Patch Step 3	Nicotine 7mg/24 hr	*Adults:* If smoking >10 cigarettes/day. **Weeks 1 to 4:** Apply one 21mg patch/day. **Weeks 5 to 6:** Apply one 14mg patch/day. **Weeks 7 to 8:** Apply one 7mg patch/day. If smoking <10 cigarettes/day. **Weeks 1 to 6:** Apply one 14mg patch/day. **Weeks 7 to 8:** Apply one 7mg patch/day.
Nortriptyline HCl†* (Pamelor)	Cap: 10mg, 25mg, 50mg, 75mg; Sol: 10mg/5mL	*Adults:* 25mg tid-qid. **Max:** 150mg/day. Total daily dose may be given once a day. Monitor serum levels if dose >100mg/day. **Elderly/Adolescents:** 30-50mg/day in single or divided doses.
Varnicline tartrate† (Chantix)	Tab: 0.5mg, 1mg	*Adults:* ≥18 yrs: Days 1-3: 0.5mg qd. Days 4-7: 0.5mg bid. Day 8 to End of Treatment: 1mg bid. **Duration:** 12 weeks with an additional 12 weeks after successful completion to ensure long-term abstinence. **Severe Renal Impairment: Initial:** 0.5mg qd. **Titrate: Max:** 0.5mg bid. **End Stage Renal Disease: Max:** 0.5mg qd.

† Available only by prescription.
* Not FDA-approved for smoking cessation.

Table 16.4. Drug Interactions for Smoking Cessation Agents

Bupropion HCl (Zyban)

Alcohol	Excessive use or abrupt discontinuation of alcohol increases the risk of seizures; use of alcohol should be minimized or avoided.
Amantadine	Caution, use low initial dose and gradually titrate buproprion.
Anoretics	Increased risk of seizures with concomitant use.
Antiarrhythmics (type 1C)	Caution, use low initial dose and gradually titrate the concomitant medication.
Antidepressants	Extreme caution with concomitant use.
Antidiabetic drugs, oral	Increased risk of seizures with concomitant use.
Antipsychotics	Extreme caution with concomitant use; use low initial dose and gradually titrate the concomitant medication.
Benzodiazepines	Excessive use or abrupt discontinuation of sedatives increases the risk of seizures.
Beta-blockers	Caution, use low initial dose and gradually titrate the concomitant medication.
Bupropion-containing drugs	Avoid concomitant use with other drugs containing bupropion.
Carbamazepine	Concomitant use may induce the metabolism of bupropion.
Cimetidine	Concomitant use may inhibit the metabolism of bupropion.
Cocaine	Increased risk of seizures in patients addicted to cocaine.
Cyclophosphamide	Caution with concomitant use.
CYP2B6 substrates or inhibitors	Caution with concomitant use.
CYP2D6 metabolized drugs	Caution, use low initial dose and gradually titrate the concomitant medication.
Insulin	Increased risk of seizures with concomitant use.
Levodopa	Caution, use low initial dose and gradually titrate buproprion.
MAO inhibitors	Concomitant use is contraindicated; at least 14 days should elapse between discontinuation of an MAOI and initiation of treatment with bupropion.
Nicotine Transdermal System	Monitor for signs and symptoms of hypertension.
Opioids	Increased risk of seizures in patients addicted to opioids.
Orphenadrine	Caution with concomitant use.
Phenobarbital	Concomitant use may induce the metabolism of bupropion.
Phenytoin	Concomitant use may induce the metabolism of bupropion.
Sedatives (eg, benzodiazepines)	Excessive use or abrupt discontinuation of sedatives increases the risk of seizures.
Seizure threshold-lowering drugs	Extreme caution with concomitant use.
SSRIs	Caution, use low initial dose and gradually titrate the concomitant medication.
Steroids (systemic)	Extreme caution with concomitant use.
Stimulants	Increased risk of seizures in patients addicted to stimulants or who are using OTC stimulants.

Table 16.4. Drug Interactions for Smoking Cessation Agents

TCAs	Caution, use low initial dose and gradually titrate the concomitant medication.
Theophylline	Extreme caution with concomitant use.
Clonidine (Catapres, Catapres-TTS)	
Alcohol	Concomitant use may potentiate CNS depression.
Barbiturates	Concomitant use may potentiate CNS depression.
Beta-blockers	Concomitant use may produce additive bradycardia and AV block.
Calcium channel blockers	Concomitant use may produce additive bradycardia and AV block.
Digitalis	Concomitant use may produce additive bradycardia and AV block.
Sedatives	Concomitant use may potentiate CNS depression.
TCAs	May reduce the hypotensive effect of clonidine.
Nicotine (Commit, Habitrol, Nicoderm CQ, Nicorette, Nicotrol Inhaler, Nicotrol Nasal Spray)	
Acetaminophen	May require dosage reduction of acetaminophen following smoking cessation.
Adrenergic antagonists (eg, prazosin)	May require dosage reduction of the adrenergic antagonist following smoking cessation.
Antiasthmatic agents	Concomitant use may require dosage adjustment of the antiasthmatic agent.
Antidepressants (eg, TCAs)	Concomitant use may require dosage adjustment of the antidepressant.
Beta-blockers (eg, propranolol)	May require dosage reduction of the beta-blocker following smoking cessation.
Caffeine	May require dosage reduction of caffeine following smoking cessation.
Coffee	Concomitant use reduces the effects of nicotine.
Insulin	Concomitant use may require dosage adjustment of insulin.
Juices	Concomitant use reduces the effects of nicotine.
Nicotine	Avoid concomitant use with other products containing nicotine (eg, smoking, chewing tobacco).
Oxazepam	May require dosage reduction of oxazepam following smoking cessation.
Pentazocine	May require dosage reduction of pentazocine following smoking cessation.
Prazosin	May require dosage reduction of the adrenergic antagonist following smoking cessation.
Propranolol	May require dosage reduction of the beta-blocker following smoking cessation.
Soft drinks	Concomitant use reduces the effects of nicotine.
Theophylline	May require dosage adjustment of theophylline following smoking cessation.
TCAs	Concomitant use may require dosage adjustment of the antidepressant.
Wine	Concomitant use reduces the effects of nicotine.
Nortriptyline HCl (Pamelor)	
Alcohol	May potentiate effects of alcohol.
Anticholinergic drugs	Monitor closely if using concomitantly.

Table 16.4. Drug Interactions for Smoking Cessation Agents

Antidepressants	Concomitant use increases the plasma levels of nortriptyline.
Chlorpropamide	Caution, may cause hypoglycemia.
Cimetidine	Increases plasma levels of nortriptyline.
Citalopram	Caution when switching to or from an SSRI.
CYP2D6 inhibitors	Increases plasma levels of nortriptyline; dosage adjustment of nortriptyline or the other drug may be necessary.
CYP2D6 substrates	Concomitant use increases the plasma levels of nortriptyline.
Escitalopram	Caution when switching to or from an SSRI.
Flecainide	Concomitant use increases the plasma levels of nortriptyline.
Guanethidine	May block the antihypertensive effects of guanethidine.
Fluoxetine	Caution when switching to or from an SSRI; may need at least 5 wks before initiating treatment with nortriptyline following withdrawal from fluoxetine.
MAO inhibitors	Contraindicated, do not give concomitantly or within at least 2 wks of treatment with an MAO inhibitor.
Paroxetine	Caution when switching to or from an SSRI.
Phenothiazines	Concomitant use increases the plasma levels of nortriptyline.
Propafenone	Concomitant use increases the plasma levels of nortriptyline.
Quinidine	Increases plasma levels of nortriptyline; dosage adjustment of nortriptyline or the other drug may be necessary.
Reserpine	May produce a stimulating effect in depressed patients.
SSRIs	Caution when switching to or from an SSRI; may need at least 5 weeks before initiating treatment with nortriptyline following withdrawal from fluoxetine.
Sertraline	Caution when switching to or from an SSRI.
Sympathomimetic drugs	Monitor closely if using concomitantly.
Thyroid drugs	Monitor closely; cardiac arrhythmias may develop.
Varenicline tartrate (Chantix)	
Cimetidine	Concomitant use reduces the renal clearance of varenicline.
Nicotine replacement therapy (NRT)	Concomitant use may lead to an increased amount of adverse effects (eg, vomiting, headache, nausea).

Smoking and Diabetes

American Diabetes Association

BACKGROUND

As documented in the American Diabetes Association's technical review "Smoking and Diabetes" (1), a large body of evidence from epidemiological, case-control, and cohort studies provides convincing documentation of the causal link between cigarette smoking and health risks. Cigarette smoking is the leading avoidable cause of mortality in the U.S., accounting for 400,000 deaths each year. Cigarette smoking accounts for one out of every five deaths in the U.S. and is the most important modifiable cause of premature death. Cigarettes provide the delivery system for nicotine, an addictive substance related to various pharmacological, biochemical, and psychological processes that interact to support a compulsive pattern of drug use.

Much of the prior work documenting the impact of smoking on health did not discuss separately results on subsets of individuals with diabetes, suggesting the identified risks are at least equivalent to those found in the general population. Other studies of individuals with diabetes consistently found a heightened risk of morbidity and premature death associated with the development of macrovascular complications among smokers. The cardiovascular burden of diabetes, especially in combination with smoking, has not been effectively communicated to people with diabetes or to health care providers, and there is little evidence that this risk factor is being addressed as consistently and comprehensively as its importance requires. Smoking is also related to the premature development of microvascular complications of diabetes and may even have a role in the development of type 2 diabetes (1).

General smoking prevalence decreased substantially up until about 1990 because of extensive public health efforts, which included making the population aware of the health hazards of active and passive smoking, implementation of smoking cessation interventions, and policy changes. However, since then there has been very little further reduction, and about 25% of American adults continue to smoke, with variations reported by ethnic and sociodemographic groups. These figures mirror the prevalence of tobacco use among individuals with diabetes. It appears that adolescents may initiate smoking after being diagnosed with diabetes and that the prevalence of tobacco use decreases with disease duration (1–3).

Effectiveness of smoking cessation counseling

Smoking cessation is one of the few interventions that can safely and cost-effectively be recommended for all patients, and it has been identified as a gold standard against which other preventive behaviors should be evaluated. A number of large randomized clinical trials have demonstrated the efficacy and cost-effectiveness of certain forms of provider and behavioral counseling in changing smoking behavior of primary care and hospitalized patients. This work, combined with the more limited studies specific to individuals with diabetes, suggests that smoking cessation counseling is effective in reducing tobacco use in this high-risk group (3,4). This evidence has been summarized in the updated clinical practice guideline from the U.S. Public Health Service "Treating Tobacco Use and Dependence" (4).

Several treatment characteristics have been identified as critical to achieve cessation. These characteristics include brief counseling by multiple health care providers, use of individual or group counseling strategies, and use of pharmacotherapy (1). Effective pharmacotherapies now include nicotine replacement therapy in a variety of forms (gum, patch, inhaler, spray) and antidepressants (bupropion and nortriptyline). Although many large-scale well-controlled outcome studies have included patients with diabetes, few have reported results separately for patients with diabetes versus other participants. Special issues that affect successful abstinence have been identified in these studies and include weight management and depression. Postcessation weight gain may be an impediment to smoking cessation, especially among women or other people concerned with weight management (4). The presence of comorbid psychiatric conditions such as depression is associated with a greater prevalence of smoking and an increased risk of relapse after quitting. Though not reported separately, these issues are expected to be at least equally relevant for diabetic patients as for general patients (1).

Smoking cessation delivery systems
Despite demonstrated efficacy and cost-effectiveness, smoking cessation has not received the priority it deserves from health care providers. Only about half of smokers with diabetes have been advised to quit smoking by their health care providers (1). One important means of assuring systematic advice regarding the prevention and cessation of tobacco use is through the implementation of smoking cessation delivery systems in office practices and hospitals. These systems require organizational changes in clinics and hospitals to systematically identify all tobacco users at every visit, so that evaluation of smoking status becomes a routine vital sign (1,4). After tobacco users have been identified by staff, clinicians should provide a brief assessment of interest in quitting, advise those without current interest how important it is to quit, and connect those prepared to quit with those who can provide further information, assistance, and follow-up.

RECOMMENDATIONS

Substantial evidence supports inclusion of the prevention and cessation of tobacco use as an important component of state-of-the-art clinical diabetes care (4). Health care providers engaged in the care and management of individuals with diabetes should follow the approach summarized in **Table 1** and address the following primary areas.

Ask
The routine assessment of current tobacco use is a critical first step toward encouraging cessation. The nurse or medical technician who prepares patients for their visit should do this. Nonsmoking adults are unlikely to start, so a sticker on their charts can prevent having to ask them at each visit.

Assess
In those who are current tobacco users, it is important to assess their interest in quitting by asking if they are ready to quit in the next

Table 1. Recommendations Regarding Diabetes and Smoking (E)

Assessment of smoking status and history

- Systematic documentation of a history of tobacco use must be obtained from all adolescent and adult individuals with diabetes.

Counseling on smoking prevention and cessation

- All health care providers should advise individuals with diabetes not to initiate smoking. This advice should be consistently repeated to prevent smoking and other tobacco use among children and adolescents with diabetes under age 21 years.
- Among smokers, cessation counseling must be completed as a routine component of diabetes care.
- Every smoker should be urged to quit in a clear, strong, and personalized manner that describes the added risks of smoking and diabetes.
- Every diabetic smoker should be asked if he or she is willing to quit at this time.

If no, initiate brief and motivational discussion regarding need to stop using tobacco, risks of continued use, and encouragement to quit as well as support when ready.

If yes, assess preference for and initiate either minimal, brief, or intensive cessation counseling and offer pharmacological supplements as appropriate.

Effective systems for delivery of smoking cessation

- Training of all diabetes health care providers in the Public Health Service guidelines regarding smoking should be implemented.
- Follow-up procedures designed to assess and promote quitting status must be arranged for all diabetic smokers.

30 days (preparation phase) or in the next 6 months (contemplation phase). Knowledge of this readiness stage allows tailoring of the intervention to each individual (1).

Advise

Health care providers should advise all smokers with diabetes how important it is for them to quit. There is a dose-response relationship between type, intensity, and duration of treatment and smoking cessation. In general, minimal interventions are defined as <3 min of counseling, whereas brief interventions are defined as 3–10 min of counseling (4). While more intense inter-

ventions are most effective in producing long-term abstinence from tobacco, few smokers are willing to participate (1,3,4).

Assist

The keys to assistance are helping the smoker to set a quit date, providing information about how to prepare for that date, and offering counseling and/or medication assistance to those who are interested. Several pharmacological agents increase smoking cessation rates when used in conjunction with behavioral interventions. These include 4–6 weeks of nicotine replacement therapy, bupropion (150 mg p.o. q.d. or b.i.d.) or nortriptyline (25–75 mg p.o. q.h.s.).

Arrange

In addition to providing support and pharmacological assistance to smokers who are ready to quit, health care providers should also make arrangements for a follow-up phone call soon after the quit date. This can be done by clinic staff. Smokers receiving pharmacotherapy should also have a return office visit arranged.

Organize your clinic

Effective systems for implementing these guidelines should be incorporated into the routine practice of diabetes care. Recording smoking status as a vital sign increases identification of current tobacco users. Organized office information systems and delegation of cessation support and follow-up to trained office staff will greatly increase tobacco cessation rates.

Advocacy for tobacco control through public policy initiatives is also an appropriate and potentially effective way to reduce the burden of excess morbidity and mortality that tobacco use confers on those with diabetes.

FOOTNOTES

The recommendations in this paper are based on the evidence reviewed in the following publication: Smoking and diabetes (Technical Review). *Diabetes Care* 22:1887–1898, 1999.

The initial draft of this paper was prepared by Debra Haire-Joshu, PhD, Russell E. Glasgow, PhD, and Tiffany L. Tibbs, MA. The paper was peer-reviewed, modified, and approved by the Professional Practice Committee and the Executive Committee, October 2003.

REFERENCES

1. Haire-Joshu D, Glasgow RE, Tibbs TL: Smoking and diabetes (Technical Review). *Diabetes Care* 22:1887–1898, 1999.
2. U.S. Department of Health and Human Services: *Preventing Tobacco Use Among Young People: A Report of the Surgeon General*. Atlanta, GA, U. S. Department of Health and Human Services, Public Health Service, Centers for Disease Control and Prevention, National Center for Chronic Disease Prevention and Health Promotion, Office on Smoking and Health, 1994.
3. U.S. Preventive Services Task Force: Counseling to prevent tobacco use. *In Guide to Clinical Preventive Services*. 2nd ed. Baltimore, MD, Williams & Wilkins, 1996, p. 597–609.
4. Fiore M, Bailey W, Cohen S: *Treating Tobacco Use and Dependence: Clinical Practice Guideline*. Rockville, MD, U.S. Department of Health and Human Services, Public Health Service, June 2000.

Section III

Management of Microvascular Disease and Other Comorbidities

Chapter 17

Management of Microvascular Disease

R. Keith Campbell, PharmB, MBA, CDE
Stephen M. Setter, PharmD, CDE, DVM

INTRODUCTION

Sustained hyperglycemia in conjunction with postprandial elevations of blood glucose and lipids damage the small blood vessels throughout the body of a person with diabetes. Cardiovascular disease is the main cause of death in diabetes patients. Both macrovascular and microvascular diabetes complications are common in patients with diabetes over time. The long-term complications of diabetes mellitus can be classified into 3 major types: macrovascular disease, microvascular disease, and endocrine complications.

Macrovascular disease, which affects the large vessels of the body, such as the coronary or lower extremity arteries (eg, femoral, popliteal), may result in myocardial infarction, stroke, and peripheral vascular occlusive disease, respectively. Up to 80% of deaths in people with type 2 diabetes are attributed to cardiovascular disease and stroke. The increased prevalence of macrovascular disease in people with diabetes is due to many factors, including, but not limited to, obesity, lipid abnormalities, hypertension, hyperglycemia, hypercoagulation factors, platelet dysfunction, inflammation, and endothelial dysfunction.

Diabetic microvascular disease affects the small vessels, such as those supplying the retina, nerves, and kidneys. End organ damage can lead to diabetic retinopathy and blindness, diabetic neuropathy, which may result in lower limb amputation, and diabetic nephropathy, often leading to end-stage renal disease (ESRD) requiring dialysis or transplantation. It is well established that chronic hyperglycemia results in these primary chronic microvascular complications of diabetes. Diabetes is the leading cause of renal failure and adult blindness in developed countries, contributing to >33,000 new cases of ESRD and 24,000 new cases of vision loss each year in the US. The term "endocrine complications" is a bit of a misnomer. Sustained hyperglycemia does not cause damage to other endocrine organs, but there is an increased incidence of thyroid, gonad, and other endocrine organ problems in diabetes patients. For example, in men with type 2 diabetes, up to 40% have been found to have low levels of testosterone, causing hypogonadism. A recent symposium for the American Association of Diabetes Educators concluded that men with type 2 and type 1 diabetes be screened for low testosterone since men with hypogonadism have abdominal obesity with increased waist circumference, are fatigued, have low sex drive, erectile dysfunction, depression, and low bone density.

In addition to chronic hyperglycemia, diabetic microvascular complications arise from other metabolic alterations that include, but are not limited to, insulin resistance, hypertension, and dyslipidemia. Under hyperglycemic conditions, blood flow and microvascular contractility changes are seen in the retina, microvessels of peripheral nerves, and kidney.

Endocrine complications of diabetes may affect the gonads, thyroid, and other endocrine organs.

MICROVASCULAR DISEASE

One of the principles and primary goals of diabetes management is to delay and/or prevent the development of chronic complications. Numerous studies have proved that near normalization of blood glucose will significantly decrease chronic diabetes complications. This has resulted in a renewed emphasis on empowering patients to tightly manage blood glucose, lipids, and blood pressure by using whatever available drugs or combination of drugs to achieve specific objectives and decrease the risk of chronic complications.

Two landmark studies, the Diabetes Control and Complications Trial (DCCT), involving patients with type 1 diabetes, and the United Kingdom Prospective Diabetes Study, (UKPDS) involving patients with type 2 diabetes, conclusively demonstrated that improved glycemic control contributes to significant microvascular risk reduction. The DCCT demonstrated a 63% relative risk reduction in retinopathy and 54% and 60% risk reductions in nephropathy and neuropathy, respectively. The UKPDS demonstrated up to a 21% risk reduction in retinopathy and a 33% risk reduction in nephropathy. A smaller study in patients with type 2 diabetes from Japan showed relative risk reductions of developing retinopathy (69%) and nephropathy (70%) in patients achieving tighter glycemic control compared with controls.

Theories on how hyperglycemia contributes to microvascular damage are emerging, with the hope of providing additional pharmacotherapeutic interventions to prevent or slow the progression of chronic diabetes-related microvascular disease. The prominent contemporary biochemical pathway theories on how diabetes causes damage to the microvasculature include, but are not limited to: 1) increased polyol (sorbitol/aldose reductase) pathway flux; 2) production of advanced glycation end-products (AGE); 3) generation of reactive oxygen species (oxidative stress); and 4) activation of diacylglycerol and protein kinase C (PKC) isoforms. The following is a review that explores these biochemical pathways currently thought to contribute to the development of chronic diabetic microvascular complications.

The following is a list of the numerous causes and consequences of sustained hyperglycemia that result in chronic diabetes complications often involving the microvasculature:

- Increased capillary basement membrane thickening, causing microvascular disease
- Impairment of phagocytosis, resulting in impaired immunity and an inability to fight infections
- Abnormally high levels of minor (glycosylated) proteins: advanced glycosylated end products (AGE) that interfere with the protein's normal physiology
- Glucose metabolized to sorbitol via the polyol pathway with deposition in cornea and in nerves
- Increased aldose reductase
- Faulty lipid metabolism yielding increased number of small LDL particles, low HDL and hypertriglyceridemia
- Increased blood pressure
- Hemorrheologic factors affected adversely, including:
  - Increased platelet adhesiveness
  - Increased serum fibrinogen levels

– Increased blood viscosity
– Decreased red blood cell flexibility
- Increased coagulation factors like plasminogen activator inhibitor-1 (PAI-1)
- Increased lipoprotein
- Increased CRP and other inflammatory factors.
- Increased activation of some isoforms of protein kinase C (PKC) causing reduced vascular contractility
- Increased sialic acid levels in the blood
- Increased weight
- Increased incidence of cataracts, macular degeneration, glaucoma
- Increased incidence of cancer
- Increased neonatal morbidity and mortality
- Hearing disorders, dental and gum problems
- Numerous foot and lower limb problems including fungal infections
- Genetic damage to sperm
- Increased connective tissue problems
- Oxidative stress throughout the body

INCREASED POLYOL (SORBITOL/ALDOSE REDUCTASE) PATHWAY

Most cells in the body require the presence and action of insulin for glucose to gain entry into the intracellular compartment. However, vascular endothelial cells of the retina, kidney, and nervous tissue are insulin independent; therefore, there is a free interchange of glucose from the extracellular to intracellular environment regardless of insulin's presence or action. This diffusion of glucose into retinal, nerve, and kidney microvascular endothelial cells allows normal physiologic cellular functions to proceed during the euglycemic state, with any excess glucose being promptly metabolized to sorbitol by the enzyme aldose reductase. Aldose reductase has a low affinity for glucose at normal glucose concentrations (70-110 mg/dL), and metabolism of glucose by the polyol pathway accounts for a very small percentage of glucose use under euglycemic conditions. However, in the hyperglycemic state, excess glucose enters the polyol pathway, resulting in excess sorbitol production, with a concomitant decrease in nicotinamide-adenine dinucleotide phosphate (NADPH). Low levels of NADPH can decrease nitric oxide production in endothelial cells and adversely affect cellular redox balance, thereby resulting in deleterious metabolic consequences including oxidative stress.

Persistently high levels of intracellular glucose can result in significant sorbitol, fructose, and unbound cytosolic NADH accumulation. Potential mechanisms of how shunting of glucose into the polyol pathway results in microvascular damage and malfunction include: 1) sorbitol-induced osmotic stress due to accumulated sorbitol; 2) altered or decreased Na/K-ATPase activity; 3) myo-inositol depletion with impaired phosphatidylinositol metabolism; 4) increased prostaglandin production; and 5) alterations in protein kinase C (PKC) isoform activity.

At one time, diabetes-related cataract formation was proposed to primarily involve osmotic alterations due to accumulated intracellular sorbitol. The osmotic stress theory has since been abandoned. It was previously thought that, because sorbitol does not easily cross cell membranes, damage to microvascular cells resulted from increases in intracellular osmotic pressure. However, levels of sorbitol in diabetic vascular cells and nerves are too low to induce osmotic damage. **Cataracts are twice as common as is glaucoma in diabetes patients, contributing to 24,000 new cases of vision loss each year in the US.** Cataracts from diabetes patients have high levels of sorbitol deposited as crystals in the lens.

Increased flux through the polyol pathway can lead to microvascular damage by contributing to AGE formation, isospecific protein kinase C activation, and reactive oxygen species (ROS) generation. In vivo studies involving polyol pathway inhibitors have been, for the most part, disappointing. Inhibition of sorbitol dehydrogenase has been shown to prevent diabetes-induced retinopathy, nephropathy, and neuropathy. In a 52-week, randomized, placebo-controlled, double-blind clinical trial, zenarestat, a potent aldose reductase inhibitor, was studied in patients with mild to moderate diabetic peripheral neuropathy. Nerve conduction velocity and small-diameter sural nerve density were positively impacted. The aldose reductase inhibitor fidarestat was studied in a clinical trial in patients with type 1 or 2 diabetes who had diabetes-associated neuropathy. In this 52-week, placebo-controlled, double-blind parallel-group study, 279 patients received either a placebo or fidarestat 1 mg. Electrophysiologic measurements were evaluated along with subjective symptoms. Of the eight electrophysiologic measurements, five significantly improved over baseline and none demonstrated significant deterioration. In the placebo-treated patients, no measure significantly improved and one measure significantly deteriorated. While fidarestat was efficacious and well tolerated in this trial, results from most other aldose reductase inhibitor clinical trials have been negative due to inadequate efficacy and/or safety.

In summary, a variety of data support the premise that intracellular metabolism of glucose through the sorbitol pathway plays a potentially important, initiating role in the microvascular dysfunction induced by diabetes. However, most human studies to date have been unable to demonstrate a clinical benefit. Note that vitamin C in doses of 400 mg or greater is a potent aldose reductase inhibitor.

PRODUCTION OF ADVANCED GLYCATION END-PRODUCTS (AGE)

Glucose can react nonenzymatically with the amino group of proteins and other macromolecules to form Schiff bases, which are transformed into Amadori products (see **Figure 1**). As discussed below, degradation of Amadori products results in the production of highly reactive carbonyl compounds that react with unbound amino groups and, with time, form AGE, which are irreversibly cross-linked substances. This alteration of proteins by glucose is termed "glycation." It is likely that intracellular hyperglycemia is the primary initiating event in the formation of both intracellular and extracellular AGE. Intracellular AGE formation occurs within a week of endothelial cells being exposed to high glucose levels and has been shown to be present in increased amounts in retinal vessels and renal glomeruli of persons with diabetes. Furthermore, increased serum concentrations of AGE are associated with endothelial dysfunction in patients with diabetes.

AGE form from various mechanisms including: 1) intracellular auto-oxidation of glucose to glyoxal; 2) decomposition of the Amadori product glucose-derived 1-amino-1-deoxyfructose; 3) lysine adduction to 3-deoxyglucosone, a derivative of fructose, the end product of the sorbitol pathway; and 4) fragmentation of glyceraldehyde-3-phosphate, which accumulates as a result of increased sorbitol pathway activity and the alteration of dihydroxyacetone phosphate to methylglyoxal. These reactive intracellular dicarbonyls—glyoxal, methylglyoxal, and 3-deoxyglucosone—can react with amino groups of intracellular and extracellular proteins to form AGE. Oxidative and nonoxidative reactions account for carbonyl stress, which is a more appropriate term than oxidative stress. The proteins bound to the glucose

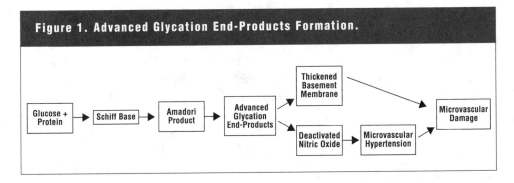

Figure 1. Advanced Glycation End-Products Formation.

do not behave in a normal physiologic manner and are known to promote microvascular abnormalities. In addition, the glycated proteins are deposited in the basement membranes of capillaries, making it difficult for oxygen and nutrients to pass into tissues. The thickened basement membranes also interfere with the ability of white blood cells to migrate into tissues to fight infections. When AGE attach to their receptors, known as advanced glycation end-product receptors (AGE-R), multiple cellular changes can occur that alter normal cellular physiology.

AGE formation can contribute to thickening of the basement membrane of various tissues (eg, renal glomeruli) and to microvascular hypertension by deactivating nitric oxide. Together, basement membrane thickening and microvascular hypertension result in the microvascular leakage and/or occlusion that underlie the development and progression of diabetic retinopathy, diabetic neuropathy, and diabetic nephropathy. Therefore, AGE can contribute to the development of hypertension and precipitate pro-thrombotic events that are common in patients with diabetes. AGE may also adversely affect vascular permeability.

Atherosclerotic lesions also contain AGE, which may play a role in macrovascular occlusive disease that is often accelerated in patients with diabetes.

In animal models, AGE inhibitors prevent chronic manifestations of diabetic microvascular disease in the retina, kidney, and nerve. Aminoguanidine, an AGE inhibitor, was studied in a randomized, double-blind, placebo-controlled trial involving patients with type 1 diabetes with overt nephropathy. Results showed that aminoguanidine lowered total urinary protein, slowed the progression of nephropathy, and reduced the progression of diabetic retinopathy. However, in general, trials involving the AGE inhibitors aminoguanidine and pimagedine have been hindered by dose-limiting toxicity that has included the development of anemia, flulike symptoms, and glomerulonephritis with concurrent antinuclear antibody formation. The most commonly known AGE is hemoglobin A_{1c} (HbA_{1c}). It results when excess glucose binds with hemoglobin to form HbA_{1c}, which is commonly used to evaluate treatment success. The hemoglobin molecule has a life cycle of 3-4 months so one can tell how the diabetes patient has managed blood glucose levels during that time. Target HbA_{1c} should be less than 7%.

GENERATION OF REACTIVE OXYGEN SPECIES

The term oxidative stress refers to the imbalance between the production of reactive oxygen species and the normal antioxidant protective mechanisms present to guard tissues from oxidative damage. Hyperglycemia can increase oxidative stress through enzymatic and nonenzymatic processes (see **Figure 2**). Glucose has pro-

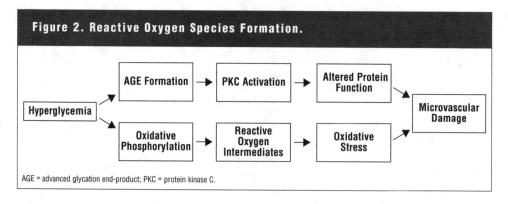

Figure 2. Reactive Oxygen Species Formation.

AGE = advanced glycation end-product; PKC = protein kinase C.

oxidant properties in the presence of heavy metals, and glycosylation of proteins further adds to the oxidative stress and the aforementioned carbonyl stress. Additionally, free radicals can form from the auto-oxidation of glucose. Additionally, hyperglycemia-stimulated reactive oxygen species formation can inactivate or reduce nitric oxide levels via the uncoupling of nitric oxide synthase activity.

Increased reactive oxygen species may involve the generation of reducing equivalents in the form of unbound cytosolic NADH linked to increased sorbitol pathway activity, thereby providing the source of electrons needed by several enzyme systems to generate superoxide. It has been proposed that overproduction of superoxide by the mitochondrial electron-transport chain links four of the common theories on how diabetic microvascular complications arise, the first three of which are discussed here: increased polyol pathway flux; increased intracellular AGE formation and activation of protein kinase C; and increased flux through the hexosamine pathway.

With regard to diabetes, free radical formation, regardless of the cause, results in damaged protein and mitochondrial DNA, which can have deleterious effects on the microvasculature. Evidence of increased oxidative stress in diabetes is equivocal. However, some data suggest that the production of reactive oxygen species is increased in the diabetic state and that reactive oxygen species may contribute to increased microvascular permeability and resultant microvascular damage. Additionally, elevated levels of reactive oxygen species can increase intracellular calcium levels in endothelial tissue culture. Increases in intracellular unbound calcium levels have been associated with increased endothelial hyperpermeability of macromolecules.

Antioxidant levels are reported to be decreased in diabetic patients. In animal models, antioxidants have shown effectiveness in attenuating diabetic microvascular complications. In humans, the effectiveness of antioxidant supplementation has not been well substantiated. However, in one study involving patients with type 1 diabetes of <10 years' duration, the antioxidant vitamin E showed effectiveness in normalizing retinal hemodynamics and improving creatinine clearance. It is clear that many of the microvascular complications of diabetes are a direct result of oxidative stress.

ACTIVATION OF DIACYLGLYCEROL AND PROTEIN KINASE C ISOFORMS

Hyperglycemia yields increased levels of diacylglycerol, which is found throughout cell membranes and is a key contributor to the activation of various protein kinase C isoforms. Diacylglycerol formation induced by glucose has been documented in cultured cells in tissues from persons with diabetes mellitus. In people with diabetes, the tissues and organs that exhibit increased diacylglycerol activity include the retina, heart, glomeruli, liver, and aorta. It is hypothesized that tight glycemic control may play a critical role in preventing protein kinase C activation by reducing diacylglycerol levels.

The protein kinase C family consists of multifunctional phosphorylating isoenzymes that are found throughout the body, where they perform important physiologic roles. There are 12 known protein kinase C isoenzymes classified into 3 subclasses (conventional or classical, novel, atypical). Protein kinase C classification is dependent on the structure of their regulatory domain and, consequently, the type of cofactors (phosphatidylserine, diacylglycerol, free fatty acids, calcium, and magnesium) required to activate and regulate enzymatic activity.

It appears that protein kinase C-β isoforms are the most sensitive to changes in diacylglycerol levels. Protein kinase C-β is present in pancreatic islet cells, monocytes, brain, and many vascular tissues including those of the retina, kidney, and heart. While the protein kinase C family of isoenzymes has wide distribution throughout the body, the effects of inhibitors specific for 1 or very few protein kinase C subclasses might be limited to specific organs or biochemical pathways. Protein kinase C-β, -β$_1$, and -β$_2$ isoenzymes are elevated in the retina during acute and chronic hyperglycemic states. In a hyperglycemic environment, protein kinase C-β displays the most significant increase within various vascular tissues. Therefore, protein kinase C-β may be a very important therapeutic target with regard to the treatment of diabetic microvascular complications.

Increased retinal permeability and retinal neovascularization may be mediated by protein kinase C activation. Furthermore, in the vasculature, protein kinase C activation increases basement matrix protein formation, activates leukocytes, and causes smooth muscle proliferation and contraction. In the glomerulus, elevated glucose levels stimulate growth factor production, resulting in increased glomerular pressures and matrix protein deposition. Protein kinase C is also involved in vascular endothelial growth factor (VEGF) formation, which is implicated in stimulating microalbuminemia as well as stimulating the growth of new fragile capillaries. Therefore, protein kinase C activation may have detrimental long-term negative sequelae in patients with diabetes.

Ruboxistaurin mesylate (LY333531) is a specific inhibitor of the protein kinase C-β isoform that has been shown to decrease endothelial cell proliferation, angiogenesis, and vascular permeability in vitro and in animal models. Ruboxistaurin (RBX) has been shown to reduce elevated glomerular filtration rate (glomerular hyperfiltration occurs in the early phase of the development of diabetic nephropathy), reduce albumin excretion, and improve retinal mean circulation time. Assessments in the retina demonstrate that local administration of RBX decreases retinal protein kinase C-β activation, decreases prolonged mean retinal circulation time, and increases retinal blood flow. It is postulated that the positive effects of protein kinase C-β inhibition on nerve conduction may be due to improved nerve blood flow. In humans, a one-month assessment of RBX was performed in 29 patients with type 1 or 2 diabetes of <10 years' duration. Significant improvements in retinal blood flow and mean circulation time were demonstrated, without alterations to HbA$_{1c}$ or fasting blood glucose levels. Clinical research is ongoing to establish the effect of blocking protein kinase C action on the development and progression of the major diabetic microvascular complications of diabetes, namely retinopathy, neuropathy, and nephropathy.

RBX has been studied in diabetes patients with moderately severe to very severe non-proliferative retinopathy. The drug was well tolerated and reduced the risk of moderate visual loss, but did not prevent diabetic retinopathy progression. RBX was also studied in diabetes patients with nephropathy. After one year, the amount of the protein albumin in the urine was lowered in the patients who took RBX; this effect was seen after one month. RBX may help patients with type 2 diabetes who are taking medications to treat kidney damage. Larger studies are needed to see how safe and effective it is over long periods. RBX has been reviewed by the FDA but has NOT been approved, with recommendations that further studies are needed.

SUMMARY

Microvascular dysfunction and damage related to diabetes is often the result of microvascular endothelial compromise. Endothelial damage underlies the chronic microvascular complications experienced by people with diabetes mellitus. Multiple separate, but potentially interconnected biochemical pathways and pathophysiologic mechanisms are thought to contribute to endothelial dysfunction. Biochemical pathways including increased flux through the polyol pathway, generation of reactive oxygen species, the formation of AGE, diacylglycerol generation, and protein kinase C activation, as well as other pathophysiologic events (eg, dyslipidemia, atherosclerosis, hypertension, inflammation) appear to contribute to damaged and dysfunctional endothelium.

In addition to the benefits of achieving tight glycemic and blood pressure control, the potential role of inhibiting specific biochemical and pathophysiologic pathways with the goal of preventing or ameliorating diabetic retinopathy, diabetic neuropathy, and diabetic nephropathy affords promise for the many patients at risk for or currently experiencing diabetes-associated microvascular disease.

In addition to chronic hyperglycemia, diabetic microvascular complications arise from other metabolic alterations that include, but are not limited to, insulin resistance, hypertension, and dyslipidemia. Under hyperglycemic conditions, blood flow and microvascular contractility changes are seen in the retina, microvessels of peripheral nerves, and kidneys.

The three major microvascular complications of diabetes are retinopathy, nephropathy, and neuropathy. Each is significantly influenced by sustained hyperglycemia. Remember that diabetes equals cardiovascular disease. The care and treatment of diabetes must therefore include near normalization of blood pressure, blood lipids, coagulation factors, blood glucose levels while encouraging the patient to take charge of his or her diabetes and maintain a normal, satisfying lifestyle.

For retinopathy, the proven treatment protocol is to try to normalize blood glucose levels and have at least annual pupil-dilated eye exams by a retinal specialist. If microvascular changes are found, pan-retinal photocoagulation administered via laser therapy significantly reduces progression to visual loss. Other treatment options include a vitrectomy for patients who have had a retinal bleed into the vitreous. Being checked for glaucoma and cataracts is also essential with appropriate treatments prescribed if these problems occur.

For neuropathy, once again, normalization of blood glucose levels is the treatment of choice to prevent as well as treat the many forms of this debilitating complication. See chapter 18 for medications used to treat diabetic neuropathic disorders.

Nephropathy is also prevented by normalizing blood glucose levels. Renal protection can also take place if angiotensin converting enzyme inhibitors (ACEIs) or angiotensin receptor blockers (ARBs) are given to diabetes patients. Normalizing blood pressure is a must. See chapter 13 for medications used to treat hypertension.

SUGGESTED READING

Aiello LP, Gardner TW, King GL, et al. Diabetic retinopathy: technical review. *Diabetes Care*. 1998;21:143-156.

Aiello, etal. The effect of ruboxistaurin on visual loss in patients with moderately severe to very severe DR. *Diabetes*. 2005; 54:2188-2197.

Beckman JA, Goldfine AB, Gordon MB, et al. Inhibition of protein kinase Cß prevents impaired endothelium-dependent vasodilation caused by hyperglycemia in humans. *Circ Res* 2002;90(1):107-111.

Brownlee M. Advanced products of nonenzymatic glycosylation and the pathogenesis of diabetic complications. In Rifkin H, Porte D Jr, eds. Diabetes Mellitus: Theory and Practice. New York: Elsevier, 1990:279-291.

Brownlee M. Advanced protein glycosylation in diabetes and aging. *Annual Rev Med*. 1995;46:223-234.

Brownlee M. Biochemistry and molecular cell biology of diabetic complications. *Nature*. 2001;414:813-820.

Feldman EL. Oxidative stress and diabetic neuropathy: a new understanding of an old problem. *J Clin Invest*. 2003;111:431-433.

Forbes JM, Cooper ME, Oldfield MD, et al. Role of advanced glycation end products in diabetic nephropathy. *J Am Soc Nephrol*. 2003;14:S254-S258.

Kles KA, Vinik AI. Pathophysiology and treatment of diabetic peripheral neuropathy: the case for diabetic neurovascular function as an essential component. *Curr Diabetes Rev*. 2006;2:131-145.

King G, Brownlee M. The cellular and molecular mechanisms of diabetic complications. *Endocrinol Metab Clin North Am*. 1996;2:255-270.

Koya D, King GL. Protein kinase C activation and the development of diabetic complications. *Diabetes*. 1998;47:859-866.

Krolewski AS, Laffel LM, Krolewski M, et al. Glycosylated hemoglobin and the risk of mircroalbuminuria in patients with insulin-dependent diabetes mellitus. *N Engl J Med.* 1995;332:1251-1255.

Shore AC, Tooke JE. Microvascular function and haemodynamic disturbances in diabetes mellitus and its complications. In Pickup J, Williams G, eds. Textbook of Diabetes, Vol 1. Oxford, UK: Blackwell Scientific, 1997:43.1-43.13.

Tuttle KR, et al. Effect of ruboxistaurin on nephropathy in type 2 diabetes. *Diabetes Care.* 2005;28:2686-2690.

Vinik A. Diabetic neuropathy: pathogenesis and therapy. *Am J Med.* 1999;107:17S-26S.

Vinik A, Bril V, Kempler, et al. For the MBBQ Study: Treatment of symptomatic diabetic peripheral neuropathy with protein kinase Cß inhibitor ruboxistaurin mesylate during a 1-year randomized, placebo-controlled, double-blind clinical trial. *Clin Ther.* 2005;27: 1164s-1180s.

Wassef L, Langham RG, Kelly DJ. Vasoactive renal factors and the progression of diabetic nephropathy. *Curr Pharm Des.* 2004;10:3373-3384.

Williams ME, Tuttle KR. The next generation of diabetic nephropathy therapies: an update. *Adv Chronic Kidney Dis.* 2005;12:212-222.

Witzke KA, Vinik AI. Diabetic neuropathy in older adults. *Rev Endocrin Metab Disord.* 2005;6:117-127.

Yamagishi S, Edelstein D, Du XD, Brownlee M. Hyperglycemia potentiates platelet-derived growth factor induced proliferation of smooth muscle cells through mitochondrial superoxide overproduction. *Diabetes.* 2001;50:1491-1494.

Nephropathy in Diabetes

American Diabetes Association

INTRODUCTION

Diabetes has become the most common single cause of end-stage renal disease (ESRD) in the U.S. and Europe; this is due to the facts that 1) diabetes, particularly type 2, is increasing in prevalence; 2) diabetes patients now live longer; and 3) patients with diabetic ESRD are now being accepted for treatment in ESRD programs where formerly they had been excluded. In the U.S., diabetic nephropathy accounts for about 40% of new cases of ESRD, and in 1997, the cost for treatment of diabetic patients with ESRD was in excess of $15.6 billion. About 20–30% of patients with type 1 or type 2 diabetes develop evidence of nephropathy, but in type 2 diabetes, a considerably smaller fraction of these progress to ESRD. However, because of the much greater prevalence of type 2 diabetes, such patients constitute over half of those diabetic patients currently starting on dialysis. There is considerable racial/ethnic variability in this regard, with Native Americans, Hispanics (especially Mexican-Americans), and African-Americans having much higher risks of developing ESRD than non-Hispanic whites

with type 2 diabetes. Recent studies have now demonstrated that the onset and course of diabetic nephropathy can be ameliorated to a very significant degree by several interventions, but these interventions have their greatest impact if instituted at a point very early in the course of the development of this complication. This position statement is based on recent review articles that discuss published research and issues that remain unresolved and provides recommendations regarding the detection, prevention, and treatment of early nephropathy.

NATURAL HISTORY OF DIABETIC NEPHROPATHY

The earliest clinical evidence of nephropathy is the appearance of low but abnormal levels ($\geq$30 mg/day or 20 μg/min) of albumin in the urine, referred to as microalbuminuria, and patients with microalbuminuria are referred to as having incipient nephropathy. Without specific interventions, ~80% of subjects with type 1 diabetes who develop sustained microalbuminuria have their urinary albumin excretion increase at a rate of

Abbreviations: ACE, angiotensin-converting enzyme; ARB, angiotensin receptor blocker; DCCB, dihydropyridine calcium channel blocker; ESRD, end-stage renal disease; GFR, glomerular filtration rate; UKPDS, United Kingdom Prospective Diabetes Study

~10–20% per year to the stage of overt nephropathy or clinical albuminuria (≥300 mg/24 h or ≥200 µg/min) over a period of 10–15 years, with hypertension also developing along the way. Once overt nephropathy occurs, without specific interventions, the glomerular filtration rate (GFR) gradually falls over a period of several years at a rate that is highly variable from individual to individual (2–20 mL/min/year). ESRD develops in 50% of type 1 diabetic individuals with overt nephropathy within 10 years and in >75% by 20 years.

A higher proportion of individuals with type 2 diabetes are found to have microalbuminuria and overt nephropathy shortly after the diagnosis of their diabetes, because diabetes is actually present for many years before the diagnosis is made and also because the presence of albuminuria may be less specific for the presence of diabetic nephropathy, as shown by biopsy studies. Without specific interventions, 20–40% of type 2 diabetic patients with microalbuminuria progress to overt nephropathy, but by 20 years after onset of overt nephropathy, only ~20% will have progressed to ESRD. Once the GFR begins to fall, the rates of fall in GFR are again highly variable from one individual to another, but overall, they may not be substantially different between patients with type 1 and patients with type 2 diabetes. However, the greater risk of dying from associated coronary artery disease in the older population with type 2 diabetes may prevent many with earlier stages of nephropathy from progressing to ESRD. As therapies and interventions for coronary artery disease continue to improve, however, more patients with type 2 diabetes may be expected to survive long enough to develop renal failure.

In addition to its being the earliest manifestation of nephropathy, albuminuria is a marker of greatly increased cardiovascular morbidity and mortality for patients with either type 1 or type 2 diabetes. Thus, the finding of microalbuminuria is an indication for screening for possible vascular disease and aggressive intervention to reduce all cardiovascular risk factors (e.g., lowering of LDL cholesterol, antihypertensive therapy, cessation of smoking, institution of exercise, etc.). In addition, there is some preliminary evidence to suggest that lowering of cholesterol may also reduce the level of proteinuria.

SCREENING FOR ALBUMINURIA

A test for the presence of microalbumin should be performed at diagnosis in patients with type 2 diabetes. Microalbuminuria rarely occurs with short duration of type 1 diabetes; therefore, screening in individuals with type 1 diabetes should begin after 5 years' disease duration. Some evidence suggests that the prepubertal duration of diabetes may be important in the development of microvascular complications; therefore, clinical judgement should be exercised when individualizing these recommendations. Because of the difficulty in precise dating of the onset of type 2 diabetes, such screening should begin at the time of diagnosis. After the initial screening and in the absence of previously demonstrated microalbuminuria, a test for the presence of microalbumin should be performed annually.

Screening for microalbuminuria can be performed by three methods: 1) measurement of the albumin-to-creatinine ratio in a random spot collection; 2) 24-h collection with creatinine, allowing the simultaneous measurement of creatinine clearance; and 3) timed (e.g., 4-h or overnight) collection. The first method is often found to be the easiest to carry out in an office setting, generally provides accurate information, and is therefore preferred; first-void or other morning collections are best because of the known diurnal

Table 1: Definitions of Abnormalities in Albumin Excretion			
Category	Spot collection (µg/mg creatinine)	24-h collection (mg/24 h)	Timed collection (µg/min)
Normal	<30	<30	<20
Microalbuminuria	30–299	30–299	20–199
Clinical albuminuria	≥300	≥300	≥200

variation in albumin excretion, but if this timing cannot be used, uniformity of timing for different collections in the same individual should be employed. Specific assays are needed to detect microalbuminuria because standard hospital laboratory assays for urinary protein are not sufficiently sensitive to measure such levels. Microalbuminuria is said to be present if urinary albumin excretion is ≥30 mg/24 h (equivalent to 20 µg/min on a timed specimen or 30 mg/g creatinine on a random sample) (**Table 1**). Short-term hyperglycemia, exercise, urinary tract infections, marked hypertension, heart failure, and acute febrile illness can cause transient elevations in urinary albumin excretion. If assays for microalbuminuria are not readily available, screening with reagent tablets or dipsticks for microalbumin may be carried out, since they show acceptable sensitivity (95%) and specificity (93%) when carried out by trained personnel. Because reagent strips only indicate concentration and do not correct for creatinine as the spot urine albumin-to-creatinine ratio does, they are subject to possible errors from alterations in urine concentration. All positive tests by reagent strips or tablets should be confirmed by more specific methods. There is also marked day-to-day variability in albumin excretion, so at least two of three collections done in a 3- to 6-month period should show elevated levels before designating a patient as having microalbuminuria. An algorithm for microalbuminuria screening is given in **Fig. 1**.

Because of variability in urinary albumin excretion, two of three specimens collected within a 3- to 6-month period should be abnormal before considering a patient to have crossed one of these diagnostic thresholds. Exercise within 24 h, infection, fever, congestive heart failure, marked hyperglycemia, marked hypertension, pyuria, and hematuria may elevate urinary albumin excretion over baseline values.

EFFECT OF GLYCEMIC CONTROL

The Diabetes Control and Complications Trial (DCCT) and the United Kingdom Prospective Diabetes Study (UKPDS) have definitively shown that intensive diabetes therapy can significantly reduce the risk of the development of microalbuminuria and overt nephropathy in people with diabetes. The glycemic control recommendations for all patients with diabetes in the American Diabetes Association's "Standards of Medical Care for Patients with Diabetes Mellitus" should be followed in this regard.

HYPERTENSION CONTROL

In patients with type 1 diabetes, hypertension is usually caused by underlying diabetic nephropathy and typically manifests about the time that patients develop microalbuminuria. In patients with type 2 diabetes, hypertension is present at the time of diagnosis of diabetes in about one-third of patients. The common coexistence of glucose intolerance, hypertension, elevated LDL cholesterol and

Figure 1. Screening for Microalbuminuria

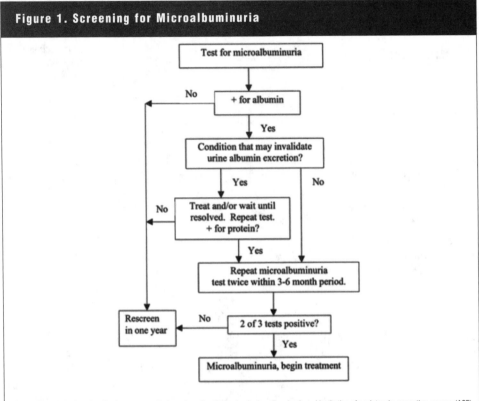

The role of annual microalbuminuria assessment is less clear after diagnosis of microalbuminuria and institution of angiotensin-converting enzyme (ACE) inhibitor or angiotensin receptor blocker (ARB) therapy and blood pressure control. Many experts recommend continued surveillance to assess both response to therapy and progression of disease. In addition to assessment of urinary albumin excretion, assessment of glomerular function is important in patients with diabetic kidney disease.

triglycerides, and a reduction in HDL cholesterol, obesity, and susceptibility to cardiovascular disease suggests that they may relate to common underlying mechanisms, such as insulin resistance; and this complex is often referred to as syndrome X and/or the metabolic syndrome. Hypertension in type 2 diabetic patients may also be related to underlying diabetic nephropathy, be due to coexisting "essential" hypertension, or be due to a myriad of other secondary causes, such as renal vascular disease. Isolated systolic hypertension has been attributed to the loss of elastic compliance of atherosclerotic large vessels. In general, the hypertension in patients with both types of diabetes is associated with an expanded plasma volume, increased peripheral vascular resistance, and low renin activity.

Both systolic and diastolic hypertension markedly accelerate the progression of diabetic nephropathy, and aggressive antihypertensive management is able to greatly decrease the rate of fall of GFR. Appropriate antihypertensive intervention can significantly increase the median life expectancy in patients with type 1 diabetes, with a reduction in mortality from 94% to 45% and a reduction in the need for dialysis and transplantation from 73% to 31% 16 years after the development of overt nephropathy.

In accordance with the "Standards of Medical Care in Diabetes Mellitus," the position statement on "Hypertension Management in Adults With Diabetes," and other recommendations, the primary goal of therapy for nonpregnant diabetic patients ≥18 years of age is to decrease blood pressure to and maintain it at <130 mmHg systolic and <80 mmHg diastolic. For patients with isolated systolic hypertension with a systolic pressure of ≥180 mmHg, the initial goal of treatment is to gradually lower the systolic blood pressure in stages. If initial goals are met and well tolerated, further lowering may be indicated.

A major aspect of initial treatment should consist of lifestyle modifications, such as weight loss, reduction of salt and alcohol intake, and exercise, as outlined in the "Standards of Medical Care for Patients with Diabetes Mellitus" and the position statement on "Treatment of Hypertension in Adults with Diabetes." In patients with underlying nephropathy, treatment with ACE inhibitors or ARBs is also indicated as part of initial therapy (see below). If after 4–6 weeks sufficient blood pressure reduction has not occurred, additional pharmacological therapy is indicated. (See the American Diabetes Association position statement "Treatment of Hypertension in Adults with Diabetes" for a complete discussion on this subject.) In general, these medications may be added in stepwise fashion and their individual use may depend on other factors such as fluid overload and vascular disease.

USE OF ANTIHYPERTENSIVE AGENTS

The positive response to antihypertensive treatment coupled with the concept that often there is a progressive deterioration of renal function regardless of the underlying etiology gave rise to the idea that hemodynamic factors may be critical in furthering the fall in GFR. In this hypothesis, damage to glomeruli causes changes in the microcirculation that result in hyperfiltration occurring in the remaining glomeruli with increased intraglomerular pressure and increased sensitivity to angiotensin II; the single-nephron

hyperfiltration with intraglomerular hypertension is itself damaging. Many studies have shown that in hypertensive patients with type 1 diabetes, ACE inhibitors can reduce the level of albuminuria and the rate of progression of renal disease to a greater degree than other antihypertensive agents that lower blood pressure by an equal amount. Other studies have shown that there is benefit in reducing the progression of microalbuminuria in normotensive patients with type 1 diabetes and normotensive and hypertensive patients with type 2 diabetes.

Use of ACE inhibitors or ARBs may exacerbate hyperkalemia in patients with advanced renal insufficiency and/or hyporeninemic hypoaldosteronism. In older patients with bilateral renal artery stenosis and in patients with advanced renal disease even without renal artery stenosis, ACE inhibitors may cause a rapid decline in renal function. Whether this occurs with ARBs is unknown. Cough may also occur with ACE inhibitors. ACE inhibitors are contraindicated in pregnancy and therefore should be used with caution in women of childbearing potential. There is no data on ARB use in pregnancy, but they are classified as class C/D.

Because of the high proportion of patients who progress from microalbuminuria to overt nephropathy and subsequently to ESRD, use of ACE inhibitors or ARBs is recommended for all patients with microalbuminuria or advanced stages of neuropathy. The effect of ACE inhibitors appears to be a class effect, so choice of agent may depend on cost and compliance issues.

The recent UKPDS compared antihypertensive treatment with an ACE inhibitor to that with a β-blocker. Both drugs were equally effective in lowering blood pressure and there were no significant differences in the incidence of microalbuminuria or proteinuria. However, because of the low prevalence of nephropathy in the population studied, it is unclear whether there were sufficient events to observe a protective effect of either drug on the progression of nephropathy. Some studies have demonstrated that the non-dihydropyridine calcium channel blocker (NDCCB) classes of calcium-channel blockers can reduce the level of albuminuria, but no studies to date have demonstrated a reduction in the rate of fall of GFR with their use.

See Chapter 13 for more information on antihypertensive agents.

PROTEIN RESTRICTION

Animal studies have shown that restriction of dietary protein intake also reduces hyperfiltration and intraglomerular pressure and retards the progression of several models of renal disease, including diabetic glomerulopathy: Several small studies in humans with diabetic nephropathy have shown that a prescribed protein-restricted diet of 0.6 g/kg/day (subjects actually only achieved a restriction of 0.8 g/kg/day) retards the rate of fall of GFR modestly. However, the Modified Diet in Renal Disease Study, in which only 3% of the patients had type 2 diabetes and none had type 1 diabetes, failed to show a clear benefit of protein restriction.

At this point in time, the general consensus is to prescribe a protein intake of approximately the adult Recommended Dietary Allowance (RDA) of 0.8 g/kg/day (~10% of daily calories) in the patient with overt nephropathy. However, it has been suggested that once the GFR begins to fall, further restriction to 0.6 g/kg/day may prove useful in slowing the decline of GFR in selected patients. On the other hand, nutrition deficiency may occur in some individuals and may be associated with muscle weakness. Protein-restricted meal plans should be designed by a registered dietitian familiar with all components of the dietary management of diabetes.

OTHER ASPECTS OF TREATMENT

Other standard modalities for the treatment of progressive renal disease and its complications (e.g., osteodystrophy) must also be used when indicated, such as sodium and phosphate restriction and use of phosphate binders. When the GFR begins to decline substantially, referral to a physician experienced in the care of such patients is indicated. Radiocontrast media are particularly nephrotoxic in patients with diabetic nephropathy, and azotemic patients should be carefully hydrated before receiving any procedures requiring contrast that cannot be avoided.

General recommendations
- To reduce the risk and/or slow the progression of nephropathy, optimize glucose control. (A)
- To reduce the risk and/or slow the progression of nephropathy, optimize blood pressure control. (A)

Screening
- Perform an annual test for the presence of microalbuminia in 1) type 1 diabetic patients who have had diabetes >5 years and 2) all type 2 diabetic patients starting at diagnosis. (E)

Treatment
- In the treatment of albuminuria/ nephropathy both ACE inhibitors and ARBs can be used:
  - In hypertensive type 1 diabetic patients with any degree of albuminuria, ACE inhibitors have been shown to delay the progression of nephropathy. (A)
  - In hypertensive type 2 diabetic patients with microalbuminuria, ACE inhibitors and ARBs have been shown to delay the progression to macroalbuminuria. (A)

– In patients with type 2 diabetes, hypertension, macroalbuminuria, and renal insufficiency (serum creatinine >1.5 mg/dL), ARBs have been shown to delay the progression of nephropathy. (A)

- If one class is not tolerated, the other should be substituted. (E)
- With regards to slowing the progression of nephropathy, the use of DCCBs as initial therapy is not more effective than placebo. Their use in nephropathy should be restricted to additional therapy to further lower blood pressure in patients already treated with ACE inhibitors or ARBs. (B)
- In the setting of the albuminuria or nephropathy, in patients unable to tolerate ACE inhibitors and/or ARBs, consider the use of non-DCCBs, β-blockers, or diuretics for the management of blood pressure. (E)
- With the onset of overt nephropathy, initiate protein restriction to 0.8 g/kg/day (~10% of daily calories), the current adult RDA for protein. Further restriction may be useful in slowing the decline of GFR in selected patients. (B)
- If ACE inhibitors or ARBs are used, monitor serum potassium levels for the development of hyperkalemia. (B)
- Consider referral to a physician experienced in the care of diabetic renal disease when either the GFR has fallen to <60 mL/min/m² or difficulties have occurred in the management of hypertension or hyperkalemia. (B)

SUMMARY

Annual screening for microalbuminuria will allow the identification of patients with nephropathy at a point very early in its course. Improving glycemic control, aggressive antihypertensive treatment, and the use of ACE inhibitors or ARBs will slow the rate of progression of nephropathy. In addition, protein restriction and other treatment modalities such as phosphate lowering may have benefits in selected patients.

FOOTNOTES

The recommendations in this paper are based on the evidence reviewed in the following publications: Diabetic nephropathy: etiologic and therapeutic considerations. *Diabetes Rev* 3:510–564, 1995; and Prevention of diabetic renal disease with special reference to microalbuminuria. *Lancet* 346:1080–1084, 1995.

The initial draft of this paper was prepared by Mark E. Molitch, MD (chair); Ralph A. DeFronzo, MD; Marion J. Franz, MS, RD, CDE; William F. Keane, MD; Carl Erik Mogensen, MD; Hans-Henrik Parving, MD; and Michael W. Steffes, MD, PhD. The paper was peer-reviewed, modified, and approved by the Professional Practice Committee and the Executive Committee, November 1996. Most recent review/revision, October 2001.

REFERENCES

1. American Diabetes Association. *Diabetes 2001 Vital Statistics.* Alexandria, VA, ADA, 2001
2. American Diabetes Association: Standards of medical care in diabetes (Position Statement). *Diabetes Care* 27: (Suppl. 1):S15–S35, 2004.
3. American Diabetes Association: Hypertension management in adults with diabetes (Position Statement). *Diabetes Care* 27 (Suppl. 1):S65–S67, 2004
4. Bakris GL, Williams M, Dworkin L, Elliott WJ, Epstein M, Toto R, Tuttle K, Douglas J, Hsueh W, Sowers J: Preserving renal function in adults with hypertension and diabetes: a consensus approach. *Am J Kid Dis* 36:646–661, 2000.
5. Brenner BM, Cooper ME, de Zeeuw D, Keane WF, Mitch WE, Parving HH, Remuzzi G, Snapinn SM, Zhang Z, Shahinfar S: Effects of losartan on renal and cardiovascular outcomes in patients with type 2 diabetes and nephropathy. *N Engl J Med* 345:861–869, 2001.
6. DeFronzo RA: Diabetic nephropathy: etiologic and therapeutic considerations. *Diabetes Rev* 3:510–564, 1995
7. Diabetes Control and Complications Trial Research Group: The effect of intensive treatment of diabetes on the development and progression of long-term complications in insulin-dependent diabetes mellitus. *N Engl J Med* 329:977–986, 1993.
8. Lewis EJ, Hunsicker LG, Clarke WR, Berl T, Pohl MA, Lewis JB, Ritz E, Atkins RC, Rohde BS, Raz I: Renoprotective effect of the angiotensin-receptor antagonist irbesartan in patients with nephropathy due to type 2 diabetes. *N Eng J Med* 345:851–860, 2001.

9. Lewis EJ, Hunsicker LG, Bain RP, and Rohde RD. The effect of angiotensin-converting-enzyme inhibition on diabetic nephropathy. The Collaborative Study Group. *N Engl J Med* 329:1456–1462, 1993.

10. Mogensen CE, Keane WF, Bennett PH, Jerums G, Parving H-H, Passa P, Steffes MW, Striker GE, Viberti GC: Prevention of diabetic renal disease with special reference to microalbuminuria. *Lancet* 346:1080–1084, 1995.

11. Mogensen CE, Neldam S, Tikkanen I, Oren S, Viskoper R, Watts RW, Cooper ME: Randomised controlled trial of dual blockade of renin-angiotensin system in patients with hypertension, microalbuminuria, and non-insulin dependent diabetes: the Candesartan and Lisinopril Microalbuminuria (CALM) Study. *BMJ* 1440–1444, 2000.

12. Parving HH, Lehnert H, Brochner-Mortensen J, Gomis R, Andersen S, Arner P: The effect of irbesartan on the development of diabetic nephropathy in patients with type 2 diabetes. *N Engl J Med* 345:870–878, 2001.

13. UK Prospective Diabetes Study Group: Efficacy of atenolol and captopril in reducing the risk of macrovascular complications in type 2 diabetes (UKPDS 39). *BMJ* 317:713–720, 1998.

14. UK Prospective Diabetes Study Group: Intensive blood glucose control with sulphonylureas or insulin compared with conventional treatment and risk of complications in patients with type 2 diabetes (UKPDS 33). *Lancet* 352:837–853, 1998.

15. UK Prospective Diabetes Study Group: Tight blood pressure control and risk of macrovascular and microvascular complications in type 2 diabetes (UKPDS 38). *BMJ* 317:703–713, 1998.

Retinopathy in Diabetes

Donald S. Fong, MD, MPH, Lloyd Aiello, MD, PHD, Thomas W. Gardner, MD, George L. King, MD, George Blankenship, MD, Jerry D. Cavallerano, OD, PHD, Fredrick L. Ferris, III, MD and Ronald Klein, MD, MPH for the American Diabetes Association

INTRODUCTION

Diabetic retinopathy is the most frequent cause of new cases of blindness among adults aged 20–74 years. During the first two decades of disease, nearly all patients with type 1 diabetes and >60% of patients with type 2 diabetes have retinopathy. In the Wisconsin Epidemiologic Study of Diabetic Retinopathy (WESDR), 3.6% of younger-onset patients (type 1 diabetes) and 1.6% of older-onset patients (type 2 diabetes) were legally blind. In the younger-onset group, 86% of blindness was attributable to diabetic retinopathy. In the older-onset group, in which other eye diseases were common, one-third of the cases of legal blindness were due to diabetic retinopathy.

NATURAL HISTORY OF DIABETIC RETINOPATHY

Diabetic retinopathy progresses from mild nonproliferative abnormalities, characterized by increased vascular permeability, to moderate and severe nonproliferative diabetic retinopathy (NPDR), characterized by vascular closure, to proliferative diabetic retinopathy (PDR), characterized by the growth of new blood vessels on the retina and posterior surface of the vitreous. Macular edema, characterized by retinal thickening from leaky blood vessels, can develop at all stages of retinopathy. Pregnancy, puberty, blood glucose control, hypertension, and cataract surgery can accelerate these changes.

Vision-threatening retinopathy is rare in type 1 diabetic patients in the first 3–5 years of diabetes or before puberty. During the next two decades, nearly all type 1 diabetic patients develop retinopathy. Up to 21% of patients with type 2 diabetes have retinopathy at the time of first diagnosis of diabetes, and most develop some degree of retinopathy over time. Vision loss due to diabetic retinopathy results from several mechanisms. Central vision may be impaired by macular edema or capillary nonperfusion. New blood vessels of PDR and contraction of the accompanying fibrous tissue can distort the retina and lead to tractional retinal detachment, producing severe and often irreversible vision loss. In addition, the new blood vessels may bleed, adding the further

Abbreviations: DCCT, Diabetes Control and Complications Trial, ETDRS, Early Treatment Diabetic Retinopathy Study, HRC, high-risk characteristic, NPDR, nonproliferative diabetic retinopathy, PDR, proliferative diabetic retinopathy, UKPDS, U.K. Prospective Diabetes Study, WESDR, Wisconsin Epidemiologic Study of Diabetic Retinopathy

complication of preretinal or vitreous hemorrhage. Finally, neovascular glaucoma associated with PDR can be a cause of visual loss.

RISK FACTORS AND TREATMENTS

Duration of disease
The duration of diabetes is probably the strongest predictor for development and progression of retinopathy. Among younger-onset patients with diabetes in the WESDR, the prevalence of any retinopathy was 8% at 3 years, 25% at 5 years, 60% at 10 years, and 80% at 15 years. The prevalence of PDR was 0% at 3 years and increased to 25% at 15 years (1). The incidence of retinopathy also increased with increasing duration. The 4-year incidence of developing proliferative retinopathy in the WESDR younger-onset group increased from 0% during the first 5 years to 27.9% during years 13–14 of diabetes. After 15 years, the incidence of developing PDR remained stable.

GLYCEMIC CONTROL

The Diabetes Control and Complications Trial (DCCT) investigated the effect of hyperglycemia in type 1 diabetic patients, as well as the incidence of diabetic retinopathy, nephropathy, and neuropathy. A total of 1,441 patients who had either no retinopathy at baseline (primary prevention cohort) or minimal-to-moderate NPDR (secondary progression cohort) were treated by either conventional treatment (one or two daily injections of insulin) or intensive diabetes management with three or more daily insulin injections or a continuous subcutaneous insulin infusion. In the primary prevention cohort, the cumulative incidence of progression in retinopathy over the first 36 months was quite similar between the two groups.

After that time, there was a persistent decrease in the intensive group. Intensive therapy reduced the mean risk of retinopathy by 76% (95% CI 62–85). In the secondary intervention cohort, the intensive group had a higher cumulative incidence of sustained progression during the first year. However, by 36 months, the intensive group had lower risks of progression. Intensive therapy reduced the risk of progression by 54% (95% CI 39–66).

The protective effect of glycemic control has also been for confirmed patients with type 2 diabetes. The U.K. Prospective Diabetes Study (UKPDS) demonstrated that improved blood glucose control reduced the risk of developing retinopathy and nephropathy and possibly reduces neuropathy. The overall rate of microvascular complications was decreased by 25% in patients receiving intensive therapy versus conventional therapy. Epidemiological analysis of the UKPDS data showed a continuous relationship between the risk of microvascular complications and glycemia, such that for every percentage point decrease in HbA_{1c} (e.g., from 8 to 7%), there was a 35% reduction in the risk of microvascular complications.

BLOOD PRESSURE CONTROL

The UKPDS also investigated the influence of tight blood pressure control (2). A total of 1,148 hypertensive patients with type 2 diabetes were randomized to less tight (<180/105 mmHg) and tight blood pressure control (<150/85 mmHg) with the use of an ACE inhibitor or a β-blocker. With a median follow-up of 8.4 years, patients assigned to tight control had a 34% reduction in progression of retinopathy and a 47% reduced risk of deterioration in visual acuity of three lines in association with a 10/5 mmHg reduction in blood pressure. In addition, there were reductions in deaths related to diabetes and strokes.

To determine whether intensive blood pressure control offers additional benefit over moderate control, the Appropriate Blood Pressure Control in Diabetes (ABCD) Trial (3) randomized patients to either intensive or moderate blood pressure control. Hypertensive subjects, defined as having a baseline diastolic blood pressure of ≥90 mmHg, were randomized to intensive blood pressure control (diastolic blood pressure goal of 75 mmHg) versus moderate blood pressure control (diastolic blood pressure goal of 80–89 mmHg). A total of 470 patients were randomized to either nisoldipine or enalapril and followed for a mean of 5.3 years. The mean blood pressure achieved was 132/78 mmHg in the intensive group and 138/86 mmHg in the moderate control group. Although intensive therapy demonstrated a lower incidence of deaths (5.5 vs. 10.7%, $P=0.037$), there was no difference between the intensive and moderate groups with regard to the progression of diabetic retinopathy and neuropathy.

To determine whether inhibitors of ACE can slow progression of nephropathy in patients without hypertension, the EURO-DIAB Controlled Trial of Lisinopril in Insulin Dependent Diabetes (EUCLID) study group investigated the effect of lisinopril on retinopathy in type 1 diabetes. Eligible patients were not hypertensive, and were normoalbuminuric (85%) or microalbuminuric. The proportion of patients with retinopathy at baseline was similar, but patients assigned to lisinopril had significantly lower HbA_{1c} at baseline. Treatment reduced the development of retinopathy, but the effect may have been due to its pressure-lowering effect in patients who had undetected hypertension. Until these issues are addressed, these findings need to be confirmed before changes to clinical practice can be advocated.

ASPIRIN TREATMENT

The Early Treatment Diabetic Retinopathy Study (ETDRS) investigated whether aspirin (650 mg/day) could retard the progression of retinopathy. After examining progression of retinopathy, development of vitreous hemorrhage, or duration of vitreous hemorrhage, aspirin was shown to have no effect on retinopathy. With these findings, there are no ocular contraindications to the use of aspirin when required for cardiovascular disease or other medical indications.

LASER PHOTOCOAGULATION

The Diabetic Retinopathy Study (DRS) investigated whether scatter (panretinal) photocoagulation, compared with indefinite deferral, could reduce the risk of vision loss from PDR. After only 2 years, photocoagulation was shown to significantly reduce severe visual loss (i.e., best acuity of 5/200 or worse). The benefit persisted through the entire duration of follow-up and was greatest among patients whose eyes had high-risk characteristics (HRCs; disc neovascularization or vitreous hemorrhage with any retinal neovascuariztion). The treatment effect was much smaller for eyes that did not have HRCs.

To determine the timing of photocoagulation, the ETDRS examined the effect of treating eyes with mild NPDR to early PDR. The rates of visual loss were low with either treatment applied early or delayed until development of HRCs. Because of this low rate and the risk of complications, the report suggested that scatter photocoagulation be deferred in eyes with mild-to-moderate NPDR. The ETDRS also demonstrated the effectiveness of focal photocoagulation in eyes with macular edema. In patients with clinically significant macular edema, 24% of untreated eyes, compared with 12% of treated eyes, developed doubling of the visual angle.

EVALUATION OF DIABETIC RETINOPATHY

An important cause of blindness, diabetic retinopathy has few visual or ophthalmic symptoms until visual loss develops. At present, laser photocoagulation for diabetic retinopathy is effective at slowing the progression of retinopathy and reducing visual loss, but the treatment usually does not restore lost vision. Because these treatments are aimed at preventing vision loss and retinopathy can be asymptomatic, it is important to identify and treat patients early in the disease. To achieve this goal, patients with diabetes should be routinely evaluated to detect treatable disease.

Dilated indirect ophthalmoscopy coupled with biomicroscopy and seven-standard field stereoscopic 30° fundus photography are both accepted methods for examining diabetic retinopathy. Stereo fundus photography is more sensitive at detecting retinopathy than clinical examination, but clinical examination is superior for detecting retinal thickening from macular edema and for early neovascularization. Fundus photography also requires both a trained photographer and a trained reader.

The use of film and digital nonmydriatic images to examine for diabetic retinopathy has been described. Although they permit undilated photographic retinopathy screening, these techniques have not been fully evaluated. The use of the nonmydriatic camera for follow-up of patients with diabetes in the physician's office might be considered in situations where dilated eye examination cannot be obtained.

Guidelines for the frequency of dilated eye examinations have been largely based on the severity of the retinopathy (1,4). For patients with moderate-to-severe NPDR, frequent eye examinations are necessary to determine when to initiate treatment. However, for patients without retinopathy or with only few microaneurysms, the need for annual dilated eye examinations is not as well defined. For these patients, the annual incidence of progression to either proliferative retinopathy or macular edema is low; therefore, some have suggested a longer interval between examinations (5). Recently, analyses suggested that annual examination for some patients with type 2 diabetes may not be cost-effective and that consideration should be given to increasing the screening interval (6). However, these analyses may not have completely considered all the factors: 1) The analyses assumed that legal blindness was the only level of visual loss with economic consequences, but other visual function outcomes, such as visual acuity worse than 20/40, are clinically important, occur much more frequently, and have economic consequences. 2) The analyses used NPDR progression figures from newly diagnosed patients with diabetes (7). Although rates of progression are stratified by HbA_{1c} levels, newly diagnosed patients are different from those with the same level of retinopathy and have a longer diabetes duration. While rates of progression correlate with HbA_{1c} levels, newly diagnosed patients with the same level of retinopathy progress differently than those with longer duration of disease. A person with a longer duration of diabetes is more likely to progress during the next year of observation (8). 3) The rates of progression were derived from diabetic individuals of northern European extraction and are not applicable to other ethnic and racial groups who have higher rates of retinopathy progression, such as African- and Hispanic-Americans (9,10).

In determining the examination interval for an individual patient, the eye care

Table 1. Ophthalmologic Examination Schedule

Patient group	Recommended first examination	Minimum routine follow-up*
Type 1 diabetes	Within 3–5 years after diagnosis of diabetes once patient is age 10 years or older†	Yearly
Type 2 diabetes	At time of diagnosis of diabetes	Yearly
Pregnancy in preexisting diabetes	Prior to conception and during first trimester	Physician discretion pending results of first trimester exam

* Abnormal findings necessitate more frequent follow-up.

† Some evidence suggests that the prepubertal duration of diabetes may be important in the development of microvascular complications; therefore, clinical judgment should be used when applying these recommendations to individual patients.

provider should also consider the implications of less frequent eye examinations. Older people are at higher risk for cataract, glaucoma, age-related macular degeneration, and other potentially blinding disorders. Detection of these problems adds value to the examination but is rarely considered in analyses of screening interval. Patient education also occurs during examinations. Patients know the importance of controlling their blood glucose, blood pressure, and serum lipids, and this importance can be reinforced at a time when patients are particularly aware of the implications of vision loss. In addition, long intervals between follow-up visits may lead to difficulties in maintaining contact with patients. Patients may be unlikely to remember that they need an eye examination after several years have passed.

After considering these issues, and in the absence of empirical data showing otherwise, persons with diabetes should have an annual eye examination.

SUMMARY AND RECOMMENDATIONS

Treatment modalities exist that can prevent or delay the onset of diabetic retinopathy, as well as prevent loss of vision, in a large proportion of patients with diabetes. The DCCT and the UKPDS established that glycemic and blood pressure control can prevent and delay the progression of diabetic retinopathy in patients with diabetes. Timely laser photocoagulation therapy can also prevent loss of vision in a large proportion of patients with severe NPDR and PDR and/or macular edema. Because a significant number of patients with vision-threatening disease may not have symptoms, ongoing evaluation for retinopathy is a valuable and required strategy.

The recommendations for initial and subsequent ophthalmologic evaluation of patients with diabetes are stated below and summarized in **Table 1**.

GUIDELINES

Patients with type 1 diabetes should have an initial dilated and comprehensive eye examination by an ophthalmologist or optometrist within 3–5 years after the onset of diabetes. In general, evaluation for diabetic eye disease is not necessary before 10 years of age. However, some evidence suggests that the prepubertal duration of diabetes may be important in the development of microvascular complications; therefore, clinical judgment should be used when applying these recommendations to individual patients. (B)

Patients with type 2 diabetes should have an initial dilated and comprehensive eye examination by an ophthalmologist or optometrist shortly after diabetes diagnosis. (B)

Subsequent examinations for both type 1 and type 2 diabetic patients should be repeated annually by an ophthalmologist or optometrist who is knowledgeable and experienced in diagnosing the presence of diabetic retinopathy and is aware of its management. Less frequent exams (every 2–3 years) may be considered with the advice of an eye care professional in the setting of a normal eye exam. Examinations will be required more frequently if retinopathy is progressing. This follow-up interval is recommended recognizing that there are limited data addressing this issue. (B)

When planning pregnancy, women with preexisting diabetes should have a comprehensive eye examination and should be counseled on the risk of development and/or progression of diabetic retinopathy. Women with diabetes who become pregnant should have a comprehensive eye examination in the first trimester and close follow-up throughout pregnancy (**Table 1**). This guideline does not apply to women who develop gestational diabetes, because such individuals are not at increased risk for diabetic retinopathy. (B)

Patients with any level of macular edema, severe NPDR, or any PDR require the prompt care of an ophthalmologist who is knowledgeable and experienced in the management and treatment of diabetic retinopathy. Referral to an ophthalmologist should not be delayed until PDR has developed in patients who are known to have severe nonproliferative or more advanced retinopathy. Early referral to an ophthalmologist is particularly important for patients with type 2 diabetes and severe NPDR, since laser treatment at this stage is associated with a 50% reduction in the risk of severe visual loss and vitrectomy. (E)

Patients who experience vision loss from diabetes should be encouraged to pursue visual rehabilitation with an ophthalmologist or optometrist who is trained or experienced in low-vision care. (E)

ACKNOWLEDGEMENTS

This manuscript was developed in cooperation with the American Optometric Association (Michael Duneas, OD), and the American Academy of Ophthalmology (Donald S. Fong, MD, MPH). We gratefully acknowledge the invaluable assistance of these associations and their designated representatives.

FOOTNOTES

The recommendations in this paper are based on the evidence reviewed in the following publication: Diabetic retinopathy (Technical Review). *Diabetes Care* 21:143–156, 1998. Most recent review/revision, 2002

REFERENCES

1. Klein R, Klein BE, Moss SE, Davis MD, DeMets DL: The Wisconsin Epidemiologic Study of Diabetic Retinopathy. II. Prevalence and risk of diabetic retinopathy when age at diagnosis is less than 30 years. *Arch Ophthalmol* 102: 520–526, 1984.

2. UK Prospective Diabetes Study Group: Tight blood pressure control and risk of macrovascular and microvascular complications in type 2 diabetes: UKPDS 38. *BMJ* 317: 708–713, 1998.

3. Estacio RO, Jeffers BW, Gifford N, Schrier RW: Effect of blood pressure control on diabetic microvascular complications in patients with hypertension and type 2 diabetes. *Diabetes Care* 23 (Suppl. 2): B54–B64, 2000.

4. Klein R, Klein BE, Moss SE, Davis MD, DeMets DL: The Wisconsin Epidemiologic Study of Diabetic Retinopathy. III. Prevalence and risk of diabetic retinopathy when age at diagnosis is 30 or more years. *Arch Ophthalmol* 102: 527–532, 1984.

5. Batchelder T, Barricks M: The Wisconsin Epidemiologic Study of Diabetic Retinopathy (Letter) *Arch Ophthalmol* 113: 702–703, 1995.

6. Vijan S, Hofer TP, Hayward RA: Cost-utility analysis of screening intervals for diabetic retinopathy in patients with type 2 diabetes mellitus. *JAMA* 283: 889–896, 2000.

7. UK Prospective Diabetes Study (UKPDS) Group: Effect of intensive blood-glucose control with metformin on complications in overweight patients with type 2 diabetes (UKPDS 34). *Lancet* 12:352: 854–865, 1998.

8. Klein R, Klein BE, Moss SE, Cruickshanks KJ: The Wisconsin Epidemiologic Study of Diabetic Retinopathy. XIV. Ten-year incidence and progression of diabetic retinopathy. *Arch Ophthalmol* 112: 1217–1228, 1994.

9. Harris MI, Klein R, Cowie CC, Rowland M, Byrd-Holt DD: Is the risk of diabetic retinopathy greater in non-Hispanic blacks and Mexican Americans than in non-Hispanic whites with type 2 diabetes? A U.S. population study. *Diabetes Care* 21: 1230–1235, 1998.

10. Haffner SM, Fong D, Stern MP, Pugh JA, Hazuda HP, Patterson JK, van Heuven WA, Klein R: Diabetic retinopathy in Mexican Americans and non-Hispanic whites. *Diabetes* 37: 878–884, 1988.

Chapter 18

Diabetic Neuropathic Disorders

Travis E. Sonnett, PharmD

OVERVIEW

Diabetes and neuropathy have been associated for over a century, with the first structural classification performed by Leyden in 1893. The term "diabetic neuropathy" encompasses several different forms of neuropathy, and several different origins of neuropathy in the diabetic patient, from metabolic to immune. The two most common forms of neuropathy in the diabetic patient are diabetic peripheral neuropathy (DPN), and diabetic autonomic neuropathy (DAN).

DPN occurs in both type 1 and type 2 diabetic patients, and may result from several different damaged pathways. Chronic hyperglycemia, resulting in microvascular and neuronal damage, is the main mechanism by which DPN is considered to develop. Nerve biopsies of diabetic patients diagnosed with DPN have shown a thickening of the basement membranes of vessels feeding damaged neurons, and a greater variation overall of vessel lumen thickness. Damaged blood vessels display a poor vasodilatory response to nitric oxide, and ischemia is prominent in the microvasculature. Following this cascade, hypoxia will eventually follow, leading to neuronal starvation and death. Increased influx of glucose and other sugar molecules may increase basement membrane thickening through the polyol flux pathway. This pathway may also be responsible for destruction

of neuronal supporting cells, leading to eventual axonal changes. These changes may include an increase of intraneuronal sodium, slowing nerve conduction in both sensory and motor neurons. Oxidative stress in tandem with the polyol pathway is another mechanism by which neuronal damage, and ultimately DPN, is theorized to occur, with free radicals damaging neuronal tissue. Antioxidant levels in the diabetic patient are depleted, allowing formation of free radicals through the oxidation of glucose and other cellular mechanisms. Free radicals such as peroxynitrite and superoxide form, and the damage produced can ultimately lead to neuronal cell death. Through these mechanisms, microvascular damage and neuronal cell death occur, leading to neurodegeneration and the development of DPN. Clinical manifestations of this complication arise as a change in sensation in the extremities, most commonly beginning in the toes and feet. The sensation is identified as a sensory anomaly (eg, tingling, burning, or crawling) of the affected area, or can be a loss of sensation. Progression of sensory loss may occur, increasing the patient's risk of complications such as diabetic foot ulceration or Charcot joints. Treatment is available for the symptoms associated with DPN.

Diabetic autonomic neuropathy is the most significant form of neuropathy affecting the diabetic patient, as this can involve the cardiovascular, gastrointestinal, and genitourinary systems. Autonomic neuropathy does not require the involvement of large nerve fibers, and is considered by some to be a larger category of DPN. Cardiovascular complications associated with DAN can lead to hypotensive episodes, irregular heartbeat, and instability related to anesthetic administration, and increased risk of myocardial infarction and sudden death. Gastrointestinal neuropathy can involve the GI tract as a whole, and is commonly identified by gastroparesis and esophageal difficulties. Genitourinary neuropathy occurs through loss of coordination of smooth muscle, and often results in urinary incontinence issues and sexual dysfunction in both men and women. Therapies are available to treat all forms of DAN, although most involve intensive glucose control, coupled with medications addressing the symptoms associated with the affected organ system.

GABA ANALOGS (GABAPENTIN, PREGABALIN)

Gabapentin and pregabalin are structurally related GABA analogs available for the treatment of neuropathic pain associated with DPN and post-herpetic neuralgia. Initially available in 1993 for adjunctive treatment of partial seizures, gabapentin has since been studied for neuropathy, while pregabalin was FDA-approved in 2004 for treatment of diabetic-associated neuropathy and post-herpetic neuralgia. While gabapentin and pregabalin may share the same mechanism of action, kinetic differences between these agents warrant review prior to prescribing DPN therapy.

Pharmacology
Gabapentin and pregabalin are structurally related to the neurotransmitter gamma-aminobutyric acid (GABA), but do not influence receptors or utilize this pathway as

a mechanism of action. These agents bind to the α_2-Δ subunit of neural presynaptic voltage-gated calcium channels, decreasing calcium flow. Decreased neurotransmitter release from these neurons occurs, thus limiting neuronal excitation. This mechanism is theorized to account for the analgesic effect and decrease in neuropathic pain produced through administration of pregabalin or gabapentin. Suppression of neuronal peptides such as substance P, glutamate, and upregulation of GABA transporters are other pathways by which GABA analogs are theorized to impact neuronal pain transmission.

Pregabalin follows a linear kinetics model, with peak concentrations achieved 1.5 hours after administration, and steady state concentrations achieved after 1-2 days of continuous dosing. Gabapentin is a nonlinear agent, with bioavailability varying based on dose of the medication. Neither medication is significantly protein bound, or metabolized by the CYP450 system. Both medications are primarily cleared by the renal system; dosing adjustments based on renal impairment may be required, while both agents are dialyzable. Dosing adjustments in the elderly may be necessary based on renal function as well. The half-life for these agents is 5-7 hours, and may increase in patients with impaired renal function.

Clinical Advantages
Pregabalin has been found to exhibit linear kinetics during clinical trials, and may have a more predictable dose/response expectation when compared to gabapentin. While gabapentin does have an FDA-approved maximum dose, it has been studied at doses in excess of 3200mg with successful response. Tolerance may develop with continued gabapentin use, and dose escalation may be required to alleviate pain. Pregabalin has not been reported to develop tolerance at this time; continued monitoring to ensure successful therapy is still recommended.

Therapeutic Considerations

Precaution is warranted in patients with a true hypersensitivity reaction to one of these agents when considering use of the other; while true cross-reactivity is not known, the chemical relation may predispose a patient to allergy. Risk of suicidal ideation and self-harm has also been found in clinical trials with anticonvulsants, and this warning is extended to use of GABA analogs as well. Common side effects of GABA analogs include, but are not limited to: sedation, dizziness, CNS depression, blurred vision, balance issues, tremor, and confusion. A more detailed list is provided in **Table 18.1** for these medications. GABA analogs are classified pregnancy risk category C, and should only be used in breast-feeding patients where the benefit outweighs any risk; it is unknown if either of these agents is excreted in breast milk. Administration of GABA analogs with other CNS depressants may increase risk of sedation and other like side effects. Pregabalin should be administered with thiazolidinediones with caution, as these agents combined may increase the risk of weight gain and edema. Gabapentin should be administered at least 2 hours before or after antacid therapy, as antacids (eg, aluminum hydroxide, magnesium hydroxide) may decrease the bioavailability of gabapentin by 20%. Discontinuation of either agent should be performed in a downward titration, as withdrawal-like symptoms may occur with abrupt discontinuation of therapy. (See **Table 18.2** for more information on drug interactions.) Pregabalin is a schedule C-V controlled substance, and appropriate monitoring for misuse must be undertaken when prescribing this medication.

DULOXETINE

Duloxetine is a serotonin-norepinephrine reuptake inhibitor (SNRI), and the first agent approved for treatment of DPN. While sharing distinction with another SNRI, venlafaxine, duloxetine is the only medication in the SNRI class that is approved for use in both major depressive disorder and DPN.

Pharmacology

Duloxetine is a dual-acting SNRI, and is considered to maintain its analgesic effect through this mechanism. Serotonin and norepinephrine elicit neurogenic transmission in the brainstem and spinal column, and are theorized to minimize pain transmission from the periphery to the CNS via these pathways. Duloxetine has no effect at H_1-histaminergic, α-adrenergic, dopaminergic, or opioid receptors. Sodium channel activity also occurs minimally with this medication.

Duloxetine is provided as an encapsulated form, which contains enteric coated pellets; duloxetine degrades in an acidic environment, and requires enteric coating to survive the stomach and pass into the small intestine for absorption. Upon administration, duloxetine absorption occurs in approximately 2 hours, achieving peak in 6 hours. Steady state plasma concentrations are achieved in approximately 3 days. Duloxetine is over 90% protein bound, and interactions between other highly protein bound medications may occur. Duloxetine metabolism occurs via CYP450 2D6 and 1A2, with a half-life of 8-17 hours. Elimination occurs primarily through the urine (70%), with secondary elimination though the feces (20%).

Clinical Advantages

Duloxetine is a dual-acting antidepressant, and may be an optimal choice for the diabetic patient with both neuropathy and depression. Fixed dosing and lack of tolerance are positive considerations for duloxetine when considering DPN therapy.

Therapeutic Considerations

Duloxetine is a substrate of CYP2D6 and 1A2, and as such can be affected by medications acting as both inhibitors and inducers of these isoenzymes. Studies with fluvoxamine, an inhibitor of CYP1A2, displayed an increase in concentration and half-life of duloxetine; other CYP1A2 inhibitors may have the same effect. Inhibitors of CYP2D6 may have a like effect; paroxetine has been shown to increase concentrations and half life of duloxetine. Duloxetine is also an inhibitor of CYP2D6, and has been shown to increase levels of medications such as flecainide and propafenone. **Table 18.2** shows an extensive list of medications known to interact with duloxetine, and medications that should be co-administered with caution. Patients should be monitored for cardiovascular changes when duloxetine is first initiated, as increases in blood pressure and heart rate may occur. Common side effects with duloxetine include, but are not restricted to: nausea and vomiting, dizziness, fatigue, and somnolence. **Table 18.1** illustrates a more thorough adverse effect profile. Adverse effects may occur within the first eight weeks of treatment initiation or at a dosage increase, but typically dissipate with time. Duloxetine has been shown in study to be well tolerated by the elderly, while dose adjustments for hepatic and renally impaired patients are not necessary. Discontinuation of duloxetine is recommended through a downward dose titration, while cross-titration of other agents may occur.

TRICYCLIC ANTIDEPRESSANTS

Tricyclic antidepressants (TCAs) have been available for more than 40 years, and have been used to treat a number of conditions, from depression to neuropathic pain. TCAs were the first medication class used in placebo-controlled trials for neuropathic pain, while several clinical trials performed investigated the effectiveness of TCAs as a

primary treatment for DPN. Regardless of these trials, there is not an FDA-approved TCA for treatment of neuropathic pain. While these medications are considered first-line agents by many healthcare professionals for the treatment of DPN, there are several factors to take into consideration when selecting a TCA as a treatment.

Pharmacology
The primary mechanism of action of TCAs occurs through inhibition of serotonin and norepinephrine reuptake. Analgesic effect is considered to be independent of the primary antidepressant effect, and is theorized to be related to a secondary mechanism such as α-adrenergic, H_1-histaminergic, and muscarinic receptor blockade, sodium-channel blockade, or possibly N-methyl-D-aspartate blockade. Dopamine is not directly affected by this class of medications, although reuptake may fluctuate through indirect effects on adrenergic receptors.

Distribution of TCAs occurs in every organ system of the body, primarily in the brain, heart, liver, and lung tissues. While peak plasma levels may occur within 24 hours, peak effect may not be seen until two to four weeks. TCAs are also highly protein bound, and interactions with other protein bound medications (eg, warfarin) need to monitored. Elimination half-lives for these medications vary between agents, and can last from 6-100 hours. Metabolism occurs mainly in the liver, with excretion of these medications occurring in both the urine and feces.

Clinical Advantages
While TCAs are not FDA-approved for the treatment of DPN, success has been reported in treatment of DPN with every one of the covered agents. Side effect profiles limit the usefulness of these medications, however; nortriptyline and desipramine are the preferred agents in this class, as the side effect frequency and profile are considered to be

less severe. TCAs may also aid in patients diagnosed with other disease states, such as depression, sleep disorders, urinary incontinence, and behavioral disorders.

Therapeutic Considerations

TCAs are separated into two categories: secondary amines (eg, amitriptyline, imipramine) and tertiary amines (eg, nortriptyline, desipramine). While the mechanisms of each category remain the same, the side effect comparison varies. Secondary amines have been shown to produce a markedly lower incidence of adverse effects when compared to tertiary amines, and are considered the more favorable selection for treatment of neuropathic disorders. Anticholinergic effects are considered the most common ADR experienced with this class of medications, while **Table 18.1** will provide a comprehensive list. Patients with a history of suicidal ideation must be monitored when using these medications, as TCAs can produce toxicity and death when taken inappropriately. Elderly patients should be monitored closely for adverse events, as this class of medications can produce confusion, delirium, and acute dementia in aged patients. Use during pregnancy is not recommended, as TCAs are a pregnancy risk Category C or D, depending upon the agent. TCAs are also not recommended for use in nursing mothers, as they actively cross through breast milk. Patients already taking antidepressant therapy must be monitored for the possibility of serotonin syndrome when started on a TCA. There are also significant interactions between TCAs and monoamine oxidase inhibitors; concurrent use of these two medication classes is not recommended. (See **Table 18.2** for a more extensive list of drug interactions.) Dosages of TCAs vary greatly between agents, and can have a large variation within the medication itself. **Table 18.1** provides a list of recommended dosages for treatment of DPN. Titration of TCAs is recommended, and may take several weeks to months to reach the target

dose; patients are also advised that these medications may take two to four weeks to reach peak effect, even after a dosage change, and must remain compliant to maximize success. TCAs can also be used with other DPN medications, such as pregabalin and gabapentin, but monitoring for ADR must be maintained to ensure patient safety and success.

CARBAMAZEPINE

Carbamazepine is one of the oldest medications studied and used to treat forms of neuropathy, specifically trigeminal neuralgia and DPN. Clinical trials dating from the early 1960s to the present have found carbamazepine to be effective in treating both DPN and trigeminal neuralgia, although the risks of adverse events may outweigh the benefits when compared to newer medications. Although not FDA-approved for DPN, cumulative clinical trial data rank carbamazepine as a first-line agent for treatment of trigeminal neuralgia, and a third line agent for treatment of DPN.

Pharmacology

Carbamazepine is classified as an iminostilbene derivative, related to the tricyclic antidepressants in chemical structure. The mechanism of action for carbamazepine is related to its ability to block voltage-dependent sodium channels, thus reducing ectopic nerve discharge and stabilizing neural membranes while minimizing effect on normal nerve conductance. Although chemically related to the TCAs, carbamazepine is not considered to have a mechanistic effect on neural transmitters.

The kinetics of carbamazepine can make it a difficult medication to manage. The therapeutic window for treatment of seizure disorders is 4-12 mcg/mL; however, a standard range for the treatment of neuropathic pain has not been established. Oral carbamazepine has a bioavailability of 70% to 80%, which is increased in the presence of food, and is 76% protein bound. Carbamazepine is 98% metabolized by the CYP450 system by isoenzyme 3A4. During prolonged therapy or higher dosing, carbamazepine autoinduction may occur through the CYP450 system; accumulation of the active metabolite of carbamazepine plays a role in the development of toxicity. Concomitant use of lamotrigine or valproic acid may increase risk of toxicity. Carbamazepine has a half-life of 25-65 hours, and is excreted through both the urine and feces.

Clinical Advantages

Carbamazepine is considered a third-line agent in the treatment of DPN. Side effects may limit its use, but reports have shown success with carbamazepine therapy when other treatment classes have failed. Carbamazepine does have a unique mechanism of action, which allows it consideration when compared to other agents.

Therapeutic Considerations

Adverse events are common with carbamazepine use, with a reported 50% occurrence rate. Common events include, but are not limited to, dizziness, drowsiness, blurred vision, and nausea (see **Table 18.1**). Rare blood disorders can occur with carbamazepine use, and can occur even after established use; monitoring throughout therapy is advised. Carbamazepine has also been identified to increase suicidal ideation and behavior in patients using them for all indications, with actions occurring at any point during therapy. Monitoring for signs or symptoms of depression, behavioral change, and suicidal ideation should be maintained through therapy. Patients with a history of barbiturate, hydantoin, or tricyclic antidepressant hypersensitivity are not considered candidates for

carbamazepine therapy, as cross-sensitivity can occur in 30% to 80% of patients. Caution is warranted in patients with existing liver or cardiac disease. Elderly patients should be monitored closely for adverse events, as this class of medications can produce confusion, delirium, and acute dementia in aged patients. Carbamazepine is classified as a pregnancy category D, and is not recommended in patients that are breastfeeding, although the American Pediatrics Association has deemed it acceptable if necessary. Starting dosages are recommended in **Table 18.1**, with titration to effective dose recommended.

LIDOCAINE

Topical lidocaine patches have been clinically studied for use in the treatment of DPN. Lidocaine works through inhibition of voltage-gated sodium channels, which are theorized to spontaneously activate in damaged neurons. Lidocaine has been shown to decrease pain levels in diabetic polyneuropathy, as well as increase quality of life and reduce the negative impact neuropathy may have on activities of daily living.

Pharmacology

Lidocaine topical patches have been studied in a variety of fashions, and are found to reach effect in 5-15 minutes, peak plasma levels after 18 hours, and decreased to minimal levels 12 hours after each application for a studied three-day period. Topical lidocaine reaches systemic levels equal to $^1/_{10}$ the level necessary to treat cardiac arrhythmias, and is not considered to have an appreciable effect on the cardiovascular system. Distribution of topical lidocaine is negligible, metabolism occurs primarily in the liver, while excretion is primarily through the kidneys.

Clinical Advantages

Lidocaine patches can be used as an adjunct to oral therapy, and are not considered a primary therapy. While successful in limited trials, lidocaine has not been shown to have the same rate of pain reduction as oral therapy, and is limited as a secondary therapy at this time.

Therapeutic Considerations

Common side effects associated with topical lidocaine use include, but are not restricted to skin site reactions, irritations, and discoloration. These reactions usually resolve within minutes to hours, and are considered mild. Systemic reactions are extremely rare, as topical lidocaine preparations are not systemically absorbed in concentrations that would elicit a systemic response. Adjustments for the elderly are not recommended, as changes in effect due to age have not been noted.

CAPSAICIN

Topical capsaicin cream has been successfully utilized in the treatment of neuropathic pain associated with both post-herpetic neuralgia and diabetic polyneuropathy. Capsaicin is an alkaloid derived from the herb *Capsicum officinalis*, and is believed to stimulate sensory afferent C-fibers, depleting substance P and desensitizing receptors.

Pharmacology

Capsaicin cream lasts four to six hours after application, and must be applied three to four times daily to achieve maximal effect. Pain management with capsaicin may begin as soon as two weeks, but takes six to eight weeks to reach maximal effect.

Clinical Advantages

Capsaicin can be used as an adjunct to oral therapy, and is not considered a primary agent. Limited studies have shown reductions in pain, although intolerance to the adverse effects of capsaicin reduced study populations and results. Capsaicin is limited to secondary therapy at this time.

Therapeutic Considerations

Initial application of capsaicin may result in an unpleasant burning sensation, which may persist for days after initial use. This effect may lead to discontinuation by many patients, as toleration and continuation of therapy may be difficult. Other side effects are related to application to the skin, and may be described as tingling, stinging, redness, or irritation. Applying heat with capsaicin therapy may increase the effect and intensify sensation. No special instructions are necessary when used with the elderly.

DIABETIC GASTROPARESIS

Gastroparesis is defined as a delay in gastric emptying without an obstruction of the stomach, and occurs in 30% to 50% of patients with type 1 or type 2 diabetes. Chronically elevated blood glucose and HBA_{1c} levels are associated with an increased risk of gastrointestinal symptoms associated with gastroparesis. The mechanism by which diabetic gastroparesis occurs is mainly associated with central autonomic neuropathy affecting the vagus nerve, and a decrease in the number of inhibitory neurons associated with gastrointestinal motor control. Increased levels of glucagon are also considered a factor in gastroparesis, and slow the rate at which food is delivered for digestion in the small intestine. These mechanisms lead to a decrease in fundic and antral motor activity, a reduction of interdigestive migration control, and an increase in digestive and gastric spasmodic disorders.

The common symptoms associated with diabetic gastroparesis are early satiety, nausea, vomiting, abdominal pain, and bloating. Diabetic gastroparesis can have a negative impact on the patient's quality of life, and may impact the psychological health of the patient. Other sources of delayed gastric emptying may include infection, thyroid disorders, psychological disorders, visceral nerve hypersensitivity, disordered gastric activity or mechanical disorder, or medication-induced gastroparesis. The cause of delayed gastric emptying must be identified prior to treatment, to ensure the success of chosen therapy for the patient. Several therapies are available for treatment of diabetic gastroparesis, although a combination of strict glycemic control, dietary changes, and medication therapy may result in the best outcome for the patient.

Metoclopramide

Metoclopramide was first approved for prescription usage in 1979, and is FDA-approved for the treatment of diabetic gastroparesis. It was originally investigated for treatment of pregnancy-associated nausea and vomiting, but since coming into the market, has been found to be useful in several emetic- and gastrointestinal-associated conditions.

Pharmacology

Metoclopramide acts on many neurotransmitters; it is a 5HT4 agonist, a 5HT3 antagonist, a central and peripheral dopamine D2 antagonist, as well as a cholinesterase inhibitor. Metoclopramide acts as a 5HT4 receptor agonist and peripheral dopamine D2 receptor antagonist to decrease fundal relaxation and increase antral contractions, thus improving gastric emptying. It also acts as an anti-emetic, through antagonism of central dopamine D2 receptors in the area postrema and antagonism of 5HT3 receptors.

Metoclopramide is available in oral and parenteral forms; onset of action is 30-60 minutes for oral, 10-15 minutes for IM, and 1-3 minutes for IV. Metoclopramide is only 30% protein bound, and crosses the blood brain barrier. The half-life for metoclopramide is 2.5-6 hours, allowing for dosing multiple times a day with meals. Metabolism occurs through conjugation, and the medication is primarily excreted through the urine (85%).

Clinical Advantages

Metoclopramide, through actions in the central dopaminergic system, acts as an antiemetic as well as a prokinetic agent. Metoclopramide is also available as intravenous, intramuscular, and subcutaneous injections. QT interval prolongation is also a nonissue with metoclopramide, when compared to other agents.

Therapeutic Considerations

Metoclopramide is an effective therapy for treatment of diabetic gastroparesis, but there are several notable issues with this medication that are worth discussion. Metoclopramide is available in several forms, from oral to parenteral, making it available for use in all patient settings. It is not as effective as cisapride at improving gastric emptying, and may be limited by its side effect profile. Also, after one month of oral therapy metoclopramide is not shown to improve gastric emptying of liquids, while cisapride and erythromycin have been shown to maintain improved emptying of both liquids and solids. Side effects center on the central nervous system, and include dizziness, drowsiness, motor and coordination impairment, and extrapyramidal symptoms. Due to its effects on dopamine, metoclopramide may also cause neuroendocrine effects such as lactation, gynecomastia, and impotence. A more extensive side effect profile is available in **Table 18.1**. Increasing gastric emptying may also increase or decrease the absorption of co-administered medications (eg, lithium, digoxin); plasma levels should be monitored initially for drugs with a narrow therapeutic index to ensure safety and efficacy. Use of metoclopramide in Parkinson's disease patients may lead to exacerbation of symptoms and/or complications due to metoclopramide's dopamine antagonism; close monitoring is recommended for success in Parkinson's disease therapy. Metoclopramide is renally cleared, and adjustment of metoclopramide dosing may be necessary in the renally impaired patient, as accumulation and toxicity may occur. Metoclopramide is a pregnancy Category B, and does cross in breast milk; caution is warranted when using in a breastfeeding patient.

Cisapride

Cisapride is an oral prokinetic agent that is structurally similar to metoclopramide, but lacks the CNS effects and dopamine antagonism that is part of metoclopramide's function. It was originally approved in 1993 for the treatment of GERD, and has since been used to treat diabetic gastroparesis, although this indication is not FDA approved. In 2000, cisapride was withdrawn from widespread use due to the risk of life threatening arrhythmias. It is only available through special access programs with registered physicians, with required cardiac screening, electrolytes, and monitoring prior to and during use.

Pharmacology

Cisapride increases acetylcholine release from the postganglionic nerve endings of the myenteric plexus of the stomach through agonistic activity on the 5HT4 receptor. This activity decreases gastric acid exposure of the esophagus, increases esophageal sphincter pressure and motility, increases antral contractions and improves gastric emptying of both solids and liquids, and decreases colonic transit time. Symptomatic relief with cisapride has been seen in therapy lasting >1 year. Cisapride does not cross the blood brain barrier, and is not known to cause CNS or dopamine-related adverse effects.

Administered orally, cisapride onset occurs in 30-60 minutes, while peak plasma concentrations occur in 1-2 hours. Cisapride is 98% protein bound, and is metabolized by the CYP450 isoenzyme 3A4. The half-life for cisapride is about 10 hours, although that may increase in hepatically impaired patients and the elderly. Cisapride may also prolong the cardiac QT interval, and is not recommended for use in patients with a QT interval greater than 450 ms.

Clinical Advantages

Cisapride was considered the drug of choice for treatment of diabetic gastroparesis, until reports of severe, life-threatening adverse effects led to its limited-use restriction. Long-term studies have shown continued improvement and maintenance of symptoms, with minimal side effects. Cisapride is also effective at improving gastric emptying of both solids and liquids, where metoclopramide only has effect on solids after one month.

Therapeutic Considerations

Cisapride is only available through prescribers registered with the manufacturer to provide the medication to individuals who have failed on other approved therapies. These investigational protocols are specific to adults with GERD, diabetic gastroparesis, pseudo-obstruction, or severe chronic constipation, and children with GERD or pseudo-obstruction. Cisapride has class III antiarrhythmic properties, and is known to prolong the QT interval and cause cardiac arrhythmias and torsades de pointes. When used in combination with CYP3A4 inhibitors (eg, azole antifungals, macrolide antibiotics), cisapride plasma levels and risk of arrhythmia may increase. Cisapride is also not recommended for use with other antiarrythmic medications (eg, amiodarone, sotalol), as this may increase the risk of QT prolongation and arrhythmia. Use of grapefruit juice with cisapride is not recommended, and may increase plasma levels of the medication by as much as 50%. Increasing gastric emptying may also increase or decrease the absorption of coadministered medications (eg, lithium, digoxin); plasma levels should be monitored initially for drugs with a narrow therapeutic index to ensure safety and efficacy. Common side effects associated with cisapride use include headache, nausea and vomiting, abdominal pain, diarrhea, and constipation. **Table 18.1** provides a more extensive list of adverse effects. Patients must undergo a 12-point ECG, electrolyte panel, and extensive physical and history prior to beginning cisapride therapy to rule out arrhythmia risk, electrolyte imbalance, and medication interactions that would predispose the patient to arrhythmia. Cisapride is considered the optimal prokinetic for use in the treatment of diabetic gastroparesis; however the risks of serious adverse events have limited its use in treatment.

Erythromycin

Erythromycin was first introduced in the U.S. in 1952, after FDA approval for use as an anti-infective agent. A macrolide antibiotic, erythromycin was found to have other uses through clinical trials, such as a treatment for diabetic gastroparesis, gastritis, and bowel preparation for colonoscopy. While erythromycin is FDA-approved for many bacterial strains, it has not gained FDA approval for treating diabetic gastroparesis, and its use is considered off-label. The usual dose is 150-250 mg po tid-qid 30 minutes prior to meals.

Pharmacology

Unlike metoclopramide and cisapride, erythromycin's mechanism of action does not affect dopamine or acetylcholine. Erythromycin binds to motilin receptors in the gastric antrum and proximal duodenum, mimicking the effect of the polypeptide motilin. This action increases motility and improves gastric emptying of both liquids and solids.

Erythromycin is available in both oral and parenteral forms, although the bioavailability of oral erythromycin is extremely poor. Peak concentrations of oral erythromycin are achieved in 1-4 hours, and can be influenced by food, gastric emptying rate, and the salt form administered. Erythromycin is metabolized primarily in the liver, and excreted through the feces. Hepatic impairment may increase plasma concentrations and the half-life of the medication.

Clinical Advantages

Erythromycin is available in oral and intravenous form, and is the most potent agent for treatment of diabetic gastroparesis when given intravenously. The oral suspension has been found to be more effective than the oral tablets in study. Erythromycin's absorption and therapeutic efficacy are decreased by hyperglycemia, and controlled blood glucose must be established to maximize therapeutic effect.

Therapeutic Considerations

Of all available agents for treatment of diabetic gastroparesis, erythromycin is the most potent when administered intravenously. Erythromycin is another agent that can be used successfully as a long-term therapy, although down-regulation of motilin receptors may be of concern. Long-term exposure to antibiotic therapy is another concern with this agent, and needs to be monitored when infection is present. Common adverse effects of erythromycin include, but are not limited to, nausea and vomiting, diarrhea, abdominal pain, headache, rash, and possible cardiac QT interval prolongation. For a more extensive list, please see **Table 18.1**. Erythromycin is an inhibitor of CYP450 isoenzyme 3A4, and has many drug interactions to monitor, such as theophylline, benzodiazepines, and carbamazepine; **Table 18.2** has an extensive list of drug interactions with erythromycin. Grapefruit juice is not recommended for use with erythromycin, as the serum concentrations of erythromycin may increase with coadministration. Erythromycin is a known cardiac QT interval prolonging agent, and coadministration with other antiarrhythmics may increase the risk of cardiac events. Monitoring is advised with coadministration of these agents. Use of erythromycin in patients with hepatic dysfunction requires caution due to an increased risk of adverse events. Patients with a diagnosed arrhythmia disorder or prolonged QT interval should receive erythromycin with caution, as this medication has been shown to cause ventricular arrhythmias of the torsades de pointes type. Erythromycin is a pregnancy Category B, and is considered safe for use in breastfeeding patients.

ERECTILE DYSFUNCTION

Erectile dysfunction is the inability to achieve or maintain an erection sufficient for sexual intercourse. Causes for ED vary, and may relate to psychological, neurological, hormonal, vascular, medication, age-related factors, or a combination of conditions. Endothelial dysfunction is the common cause of ED, and the common link among ED, diabetes, and vascular disease. Endothelial dysfunction in the pudendal penile arteries/arterioles leads to a loss of vascular patency, and increases the risk of atherosclerosis, thrombosis, plaque formation, and occlusive artery disease. The endothelium is responsible for release of nitric oxide, which ultimately increases the release of cGMP, leading to increased relaxation of smooth vascular muscle cells. Endothelial dysfunction lowers nitric oxide formation and release, which has been identified as a key contributor to ED. Other factors related to endothelial dysfunction and ED include hypertension, hyperlipidemia, coronary artery disease, and other cardiovascular disorders.

Guidelines for treatment of ED recommend a thorough patient history, as a necessity to identify any underlying condition that may account for symptoms associated with ED. Patient interviewing may also identify specific problems with the sexual process of the patient; these details may also identify any psychological concerns, or basis for sexual dysfunction. Testing of A1C, lipids, prostate specific antigen, and testosterone levels may rule out any hormonal or organic concerns as well. Erectile dysfunction may be present without a current diagnosis of cardiovascular disease; a thorough physical is recommended to rule out any undiagnosed cardiovascular disease, as ED is often preceded by PVD or atherosclerosis. While therapy may be initiated to treat ED, it is also recommended to educate the patient regarding underlying conditions (eg, diabetes, CVD), and make sure that control of these conditions is established to reduce any risk of further damage and worsening ED.

Sildenafil

Sildenafil is a phosphodiesterase inhibitor used in the treatment of erectile dysfunction and pulmonary arterial hypertension. Initial development of sildenafil was aimed at treatment of angina pectoris, but trials moved the development of sildenafil into the ED market. Sildenafil was the first drug in its class to be developed and approved, and has been tested in over 4,000 patients in clinical trials. Sildenafil was FDA-approved for treatment of ED in 1998, and was later approved for treatment of pulmonary arterial hypertension in 2005.

Pharmacology

Phosphodiesterase inhibitors such as sildenafil exert their action through a blockade of cGMP-specific phosphodiesterase-5. Initially the endothelium of the corpus cavernosum releases nitric oxide during sexual stimulation; nitric oxide stimulates the release of cGMP, which relaxes the smooth muscle of the corpus cavernosum and allows blood flow to occur. In erectile dysfunction, cGMP levels are decreased, and smooth muscle relaxation may not occur, leading to failure of erection. By inhibiting phosphodiesterase-5, sildenafil raises levels of cGMP, and improves smooth muscle relaxation in the corpus cavernosum, improving erectile function. Sildenafil also has a minor affinity for the phosphodiesterase-6 enzyme, and can cause abnormalities in color visualization when administered in high doses.

Sildenafil is administered orally, is 40% bioavailable, and reaches peak plasma concentrations in 30-120 minutes. High fat content in meals can reduce the absorption of sildenafil, and delay onset of action. Protein binding is upward of 96%, and metabolism occurs primarily through the CYP450 isoenzyme 3A4. Active metabolites of sildenafil exert the same activity as sildenafil, and account for about 20% of pharmacologic activity. Excretion occurs primarily through the feces, with a small percentage excreted through urine. The half-life of sildenafil is approximately 4 hours. Dose adjustments in both hepatic and renal impairment may be necessary, as plasma concentrations of sildenafil were significantly higher in patients studied with these disease states.

Clinical Advantages

Sildenafil is one of the most studied medications for use in the treatment of ED. Onset of action occurs within 60 minutes, and duration can last up to 4 hours, minimizing adverse effects but allowing the patient time to engage in activity. A wide range of dosing is available, allowing for use in patients with other possible disease states (eg, hepatic impairment).

Therapeutic Considerations

Sildenafil is not recommended for use in patients utilizing nitrate therapy, as the combination may increase the risk of a hypotensive crisis or event. Use of sildenafil in the elderly, hepatically impaired, and renally impaired all warrant caution, as plasma concentrations of sildenafil in these patients is increased when compared to younger healthy individuals. Combined use of sildenafil with known CYP3A4 inhibitors (eg, erythromycin, ketoconazole) may increase plasma concentrations of sildenafil through inhibition of metabolism; monitoring for adverse events is advised. Caution should also be exercised when using sildenafil in patients with past history of cardiovascular events (eg, MI, stroke). Due to its effect on the phosphodiesterase-6 enzyme, any visual disturbance or change in color perception should be reported, as this may be caused by sildenafil use. Common adverse effects associated with sildenafil use include, but are not limited to headache, flushing, dizziness, and rash. **Table 18.1** has a more extensive list of adverse effects associated with sildenafil. Repeated dosing is recommended, continued exposure has been shown to improve response to sildenafil. Recommended dosing for patients aged ≥65 years is initiated at 25 mg per dose, with escalation based on tolerance and results.

Vardenafil

Vardenafil is the second phosphodiesterase inhibitor approved for use in the treatment of ED. Unlike other agents, vardenafil has been approved only for treatment of ED, and has not been evaluated for use in pulmonary hypertension or other like conditions. Vardenafil has been studied in larger population trials, and gained FDA approval in 2003.

Pharmacology

Selective phosphodiesterase inhibitors such as vardenafil exert their action through a blockade of cGMP-specific phosphodiesterase-5. In normal erectile function, cGMP causes smooth muscle relaxation of the corpus cavernosum, allowing increased blood flow into the corpus cavernosum and normal erectile function. Decreased levels of cGMP lead to failure of the corpus cavernosum to relax, resulting in erectile dysfunction. Through inhibition of phosphodiesterase-5, vardenafil raises levels of cGMP, and improves smooth muscle relaxation in the corpus cavernosum, improving erectile function. Vardenafil is also selective for phosphodiesterase-5, and does not affect phosphodiesterase isoenzymes in other organ systems (eg, phosphodiesterase-6 in the retina).

After oral administration of vardenafil, onset of action occurs within 60 minutes. Bioavailability is about 15%, while peak plasma concentrations occur in 30-120 minutes. High fat content in meals reduces maximal concentration by as much as 50%. Protein binding of vardenafil is 95%, and vardenafil is primarily metabolized through the CYP450 isoenzyme 3A4. Vardenafil metabolites may exert the same effect as the parent compound, and accounts for 7% of activity. Vardenafil is primarily excreted through the feces, with a half-life of 4-5 hours. Lower dosing should be considered for the elderly and the hepatically impaired, as plasma concentrations were significantly higher versus younger, healthy individuals.

Clinical Advantages

Vardenafil has been extensively studied, albeit not in as great a population as sildenafil, for use in the treatment of ED. Onset of action occurs within 60 minutes, and duration can last up to 5 hours, allowing the patient time to engage in activity after administration. A wide range of dosing is available, allowing for use in patients with other possible disease states (eg, hepatic impairment). Vardenafil does not affect the phosphodiesterase-6 enzyme, and has not been reported to have effect on color visualization or other visual disturbances.

Therapeutic Considerations

Vardenafil is not recommended for use in patients utilizing nitrate therapy, as the combination may increase the risk of a hypotensive crisis or event. Use of vardenafil in the elderly and hepatically impaired all warrant caution, as plasma concentrations of vardenafil in these patients is increased when compared to younger, healthy individuals. Use of vardenafil in patients with a known cardiac QT interval prolongation, or known use of antiarrhythmics is not recommended, as vardenafil has been shown in clinical study to increase the QT interval. Combined use of vardenafil with known CYP3A4 inhibitors (eg, erythromycin, ketoconazole) may increase plasma concentrations of vardenafil through inhibition of metabolism; monitoring for adverse effects such as hypotension is advised. Caution should also be exercised when using vardenafil in a patient with past history of cardiovascular events (eg, MI, stroke). Common adverse effects associated with vardenafil use include, but are not limited to headache, flushing, rhinitis, dyspepsia, dizziness, and rash. **Table 18.1** has a more extensive list of adverse effects associated with vardenafil. Repeated dosing is recommended; continued exposure has been shown to improve response to vardenafil. Recommended dosing for patients aged ≥65 years is initiated at 5 mg per dose, with escalation based on tolerance and results.

Tadalafil

Tadalafil is a selective phosphodiesterase-5 inhibitor approved for the treatment of ED. Tadalafil was originally FDA-approved in 2003 for treatment of male ED, but has since gained a broader timing designation due to its longer half-life and extended duration of action.

Pharmacology

Tadalafil, a selective phosphodiesterase inhibitor, exerts its action through a blockade of cGMP-specific phosphodiesterase-5. In normal erectile function, cGMP causes smooth muscle relaxation of the corpus cavernosum, allowing increased blood flow into the corpus cavernosum and normal erectile function. Decreased levels of cGMP lead to failure of the corpus cavernosum to relax, resulting in erectile dysfunction. Through inhibition of phosphodiesterase-5, tadalafil raises levels of cGMP, and improves smooth muscle relaxation in the corpus cavernosum, improving erectile function. Tadalafil is specific to phosphodiesterase-5, and does not affect phosphodiesterase isoenzymes in other organ systems (eg, phosphodiesterease-6 in the retina).

Tadalafil is administered orally with an onset of action of 30-45 minutes, and peak plasma concentrations reached in 30-360 minutes. Administration with food has not been shown to affect the absorption or levels of tadalafil. Protein binding of tadalafil is 94%, and tadalafil is primarily metabolized through the CYP450 isoenzyme 3A4. Tadalafil metabolites have not been shown to influence ED at this time, and tadalafil is regarded as the only component exerting therapeutic effects. Tadalafil is primarily excreted through the feces (61%) and secondarily through the urine (36%), with a half-life of 17.5 hours in healthy individuals. Lower dosing should be considered for the elderly and the hepatically impaired, as plasma concentrations were significantly higher versus younger, healthy individuals. A decrease in the initial and continued dose is recommended for those with moderate to severe renal impairment, as drug concentrations have been shown to increase in individuals with this disease state.

Clinical Advantages

Tadalafil has been extensively studied and is approved for use in the treatment of ED.

Onset of action occurs within 45 minutes, and duration can last up to 36 hours, allowing the largest window of action for the patient to engage in sexual activity. A wide range of dosing is available, allowing for use in patients with other possible disease states (eg, renal impairment). Tadalafil does not affect the phosphodiesterase-6 enzyme, and has not been reported to have effect on color visualization or other visual disturbances.

Therapeutic Considerations

Tadalafil is not recommended for use in patients utilizing nitrate therapy, as the combination may increase the risk of a hypotensive crisis or event. Caution is recommended with use of tadalafil in the renally impaired, as plasma concentrations of tadalafil in these patients is increased when compared to healthy individuals. Dose adjustments based on age or hepatic impairment are not necessary, although doses higher than 10 mg daily are not recommended in the hepatically impaired. Combined use of tadalafil with known CYP3A4 inhibitors (eg, erythromycin, ketoconazole) may increase plasma concentrations of tadalafil through inhibition of metabolism; monitoring for adverse effects such as hypotension is advised. Use of grapefruit juice with tadalafil is also not recommended, as increases in tadalafil plasma levels may be seen with combined grapefruit use. Caution should also be exercised when using tadalafil in patients with a past history of cardiovascular events (eg, MI, stroke). Common adverse effects associated with tadalafil use include, but are not limited to headache, flushing, rhinitis, dyspepsia, dizziness, and rash. **Table 18.1** has a more extensive list of adverse effects associated with tadalafil. Due to tadalafil's extended half-life and duration of action, initiation with a low starting dose (5 mg) and titration based on results is recommended, to minimize adverse events should they occur. Repeated dosing is recommended; continued exposure has been shown to improve response to tadalafil. Recommended dosing for patients aged ≥65 years is initiated at 10 mg per dose, with escalation based on tolerance and results.

Alprostadil

Alprostadil is a naturally occurring prostaglandin E found in the seminal vesicles and cavernous tissues of the penis. Available in multiple delivery systems, alprostadil is an effective treatment that is approved by the FDA for ED. Alprostadil was first released for FDA-approved use in 1981 for treatment of patent ductus arteriosis, was later approved in 1995 as in intracavernosal injection, and was approved in 1996 as an intraurethral tablet.

Pharmacology

Alprostadil acts upon the smooth muscle of the corpus cavernosum, stimulating activity of adenylate cyclase. Through this mechanism, an increase of intracellular cyclic adenosine monophosphate (cAMP) occurs, and decreases intracellular calcium. A decrease in norepinephrine also occurs through this mechanism, leading to smooth muscle relaxation and increased blood flow. Through this mechanism, alprostadil dilates cavernosal arteries, increases arterial blood flow, and enhances erectile function.

Administration of alprostadil occurs through intracavernosal injection or intraurethral tablet application. Upon administration, onset of action occurs in 5-10 minutes with duration of action in 30-60 minutes. The outcome of a successful erection occurs within 2-25 minutes of administration, and lasts up to several hours. The majority of alprostadil is absorbed locally with minimal systemic absorption, with no reported development of tolerance. Alprostadil is metabolized to inactive metabolites, and primarily excreted in the urine.

Clinical Advantages

Alprostadil is available as an intracavernosal injection, and an intraurethrally applied tablet, allowing for administration of an ED medication in individuals unable to take phosphodieserase-5 inhibitors. Concurrent use with nitrates or other antianginal medications is not contraindicated, as with other ED medications. Systemic absorption is minimal, with little to no adverse effects associated with the medication. No dosing adjustments are necessary for known disease states, such as hepatic or renal impairment.

Therapeutic Considerations

Alprostadil is not recommended for use in patients who are at risk of experiencing or who have experienced priapism (eg, erection ≥6 hours). Intraurethral tablet administration is not recommended for use in patients with penile deformities or structural abnormalities. Discontinuation of the medication is recommended if injection site reactions occur. Other side effects noted during use include hypotension and syncope (See **Table 18.1**). There have been no reported interactions between alprostadil and other medications, although it is noted that concurrent use of antihypertensives and alprostadil may increase risk of hypotensive events. Although no dosing recommendations have been outlined, initial dosing is recommended to begin at 1.25 mcg for injection and 125 mcg per intraurethral tablet, with titration based on physiological response. Injections should be given no more than 3 times per week, with at least a 24-hour period between doses.

SUGGESTED READING

Backonja M. Use of anticonvulsants for treatment of neuropathic pain. *Neurology.* 2002;59(Suppl 2):S14-S17.

Backonja M, Glanzman R. Gabapentin dosing for neuropathic pain: evidence from randomized, placebo-controlled trials. *Clin Ther.* 2003;25(1):81-104.

Barbano R, Herrmann D, et al. Effectiveness, tolerability, and impact on quality of life of the 5% lidocaine patch in diabetic polyneuropathy. *Arch Neurol.* 2004;61:914-918.

Camilleri M. Diabetic gastroparesis. *N Engl J Med.* 2007;356:820-829.

Chong M, Hester J. Diabetic painful neuropathy: current and future treatment options. *Drugs.* 2007;67(4):569-585.

De Block C, De Leeuw I, et al. Current concepts in gastric motility in diabetes mellitus. *Curr Diabet Rev.* 2006;2:113-130.

Dugan S, Fuller M. Duloxetine: a dual reuptake inhibitor. *Ann Pharmacother.* 2004;38:2078-2085.

Dworkin R, Backonja M, et al. Advances in neuropathic pain. *Arch Neurol.* 2003;60:1524-1534.

Eisenberg E, River Y, et al. Antiepileptic drugs in the treatment of neuropathic pain. *Drugs.* 2007;67(9):1265-1289.

Hellstrom W. Current safety and tolerability issues in men with erectile dysfunction receiving PDE5 inhibitors. *Int J Clin Pract.* 2007;61(9):1547-1554.

Head K. Peripheral neuropathy: pathogenic mechanisms and alternative therapies. *Alter Med Rev.* 2006;11(4):294-329.

Jackson K. Pharmacotherapy for neuropathic pain. *Pain Pract.* 2006;6(1):27-33.

Kajdasz D, Iyengar S, et al. Duloxetine for the management of diabetic peripheral neuropathic pain: evidence-based findings from post hoc analysis of three multicenter, randomized, double-blind, placebo-controlled, parallel-group studies. *Clin Ther.* 2007;29:2536-2546.

Kuo P, Rayner C, et al. Pathophysiology and management of diabetic gastropathy: a guide for endocrinologists. *Drugs.* 2007;67(12):1671-1687.

Mellegers M, Furlan A, et al. Gabapentin for neuropathic pain: systematic review of controlled and uncontrolled literature. *Clin J Pain.* 2001;17(4):284-295.

Parkman HP, Hasler WL, Fisher RS. American Gastroenterological Association technical review on the diagnosis and treatment of gastroparesis. *Gastroenterology.* 2004;127:1592-1622.

Pasquale P. Metabolic risk factors, endothelial dysfunction, and erectile dysfunction in men with diabetes. *Am J Med Sci*. 2007;334(6):466-480.

Perkins B, Bril V. Emerging therapies for diabetic neuropathy: a clinical overview. *Curr Diabetes Rev*. 2005;1(3):271-280.

Setter S, Iltz J, et al. Phosphodiesterase 5 inhibitors for erectile dysfunction. *Ann Pharmacother*. 2005;39:1286-1295.

Sindrup S, Otto M, et al. Antidepressants in the treatment of neuropathic pain. *Basic Clin Pharmacol Toxicol*. 2005;96(6):399-409.

Sivalingam S, Hashim H, et al. An overview of the diagnosis and treatment of erectile dysfunction. *Drugs*. 2006;66(18):2339-2355.

Smith T. Duloxetine in diabetic neuropathy. *Expert Opin Pharmacother*. 2006;7(2):215-223.

Sonnett T, Setter S, et al. Pregabalin for the treatment of painful neuropathy. *Expert Rev Neurotherapeutics*. 2006;6(11):1629-1635.

Tassone D, Boyce E, et al. Pregabalin: a novel gamma-aminobutyric acid analogue in the treatment of neuropathic pain, partial-onset seizures, and anxiety disorders. *Clin Ther*. 2007;29(1):26-48.

Tracy J, Dyck P. The spectrum of diabetic neuropathies. *Phys Med Rehabil Clin N Am*. 2008; 19(1):1-26.

Vinik A, Freeman R, et al. Diabetic autonomic neuropathy. *Semin Neurol*. 2003;23(4):365-372.

Zin C, Nissen L, et al. An update on the pharmacological management of post-herpetic neuralgia and painful diabetic neuropathy. *CNS Drugs*. 2008;22(5):417-442.

Zochodne D. Diabetes mellitus and the peripheral nervous system: manifestations and mechanisms. *Muscle Nerve*. 2007;36(2):144-166.

Table 18.1. Prescribing Information for Neuropathic Therapies

GENERIC (BRAND)	FORM/ STRENGTH	DOSAGE	WARNINGS/PRECAUTIONS & CONTRAINDICATIONS	ADVERSE REACTIONS
Management of Peripheral Neuropathy				

Management of Peripheral Neuropathy

ANTICONVULSANT

GENERIC (BRAND)	FORM/ STRENGTH	DOSAGE	WARNINGS/PRECAUTIONS & CONTRAINDICATIONS	ADVERSE REACTIONS
Carbamazepine (Tegretol, Tegretol-XR)	**Sus:** 100mg/5mL [450mL]; **Tab:** (Tegretol) 200mg*; **Tab, Chewable:** 100mg*; **Tab, Extended-Release:** (Tegretol-XR) 100mg, 200mg, 400mg. *scored	***Adults: Epilepsy:*** Initial: **(Immediate- or Extended-Release Tabs)** 200mg bid or **(Sus)** 100mg qid. Titrate: **(Immediate-Release Tabs/Sus)** Increase weekly by 200mg/day given tid-qid. **(Extended-Release Tabs)** Increase weekly by 200mg/day given bid. Maint: 800-1200mg/day. Max: 1200mg/day. **Trigeminal Neuralgia:** Initial (Day 1): **(Immediate- or Extended-Release Tabs)** 100mg bid or **(Sus)** 50mg qid. Titrate: May increase by 100mg q12h **(Tabs)** or 50mg qid **(Sus).** Maint: 400-800mg/day. Max: 1200mg/day. Re-evaluate every 3 months. ***Pediatrics: Epilepsy:*** **>12 yrs:** Initial: **(Immediate- or Extended-Release Tabs)** 200mg bid or **(Sus)** 100mg qid. Titrate: **(Immediate-Release Tabs/Sus)** Increase weekly by 200mg/day given tid-qid. **(Extended-Release Tabs)** Increase weekly by 200mg/day given bid. Max: **12-15 yrs:** 1000mg/day. **>15 yrs:** 1200mg/day. **6-12 yrs:** Initial: **(Immediate- or Extended-Release Tabs)** 100mg bid or **(Sus)** 50mg qid. Titrate: **(Immediate-Release Tabs/Sus)** Increase weekly by 100mg/day given tid-qid. **(Extended-Release Tabs)** Increase weekly by 100mg/day given bid. Maint: 400-800mg/day. Max: 1000mg/day. **6 months-6 yrs:** Initial: **(Immediate-Release Tabs)** 10-20mg/kg/day given bid-tid or **(Sus)** 10-20mg/kg/day given qid. Titrate: **(Immediate-Release Tabs/Sus)** Increase weekly tid-qid. Max: 35mg/kg/day. Extended-Release tabs should be swallowed whole and not crushed or chewed.	**BB:** Serious and fatal dermatologic reactions, including toxic epiderml necrolysis (TEN), Stevens-Johnson syndrome (SJS), and presence of HLA-B* 1502 allele reported. Aplastic anemia and agranulocytosis reported. Obtain complete pretreatment hematological testing as a baseline. D/C if evidence of bone marrow depression develops. **W/P:** Lyell's syndrome, Stevens-Johnson syndrome, multi-organ hypersensitivity reactions, and presence of HLA-B*1502 reported. Caution with history of adverse hematologic reaction to any drug, increased IOP, the elderly, mixed seizure disorder with atypical absence seizure. Fetal harm with pregnancy. May activate latent psychosis. Caution with cardiac (eg, conduction disturbance including second and third degree AV block), hepatic, or renal damage. Perform eye exam and monitor LFTs and renal function at baseline and periodically. Suspension produces higher peak levels than the tablet. Avoid in hepatic porphyria (eg, acute intermittent porphyria, variegate porphyria, porphyria cutanea tarda). Withdraw gradually to minimize the potential of increased seizure frequency. **Contra:** History of bone marrow depression, MAOI use within 14 days, hypersensitivity to TCAs. Co-administration with nefazodone. **P/N:** Category D, not for use in nursing.	Dizziness, drowsiness, unsteadiness, nausea, vomiting, bone marrow depression, rash, urticaria, photosensitivity reactions, CHF, edema, HTN, hypotension, Stevens-Johnson syndrome, toxic epidermal necrolysis.

GABA ANALOGS

GENERIC (BRAND)	FORM/ STRENGTH	DOSAGE	WARNINGS/PRECAUTIONS & CONTRAINDICATIONS	ADVERSE REACTIONS
Gabapentin (Neurontin)	**Cap:** 100mg, 300mg, 400mg; **Sol:** 250mg/ 5mL; **Tab:** 600mg*, 800mg* *scored	***Adults: Epilepsy:*** Initial: 300mg tid. Titrate: Increase up to 1800mg/day. Max: 3600mg/ day. **Postherpetic Neuralgia:** 300mg single dose on Day 1, then 300mg bid on Day 2, and 300mg tid on Day 3. Increase further prn for pain. Max: 600mg tid. **Renal Impairment: CrCl 30-59mL/min:** 400-1400 mg/day. **CrCl 15-29mL/min:** 200-700 mg/day. **CrCl 15mL/min:** 100-300mg/day. **CrCl <15 mL/min:** Reduce dose in proportion toCrCl. **Hemodialysis:** Maint: Base on CrCl. Give supplemental dose (125-350mg) after 4 hrs of hemodialysis. Refer to prescribing information for dose-adjustment. ***Pediatrics: Epilepsy:* >12 yrs:** Initial: 300mg tid. Titrate: Increase up to 1800mg/day. Max: 3600mg/day. **3-12 yrs:** Initial: 10-15mg/kg/day given tid. Titrate: Increase over 3 days. 3-4 yrs: Usual: 40mg/kg/day given tid. ≥5 yrs: 25-35mg/kg/day given tid. Max: 50mg/kg/day. **Renal Impairment: ≥12 yrs: CrCl 30-59mL/min:** 400-1400 mg/day. **CrCl 15-29mL/min:** 200-700 mg/day. **CrCl 15mL/min:** 100-300mg/day. **CrCl <15 mL/min:** Reduce dose in proportion to CrCl. **Hemodialysis:** Maint: Base on CrCl. Give supplemental dose (125-350 mg) after 4 hrs of hemodialysis. Refer to prescribing information for dose-adjustment.	**W/P:** Avoid abrupt withdrawal. Possible tumorigenic potential. Sudden and unexplained deaths reported. Neuropsychiatric adverse events in pediatrics (3-12 yrs). **P/N:** Category C, caution in nursing.	Somnolence, dizziness, ataxia, nystagmus, fatigue, tremor, rhinitis, weight gain, nausea, vomiting, viral infection, fever, dysarthria, diplopia.

BB = black box warning; **W/P** = warnings/precautions; **Contra** = contraindications; **P/N** = pregnancy category rating and nursing considerations.

Table 18.1. Prescribing Information for Neuropathic Therapies

GENERIC (BRAND)	FORM/ STRENGTH	DOSAGE	WARNINGS/PRECAUTIONS & CONTRAINDICATIONS	ADVERSE REACTIONS
GABA ANALOGS *(Cont.)*				
Pregabalin (Lyrica)	**Cap:** 25mg, 50mg, 75mg, 100mg, 150mg, 200mg, 225mg, 300mg	***Adults:* Neuropathic Pain:** Initial: 50mg tid (150mg/day). Titrate: May increase to 300mg/day within 1 week. Max: 100mg tid (300mg/day). **Post-Herpetic Neuralgia:** Max: Initial: 150mg/day divided bid or tid. 600mg/day divided bid or tid. **Epilepsy:** Initial: 150mg/day divided bid-tid. Max: 600mg/day. **Fibromyalgia:** Initial: 75mg bid (150mg/day). Titrate: May increase to 150mg bid (300mg/day) within 1 week based on efficacy and tolerability. May further increase to 225mg bid (450mg/day) if needed. Max: 450mg/day. **Renal Impairment: CrCl 30-60 mL/min:** 75-300mg/day divided bid or tid. **CrCl 15-30 mL/min:** 25-150mg/day divided qd or bid. **CrCl <15mL/min:** 25-75mg/day given qd. Give supplemental dose (25-150mg) immediately after every 4-hr hemodialysis treatment. Refer to prescribing information for further details. **D/C:** Taper over minimum of 1 week.	**W/P:** Avoid abrupt withdrawal. Gradually taper over 1 week. Possible tumorigenic potential. May impair physical/mental potential. May impair physical/mental vision, monitor for ophthalmic changes; peripheral edema, caution in heart failure; elevated creatine kinase, d/c if myopathy or markedly elevated creatine kinase levels occur; decreased platelet count; and mild PR-interval prolongation. Angioedema reported in initial and chronic treatment. **P/N:** Category C, not for use in nursing.	Somnolence, dizziness, dry mouth, edema, blurredvision, weight gain, abnormal thinking (difficulty with concentration/attention), headache, nausea, diarrhea.
SEROTONIN/NOREPINEPHRINE REUPTAKE INHIBITOR (SNRI)				
Duloxetine HCl (Cymbalta)	**Cap, Delayed-Release:** 20mg, 30mg, 60mg	***Adults:* MDD:** Initial: 40mg/day (given as 20mg bid) to 60mg/day (given qd or as 30mg bid). Re-evaluate periodically. **Diabetic Peripheral Neuropathic Pain:** 60mg/day given qd. May lower starting dose if tolerability a concern. **Renal Impairment:** Consider lower starting dose with gradual increase. **GAD:** Initial: 60mg qd or 30mg qd for 1 week to adjust before increasing to 60mg qd. Titrate: May increase by increments of 30mg qd if needed. Max: 120 mg qd. Do not chew or crush.	**BB:** Antidepressants increased the risk of suicidal thinking and behavior (suicidality) in short-term studies in children, adolescents, and young adults with major depressive disorder (MDD) and other psychiatric disorders. Not approved for use in pediatric patients. **W/P:** Monitor for clinical worsening and/or suicidality. May increase risk of serum transaminase elevations. May cause hepatotoxicity. Avoid with chronic liver disease. May increase BP; obtain baseline and monitor periodically. Orthostatic hypotension and syncope reported. Avoid abrupt cessation and with severe renal impairment/ESRD or hepatic insufficiency. Caution with conditions that may slow gastric emptying, history of mania or seizures. May increase risk of mydriasis; caution in patients with controlled narrow-angle glaucoma. Serotonin syndrome may occur; caution with concomitant use of serotonergic drugs. Hyponatremia reported. May affect urethral resistance. May increase risk of abnormal bleeding; caution with aspirin, NSAIDs, warfarin. Increases the risk of elevation of serum transaminase levels. **Contra:** Concomitant use of MAOIs, uncontrolled narrow-angle glaucoma. **P/N:** Category C, not for use in nursing.	Nausea, dry mouth, constipation, diarrhea, vomiting, decreased appetite, fatigue, dizziness, somnolence, increased sweating, blurred vision, insomnia, agitation, erectile dysfunction.
TOPICAL AGENT				
Lidocaine (Lidoderm Patch)	**Patch:** 5% [30°]	***Adults:*** Apply to intact skin, cover most painful area. Apply up to 3 patches, once for up to 12 hrs within 24-hr period. May cut patches into smaller sizes before removal of the release liner. **Debilitated/ Impaired Elimination:** Treat smaller areas. Remove if irritation or burning occurs; may reapply when irritation subsides.	**W/P:** Serious adverse events may occur in children or pets if ingested. Increased risk of toxicity in severe hepatic disease. Avoid broken or inflamed skin, eye contact, larger area or longer duration than recommended. Increased levels with application of >3 patches, small patients. **P/N:** Category B, caution in nursing.	Application site reactions such as: erythema, edema, bruising, papules, vesicles, discoloration, depigmentation, burning sensation, pruritus, dermatitis, petechia, blisters, exfoliation, abnormal sensation, irritation, allergic reactions (rare).

BB = black box warning; **W/P** = warnings/precautions; **Contra** = contraindications; **P/N** = pregnancy category rating and nursing considerations.

Table 18.1. Prescribing Information for Neuropathic Therapies

GENERIC (BRAND)	FORM/ STRENGTH	DOSAGE	WARNINGS/PRECAUTIONS & CONTRAINDICATIONS	ADVERSE REACTIONS
TRICYCLIC ANTIDEPRESSANTS				
Amitriptyline HCl (Elavil*)	**Inj:** 10mg/mL; **Tab:** 10mg, 25mg, 50mg, 75mg, 100mg, 150mg	**Adults: PO:** Initial: (Outpatient) 75mg/day in divided doses or 50-100mg qhs. (Inpatient) 100mg/day. Titrate: (Outpatient) Increase by 25-50mg qhs. (Inpatient) Increase to 200mg/day. Maint: 50-100mg qhs. Max: (Outpatient) 150mg/day. (Inpatient) 300mg/day. **IM:** Initial: 20-30mgqid. **Elderly:** 10mg tid or 20mg qhs.	**BB:** Antidepressants increased the risk of suicidal thinking and behavior (suicidality) in short-term studies in children, adolescents, and young adults with Major Depressive Disorder (MDD) and other psychiatric disorders. **W/P:** Caution with history of seizures, urinary retention, angle-closure glaucoma, increased IOP, hyperthyroidism, cardiovascular disorders, liver dysfunction. Increases symptoms with schizophrenia and manic-depression. D/C several weeks before elective surgery. May alter blood glucose levels. **Contra:** MAOI use or within 14 days, acute recovery period following MI. **P/N:** Category C, not for use in nursing.	MI, stroke, seizure, paralytic ileus, urinary retention, constipation, blurred vision, dry mouth, hyperpyrexia, rash, bone marrow depression, testicular swelling, gynecomastia (male), breast enlargement (female), alopecia, edema.
Desipramine HCl (Norpramin)	**Tab:** 10mg, 25mg, 50mg, 75mg, 100mg, 150mg	**Adults:** Usual: 100-200mg/day given qd or in divided doses. Max: 300mg/day. **Elderly/Adolescents:** Usual: 25-100mg/day given qd or in divided doses. Max: 150mg/day.	**BB:** Antidepressants increased the risk of suicidal thinking and behavior (suicidality) in short-term studies in children, adolescents, and young adults with Major Depressive Disorder (MDD) and other psychiatric disorders. Desipramine is not approved for use in pediatric patients. **W/P:** Hypomania with manic-depressive disease. D/C prior to elective surgery. Do not withdraw abruptly. Extreme caution with urinary retention, glaucoma, seizure disorders, cardiovascular disease, thyroid disease, alcohol abuse. May exacerbate psychosis; caution with schizophrenia. May impair mental or physical abilities. May alter blood glucose levels. **Contra:** MAOI use within 14 days, acute recovery period following MI. **P/N:** Safety in pregnancy and nursing not known.	Arrhythmias, hypotension, HTN, tachycardia, confusion, hallucination, dizziness, anxiety, numbness, tingling, ataxia, tremors, dry mouth, urinary retention, urticaria, photosensitivity, SIADH, altered libido.
Doxepin HCl (Sinequan)	**Cap:** 10mg, 25mg, 50mg, 75mg, 100mg, 150mg; **Sol, Concentrate:** 10mg/mL [120mL]	**Adults: Very Mild Illness:** Usual: 25-50mg/day. Titrate: **Mild to Moderate Severity:** Initial: 75mg/day. Usual: 75-150mg/day. **Severely Ill:** May increase up to 300mg/day. Dilute solution with 120mL of water, milk or juice. Give once daily or in divided doses. Divide dose if >150mg. **Elderly:** Use lower doses and monitor closely.	**BB:** Antidepressants increased the risk of suicidal thinking and behavior (suicidality) in short-term studies in children, adolescents, and young adults with Major Depressive Disorder (MDD) and other psychiatric disorders. Doxepin is not approved for use in pediatric patients. **W/P:** Monitor for suicidal tendencies and increased symptoms of psychosis. Avoid abrupt discontinuation. **Contra:** Glaucoma, urinary retention. **P/N:** Safety in pregnancy and nursing not known.	Drowsiness, dry mouth, blurred vision, constipation, urinary retention, hypotension, tachycardia, rash, edema, photosensitization, pruritus, eosinophilia, nausea, dizziness.
Imipramine HCl (Tofranil)	**Tab:** 10mg, 25mg, 50mg	**Adults: Depression:** Initial: (Inpatient) 100mg/day in divided doses. Increase to 200mg/day; up to 250-300mg/day after 2 weeks if needed. (Outpatient) 75mg/day. Titrate: Increase to 150mg/day. Maint: 50-150mg/day. Max: 200mg/day. **Elderly/Adolescents:** Initial: 30-40mg/day. Max: 100mg/day. **Pediatrics: Depression: Adolescents:** Initial: 30-40mg/day. Max: 100mg/day. **Enuresis:** ≥6 yrs: Initial: 25mg/day 1 hour before bedtime. Titrate: **6-12 yrs:** If inadequate response in 1 week, increase to 50mg before bedtime. ≥**12 yrs:** Increase to 75mg before bedtime after 1 week if needed. Max: 2.5mg/kg/day.	**BB:** Antidepressants increased the risk of suicidal thinking and behavior (suicidality) in short-term studies in children, adolescents, and young adults with Major Depressive Disorder (MDD) and other psychiatric disorders. Imipramine HCl is not approved for use in pediatric patients except for patients with nocturnal enuresis. **W/P:** Caution with elderly, serious depression, cardiovascular disease, hyperthyroidism, urinary retention, narrow-angle glaucoma, increased IOP, seizure disorders, renal and hepatic impairment. May activate psychosis in schizophrenia; reduce dose. Limit electroshock therapy. May alter blood glucose levels. Photosensitivity reported.	Orthostatic hypotension, HTN, confusion, hallucinations, numbness, tremors, dry mouth, urticaria, nausea, vomiting, diarrhea, gynecomastia (male), breast enlargement (female), galactorrhea.

* Brand name discontinued; generic version is still available.
BB = black box warning; **W/P** = warnings/precautions; **Contra** = contraindications; **P/N** = pregnancy category rating and nursing considerations.

Table 18.1. Prescribing Information for Neuropathic Therapies

GENERIC (BRAND)	FORM/ STRENGTH	DOSAGE	WARNINGS/PRECAUTIONS & CONTRAINDICATIONS	ADVERSE REACTIONS
TRICYCLIC ANTIDEPRESSANTS *(Cont.)*				
Imipramine HCl (Tofranil) *(Cont.)*			D/C prior to elective surgery, or with hypomanic or manic episodes. D/C with pathological neutrophil depression. **Contra:** Within 14 days of MAOI therapy, or during acute recovery period following MI. **P/N:** Safety in pregnancy not known; not for use in nursing.	
Nortriptyline HCl (Pamelor) (	**Cap:** 10mg, 25mg, 50mg, 75mg; **Sol:** 10mg/5mL	**Adults:** 25mg tid-qid. Max: 150mg/day. Total daily dose may be given once a day. Monitor serum levels if dose >100mg/day. **Elderly/Adolescents:** 30-50mg/day in single or divided doses.	**BB:** Antidepressants increased the risk of suicidal thinking and behavior (suicidality) in short-term studies in children, adolescents, and young adults with Major Depressive Disorder (MDD) and other psychiatric disorders. Nortriptyline is not approved for use in pediatric patients. **W/P:** MI, arrhythmia, strokes have occurred. Caution with cardiovascular disease, glaucoma, history of urinary retention, hyperthyroidism. May lower seizure threshold, exacerbate psychosis or activate schizophrenia, cause symptoms of mania in bipolar disease, or alter glucose levels. D/C several days prior to elective surgery. **Contra:** MAOI use within 14 days, acute recovery period following MI. **P/N:** Safety during pregnancy and nursing not known.	Arrhythmias, hypotension, HTN, tachycardia, MI, heart block, stroke, confusion, hallucination, insomnia, tremors, ataxia, anxiety, dry mouth, blurred vision, skin rash, extrapyramidal symptoms, photosensitivity, SIADH, anorexia.

Management of Central Neuropathy

GENERIC (BRAND)	FORM/ STRENGTH	DOSAGE	WARNINGS/PRECAUTIONS & CONTRAINDICATIONS	ADVERSE REACTIONS
BLADDER DYSFUNCTION				
Darifenacin (Enablex)	**Tab, Extended-Release:** 7.5mg, 15mg	**Adults:** Initial: 7.5mg qd with liquid. Max: 15mg qd. **Moderate Hepatic Impairment/Concomitant Potent CYP3A4 Inhibitors:** Do not exceed 7.5mg/d. **Severe Hepatic Impairment:** Avoid use. Tabs should be swallowed whole; do not chew, divide or crush.	**W/P:** Risk of urinary retention; caution with significant bladder outflow obstruction. Risk of gastric retention; caution with GI obstructive disorders. May decrease GI motility; caution with severe constipation, ulcerative colitis, and myasthenia gravis. Caution with moderate hepatic impairment and narrow-angle glaucoma. Avoid use with severe hepatic impairment. May produce blurred vision or dizziness. **Contra:** Urinary retention, gastric retention, uncontrolled narrow-angle glaucoma. **P/N:** Category C, caution in nursing.	Dry mouth, constipation, dyspepsia, abdominal pain, nausea, diarrhea, UTI, dizziness, asthenia, dry eyes.
Flavoxate HCl (Urispas)	**Tab:** 100mg	**Adults:** 100-200mg tid-qid. Reduce dose with improvement. **Pediatrics:** ≥12 yrs: 100-200mg tid-qid. Reduce dose with improvement.	**W/P:** Caution with glaucoma and while operating machinery where alertness is required. Drowsiness, blurred vision may occur. **Contra:** Pyloric or duodenal obstruction, obstructive intestinal lesions or ileus, achalasia, GI hemorrhage, and obstructive uropathies of the lower urinary tract. **P/N:** Category B, caution in nursing.	Drowsiness, dry mouth, nausea, vomiting, tachycardia, palpitations, leukopenia, vertigo, nervousness, confusion, fatigue, headache, hyperpyrexia, urticaria, blurred vision.
Oxybutynin (Oxytrol)	**Patch:** 3.9mg/day [8's]	**Adults:** Apply to dry, intact skin on the abdomen, hip, or buttock twice weekly (every 3-4 days). Rotate sites.	**W/P:** Caution with hepatic or renal impairment, bladder outflow obstruction, GI obstructive disorders, ulcerative colitis, intestinal atony, myasthenia gravis, and gastroesophageal reflux. Heat prostration may occur when used in a hot environment. **Contra:** Urinary retention, gastric retention, uncontrolled narrow-angle glaucoma, and in patients at risk for these conditions. **P/N:** Category B, caution in nursing.	Application site reactions, dry mouth, drowsiness, constipation, drowsiness, dizziness, blurred vision.
Oxybutynin chloride (Ditropan, Ditropan XL)	**Syrup:** 5mg/5mL; **Tab:** 5mg*; **Tab, Extended-Release:** 5mg, 10mg, 15mg *scored	**Adults:** (**Tab, Syrup**) Usual: 5mg bid-tid. Max: 5mg qid. **Frail Elderly:** 2.5mg bid-tid. (**Tab, Extended-Release**) Initial: 5 or 10mg qd. Titrate: May increase by 5mg weekly. Max: 30mg/day. Swallow XL whole with liquid; do not chew,	**W/P:** Caution with hepatic or renal impairment, bladder outflow obstruction, GI obstruction/narrowing, ulcerative colitis, intestinal atony, myasthenia gravis, hyperthyroidism, CHD, CHF, arrhythmias, HTN, tachycardia, prostatic hypertrophy,	Dry mouth, constipation, somnolence, headache, diarrhea, nausea, blurred vision, dyspepsia, asthenia, pain, dizziness, dry eyes, UTI, insomnia,

BB = black box warning; **W/P** = warnings/precautions; **Contra** = contraindications; **P/N** = pregnancy category rating and nursing considerations.

Table 18.1. Prescribing Information for Neuropathic Therapies

GENERIC (BRAND)	FORM/ STRENGTH	DOSAGE	WARNINGS/PRECAUTIONS & CONTRAINDICATIONS	ADVERSE REACTIONS
Oxybutynin chloride (Ditropan, Ditropan XL) *(Cont.)*		divide or crush tab. *Pediatrics:* **>5 yrs:** (**Tab, Syrup**) Usual: 5mg bid. Max: 5mg tid. **6 yrs:** (**Tab, Extended-Release**) Initial: 5mg qd. Titrate: May increase by 5mg weekly. Max: 20mg/day. Swallow XL whole with liquid; do not chew, divide, or crush tab.	and GERD. Heat prostration can occur with high environmental temperatures. Tab, Extended-Release shell may be excreted in the stool. Reduce dose or d/c if anticholinergic CNS effects occur. Caution in preexisting dementia. **Contra:** Urinary retention, gastric retention and other severe decreased GI motility conditions, uncontrolled narrow-angle glaucoma, and in patients at risk for these conditions. **P/N:** Category B, caution in nursing.	nervousness.
Solifenacin succinate (Vesicare)	Tab: 5mg, 10mg	*Adults:* Usual: 5mg qd. Max: 10mg qd. **Renal Impairment (CrCl <30mL/min)/ Moderate Hepatic Impairment (Child-Pugh B)/ Potent CYP3A4 Inhibitors:** Max: 5mg qd. Do not use in severe hepatic impairment (Child-Pugh C).	**W/P:** Caution with bladder outflow obstruction, decreased gastrointestinal motility, and narrow-angle glaucoma. Caution with renal and hepatic impairment. **Contra:** Urinary retention, gastric retention, uncontrolled narrow-angle glaucoma. **P/N:** Category C, not for use in nursing.	Dry mouth, constipation, nausea, dyspepsia, UTI, blurred vision.
Tolterodine tartrate (Detrol, Detrol LA)	Cap, Extended-Release: 2mg, 4mg; Tab: 1mg, 2mg	*Adults:* (**LA Cap**) Usual: 4mg qd, may lower to 2mg. (**Tab**) Initial: 2mg bid, may lower to 1mg bid. (**LA Cap, Tab**) **Significant Hepatic/Renal Dysfunction/Concomitant CYP3A4 Inhibitors:** 1mg bid or 2mg LA cap qd.	**W/P:** Risk of urinary retention with significant bladder outflow obstruction and risk of gastric retention with GI obstructive disorders. Caution with renal impairment and narrow-angle glaucoma. Reduce dose with significant hepatic or renal dysfunction. May cause blurred vision, drowsiness, or dizziness. **Contra:** Urinary retention, gastric retention, uncontrolled narrow-angle glaucoma. **P/N:** Category C, not for use in nursing.	Dry mouth, dizziness, headache, abdominal pain, constipation, diarrhea, dyspepsia, fatigue, somnolence, aggravation of symptoms of dementia reported.
Trospium chloride (Sanctura, Sanctura XR)	Cap, Extended-Release: 60mg; Tab: 20mg	*Adults:* (**Tab**) 20mg bid. (**Cap, Extended-Release**) 60mg qd in am. Take at least 1 hour before meals or on empty stomach. (**Tab**) CrCl <30mL/min: 20mg qhs. **Elderly ≥75 yrs:** May titrate to 20mg qd based upon tolerability.	**W/P:** (Tab,Cap) Caution with significant bladder outflow obstruction, GI obstructive disorders, ulcerative colitis, intestinal atony, myasthenia gravis, moderate or severe hepatic dysfunction. Reduce dose with severe renal insufficiency. Consider risks vs benefits with controlled narrow-angle glaucoma. (Cap) Not recommended for use with severe renal impairment (CrCl <30mL/min). Consumption of alcohol within 2 hrs is not recommended. **Contra:** Active or risk of urinary retention, gastric retention, uncontrolled narrow-angle glaucoma. **P/N:** Category C, caution in nursing.	Dry mouth, constipation, headache, rash.
ERECTILE DYSFUNCTION				
Alprostadil (Caverject)	Inj: 0.02mg/mL, (**Impulse**) 10mcg, 20mcg, (**Powder**) 5mcg, 10mcg, 20mcg, 40mcg	*Adults:* Intracavernosal Injection. Avoid visible veins; alternate site and side. Determine dose in office. If no initial response, may give next higher dose within 1 hr. If partial response, give next higher dose after 24 hrs. **Vasculogenic/ Psychogenic/Mixed Etiology:** Initial: 2.5mcg. **Partial Response:** Increase by 2.5mcg, then by 5-10mcg until desired response. **No Response:** Increase by 5mcg, then by 5-10mcg until desired response. **Neurogenic Etiology** (Spinal Cord Injury): Initial: 1.25mcg. **Partial/No Response:** May give 2nd dose of 2.5mcg, 3rd dose of 5mcg, then may increase by 5mcg until desired response. Max: 60mcg/dose. Reduce dose if erection >1 hour. Give no more than 3 times weekly; allow 24 hrs between doses.	**W/P:** Impulse device is for single use only. Treat erections lasting >4 hrs immediately. Penile fibrosis, including Peyronie's disease reported. Follow-up with patient to detect penile fibrosis. If possible, treat underlying cause of ED before therapy. Blood at injection site increases risk of blood-borne disease transmission. **Contra:** Predisposition to priapism (eg, sickle cell anemia, multiple myeloma, leukemia), penis anatomical deformation (eg, angulation, cavernosal fibrosis, Peyronie's disease), penile implants, those in whom sexual activities are contraindicated, women, children or newborns. **P/N:** Not for use in women.	Penile pain, priapism/ prolonged erection, penile fibrosis, hematoma/ bleeding at injection site.

BB = black box warning; **W/P** = warnings/precautions; **Contra** = contraindications; **P/N** = pregnancy category rating and nursing considerations.

Table 18.1. Prescribing Information for Neuropathic Therapies

GENERIC (BRAND)	FORM/ STRENGTH	DOSAGE	WARNINGS/PRECAUTIONS & CONTRAINDICATIONS	ADVERSE REACTIONS
ERECTILE DYSFUNCTION *(Cont.)*				
Sildenafil citrate (Viagra)	**Tab:** 25mg, 50mg, 100mg	**Adults:** Usual: 50mg 1 hr (range 0.5-4 hrs) prior to sexual activity at frequency of up to once daily. Titrate: May decrease to 25mg qd or increase to 100mg qd. Max: 100mg qd. **Elderly/Hepatic Impairment/CrCl <30mL/min/Concomitant CYP450 3A4 Inhibitors** (eg, ketoconazole, itraconazole, erythromycin, saquinavir): Initial: 25mg qd. **Concomitant Ritonavir:** Max: 25mg q48h. **Concomitant β-blocker:** Avoid doses >25mg sildenafil within 4 hours of an β-blocker.	**W/P:** Caution with MI, stroke or life-threatening arrhythmia within last 6 months; with resting hypotension (BP<90/50) or HTN (BP>170/110); unstable angina due to cardiac failure or CAD; anatomical penile deformation; predisposition to priapism; and retinitis pigmentosa. Avoid in men where sexual activity is inadvisable due to underlying CV status. Decrease in supine BP reported. Rare reports of nonarteritic anterior ischemic optic neuropathy (NAION) with PDE5 inhibitors. Caution when PDE5 inhibitors are given concomitantly with β-blockers. PDE5 inhibitors and α-adrenergic blocking agents are both vasodilators with BP-lowering effects; additive effect on BP may be anticipated. Cases of sudden decrease or loss of hearing reported. D/C if these symptoms occur. **Contra:** Organic nitrates taken regularly and/or intermittently. **P/N:** Category B, not for use in nursing.	Headache, flushing, dyspepsia, nasal congestion, UTI, abnormal vision (eg, color tinge, increased light sensitivity, blurred vision), diarrhea, cardiovascular events, sudden decrease or loss of hearing.
Tadalafil (Cialis)	**Tab:** 2.5mg, 5mg, 10mg, 20mg	**Adults:** Prn Use: Take prior to sexual activity. Initial: 10mg. Range: 5-20mg. **Renal Impairment: CrCl 31-50mL/min:** Initial: 5mg. Max: 10mg/48 hrs. **CrCl <30mL/min/Hemodialysis:** Max: 5mg/72 hrs. **Mild/Moderate Hepatic Impairment:** Max: 10mg. **Severe Hepatic Impairment:** Avoid use. **With Potent CYP3A4 Inhibitors** (eg, Ketoconazole, Itraconazole, Ritonavir): Max: 10mg/72 hrs. Once Daily Use: Initial: 2.5mg qd without regard to timing of sexual activity. Titrate: May increase to 5mg qd based on efficacy and tolerability. **CrCl <30mL/min/ Hemodialysis/Severe Hepatic Impairment:** Avoid use. **Mild/Moderate Hepatic Impairment:** Use with caution. **With Potent CYP3A4 Inhibitors** (eg, Ketoconazole, Itraconazole, Ritonavir): Max: 2.5mg.	**W/P:** Avoid in men for whom sexual activity is inadvisable due to underlying CV status. Increased sensitivity to vasodilatory effect with left ventricular outflow obstruction. Avoid with MI (within last 90 days); unstable angina or angina occurring during sexual intercourse; NYHA Class 2 or greater heart failure (in the last 6 months); uncontrolled arrhythmias, hypotension (<90/50mmHg); or uncontrolled HTN (>170/100mmHg); stroke within the last 6 months; severe hepatic impairment (Childs-Pugh Class C); degenerative retinal disorders, including retinitis pigmentosa. Prolonged erection reported. Substantial consumption of alcohol with tadalafil can increase HR, decrease BP, dizziness, and headache. Caution with predisposition to priapism (eg, sickle cell anemia, multiple myeloma, leukemia), anatomical deformation of the penis, bleeding disorders, or active peptic ulceration. May cause transient decrease in BP. Caution with coadministration of PDE5 inhibitors and α-blockers. May cause additive hypotensive effect. Initiate at lowest dose once patient is stable on either therapy. Rare reports of nonarteritic anterior ischemic optic neuropathy (NAION) with PDE5 inhibitors. Sudden decrease or loss of hearing, tinnitus, and dizziness reported. D/C if these symptoms occur. **Contra:** Concomitant nitrates. **P/N:** Category B, not for use in nursing.	Headache, dyspepsia, back pain, myalgia, nasal congestion, flushing, limb pain, urticaria, Stevens-Johnson syndrome, exfoliative dermatitis, migraine, visual field defect, retinal vein occlusion, retinal artery occlusion, sudden decrease or loss of hearing, tinnitus.
Vardenafil HCl (Levitra)	**Tab:** 2.5mg, 5mg, 10mg, 20mg	**Adults:** Initial: 10mg one hour prior to sexual activity at frequency of up to once daily. Titrate: May decrease to 5mg or increase to max of 20mg based on response. **Elderly: ≥65 yrs:** Initial: 5mg. **Moderate Hepatic Impairment:** Initial: 5mg; Max: 10mg. **Concomitant Ritonavir:** Max: 2.5mg/72 hrs. **Concomitant Indinavir/ Saquinavir/Atazanavir/Ketoconazole 400mg daily/Itraconazole 400mg daily:** Max: 2.5mg/24 hrs. Concomitant Ketoconazole 200mg daily/Itraconazole	**W/P:** Avoid when sexual activity is inadvisable due to underlying CV status. Increased sensitivity to vasodilation effects with left ventricular outflow obstruction. Decrease in supine BP reported. Avoid with unstable angina, hypotension (SBP<90 mmHg), uncontrolled HTN(>170/100 mmHg), recent history of stroke, life-threatening arrhythmia, MI (within last 6 months), severe cardiac failure, severe hepatic impairment (Child-Pugh C), end-stage renal disease requiring dialysis,	Headache, flushing, rhinitis, dyspepsia, sinusitis, flu syndrome, sudden decrease or loss of hearing, tinnitus.

W/P = warnings/precautions; **Contra** = contraindications; **P/N** = pregnancy category rating and nursing considerations.

Table 18.1. Prescribing Information for Neuropathic Therapies

GENERIC (BRAND)	FORM/ STRENGTH	DOSAGE	WARNINGS/PRECAUTIONS & CONTRAINDICATIONS	ADVERSE REACTIONS
Vardenafil HCl (Levitra) *(Cont.)*		200mg daily/ Erythromycin: Max: 5mg/24 hrs.	hereditary degenerative retinal disorders including retinitis pigmentosa, congenital QT prolongation. Caution with bleeding disorders, peptic ulcers, anatomical deformation of the penis, or predisposition to priapism. Rare reports of non-arteritic anterior ischemic optic neuropathy (NAION) with PDE5 inhibitors. Sudden decrease or loss of hearing accompanied by tinnitus and dizziness reported. **Contra:** Concomitant nitrates or nitric oxide donors. **P/N:** Category B, not for use in nursing.	

GASTROPARESIS

GENERIC (BRAND)	FORM/ STRENGTH	DOSAGE	WARNINGS/PRECAUTIONS & CONTRAINDICATIONS	ADVERSE REACTIONS
Erythromycin*†	**Tab:** 250mg, 500mg	*Adults:* Usual: 250mg qid or 500mg q12h without food. Max: 4g/day. Treat strep infections for at least 10 days. **Streptococcal Infection Long-Term Prophylaxis of Rheumatic Fever:** 250mg bid. **Chlamydial Urogenital Infection During Pregnancy:** 500mg qid for at least 7 days or 500mg q12h or 250mg qid for at least 14 days. **Urethral/Endocervical/ Rectal Chlamydial Infections and Nongonococcal Urethritis:** 500mg qid for at least 7 days. **Primary Syphilis:** 30-40g in divided doses over 10-15 days. **Acute PID:** 500mg (erythromycin lactobionate) IV q6h for 3 days, then 500mg PO q12h for 7 days. **Intestinal Amebiasis:** 500mg q12h or 250mg q6h for 10-14 days. **Pertussis:** 40-50mg/kg/day in divided doses for 5-14 days. **Legionnaires' Disease:** 1-4g/day in divided doses. *Pediatrics:* Usual: 30-50mg/kg/day in divided doses without food. Severe Infections: May double dose. Max: 4g/day. Treat strep infections for at least 10 days. **Streptococcal Infection Long-Term Prophylaxis of Rheumatic Fever:** 250mg bid. **Chlamydial Conjunctivitis of Newborns/Chlamydial Pneumonia in Infancy:** (Sus) 12.5mg/kg qid for 2 weeks and 3 weeks, respectively. **Intestinal Amebiasis:** 30-50mg/kg/day in divided doses for 10-14 days.	**W/P:** Pseudomembranous colitis, hepatic dysfunction reported. Caution with impaired hepatic function. May aggravate weakness of patients with myasthenia gravis. **Contra:** Concomitant terfenadine, astemizole, pimozide, or cisapride. **P/N:** Category B, caution in nursing.	NV, abdominal pain, diarrhea, anorexia, abnormal LFTs, allergic reactions, superinfection (prolonged use).
Metoclopramide HCl (Reglan)	**Inj:** 5mg/mL; **Syr:** 5mg/5mL; **Tab:** 5mg, 10mg* *scored	*Adults:* GERD: PO: 10-15mg qid 30 min ac and hs. **Elderly:** 5 mg qid. Max: 12 weeks of therapy. **Intermittent Symptoms:** Up to 20mg single dose prior to provoking situation. **Gastroparesis:** 10mg PO 30 min ac and hs for 2-8 weeks. **Severe Gastroparesis:** May give same doses IV/IM for up to 10 days if needed. **Antiemetic: (Postoperative)** 10-20mg IM near end of surgery. **(Chemotherapy-Induced)** 1-2mg/kg 30 min before chemotherapy then q2h for two doses, then q3h for three doses. Give 2mg/kg for highly emetogenic drugs for initial 2 doses. **Small Bowel Intubation/Radiological Exam:** 10mg IV single dose. **CrCl <40mL/min:** 50% of normal dose. *Pediatrics:* Small Bowel Intubation: 6-14 yrs: 2.5-5mg IV single dose. **<6 yrs:** 0.1mg/kg IV single dose. **CrCl <40mL/min:** 50% of normal dose.	**W/P:** Caution with HTN, Parkinson's disease, depression. EPS, tardive dyskinesia, Parkinsonian-like symptoms, neuroleptic malignant syndrome reported. Administer IV injection slowly. Risk of developing fluid retention and volume overload especially with cirrhosis or CHF; d/c if these occur. May increase pressure of suture lines. **Contra:** Where GI mobility stimulation is dangerous (eg, perforation, obstruction, hemorrhage), pheochromocytoma, seizure disorder, concomitant drugs that cause EPS effects. **P/N:** Category B, caution with nursing.	Restlessness, drowsiness, fatigue, EPS effects (acute dystonic reactions), galactorrhea, hyperprolactinemia, hypotension, arrhythmia, diarrhea, dizziness, urinary frequency.

Continued on next page

*Available only in generic form. †Erythromycin is not FDA-approved for gastroparesis but is commonly used as an off-label treatment.
W/P = warnings/precautions; **Contra** = contraindications; **P/N** = pregnancy category rating and nursing considerations.

Table 18.1. Prescribing Information for Neuropathic Therapies

BRAND	INGREDIENT/ STRENGTH	DOSE
Management of Constipation (OTC Products)		
BULK-FORMING		
Citrucel Caplets	Methylcellulose 500mg	*Adults:* ≥12 yrs: 2 caps qd prn. **Max:** 12 tabs q24h. *Peds:* 6-12 yrs: 1 cap qd prn. **Max:** 6 tabs q24h.
Citrucel Powder	Methylcellulose 2g/tbl	*Adults:* ≥12 yrs: 1 tbl (11.5g) qd tid. *Peds:* 6-12 yrs: 1/2 tbl (5.75g) qd.
Equalactin Chewable Tablet	Calcium Polycarbophil 625mg	*Adults & Peds:* ≥12 yrs: 2 tabs qd. **Max:** 8 tabs qd. *Peds:* 6-12 yrs: 1 tab qd. **Max:** 2 tabs qd. **2 to <6 yrs:** 1 tab qd. **Max:** 2 tabs qd.
Fibercon Caplets	Calcium Polycarbophil 625mg	*Adults & Peds:* ≥12 yrs: 2 tabs qd. **Max:** 8 tabs qd. *Peds:* 6-12 yrs: 1 tab qd. **Max:** 4 tabs qd. **2 to <6 yrs:** 1 tab qd. **Max:** 2 tabs qd.
Konsyl Easy Mix Powder	Psyllium 6g/tsp	*Adults:* ≥12 yrs: 1 tsp qd-tid. *Peds:* 6-12 yrs: 1/2 tsp qd-tid.
Konsyl Fiber Caplets	Calcium Polycarbophil 625mg	*Adults & Peds:* ≥12 yrs: 2 tabs qd. **Max:** 8 tabs qd.
Konsyl Orange Powder	Psyllium 3.4g	*Adults:* ≥12 yrs: 1 tsp qd-tid. *Peds:* 6-12 yrs: 1/2 tsp qd-tid.
Konsyl Original Powder	Psyllium 6g/tsp	*Adults:* ≥12 yrs: 1 tsp qd-tid. *Peds:* 6-12 yrs: 1/2 tsp qd-tid.
Konsyl-D Powder	Psyllium 3.4g/tsp	*Adults:* ≥12 yrs: 1 tsp qd-tid. *Peds:* 6-12 yrs: 1/2 tsp qd-tid.
Metamucil Capsules	Psyllium 0.52g	*Adults & Peds:* ≥12 yrs: 5 caps qd-tid.
Metamucil Original Texture Powder	Psyllium 3.4g/tbs	*Adults:* ≥12 yrs: 1 tbs qd-tid. *Peds:* 6-12 yrs: 1/2 tsp qd-tid.
Metamucil Smooth Texture Powder	Psyllium 3.4g/tbs	*Adults:* ≥12 yrs: 1 tbs qd-tid. *Peds:* 6-12 yrs: 1/2 tsp qd-tid.
Metamucil Wafers	Psyllium 3.4 g/dose	*Adults:* ≥12 yrs: 2 wafers qd-tid. *Peds:* 6-12 yrs: 1 wafer qd-tid.
HYPEROSMOTICS		
Fleet Children's Babylax Suppositories	Glycerin 2.3g	*Peds:* 2-5 yrs: 1 supp. ud.
Fleet Glycerin Suppositories	Glycerin 2g	*Adults & Peds:* ≥6 yrs: 1 supp ud.
Fleet Liquid Glycerin Suppositories	Glycerin 5.6g	*Adults & Peds:* ≥6 yrs: 1 supp ud.
Fleet Mineral Oil Enema	Mineral Oil 133mL	*Adults:* ≥12 yrs: 1 bottle (133mL). *Peds:* 2-12 yrs: 1/2 bottle (66.5mL)
HYPEROSMOTIC COMBINATION		
Fleet Pain Relief Pre-Moistened Anorectal Pads	Glycerin/Pramoxine HCl 12%-1%	*Adults & Peds:* ≥12 yrs: Apply to affected area up to five times daily.
OSMOTIC		
MiraLAX	Polyethylene Glycol 3350	*Adults & Peds:* ≥17 yrs: Stir and dissolve 17g in 4-8 oz of beverage and drink qd. Use no more than 7 days.
SALINES		
Ex-Lax Milk of Magnesia Liquid	Magnesium Hydroxide 400mg/5mL	*Adults & Peds:* ≥12 yrs: Take 2-4 tbs hs. *Peds:* 6-11 yrs: 1-2 tbs hs. 2-5 yrs: 1-3 tbs hs.
Fleet Children's Enema	Monobasic Sodium Phosphate/Dibasic Sodium Phosphate 9.5g-3.5g/66mL	*Peds:* 5-11 yrs: 1 bottle (66mL). 2-5 yrs: 1/2 bottle (33mL).
Fleet Enema	Monobasic Sodium Phosphate/Dibasic Sodium Phosphate 19g-7g/133mL	*Adults & Peds:* ≥12 yrs: 1 bottle (133mL).
Fleet Phospho-Soda	Monobasic Sodium Phosphate/Dibasic Sodium Phosphate 2.4g-0.9g/5mL	*Adults:* ≥12 yrs: 1 tbl in 8 oz of water. **Max:** 3 tbl. *Peds:* 10-11 yrs: 1 tbl in 8 oz of water. **Max:** 1 tbl. 5-9 yrs: 1/2 tbl in 8 oz of water. **Max:** 1/2 tbl.
Magnesium Citrate Solution	Magnesium Citrate 1.75gm/30mL	*Adults:* ≥12 yrs: 300mL. *Peds:* 6-12 yrs: 90-210mL. 2-6 yrs: 60-90mL.

Table 18.1. Prescribing Information for Neuropathic Therapies

BRAND	INGREDIENT/ STRENGTH	DOSE
Phillips Antacid/Laxative Chewable Tablets	Magnesium Hydroxide 311mg	*Adults:* ≥12 yrs: 6-8 tabs qd. *Peds:* 6-11 yrs: 3-4 tabs qd. 2-5 yrs: 1-2 tabs qd.
Phillips Soft Chews, Laxative	Magnesium/Sodium 500mg-10 mg	*Adults & Peds:* ≥12 yrs: Take 2-4 tab qd. Max: 4 tab q24h.
Phillips Cramp-Free Laxative Caplets	Magnesium 500 mg	*Adults & Peds:* ≥12 yrs: Take 2-4 tabs qd. Max: 4 tabs q24h.
Phillips Milk of Magnesia Concentrated Liquid	Magnesium Hydroxide 800mg/5mL	*Adults:* ≥12 yrs: 15-30mL qd. *Peds:* 6-11 yrs: 7.5-15mL qd. 2-5 yrs: 2.5-7.5mL qd.
Phillips Milk of Magnesia Liquid	Magnesium Hydroxide 400mg/5mL	*Adults:* ≥12 yrs: 30-60mL qd. *Peds:* 6-11 yrs: 15-30mL qd. 2-5 yrs: 5-15mL qd.
SALINE COMBINATION		
Phillips M-O Liquid	Magnesium Hydroxide/Mineral Oil 300mg-1.25mL/5mL	*Adults:* ≥12 yrs: 30-60mL qd. *Peds:* 6-11 yrs: 5-15mL qd.
STIMULANTS		
Alophen Enteric Coated Stimulant Laxative Pills	Bisacodyl 5mg	*Adults:* ≥12 yrs: Take 1-3 tabs qd. *Peds:* 6-12 yrs: Take 1 tab qd.
Carter's Laxative, Sodium Free Pills	Bisacodyl 5mg	*Adults:* qd.12 yrs: Take 1-3 tabs (usually 2 tabs) qd. *Peds:* 6-12 yrs: Take 1 tab qd.
Castor Oil	Castor Oil	*Adults:* ≥12 yrs: 15-60mL. *Peds:* 2-12 yrs: 5-15mL.
Correctol Stimulant Laxative Tablets For Women	Bisacodyl 5mg	*Adults:* ≥12 yrs: Take 1-3 tabs qd. *Peds:* 6-12 yrs: Take 1 tab qd.
Doxidan Capsules	Bisacodyl 5mg	*Adults:* ≥12 yrs: 1-3 caps (usually 2) qd. *Peds:* 6-12 yrs: 1 cap qd.
Dulcolax Overnight Relief Laxative Tablets	Bisacodyl 5mg	*Adults:* ≥12 yrs: 1-3 tabs (usually 2) qd. *Peds:* 6-12 yo: 1 tab qd.
Dulcolax Suppository	Bisacodyl 10mg	*Adults:* ≥12 yrs: 1 supp qd. *Peds:* 6-12 yrs: 1/2 supp qd.
Dulcolax Tablets	Bisacodyl 5mg	*Adults:* ≥12 yrs: 1-3 tabs (usually 2) qd. *Peds:* 6-12 yrs: 1 tab qd.
Ex-Lax Maximum Strength Tablets	Sennosides 25mg	*Adults:* ≥12 yrs: 2 tabs qd-bid. *Peds:* 6-12 yrs: 1 tab qd-bid.
Ex-Lax Tablets	Sennosides 15mg	*Adults:* ≥12 yrs: 2 tabs qd-bid. *Peds:* 6-12 yrs: 1 tab qd-bid.
Ex-Lax Ultra Stimulant Laxative Tablets	Bisacodyl 5mg	*Adults:* ≥12 yrs: 1-3 tabs qd. *Peds:* 6-12 yrs: 1 tab qd.
Fleet Bisacodyl Suppositories	Bisacodyl 10mg	*Adults:* ≥12 yrs: 1 supp. *Peds:* 6-12 yrs: 1/2 supp. qd.
Fleet Stimulant Laxative Tablets	Bisacodyl 5mg	*Adults:* ≥12 yrs: 1-3 tabs (usually 2) qd. *Peds:* 6-12 yrs: 1 tab qd.
Nature's Remedy Caplets	Aloe/Cascara Sagrada 100mg-150mg	*Adults:* ≥12 yrs: 2 tabs qd-bid. Max: 4 tabs bid. *Peds:* 6-12 yrs: 1 tab qd-bid. Max: 2 tabs bid. 2-6 yrs: 1/2 tab qd-bid. Max: 1 tab bid.
Perdiem Overnight Relief Tablets	Sennosides 15mg	*Adults:* ≥12 yrs: 2 tabs qd-bid. *Peds:* 6-12 yrs: 1 tab qd-bid.
Senokot Tablets	Sennosides 8.6mg	*Adults:* ≥12 yrs: 2 tabs qd. Max 4 tabs bid. *Peds:* 6-12 yrs: 1 tab qd. Max: 2 tabs bid. 2-6 yrs: 1/2 tab qd. Max: 1 tab bid.
STIMULANT COMBINATIONS		
Peri-Colace Tablets	Sennosides/Docusate 8.6mg-50mg	*Adults:* ≥12 yrs: 2-4 tabs qd. *Peds:* 6-12 yrs: 1-2 tabs qd. 2-6 yrs: 1 tab qd.
Senokot S Tablets	Sennosides/Docusate 8.6mg-50mg	*Adults:* ≥12 yrs: 2 tabs qd. Max: 4 tabs bid. *Peds:* 6-12 yrs: 1 tab qd-bid. Max: 2 tabs bid. 2-6 yrs: 1/2 tab qd. Max: 1 tab bid.
SURFACTANTS (STOOL SOFTENERS)		
Colace Capsules	Docusate Sodium 100mg	*Adults:* ≥12 yrs: 1-3 caps qd. *Peds:* 2-12 yrs: 1 cap qd.
Colace Capsules	Docusate Sodium 50mg	*Adults:* ≥12 yrs: 1-6 caps qd. *Peds:* 2-12 yrs: 1-3 caps qd.

Table 18.1. Prescribing Information for Neuropathic Therapies

BRAND	INGREDIENT/ STRENGTH	DOSE
Colace Liquid	Docusate Sodium 10mg/mL	*Adults:* ≥12 yrs: 5-15mL qd-bid. *Peds:* 2-12 yrs: 5-15mL qd.
Colace Syrup	Docusate Sodium 60mg/15mL	*Adults:* ≥12 yrs: 15-90mL qd. *Peds:* 2-12 yrs: 5-37.5mL qd.
Correctol Stool Softener Laxative Soft-Gels	Docusate Sodium 100mg	*Adults:* ≥12 yrs: Take 2 caps qd. *Peds:* 2-12 yrs: Take 1 cap qd.
Docusol Constipation Relief, Mini Enemas	Docusate Sodium 283mg	*Adults:* ≥12 yrs: Take 1-3 units qd. *Peds:* 6-12 yrs: Take 1 unit qd.
Dulcolax Stool Softener Capsules	Docusate Sodium 100mg	*Adults:* ≥12 yrs: 1-3 caps qd. *Peds:* 2-12 yrs: 1 cap qd.
Ex-Lax Stool Softener Tablets	Docusate Sodium 100mg	*Adults:* ≥12 yrs: 1-3 caps qd. *Peds:* 2-12 yrs: 1 cap qd.
Kaopectate Liqui-Gels	Docusate Calcium 240mg	*Adults & Peds:* ≥12 yrs: 1 cap qd until normal bowel movement.
Phillips Stool Softener Capsules	Docusate Sodium 100mg	*Adults:* ≥12 yrs: 1-3 caps qd. *Peds:* 6-12 yrs: 1 cap qd.

Management of Diarrhea (OTC Products)

ABSORBENT AGENTS

BRAND	INGREDIENT/ STRENGTH	DOSE
Equalactin Chewable Tablets	Calcium Polycarbophil 625mg	*Adults:* ≥12 yrs: 2 tabs q30min prn. **Max:** 8 tabs q24h. *Peds:* 6-12 yrs: 1 tab q30min. **Max:** 4 tabs q24h. **2 to ≤6 yrs:** 1 tab q30min. **Max:** 2 tabs q24h.
Fibercon Caplets	Calcium Polycarbophil 625mg	*Adults:* ≥12 yrs: 2 tabs qd. **Max:** 8 tabs q24h.
Konsyl Fiber Caplets	Calcium Polycarbophil 625mg	*Adults:* ≥12 yrs: 2 tabs qd. **Max:** 8 tabs q24h. *Peds:* 6-12 yrs: 1 tab qd. **Max:** 3 tabs q24h.

ANTIPERISTALTIC AGENTS

BRAND	INGREDIENT/ STRENGTH	DOSE
Imodium A-D Caplet	Loperamide HCl 2mg	*Adults:* ≥12 yrs: 2 caplets after first loose stool; 1 caplet after each subsequent loose stool. **Max:** 4 caplets q24h. *Peds:* 9-11 yrs (60-95 lbs): 1 caplet after first loose stool; 1/2 caplet after each subsequent loose stool. **Max:** 3 caplets q24h. 6-8 yrs (48-59 lbs): 1 caplet after first loose stool; 1/2 caplet after each subsequent loose stool. **Max:** 2 caplets q24h.
Imodium A-D E-Z Chews	Loperamide HCl 2mg	*Adults:* ≥12 yrs: 2 caplets after first loose stool; 1 caplet after each subsequent loose stool. **Max:** 4 caplets q24h. *Peds:* 9-11 yrs (60-95 lbs): 1 caplet after first loose stool; 1/2 caplet after each subsequent loose stool. **Max:** 3 caplets q24h. 6-8 yrs (48-59 lbs): 1 caplet after first loose stool; 1/2 caplet after each subsequent loose stool. **Max:** 2 caplets q24h.
Imodium A-D Liquid	Loperamide HCl 1mg/7.5mL	*Adults:* ≥12 yrs: 30mL (6 tsp) after first loose stool; 15mL (3 tsp) after each subsequent loose stool. **Max:** 60mL (12 tsp) q24h. *Peds:* 9-11 yrs (60-95 lbs): 15mL (3 tsp) after first loose stool; 7.5mL (11/2 tsp) after each subsequent loose stool. **Max:** 45mL (9 tsp) q24h. 6-8 yrs (48-59 lbs): 15 mL (3 tsp) after first loose stool; 7.5mL (11/2 tsp) after each subsequent loose stool. **Max:** 30mL (6 tsp) q24h.

ANTIPERISTALTIC/ANTIFLATULENT AGENTS

BRAND	INGREDIENT/ STRENGTH	DOSE
Imodium Advanced Caplet	Loperamide HCl/Simethicone 2mg-125mg	*Adults:* ≥12 yrs: 2 caplets after first loose stool; 1 caplet after each subsequent loose stool. **Max:** 4 caplets q24h. *Peds:* 9-11 yrs (60-95 lbs): 1 caplet after first loose stool; 1/2 caplet after each subsequent loose stool. **Max:** 3 caplets q24h. 6-8 yrs (48-59 lbs): 1 caplet after first loose stool; 1/2 caplet after each subsequent loose stool. **Max:** 2 caplets q24h.
Imodium Advanced Chewable Tablet	Loperamide HCl/Simethicone 2mg-125mg	*Adults:* ≥12 yrs: 2 caplets after first loose stool; 1 caplet after each subsequent loose stool. **Max:** 4 caplets q24h. *Peds:* 9-11 yrs (60-95 lbs): 1 caplet after first loose stool; 1/2 caplet after each subsequent loose stool. **Max:** 3 caplets q24h. 6-8 yrs (48-59 lbs): 1 caplet after first loose stool; 1/2 caplet after each subsequent loose stool. **Max:** 2 caplets q24h.

Table 18.1. Prescribing Information for Neuropathic Therapies

BRAND	INGREDIENT/ STRENGTH	DOSE
BISMUTH SUBSALICYLATE		
Kaopectate Caplets	Bismuth Subsalicylate 262mg	*Adults & Peds:* ≥**12 yrs:** 2 caplets q1/2-1h prn. **Max:** 8 doses q24h.
Kaopectate Extra Strength Liquid	Bismuth Subsalicylate 525mg/15mL	*Adults:* ≥**12 yrs:** 2 tbl (30mL). *Peds:* **9-12 yrs:** 1 tbl (15mL) q1h prn. **6-9 yrs:** 2 tsp (10mL) q1h prn. **3-6 yrs:** 1 tsp (5mL) q1h prn. **Max:** 8 doses q24h.
Kaopectate Liquid	Bismuth Subsalicylate 262mg/15mL	*Adults:* ≥**12 yrs:** 2 tbl (30mL). *Peds:* **9-12 yrs:** 1 tbl (15mL) q1h prn. **6-9 yrs:** 2 tsp (10mL) q1h prn. **3-6 yrs:** 1 tsp (5mL) q1h prn. **Max:** 8 doses q24h.
Pepto Bismol Chewable Tablets	Bismuth Subsalicylate 262mg	*Adults & Peds:* ≥**12 yrs:** 2 tabs q1/2-1h. **Max:** 8 doses (16 tabs) q24h.
Pepto Bismol Caplets	Bismuth Subsalicylate 262mg	*Adults & Peds:* ≥**12 yrs:** 2 tabs q1/2-1h. **Max:** 8 doses (16 caps) q24h.
Pepto Bismol Liquid	Bismuth Subsalicylate 262mg/15mL	*Adults & Peds:* ≥**12 yrs:** 2 tbl (30mL) q1/2-1h prn. **Max:** 8 doses (16 tbl) q24h.
Pepto Bismol Maximum Strength	Bismuth Subsalicylate 525mg/15mL	*Adults:* ≥**12 yrs:** 2 tbl (30mL) q1h prn. **Max:** 4 doses (8 tbl) q24h.

Table 18.2. Drug Interactions for Neuropathic Therapies

Management of Peripheral Neuropathy

ANTICONVULSANT

Carbamazepine (Tegretol, Tegretol XR)

Acetaminophen	Decreases plasma levels of acetaminophen.
Alprazolam	Decreases plasma levels of alprazolam.
Carbamazepine Suspension	Do not administer suspension form with other medicinal liquids or diluents.
Clomipramine	Increases plasma levels of clomipramine.
Clonazepam	Decreases plasma levels of clonazepam.
Clozapine	Decreases plasma levels of clozapine.
Contraceptives, hormonal (eg, oral, levonorgestrel subdermal implant)	May decrease plasma levels of hormonal contraceptives and decrease contraceptive effectiveness; consider alternative or back-up methods of contraception.
CYP3A4 inducers (eg, rifampin)	May increase the rate of carbamazepine metabolism.
CYP3A4 inhibitors (eg, cimetidine, macrolides)	Inhibits metabolism of carbamazepine.
Dicumarol	Decreases plasma levels of dicumarol.
Doxycycline	Decreases plasma levels of doxycycline.
Ethosuximide	Decreases plama levels of ethosuximide.
Haloperidol	Decreases plasma levels of haloperidol.
Lamotrigine	Decreases plasma levels of lamotrigine.
Lithium	Concomitant use may increase the risk of neurotoxic side effects.
MAO inhibitors	Do not use concomitantly; MAO inhibitors should be discontinued for at least 14 days prior to carbamazepine use.
Methsuximide	Decreases plasma levels of methsuximide.
Nefazodone	Contraindicated; do not administer concomitantly; decreases plasma levels of nefazodone.
Phensuximide	Decreases plasma levels of phensuximide.
Phenytoin	May increase or decrease plasma levels of phenytoin.
Primidone	Increases plasma levels of primidone
Theophylline	Decreases plasma levels of theophylline.
Tiagabine	Decreases plasma levels of tiagabine.
Topiramate	Decreases plasma levels of topiramate.
Valproate	Decreases plasma levels of valproate.
Warfarin	Decreases plasma levels of warfarin.

Table 18.2. Drug Interactions for Neuropathic Therapies

GABA ANALOGS

Gabapentin (Neurontin)

Antacids	Take gabapentin at least 2 hrs following antacid administration.
Morphine	Increases gabapentin levels when controlled release morphine is concomitantly used.

Pregabalin (Lyrica)

Alcohol	Potentiates the effects on cognitive and gross motor functioning when used concomitantly; avoid consumption of alcohol during therapy.
CNS depressants (eg, opiates, benzodiazepines)	Potentiates the effects on cognitive and gross motor functioning when used concomitantly.

SEROTONIN/NOREPINEPHRINE REUPTAKE INHIBITOR (SNRI)

Duloxetine HCl (Cymbalta)

Alcohol	Avoid substantial alcohol use.
CNS-active drugs	Caution with concomitant use.
CYP1A2 inhibitors (eg, fluvoxamine, quinolone antibiotics)	Avoid concomitant use.
CYP2D6 inhibitors (eg, paroxetine, fluoxetine, quinidine)	Increases duloxetine levels.
CYP2D6 substrates (eg, TCAs, phenothiazines, type 1C antiarrhythmics)	Caution with concomitant use.
Gastric acidity-affecting drugs	May interact; caution with concomitant use.
MAO inhibitors	Warning, do not use concomitantly; at least 14 days should elapse between discontinuation of an MAO inhibitor and initiation of therapy with duloxetine; at least 5 days should be allowed before stopping Cymbalta and starting an MAO inhibitor.
Protein-bound drugs (highly)	May increase free concentration levels of highly protein-bound drugs.
Serotonergic drugs (SSRIs, SNRIs, tramadol)	Avoid concomitant use.
Thioridazine	Avoid concomitant use.
Triptans	Avoid concomitant use; monitor patient closely.

TOPICAL AGENT

Lidocaine (Lidoderm Patch)

Anesthetics, local	If using concomitantly with other local anesthetics, consider amount of anesthetic absorbed from all agents.
Antiarrhythmics, class I (eg, tocainide, mexiletine)	Caution with concomitant use; toxic effects may be additive and potentially synergistic.

Table 18.2. Drug Interactions for Neuropathic Therapies

TRICYCLIC ANTIDEPRESSANTS

Amitriptyline HCI (Elavil*)

Alcohol	Potentiates effects of alcohol.
Anticholinergic drugs	Monitor closely for increased anticholinergic effects; may cause paralytic ileus and hyperpyrexia.
Barbiturates	Potentiates effects of barbiturates.
CNS depressants	Potentiates effects of CNS depressants.
CYP2D6 inhibitors (eg, quinidine, cimetidine)	Increases plasma levels of amitriptyline.
CYP2D6 substrates (eg, phenothiazines, propafenone, flecainide)	Increases plasma levels of amtriptyline.
Disulfiram	Caution, delirium reported with concomitant use.
Ethchlorvynol	Caution, delirium reported with concomitant use.
Guanethidine	May block antihypertensive effects of guanethidine.
MAO inhibitors	Warning, do not give concomitantly or within at least 2 weeks of treatment with an MAO inhibitor.
Neuroleptics	Monitor patients closely who are receiving concomitant therapy; hyperpyrexia reported.
SSRIs (eg, fluoxetine, citalopram, escitalopram, sertraline, paroxetine)	Caution when switching to or from an SSRI; ≥5 weeks may be needed before initiating treatment with amitriptyline following withdrawal from fluoxetine.
Sympathomimetic drugs	Monitor closely if using concomitantly.
Thyroid drugs	Monitor closely if using concomitantly.

Desipramine HCI (Norpramin)

Alcohol	Potentiates effects of alcohol.
Anticholinergic drugs	Monitor closely for increased anticholinergic effects.
Benzodiazepines (eg, diazepam, chlordiazepoxide)	Caution, additive sedative effects.
CNS depressants (eg, sedatives/hypnotics, psychotropics)	Caution, additive sedative effects.
CYP2D6 inhibitors (eg, quinidine, cimetidine)	Increases plasma levels of desipramine.
CYP2D6 substrates (eg, antidepressants, phenothiazines, propafenone, flecainide)	Increases plasma levels of desipramine.

*Brand name discontinued, generic version is still available.

Table 18.2. Drug Interactions for Neuropathic Therapies

Guanethidine	May block antihypertensive effects of guanethidine.
MAO inhibitors	Warning; do not give concomitantly or within at least 2 weeks of treatment with an MAO inhibitor.
SSRIs (eg, fluoxetine, citalopram, escitalopram, sertraline, paroxetine)	Caution with when switching to or from an SSRI; ≥5 weeks may be needed before initiating treatment with desipramine following withdrawal from fluoxetine.
Sympathomimetic drugs	Monitor closely if using concomitantly.
Thyroid drugs	Monitor closely; may cause cardiac arrhythmias.
Doxepin HCl (Doxepin, Sinequan)	
Alcohol	Warning, increased risk of doxepin overdose; potentiates effects of alcohol.
Anticholinergic drugs	Monitor closely for increased anticholinergic effects.
CYP2D6 inhibitors (eg, cimetidine, quinidine)	Increases plasma levels of doxepin.
CYP2D6 substrates (eg, antidepressants, phenothiazines, propafenone, flecainide)	Increases plasma levels of doxepin.
MAO inhibitors	Warning, do not give concomitantly or within at least 2 weeks of treatment with an MAO inhibitor.
SSRIs (eg, fluoxetine, citalopram, escitalopram, sertraline, paroxetine)	Caution when switching to or from an SSRI; ≥5 weeks may be needed before initiating treatment with doxepin following withdrawal from fluoxetine.
Tolazamide	Warning, hypoglycemia reported with concomitant use.
Imipramine HCl (Tofranil)	
Alcohol	Potentiates effects of alcohol.
Anticholinergics	Monitor closely for increased anticholinergic effects; risk of paralytic ileus.
Blood pressure-lowering drugs	Caution with concomitant use.
Clonidine	May block the effects of clonidine.
CNS depressants	Potentiates effects of CNS depressants.
CYP2D6 inhibitors (eg, quinidine, cimetidine)	Increases imipramine plasma levels.
CYP2D6 substrates (eg, phenothiazines, antidepressants, propafenone, flecainide)	Increases imipramine plasma levels.
Guanethidine	May block the effects of guanethidine.
Hepatic enzyme inducers (eg, barbiturates, phenytoin)	May decrease imipramine plasma levels.
MAO inhibitors	Warning, do not give concomitantly or within at least 2 weeks of treatment with an MAO inhibitor.

Table 18.2. Drug Interactions for Neuropathic Therapies

Methylphenidate	May increase imipramine plasma levels.
SSRIs (eg, fluoxetine, citalopram, escitalopram, sertraline, paroxetine)	Caution when switching to or from an SSRI; >5 weeks may be needed before initiating treatment with imipramine following withdrawal from fluoxetine.
Sympathomimetic amines (eg, epinephrine, norepinephrine)	Caution, avoid use; may potentiate catecholamine effects.
Thyroid drugs	Monitor closely; risk of cardiovascular toxicity.
Nortriptyline HCl (Pamelor)	
Alcohol	May potentiate effects of alcohol.
Anticholinergic drugs	Monitor closely if using concomitantly.
Chlorpropamide	Caution, may cause hypoglycemia.
Cimetidine	Increases plasma levels of nortriptyline.
CYP2D6 inhibitors (eg, quinidine)	Increases plasma levels of nortriptyline.
CYP2D6 substrates (eg, phenothiazines, antidepressants, propafenone, flecainide)	Increases plasma levels of nortriptyline.
Guanethidine	May block the antihypertensive effects of guanethidine.
MAO inhibitors	Warning, do not give concomitantly or within at least 2 weeks of treatment with an MAO inhibitor.
Reserpine	May produce a stimulating effect in depressed patients.
SSRIs (eg, fluoxetine, citalopram, escitalopram, sertraline, paroxetine)	Caution when switching to or from an SSRI; >5 weeks may be needed before initiating treatment with nortriptyline following withdrawal from fluoxetine.
Sympathomimetic drugs	Monitor closely if using concomitantly.
Thyroid drugs	Monitor closely; cardiac arrhythmias may develop.

Management of Central Neuropathy

BLADDER DYSFUNCTION AGENTS

Darifenacin (Enablex)	
Anticholinergic drugs	Concomitant use may increase the frequency and/or severity of anticholinergic effects (eg, dry mouth, constipation, blurred vision).
CYP3A4 inhibitors	Dose should not exceed 7.5mg/day with concomitant potent CYP3A4 inhibitors (eg, ketoconazole, itraconazole, ritonavir, nelfinavir, clarithromycin, nefazodone).
CYP2D6 substrates	Caution with concomitant use.
Oxybutynin (Oxytrol)	
Alcohol	May potentiate drowsiness effects.

Table 18.2. Drug Interactions for Neuropathic Therapies

Anticholinergic drugs	Concomitant use may increase the frequency and/or severity of anticholinergic effects (eg, dry mouth, constipation).
Bisphosphonates	Caution with concomitant use of drugs that can potentiate or cause esophagitis.
Concominantly used drugs	May alter GI absorption of concomitantly administered drugs due to anticholinergic effects on GI motility.

Oxybutynin chloride (Ditropan, Ditropan XL)

Alcohol	May potentiate drowsiness effects.
Anticholinergic drugs	Concomitant use may increase the frequency and/or severity of anticholinergic effects (eg, dry mouth, constipation).
Bisphosphonates	Caution with concomitant use of drugs that can potentiate or cause esophagitis.
Concomitantly used drugs	May alter GI absorption of concomitantly administered drugs due to anticholinergic effects on GI motility.
CYP3A4 inhibitors (eg, antimycotics, macrolides)	Caution with concomitant use of drugs that can potentiate or cause esophagitis.
Ketoconazole	Increases plasma levels of oxybutynin.
Sedatives	May potentiate drowsiness effects.

Solifenacin succinate (VESIcare)

CYP3A4 inhibitors	Caution with use; solifenacin dose should not exceed 5mg/day with concomitant use of a potent CYP3A4 inhibitor.
Ketoconazole	Caution with use; solifenacin dose should not exceed 5mg/day.

Tolterodine tartrate (Detrol, Detrol LA)

CYP3A4 inhibitors (eg, erythromycin, clarithromycin, ketoconazole, itraconazole, miconazole, cyclosporine, vinblastine)	Tolterodine dosing should be reduced with concomitant use.

Trospium chloride (Sanctura, Sanctura XR)

Anticholinergics	Concomitant use may increase the frequency and/or severity of anticholinergic effects.
Metformin	Caution with concomitant use; monitor closely.
Morphine	Caution with concomitant use; monitor closely.
Pancuronium	Caution with concomitant use; monitor closely.
Procainamide	Caution with concomitant use; monitor closely.
Tenofovir	Caution with concomitant use; monitor closely.
Vancomycin	Caution with concomitant use; monitor closely.

ERECTILE DYSFUNCTION AGENTS

Alprostadil (Caverject, Caverject Impulse, Muse)

Anticoagulants (eg, warfarin, heparin)	May increase bleeding risk at site of alprostadil injection.

Table 18.2. Drug Interactions for Neuropathic Therapies

Vasoactive agents	Avoid concomitant use with other vasoactive agents.
Sildenafil citrate (Viagra)	
Alpha-blockers	Caution with concominant use; may produce an additive blood pressure-lowering effect.
Amlodipine	May cause an additional reduction in supine blood pressure when used concomitantly.
CYP2C9 inhibitors	May reduce sildenafil clearance.
CYP3A4 inducers (eg, rifampin)	May decrease sildenafil levels.
CYP3A4 inhibitors (eg, cimetidine, ketoconazole, itraconazole, erythromycin, saquinavir)	Increases sildenafil levels.
Erectile dysfunction treatments, other	Avoid concomitant use with other erectile dysfunction therapies.
Nitrates	Concomitant use is contraindicated; potentiates the hypotensive effects of nitrates.
Protease inhibitors (eg, ritonavir)	Increases sildenafil levels.
Tadalafil (Cialis)	
Alcohol	May produce additive hypotensive effects when used concomitantly.
Alpha-blockers (eg, tamsulosin, doxazosin, alfuzosin)	Caution with concomitant use, may produce an additive blood pressure-lowering effect.
Antihypertensives (eg, amlodipine, metoprolol, bendrofluazide, enalapril, angiotensin-II receptor blockers)	Caution with concomitant use, may produce additive blood pressure-lowering effect.
CYP3A4 inducers (eg, rifampin, carbamazepine, phenytoin, phenobarbital)	Decreases levels of tadalafil.
CYP3A4 inhibitors (eg, ketoconazole, HIV-protease inhibitors, erythromycin, itraconazole, grapefruit juice)	Increases levels of tadalafil.
Nitrates	Concomitant use is contraindicated; potentiates the hypotensive effects of nitrates.
Vardenafil HCl (Levitra)	
Alpha-blockers	Caution with concomitant use; may produce an additive blood pressure-lowering effect.
Antiarrhythmics, class IA (eg, quinidine, procainamide)	Avoid concomitant use.

Table 18.2. Drug Interactions for Neuropathic Therapies

Antiarrhythmics, class III (eg, amiodarone, sotalol)	Avoid concomitant use.
CYP2C9 inhibitors	May reduce clearance of vardenafil.
CYP3A4 inhibitors (eg, saquinavir, atazanavir, ketoconazole, clarithromycin, erythromycin)	Increases levels of vardenafil.
Erectile dysfunction treatments, other	Avoid concominant use with other erectile dysfunction therapies.
Indinavir	Substantially increases plasma concentrations of vardenafil.
Nifedipine	May produce additive hypotensive effect when used concomitantly.
Nitrates	Concomitant use is contraindicated; potentiates the hypotensive effects of nitrates.
Ritonavir	Substantially increases plasma concentrations of vardenafil.

GASTROPARESIS AGENTS

Erythromycin*

Anticoagulants, oral	Increases the effects of oral anticoagulants.
Astemizole	Contraindicated; avoid concomitant use.
Cisapride	Contraindicated; avoid concomitant use.
Digoxin	Increases serum levels of digoxin.
Dihydroergotamine	Caution, risk of acute ergot toxicity with concomitant use.
CYP450 substrates (eg, carbamazepine, cyclosporine, phenytoin)	May increase serum levels of drugs metabolized by CYP450.
Ergotamine	Caution, risk of acute ergot toxicity with concomitant use.
HMG-CoA reductase inhibitors (eg, simvastatin, lovastatin)	May increase concentrations of HMG-CoA reductase inhibitors; rhabdomyolysis reported.
Midazolam	Increases the effects of midazolam.
Pimozide	Contraindicated; avoid concomitant use.
Sildenafil	May potentiate sildenafil effects; consider dose reduction of sildenafil.
Terfenadine	Contraindicated; avoid concomitant use.
Theophylline	May increase serum theophylline levels.
Triazolam	Increases the effects of triazolam.

Metoclopramide HCl (Reglan, Reglan Injection)

Acetaminophen	May increase rate and/or extent of intestinal absorption of acetaminophen.
Alcohol	May produce additive sedative effects when used concomitantly.
Anticholinergic drugs	Antagonizes the effects of metoclopramide on GI motility.
Cyclosporine	May increase rate and/or extent of intestinal absorption of ethanol.

* Available only in generic form.

Table 18.2. Drug Interactions for Neuropathic Therapies

Digoxin	May decrease gastric absorption.
Ethanol	May increase rate and/or extent of intestinal absorption of ethanol.
Extrapyramidal reaction-producing drugs	May increase the frequency and severity of extrapyramidal reactions.
Hypnotics	May produce additive sedative effects when used concomitantly.
Insulin	Insulin dose or timing of dose may need adjustment to prevent hypoglycemia.
Levodopa	May increase rate and/or extent of intestinal absorption of levodopa.
MAO inhibitors	Caution with concomitant use.
Narcotics	Antagonizes the effects of metoclopramide on GI motility; may produce additive sedative effects when used concomitantly.
Tetracycline	May increase rate and/or extent of intestinal absorption of tetracycline.
Tranquilizers	May produce additive sedative effects when used concomitantly.

Diabetic Neuropathies

American Diabetes Association

Andrew J.M. Boulton, MD, FRCP[1,2], Arthur I. Vinik, MD, PHD[3],
Joseph C. Arezzo, PHD[4], Vera Bril, MD[5], Eva L. Feldman, MD, PHD[6],
Roy Freeman, MB, CHB[7], Rayaz A. Malik, PHD, MRCP[1], Raelene E. Maser, PHD[8],
Jay M. Sosenko, MS, MD[2] and Dan Ziegler, MD, FRCP[9]

The diabetic neuropathies are heterogeneous, affecting different parts of the nervous system that present with diverse clinical manifestations. They may be focal or diffuse. Most common among the neuropathies are chronic sensorimotor distal symmetric polyneuropathy (DPN) and the autonomic neuropathies. DPN is a diagnosis of exclusion. The early recognition and appropriate management of neuropathy in the patient

1 Department of Medicine, Manchester Royal Infirmary, Manchester, U.K.
2 Division of Endocrinology, Diabetes & Metabolism, University of Miami School of Medicine, Miami, Florida
3 The Strelitz Diabetes Institute, Eastern Virginia Medical School, Norfolk, Virginia
4 Department of Neuroscience, Albert Einstein College of Medicine of Yeshiva University, Bronx, New York
5 Department of Medicine (Neurology), University Health Network, University of Toronto, Toronto, Canada
6 Department of Neurology, University of Michigan, Ann Arbor, Michigan
7 Department of Neurology, Harvard University, Boston, Massachusetts
8 Department of Medical Technology, University of Delaware, Newark, Delaware
9 German Diabetes Clinic, German Diabetes Center, Leibniz Institute at the Heinrich Heine University, Düsseldorf, Germany

Address correspondence and reprint requests to (somatic) Prof. A.J.M. Boulton, Department of Medicine, Manchester Royal Infirmary, Oxford Road, Manchester, M13 9WL, U.K. E-mail: aboulton@med.miami.edu . Or (autonomic) Dr. Aaron Vinik, Director, Strelitz Diabetes Research Institute, 855 W. Brambleton Ave., Norfolk, VA 23510. E-mail: vinikai@evms.edu

Abbreviations: CAN, cardiovascular autonomic neuropathy • CIDP, chronic inflammatory demyelinating polyneuropathy • DAN, diabetic autonomic neuropathy • DPN, distal symmetric polyneuropathy • HRV, heart rate variability

with diabetes is important for a number of reasons. 1) Nondiabetic neuropathies may be present in patients with diabetes. 2) A number of treatment options exist for symptomatic diabetic neuropathy. 3) Up to 50% of DPN may be asymptomatic, and patients are at risk of insensate injury to their feet. As >80% of amputations follow a foot ulcer or injury, early recognition of at-risk individuals, provision of education, and appropriate foot care may result in a reduced incidence of ulceration and consequently amputation. 4) Autonomic neuropathy may involve every system in the body. 5) Autonomic neuropathy causes substantial morbidity and increased mortality, particularly if cardiovascular autonomic neuropathy (CAN) is present. Treatment should be directed at underlying pathogenesis. Effective symptomatic treatments are available for the manifestations of DPN and autonomic neuropathy.

This statement is based on two recent technical reviews (1,2), to which the reader is referred for detailed discussion and relevant references to the literature.

DEFINITIONS AND CLASSIFICATION

An internationally agreed simple definition of DPN for clinical practice is "the presence of symptoms and/or signs of peripheral nerve dysfunction in people with diabetes after the exclusion of other causes" (3). However, the diagnosis cannot be made without a careful clinical examination of the lower limbs, as absence of symptoms should never be assumed to indicate an absence of signs. This definition conveys the important message that not all patients with peripheral nerve dysfunction have a neuropathy caused by diabetes. Confirmation can be established with quantitative electrophysiology, sensory, and autonomic function testing.

Numerous classifications of the variety of syndromes affecting the peripheral nervous system in diabetes have been proposed in recent years. The classification shown in **Table 1** is based on that originally proposed by Thomas (4).

Table 1. Classification of Diabetic Neuropathy
Generalized symmetric polyneuropathies
• Acute sensory
• Chronic sensorimotor
• Autonomic
Focal and multifocal neuropathies
• Cranial
• Truncal
• Focal limb
• Proximal motor (amyotrophy)
• Coexisting CIDP

Adapted from Thomas (4). Note: Clinicians should be alert for treatable neuropathies (CIDP, monoclonal gammopathy, vitamin B$_{12}$ deficiency, etc.) occurring in patients with diabetes.

DIAGNOSTIC CRITERIA AND BRIEF CLINICAL ASPECTS

A) Sensory neuropathies: clinical features

1) Acute sensory neuropathy

Acute sensory neuropathy is rare, tends to follow periods of poor metabolic control (e.g., ketoacidosis) or sudden change in glycemic control (e.g., "insulin neuritis"), and is characterized by the acute onset of severe sensory symptoms (as detailed below) with marked nocturnal exacerbation but few neurologic signs on examination of the legs.

2) Chronic sensorimotor DPN

This is the most common presentation of neuropathy in diabetes, and up to 50% of patients may experience symptoms, most frequently burning pain, electrical or stabbing sensations, parasthesiae, hyperasthesiae, and deep aching pain. Neuropathic pain is typically worse at night, and the symptoms are most commonly experienced in the feet and lower limbs, although in some cases the hands may also be affected. As up to half of the patients may be asymptomatic, a diagnosis may only be made on examination or, in some cases, when the patient presents with a painless foot ulcer. Other patients may not volunteer symptoms but on inquiry admit that their feet feel numb or dead. Examination of the lower limb usually reveals sensory loss of vibration, pressure, pain, and temperature perception (mediated by small and large fibers) and absent ankle reflexes. Signs of peripheral autonomic (sympathetic) dysfunction are also frequently seen and include a warm or cold foot, sometimes with distended dorsal foot veins (in the absence of obstructive peripheral vascular disease), dry skin, and the presence of calluses under pressure-bearing areas.

3) Diagnosis

The diagnosis of DPN can only be made after a careful clinical examination, and all patients with diabetes should be screened annually for DPN by examining pinprick, temperature, and vibration perception (using a 128-Hz tuning fork), 10-g monofilament pressure sensation at the distal halluces, and ankle reflexes. Combinations of more than one test have >87% sensitivity in detecting DPN.

Loss of 10-g monofilament perception and reduced vibration perception predict foot ulcers. Indeed, longitudinal studies have shown that a simple clinical examination is a good predictor of future foot ulcer risk (5). The feet should be examined for ulcers, calluses, and deformities, and footwear should be inspected. Different scoring systems have been developed for monitoring progression or response to intervention in clinical trials.

Other forms of neuropathy, including chronic inflammatory demyelinating polyneuropathy (CIDP), B_{12} deficiency, hypothyroidism, and uremia, occur more frequently in diabetes and should be ruled out. The practitioner may wish to refer the more complex patient, or those in whom diagnosis needs confirmation, to a neurologist for specialized examination and testing.

The diagnosis of chronic DPN is therefore a clinical one and involves the exclusion of nondiabetic causes: investigations should be ordered as dictated by clinical findings and might typically include serum B_{12}, thyroid function, blood urea nitrogen, and serum creatinine. A combination of typical symptomatology and distal sensory loss with absent reflexes, or the signs in the absence of symptoms, is highly suggestive of DPN.

B) Focal and multifocal neuropathies

Mononeuropathies may have a sudden onset and can occur as a result of involvement of the median (5.8% of all diabetic neuropathies), ulnar (2.1%), radial (0.6%), and common peroneal nerves. Cranial neuropathies are extremely rare (0.05%); involve primarily cranial nerves III, IV, VI, and VII; and are thought to occur due to a microvascular "infarct," which, in the majority, resolves spontaneously over several months. Electrophysiological studies show a reduction in both nerve conduction and amplitude suggestive of underlying demyelination and axonal degeneration. In contrast, up to one-

third of patients with diabetes have an entrapment. Common nerves involved are the ulnar, median, peroneal, and medial plantar nerves. Spinal stenosis is also common in people with diabetes and needs to be distinguished from the proximal neuropathies and amyotrophy. Electrophysiological studies are most helpful in identifying blocks in conduction at the entrapment sites. Entrapments may require decompression, but initial management should be expectant with strong reassurance to the patient for recovery (6).

Diabetic amyotrophy typically occurs in older patients with type 2 diabetes, and in some cases, an immune-mediated epineurial microvasculitis has been demonstrated in nerve biopsies. Clinical features of amyotrophy include severe neuropathic pain and uni- or bilateral muscle weakness and atrophy in the proximal thigh muscles. When an unusually severe, predominantly motor neuropathy and progressive polyneuropathy develops in diabetic patients, one must consider CIDP and spinal stenosis. The diagnosis of CIDP is often overlooked and the patient simply labeled as having diabetic neuropathy: progressive symmetric or asymmetric motor deficits, progressive sensory neuropathy in spite of optimal glycemic control together with typical electrophysiological findings, and an unusually high cerebro-spinal fluid protein level all suggest the possibility of an underlying treatable demyelinating neuropathy (7). As immunomodulatory therapy with combinations of corticosteroids, plasmapheresis, and intravenous immune globulin can produce a relatively rapid and substantial improvement in neurological deficits and electrophysiology in some cases of CIDP, referral to a neurologist is indicated if this diagnosis is suspected.

C) Autonomic neuropathy (8-14)

Diabetic autonomic neuropathy (DAN) results in significant morbidity and may lead to mortality in some patients with diabetes.

Table 2. Treatment of Diabetic Neuropathy Based on the Putative Pathogenetic Mechanisms

Abnormality	Compound	Aim of treatment	Status of RCTs
Polyol pathway↑	Aldose reductase inhibitors	Nerve sorbitol↓	
	Sorbinil		Withdrawn (AE)
	Tolrestat		Withdrawn(AE)
	Ponalrestat		Ineffective
	Zopolrestat		Withdrawn (marginal effects)
	Zenarestat		Withdrawn (AE)
	Lidorestat		Withdrawn (AE)
	Fidarestat		Effective in RCTs, trials ongoing
	AS-3201		Effective in RCTs, trials ongoing
	Epalrestat		Marketed in Japan
Myo-inositol↓	*Myo*-inositol	Nerve *myo*-inositol↑	Equivocal
Oxidative stress↑	α-Lipoic acid	Oxygen free radicals↓	Effective in RCTs, trials ongoing
Nerve hypoxia↑	Vasodilators	NBF↑	
	ACE inhibitors		Effective in one RCT
	Prostaglandin analogs		Effective in one RCT
	phVEGF$_{165}$ gene transfer	Angiogenesis↑	RCTs ongoing
Protein kinase C↑	Protein kinase C-β inhibitor (ruboxistaurin)	NBF↑	RCTs ongoing
C-peptide↓	C-peptide	NBF↑	Studies ongoing
Neurotrophism↓	Nerve growth factor (NGF)	Nerve regeneration, growth↑	Ineffective
	BDNF	Nerve regeneration, growth↑	Ineffective
LCFA metabolism↓	Acetyl-L-carnitine	LCFA accumulation↓	Ineffective
GLA synthesis↓	γ-Linolenic acid (GLA)	EFA metabolism↑	Withdrawn
NEG↑	Aminoguanidine	AGE accumulation↓	Withdrawn

AE, adverse event; AGE: advanced glycation end product; BDNF, brain-derived neurotrophic factor; EFA: essential fatty acid; LCFA, long-chain fatty acid; NBF, nerve blood flow; NEG, nonenzymatic glycation; RCT, randomized clinical trial.

The most common dysautonomic features are listed in **Table 2**, together with their associated symptoms and management. The symptoms of autonomic dysfunction should be elicited carefully during the history, particularly since many of these symptoms are potentially treatable.

Major clinical manifestations of DAN include resting tachycardia, exercise intolerance, orthostatic hypotension, constipation, gastroparesis, erectile dysfunction, sudomotor dysfunction, impaired neurovascular function, "brittle diabetes," and hypoglycemic autonomic failure. CAN is the most prominent

focus of autonomic dysfunction because of the life-threatening consequences of this complication and the availability of direct tests of cardiovascular autonomic function. However, neuropathies involving other organ systems should also be considered in the optimal care of patients with diabetes.

Cardiovascular

CAN is the most studied and clinically important form of DAN. The reported prevalence of CAN varies widely depending on the cohort studied and the methods of assessment. The presence of autonomic

Table 3. Oral Symptomatic Therapy of Painful Neuropathy

Drug class	Drug	Daily dose (mg)	NNT	NNH	Side effects
Tricyclics	Amitriptyline	25-150	2.4 (2.0-3.0)	2.7 (2.1-3.9)	++++
	Imipramine	25-150	2.4 (2.0-3.0)	2.7 (2.1-3.9)	++++
SSRIs	Paroxetine	40	ND	ND	+++
	Citalopram	40	ND	ND	+++
Anticonvulsants	Gabapentin	900-1,800	3.7 (2.4-8.3)	2.7 (2.2-3.4)	++
	Pregabalin	150-600	3.3 (2.3-5.9)	3.7	++
	Carbamazepine	200-400	3.3 (2.0-9.4)	1.9 (1.4-2.8)	+++
	Topiramate	Up to 400	3.0 (2.3-4.5)	9.0	++
Opioids	Tramadol	50-400	3.4 (2.3-6.4)	7.8	+++
	Oxycodone CR	10-60	ND	ND	++++

Data are median (range) unless otherwise indicated. See refs. 2, 19, and 20. ND, not determined; NNH, number needed to treat to harm one patient; NNT, number needed to treat to achieve pain relief in one patient; SSRI, selective serotonin reuptake inhibitor.

neuropathy may limit an individual's exercise capacity and increase the risk of an adverse cardiovascular event during exercise. CAN may be indicated by resting tachycardia (>100 bpm), orthostasis (a fall in systolic blood pressure >20 mmHg upon standing) without an appropriate heart rate response, or other disturbances in autonomic nervous system function involving the skin, pupils, gastrointestinal, or genitourinary systems. Sudden death and silent myocardial ischemia have been attributed to CAN in diabetes. Resting and stress thallium myocardial scintigraphy is an appropriate noninvasive test for the presence and extent of macrovascular coronary artery disease in these individuals. Hypotension and hypertension after vigorous exercise are more likely to develop in patients with autonomic neuropathy, particularly when starting an exercise program. Because these individuals may have difficulty with thermoregulation, they should be advised to avoid exercise in hot or cold environments and to be vigilant about adequate hydration.

Observational studies have consistently documented an increased risk of mortality in subjects with autonomic neuropathy, although these associations may be related in part to the presence of other comorbid complications. A recent meta-analysis of published data demonstrated that reduced cardiovascular autonomic function, as measured by heart rate variability (HRV), was strongly (i.e., relative risk is doubled) associated with increased risk of silent myocardial ischemia and mortality (1).

A patient's history and physical examination are ineffective for early detection of CAN, and therefore noninvasive tests that have demonstrated efficacy are required. Proceedings from a consensus conference in 1992 recommended that three tests (R-R variation, Valsalva maneuver, and postural blood pressure testing) be used for longitudinal testing of the cardiovascular autonomic system (**Table 5**). Other forms of autonomic neuropathy can be evaluated with specialized tests, but these are less standardized and less available than commonly used tests of cardiovascular autonomic function, which quantify loss of HRV. The ability to interpret serial HRV testing requires accurate, precise, and reproducible procedures that use established physiologic maneuvers. The battery of three recommended tests for assessing CAN is

Table 4. Treatment of Autonomic Neuropathy

Symptoms	Tests	Treatments
Cardiac		
Exercise intolerance, early fatigue and weakness with exercise	HRV, multigated angiography (MUGA) thallium scan, 123I metaiodobenzlyguanidine (MIBG) scan	Graded supervised exercise, ACE inhibitors, ß-blockers
Postural hypotension, dizziness, lightheadedness, weakness, fatigue, syncope	HRV, measure blood pressure standing and supine, measure catecholamines	Mechanical measures, clonidine, midodrine, octreotide
Gastrointestinal		
Gastroparesis, erratic glucose control	Gastric emptying study, barium study	Frequent small meals, prokinetic agents (metoclpramide, domperidone, erythromycin)
Abdominal pain or discomfort, early satiety, nausea, vomiting, belching, bloating	Endoscopy, manometry, electrogastrogram	Antibiotics, antiemetics (phenergan, compazine, tigan, scopolamine), bulking agents, tricyclic antidepressants, pancreatic extracts, pyloric Botox, gastric pacing, enteral feeding
Constipation	Endoscopy	High-fiber diet and bulking agents, osmotic laxatives, lubricating agents and prokinetic agents used cautiously
Diarrhea, often nocturnal alternating with constipation and incontinence		Trials of soluble fiber, gluten and lactose restriction, anticholinergic agents, cholestyramine, antibiotics, clonidine, somatostatin, pancreatic enzyme supplements
Sexual dysfunction		
Erectile dysfunction	History and physical examination, HRV, penile-brachial pressure index, nocturnal penile tumescence	Sex therapy, psychological counseling, sildenafil, vardenafil, tadalafil, prostaglandin E1 injection, device or prosthesis
Vaginal dryness		Vaginal lubricants
Bladder dysfunction		
Frequency, urgency, nocturia, urinary retention, incontinence	Cystometrogram, postvoiding sonography	Bethanechol, intermittent catheterization
Sudomotor (sweating) dysfunction		
Anhidrosis, heat intolerance, dry skin, hyperhidrosis	Quantitative sudomotor axon reflex, sweat test, skin blood flow	Emollients and skin lubricants, scopolamine, glycopyrrolate, botulinum toxin, vasodilators
Pupillomotor		
Visual blurring, impaired adaptation to ambient light, impaired visceral sensation	Pupillometry, HRV	Care with driving at night, recognition of unusual presentations of myocardial infarction

readily performed in the average clinic, hospital, or diagnostic center with the use of available technology (**Table 5**).

At time of diagnosis of type 2 diabetes and within 5 years after diagnosis of type 1 diabetes (unless an individual has symptoms suggestive of autonomic dysfunction earlier), patients should be screened for CAN. Screening should comprise a history and an examination for signs of autonomic dysfunction. Tests for HRV, including expiration-to-inspiration ratio and response to the Valsalva maneuver and standing, may be indicated. Early measurement of HRV can serve as a baseline from which interval tests can be compared. Regular HRV testing provides early detection and thereby promotes timely diagnostic and therapeutic interventions. HRV testing may also facilitate differential diagnosis and the attribution of symptoms (e.g., erectile dysfunction, dyspepsia, dizziness) to autonomic dysfunction. Finally, knowledge of early autonomic dysfunction can encourage patient and physician to improve metabolic control and to use therapies, such as ACE inhibitors and β-blockers, that are proven to be effective for patients with CAN.

Orthostatic measurement of blood pressure should be performed in people with diabetes and hypotension when clinically indicated.

Cardiovascular system and exercise

Cardiac autonomic function testing should be performed when planning an exercise program for individuals with diabetes about to embark on a moderate- to high-intensity exercise program, especially those at high risk for underlying cardiovascular disease (15).

Gastrointestinal

Gastrointestinal disturbances (e.g., esophageal enteropathy, gastroparesis, constipation, diarrhea, fecal incontinence) are common, and any section of the gastrointestinal tract may be affected. Gastroparesis should be suspected in individuals with erratic glucose control. Upper-gastrointestinal symptoms should lead to consideration of all possible causes, including autonomic dysfunction. Evaluation of gastric emptying should be done if symptoms are suggestive. Barium studies or referral for endoscopy may be required. Constipation is the most common lower-gastrointestinal symptom but can alternate with episodes of diarrhea. Endoscopy may be required to rule out other causes.

Genitourinary

DAN is also associated with genitourinary tract disturbances, including bladder and/or sexual dysfunction. Evaluation of bladder dysfunction should be performed in individuals with diabetes who have recurrent urinary tract infections, pyelonephritis, incontinence, or a palpable bladder. In men, DAN may cause loss of penile erection and/or retrograde ejaculation. A complete work-up for impotence in men should include history (medical and sexual); psychological evaluation; hormone levels; measurement of nocturnal penile tumescence; tests to assess penile, pelvic, and spinal nerve function; cardiovascular autonomic function tests; and measurement of penile and brachial blood pressure.

EPIDEMIOLOGY

DPN

DPN is a common disorder. Although estimates vary, it appears that at least one manifestation of DPN is present in at least 20% of adult diabetic patients. DPN has been associated with a number of modifiable and non-modifiable risk factors, including the degree of hyperglycemia, lipid and blood pressure indexes, diabetes duration, and height. DPN has been less consistently associated with cigarette smoking and alcohol consumption.

DAN

Prevalence data for DAN range from 1.6 to 90% depending on tests used, populations examined, and type and stage of disease. Risk factors for the development of DAN

Table 5. Diagnostic Tests of CAN

- **Resting heart rate** >100 bpm is abnormal.

- **Beat-to-beat HRV*** With the patient at rest and supine (not having had coffee or a hypoglycemic episode the night before), heart rate is monitored by ECG or autonomic instrument while the patient breathes in and out at six breaths per minute, paced by a metronome or similar device. A difference in heart rate of >15 bpm is normal, <10 bpm is abnormal. The lowest normal value for the expiration-to-inspiration ratio of the R-R interval is 1.17 in people 20-24 years of age. There is a decline in the value with age†.

- **Heart rate response to standing*** During continuous ECG monitoring, the R-R interval is measured at beats 15 and 30 after standing. Normally, a tachycardia is followed by reflex bradycardia. The 30:15 ratio is >1.03.

- **Heart rate response to the Valsalva maneuver*** The subject forcibly exhales into the mouthpiece of a manometer to 40 mmHg for 15 s during ECG monitoring. Healthy subjects develop tachycardia and peripheral vasoconstriction during strain and an overshoot bradycardia and rise in blood pressure with release. The ratio of longest R-R to shortest R-R should be >1.2.

- **Systolic blood pressure response to standing** Systolic blood pressure is measured in the supine subject. The patient stands, and the systolic blood pressure is measured after 2 min. Normal response is a fall of <10 mmHg, borderline is a fall of 10-29 mmHg, and abnormal is a fall of >30 mmHg with symptoms.

- **Diastolic blood pressure response to isometric exercise** The subject squeezes a handgrip dynamometer to establish a maximum. Grip is then squeezed at 30% maximum for 5 min. The normal response for diastolic blood pressure is a rise of >16 mmHg in the other arm.

- **ECG QT/QTc intervals** The QTc should be <440 ms.

- **Spectral analysis** Very-low-frequency peak (sympathetic dysfunction) Low-frequency peak↓ (sympathetic dysfunction) High-frequency peak↓ (parasympathetic dysfunction) Low-frequency-to-high-frequency ratio↓ (sympathetic imbalance)

- **Neurovascular flow** Using noninvasive laser Doppler measures of peripheral sympathetic responses to nociception.

From Vinik A, Erbas T, Pfeifer M, Feldman E, Stevens M, Russell J: Diabetic autonomic neuropathy, 2004. In *The Diabetes Mellitus Manual: A Primary Care Companion to Ellenberg and Rifkin's 6th Edition.* Inzucchi SE, Ed. New York, McGraw Hill, 2004, p. 351.

* These can now be performed quickly (<15 min) in the practitioner's office using stand-alone devices that are operator friendly.

† Lowest normal value of expiration-to-inspiration ratio: age 20-24 years, 1.17; 25-29, 1.15; 30-34, 1.13; 35-39, 1.12; 40-44, 1.10; 45-49, 1.08; 50-54, 1.07; 55-59, 1.06; 60-64, 1.04; 65-69, 1.03; and 70-75, 1.02. ECG, electrocardiogram.

include diabetes duration, age, and long-term poor glycemic control. DAN may cosegregate with factors predisposing to macrovascular events such as raised blood pressure and dyslipidemia. Thus, in addition to good glycemic control, lipid modulation and blood pressure control may be beneficial in the prevention of DAN. There are no true population-based studies using radioisotopic techniques that quantify gastric emptying in diabetic patients, but cross-sectional studies have indicated that 50% of outpatients with long-standing diabetes have delayed gastric emptying and up to 76% of diabetic outpatients indicate that they have one or more gastrointestinal symptom, the most common of which is constipation. Both upper- and lower-gastrointestinal symptoms

occur more frequently in individuals with diabetes than in control subjects, but the symptoms are nonspecific and occur in the general population (12,13). Specific symptoms such as bloating after meals, vomiting of previously ingested food, and alternating constipation and explosive diarrhea should lead to further evaluation (**Table 4**).

Genitourinary bladder dysfunction has been shown in 43-87% of individuals with type 1 diabetes. Diabetic women have a fivefold higher risk of unrecognized voiding difficulty compared with nondiabetic women. The history and physical are generally noncontributory, and the patient should be referred to a urologist for urodynamic studies.

The prevalence of erectile dysfunction in diabetic men ranges from 27 to 75% (14).

MANAGEMENT

A) Prevention

The DCCT (Diabetes Control and Complications Trial) has shown definitively that in type 1 diabetic patients, the risk of DPN and autonomic neuropathy can be reduced with improved blood glucose control. Although data from a small number of trials are much less strong for type 2 diabetic patients, DCCT data and data from epidemiologic studies (including studies of type 2 patients) strongly suggest that optimal blood glucose control helps to prevent DPN and autonomic neuropathy in both type 1 and type 2 diabetic patients. There have been no definitely positive prevention studies of other risk factor modifications for DPN, but the improvement of lipid and blood pressure indexes, and the avoidance of cigarette smoking and excess alcohol consumption, are already recommended for the prevention of other complications of diabetes.

B) Pathogenetic treatments (16-19)

Recent experimental studies suggest a multifactorial pathogenesis of diabetic neuropathy. Studies in animal models and cultured cells provide a conceptual framework for the cause and treatment of diabetic neuropathy. However, limited translational work in diabetic patients continues to generate much debate and controversy over the cause(s) of human diabetic neuropathy, and to date we have no effective long-term treatment. A summary of the drugs that have/are being studied in clinical trials is provided in **Table 2** (19).

C) Symptomatic treatments

1) DPN (2,3,20-22)

The first step in management of patients with DPN should be to aim for stable and optimal glycemic control. Although controlled trial evidence is lacking, several observational studies suggest that neuropathic symptoms improve not only with optimization of control but also with the avoidance of extreme blood glucose fluctuations. Many patients will require pharmacological treatment for painful symptoms: several agents have efficacy confirmed in published randomized controlled trials, although with the exception of Duloxetine and Pregabalin, none of the others is specifically licensed for the management of painful DPN (**Table 3**). An algorithm for the management of symptomatic DPN is provided in **Fig. 1**.

(1). Note that nonpharmacological, topical, or physical therapies might be useful at any stage. These include acupuncture, capsaicin, glyceryl trinitrate spray/patches, etc. (2).

Although a detailed discussion of all these agents is provided in the recent technical review (2), some comment will be made on the more commonly used agents.

Tricyclic drugs. The usefulness of the tricyclic drugs, such as Amitriptyline and Imipramine, has been confirmed in several randomized controlled trials. Although inexpensive and generally efficacious in the management of neuropathic pain, side effects, particularly anticholinergic (dry mouth, urinary retention, etc.), can be troublesome and limit their use in many patients. The central side effects, such as fatigue and drowsiness, are also common, so it is advised to start at 25 mg before bed and gradually increase the dose, if necessary, to a maximum of 150 mg.

Anticonvulsants. Gabapentin is now the most commonly prescribed anticonvulsant that has been proven to be efficacious in the treatment of neuropathic pain. As most patients require at least 1.8 g/day for relief of symptoms, it is advisable to start at 300 mg at bedtime and then increase over days to the dosage that achieves symptomatic relief. This gradual titration of drug dosage until the therapeutic effect is realized is advisable, as it is felt that this may lessen the severity of side effects that may be experienced if the

Figure 1. Algorithm for Management of Symptomatic DPN

Symptomatic neuropathy

↓

Exclude nondiabetic etiologies

↓

Stabilize glycemic control
(insulin not always required in type 2 diabetes)

↓

Tricyclic drugs
(e.g., Amitriptyline 25-150 mg before bed)

↓

Anticonvulsants
(e.g., Gabapentin, typical dose 1.8 g/day)

↓

Opioid or opioid-like drug
(e.g., Tramadol, Oxycodone)

↓

Consider pain clinic referral

Figure 1 – Algorithm for management of symptomatic DPN (1). Note that nonpharmacological, topical, or physical therapies might be useful at any stage. These include acupuncture, capsaicin, glyceryl trinitrate spray/patches, etc. (2).

drug is introduced at a high dose on day 1. The structurally related compound Pregabalin has recently been confirmed to be useful in painful diabetic neuropathy in a randomized controlled trial (20). In contrast to Gabapentin, which is usually given in three daily doses, Pregabalin is effective when given twice daily. As noted in **Table 4**, all of these agents are prone to side effects, typically central in nature such as drowsiness. Finally, Topiramate, another anticonvulsant used in complex partial seizures, was recently shown to be efficacious in the management of neuropathic pain (21).

Other agents. The 5-hydroxytryptamine and Norepinephrine reuptake inhibitor Duloxetine has recently been approved by the Food and Drug Administration for the treatment of neuropathic pain. However, at the time this statement was being prepared, the evidence of efficacy of this agent was only published in abstract form (22).

In cases of severe pain, certain agents may be used in combination (e.g., an antidepressant and an anticonvulsant) or combined with a topical or nonpharmacological treatment (2) (**Fig. 1**). All patients with DPN, whether symptomatic or not, are at increased risk of foot ulceration (2) and should be considered for podiatric referral and foot care education.

2) Autonomic neuropathy

Treatment approaches to the management of autonomic neuropathy are summarized in **Table 4**.

RECOMMENDATIONS FOR SCREENING FOR AND TREATMENT OF DIABETIC NEUROPATHY

A. Tight glycemic control

For all diabetic patients, maintain aggressive control of blood glucose, HbA1c, blood pressure, and lipids with pharmacological therapy and/or lifestyle changes

B. Screening

1) Chronic sensorimotor DPN

All patients with diabetes should be screened for DPN at diagnosis of type 2 diabetes and 5 years after the diagnosis of type 1 diabetes and at least annually by examining sensory function in the feet and checking ankle reflexes. One or more of the following can be used to assess sensory function: pinprick, temperature, and vibration perception (using a 128-Hz tuning fork), or pressure sensation (using a 10-g monofilament pressure sensation at the distal halluces). Any history of neuropathic symptoms should be elicited, and a careful clinical examination of the feet and lower limbs should be performed. The feet should be examined for ulcers, calluses, and deformities, and footwear should be inspected at each diabetes care visit. All patients with DPN, whether symptomatic or not, require foot care education and consideration for podiatric referral.

2) Autonomic neuropathy

Based on expert consensus and clinical experience (level E), screening should be instituted at diagnosis of type 2 diabetes and 5 years after the diagnosis of type 1 diabetes. Screening might comprise a history and an examination for signs of autonomic dysfunction. Tests for HRV, including expiration-to-inspiration ratio and response to the Valsalva maneuver and standing, may be indicated. If screening is negative, this should be repeated annually; if positive, appropriate diagnostic tests and symptomatic treatments should be instituted (Tables 4 and 5).

REFERENCES

1. Vinik AI, Maser RE, Mitchell BD, Freeman R: Diabetic autonomic neuropathy (Technical Review). *Diabetes Care* 26:1553-1579, 2003
2. Boulton AJM, Malik RA, Arezzo JC, Sosenko JM: Diabetic somatic neuropathies (Technical Review). *Diabetes Care* 27:1458-1486, 2004
3. Boulton AJM, Gries FA, Jervell JA: Guidelines for the diagnosis and outpatient management diabetic peripheral neuropathy. *Diabet Med* 15:508-514, 1998
4. Thomas PK: Classification, differential diagnosis, and staging of diabetic peripheral neuropathy. *Diabetes* 46(Suppl. 2):S54-S57, 1997
5. Abbott CA, Carrington AL, Ashe H, Bath S, Every LC, Griffiths J, Hann AW, Hussein A, Jackson N, Johnson KE, Ryder CH, Torkington R, Van Ross ER, Whalley AM, Widdows P, Williamson S, Boulton AJM: The North-West Diabetes Foot Care Study: incidence of, and risk factors for, new diabetic foot ulceration in a community-based patient cohort. *Diabet Med* 19:377-384, 2002
6. Vinik A, Mehrabyan A, Colen L, Boulton AJM: Focal entrapment neuropathies in diabetes (Review). *Diabetes Care* 27:1783-1788, 2004
7. Ayyar DR, Sharma KR: Chronic demyelinating polyradiculoneuropathy in diabetes. *Curr Diab Rep* 4:409-412, 2004
8. Esposito K, Giugliano F, Di Palo C, Giugliano G, Marfella R, D'Andrea F, D'Armiento M, Giugliano D: Effect of lifestyle changes on erectile dysfunction in obese men: a randomized controlled trial. *JAMA* 291:2978-2984, 2004
9. Boulton AJM, Selam JL, Sweeney M, Ziegler D: Sildenafil citrate for the treatment of erectile dysfunction in men with type II diabetes mellitus. *Diabetologia* 44:1296-1301, 2001
10. Saenz de Tejada I, Anglin G, Knight JR, Emmick JT: Effects of tadalafil on erectile dysfunction in men with diabetes. *Diabetes Care* 25:2159-2164, 2002
11. Goldstein I, Young J, Fischer J, Bangerter K, Segerson T, Taylor T, the Vardenafil Diabetes Study Group: Vardenafil, a new phosphodiesterase type 5 inhibitor, in the treatment of erectile dysfunction in men with diabetes. *Diabetes Care* 26:777-783, 2003
12. Maleki D, Loche R, Camilleri M: Gastrointestinal tract symptoms among persons with diabetes mellitus in the community. *Arch Intern Med* 160:2808-2816, 2000
13. Bytzer P, Talley NJ, Leemon M, Young LJ, Jones MP, Horowitz M: Prevalence of gastrointestinal symptoms associated with diabetes mellitus: a population-based survey of 15,000 adults. *Arch Intern Med* 161:1989-1996, 2001[Abstract/Free Full Text]
14. Bacon CG, Hu FB, Giovannucci E, Glasser DB, Mittleman MA, Rimm EB: Association of type and duration of diabetes with erectile dysfunction in a large cohort of men. *Diabetes Care* 25:1458-1463, 2002
15. Zinman B, Ruderman N, Campaigne BN, Devlin JT, Schneider SH: Physical activity/exercise in diabetes (Position Statement). *Diabetes Care* 27(Suppl. 1):S58-S62, 2004
16. Ziegler D, Nowak H, Kempler P, Vargha P, Low PA: Treatment of symptomatic diabetic polyneuropathy with the antioxidant alpha-lipoic acid: a meta-analysis. *Diabet Med* 21:114-121, 2004
17. Ekberg K, Brismar T, Johansson BL, Jonsson B, Lindstrom P, Wahren J: Amelioration of sensory nerve dysfunction by C-peptide in patients with type 1 diabetes. *Diabetes* 52:536-541, 2003
18. Simovic D, Isner JM, Ropper AH, Pieczek A, Weinberg DH: Improvement in chronic ischemic neuropathy after intramuscular phVEGF165 gene transfer in patients with critical limb ischemia. *Arch Neurol* 58:761-768, 2001[Abstract/Free Full Text]
19. Vinik A, Mehrabyan A: Diabetic neuropathies. *Med Clin N Am* 88:947-999, 200
20. Rosenstock J, Tuchman M, LaMoreaux L, Sharma U: Pregabalin for the treatment of painful diabetic neuropathy: a double-blind, placebo-controlled trial. *Pain* 110:628-638, 2004[Medline]
21. Raskin P, Donofrio PD, Rosenthal NR, Hewitt DJ, Jordan DM, Xiang J, Vinik AI, the CAPSS-141 Study Group: Topiramate vs placebo in painful diabetic neuropathy: analgesic and metabolic effects. *Neurology* 63:865-873, 2004
22. Wernicke J, Rosen AS, Lu Y, Iyengar S, Lee TC: Superiority of Duloxetine over placebo in the treatment of diabetic neuropathic pain demonstrated in two studies (Abstract). *Diabetes* 53 (Suppl. 2):A24, 2004

Chapter 19

Depression

Stephen M. Setter, PharmD, CDE, DVM
Cynthia F. Corbett, PhD, RN

INTRODUCTION

Depression is twice as common in adults with diabetes when compared with persons without diabetes. The increased prevalence of depression among this group remains significant even when controlling for other covariates such as obesity, cardiovascular disease, gender, and education. Meta-analysis findings indicate that major depression, diagnosed by clinical interview, is present in approximately 11% of persons with diabetes while depressive symptoms that impact quality of life and daily functioning are present in up to 66.5% of those with diabetes.

The negative consequences of the co-occurrence of diabetes and depression have been well documented. People with depression are less likely to follow a healthy eating plan, exercise or engage in physical activity, or take medications as recommended. When studied, persons with depression had poorer glycemic control and more diabetes complications as compared to those with diabetes who were not depressed. Additionally, persons with both diabetes and depression were more likely to report symptoms suggestive of both hypoglycemia and hyperglycemia (eg, sleepiness, blurry vision, thirst, paresthesias, hunger, polyuria, feeling faint, and shakiness) even after controlling for comorbidities and HbA_{1c} levels. Depression also

had a significant negative impact on quality of life. Evidence also suggests a significant increase in mortality in adults with comorbid diabetes and depression. Patients with diabetes tend to respond to pharmacotherapy and psychotherapy in the short-term with improvements in both mood and glycemic control; however, depression tends to recur at a high rate. It is important to consider, however, that only roughly 40% of depressed patients with diabetes are depression-free 12 months after initiation of their therapy. Therefore, it is imperative that depressed patients with diabetes are routinely reassessed with modifications to therapy made in a judicious and timely manner.

As trials of antidepressants in the diabetes literature are scant, the following three major classes of antidepressants used today will be covered and include: 1) selective serotonin reuptake inhibitors (SSRIs); 2) serotonin-norepinephrine reuptake inhibitors (SNRIs); and 3) tricyclic antidepressants (TCAs). For information on specific antidepressant drug therapies in these three categories, as well as for the monoamine oxidase inhibitors (MAOIs) and miscellaneous antidepressants (eg, bupropion, mirtazapine, trazodone), please refer to **Tables 19.1 and 19.2** at the end of this chapter.

Important Factors in Antidepressant Drug Selection for Patients with Diabetes

- Specific presenting diabetes symptoms
- Effect of the medication on glycemic control
- Effect of the medication on cognitive functioning
- Other adverse events
- Pharmacokinetic profile, particularly those affecting compliance
- Drug interactions
- Concomitant disease states

Possible Benefits from Treatment of Depression in Patients with Diabetes

- Reversal of depressive symptoms
- Possible decrease in anxiety symptoms
- Improved sleep patterns
- Improved appetite regulation
- Better overall coping skills and improvement in diabetes self-management
- Improved concentration/cognition
- Improved glycemic control

SELECTIVE SEROTONIN REUPTAKE INHIBITORS (SSRIs)

SSRIs are considered first-line therapies for the pharmacologic treatment of depression. In general, SSRIs are well tolerated and efficacious and often can be dosed once daily. In one trial, the antidepressant sertraline significantly prolonged the time to depression recurrence in younger research subjects with diabetes; however, in those aged 55 and older, no treatment effect was noted.

Pharmacology

Mechanism of Action

SSRIs inhibit the neuronal reuptake of serotonin in the central nervous system (CNS), thereby enhancing the activity of serotonin in the synapse. Histamine, acetylcholine, and norepinephrine receptors are not significantly impacted by SSRIs.

Pharmacokinetics

Specific pharmacokinetic characteristics of the individual SSRIs vary depending on the agent. For specific pharmacokinetic parameters, refer to individual product information.

Treatment Advantages and Disadvantages

In general, the SSRIs are well tolerated and are conveniently dosed once daily. No one SSRI has been shown to be superior to another for the treatment of depression. SSRIs have the potential to improve both depression and glycemic control in patients with diabetes. In particular, escitalopram, sertraline, and citalopram are associated with few clinically significant drug interactions, while paroxetine and fluoxetine are associated with potentially significant drug interactions in patients on multiple other therapies due to CYP2D6 inhibition. Fluoxetine also has an extended half-life with an active metabolite, norfluoxetine, possessing a half-life of 12 days. SSRIs are relatively devoid of anticholinergic, antihistaminic, and cardiovascular side effects compared to the TCAs. One potential disadvantage of the SSRIs as a class is their propensity to contribute to weight gain with extended use. Additionally, SSRIs commonly cause gastric distress (eg, nausea, vomiting, diarrhea), CNS activation (eg, insomnia, restlessness, agitation, anxiety), and sexual dysfunction.

Therapeutic Considerations

Significant Warnings and Precautions

SSRIs should not be discontinued abruptly and should not be concomitantly administered with MAOIs. All SSRIs carry a black box warning regarding suicidal ideation and, in particular, the use of SSRIs in children, adolescents, or young adults needs to be seriously evaluated considering the potential for the development of increased suicidality. In general, SSRIs carry precautions regarding bleeding tendency, hyponatremia, pregnancy (category C or D depending on the agent), seizures, use in elderly, and driving or operating machinery.

Special Populations

In older adults, initial dosing should be low and special attention paid to patients' hepatic and renal status. As previously mentioned, the use of SSRIs requires special consideration due to suicidal ideation. Sertraline, citalopram, escitalopram, and fluoxetine are pregnancy C, with paroxetine being in pregnancy category D. Note that neonates exposed to SSRIs late in the 3rd trimester may be at increased risk of health complications post-delivery. SSRIs should be used with caution in breastfeeding mothers and are generally regarded as unsafe in this population.

Adverse Effects and Monitoring

With initial therapy, SSRIs are associated with gastrointestinal side effects that often attenuate with continued use. Ejaculatory dysfunction, decreased libido, and impotence may occur in men, with females more likely to experience anorgasmia or decreased libido. As SSRIs can contribute to increased bleeding risk, caution with concomitant use with NSAIDs, aspirin, or other drugs that inhibit clotting or coagulation is warranted. It is important to monitor response to therapy and most antidepressants require 2-4 weeks of consistent administration before a clinical response is noted. Increasing the dose rapidly after initiation of therapy will not shorten the time to response but rather merely increase the likelihood of side effects, which often results in noncompliance.

Drug Interactions

As mentioned above, sertraline, escitalopram, and citalopram are associated with few clinically relevant drug interactions. As with all antidepressants, the concomitant use with CNS depressant drugs or substances (eg, alcohol) is not recommended. Paroxetine and fluoxetine, however, are associated with significant drug interactions in patients on multidrug regimens due to CYP2D6 inhibition. See **Table 19.2** or the drug's full prescribing information for more interactions guidance.

Dosage and Administration

SSRIs are often dosed once daily with some exceptions. In general, doses should be gradually titrated with response to therapy being closely monitored and re-evaluated. See **Table 19.1** or the drug's full prescribing information for specific dosing and administration.

SEROTONIN-NOREPINEPHRINE REUPTAKE INHIBITORS (SNRIs)

SNRIs are a welcome addition to the treatment of depression in patients with diabetes. Not only are they effective for the treatment of major depression but are also frequently used to treat diabetic peripheral neuropathy (DPN). Duloxetine is specifically FDA-approved for the treatment of DPN while venlafaxine has been frequently used off-label to treat the pain associated with diabetic neuropathy.

Pharmacology

Mechanism of Action

The SNRIs block the neuronal reuptake of both serotonin and norepinephrine (NE). Venlafaxine and duloxetine are more potent inhibitors of serotonin than NE. In general, the SNRIs do not appreciably alter the activity of dopaminergic, histaminergic, muscarinic, or alpha$_1$-adrenergic receptors.

Pharmacokinetics

Specific SNRI pharmacokinetic characteristics vary depending on the specific agent and dosage form being used. For specific pharmacokinetic parameters, refer to individual product information. Note that venlafaxine is available both as an immediate-release and extended-release product.

Treatment Advantages and Disadvantages

SNRIs have the advantage of being available and tolerated as once-daily dosage forms and also for being clinically useful in patients with diabetic neuropathic pain. Additionally, due to their lack of activity at receptor sites other than serotonin and NE, SNRIs have minimal anticholinergic, sedative, and cardiovascular side effects that plague the TCA class of antidepressants. Another potential advantage of SNRIs is that they are by and large associated with fewer sexual side effects than are SSRIs. Duloxetine is also approved for the treatment of peripheral neuropathy.

Therapeutic Considerations

Significant Warnings and Precautions

Increased ocular pressure may also occur with SNRIs and patients should be monitored appropriately. SNRIs are pregnancy category C and are secreted into breast milk. Nursing infants may experience serious untoward effects of antidepressant ingestion. Therefore, careful consideration should be given to the decision to discontinue breastfeeding or to discontinue SNRI therapy. SNRIs should not be abruptly discontinued and require individualized tapering based on the dose, length of therapy, and other patient-specific factors. Withdrawal symptoms associated with SNRIs include headache, dizziness, nausea/vomiting, paresthesia, and anxiety, among others. For other significant warnings and precautions,

see **Table 19.1**. Note that duloxetine may adversely affect glycemic control in some patients.

As with all antidepressants, SNRIs carry a black box warning regarding suicidal ideation and suicidality in children, adolescents, and young adults.

Special Populations

As the use of SNRIs in patients with renal or hepatic compromise varies with the agent being used, please refer to the drug's full product label for this information.

Adverse Effects and Monitoring

SNRIs have the potential to contribute to a wide range of adverse effects. These may include, but are not limited to, nausea/vomiting, fatigue, hypertension, insomnia, anxiety, tremor, and weight gain or weight loss. As patients with diabetes are often receiving treatment for hypertension upon initiation and maintenance of SNRI therapy, routine blood pressure monitoring is prudent. Additionally, since venlafaxine may result in deleterious effects on lipid parameters, perform routine testing of the lipid profile. See **Table 19.1** or the full drug label for further discussion of adverse effects associated with individual products.

Drug Interactions

SNRIs share the propensity to significantly interact with dexfenfluramine, fenfluramine, MAOIs, nefazodone, phentermine, SSRIs, tryptophan, and St. John's wort. For further product-specific drug interaction information, please see **Table 19.2**.

Dosage and Administration

Dosing parameters vary depending on the agent used; See **Table 19.1** or refer to the full drug label for specific dosing and administration information.

TRICYCLIC ANTIDEPRESSANTS (TCAs)

TCAs have a long history of use, particularly in diabetes patients with peripheral neuropathy. This class of antidepressants demonstrates complex effects on blood glucose levels and is associated with hyperglycemia with extended use. This effect combined with these drugs' known ability to promote carbohydrate craving and weight gain makes their use in patients with both diabetes and depression challenging. However, in one study a complete remission of depression was associated with a 0.8%-1.2% improvement in HbA$_{1c}$.

Pharmacology

Mechanism of Action
TCAs as a class of antidepressants result in decreased neuronal reuptake of norepinephrine (NE) and serotonin at the presynaptic terminal, with individual TCAs affecting neuronal reuptake of these neurotransmitters to varying degrees. All TCAs possess anticholinergic activity with the tertiary amines (eg, amitriptyline, doxepin) tending to be more heavily anticholinergic than the secondary amines (eg, nortriptyline, desipramine).

Pharmacokinetics
Individual pharmacokinetic characteristics vary depending on the TCA being used. For specific pharmacokinetic parameters refer to full product information for the drug in question.

Treatment Advantages and Disadvantages
TCAs have a distinct advantage over SSRIs and many other antidepressants (eg, bupropion, mirtazapine) due to their dual role of treating both depression and diabetic peripheral neuropathy. Unlike duloxetine,

however, they are not FDA approved for treatment of peripheral neuropathy. Nortriptyline and desipramine are often preferred because they are associated with fewer anticholinergic side effects and less sedation than are the tertiary amines, such as amitriptyline and doxepin. Disadvantages of TCAs include varying degrees of peripheral and central anticholinergic side effects, cardiovascular adverse events (eg, arrhythmias, sinus tachycardia, conduction defects) and the propensity to cause weight gain. Another significant disadvantage of the TCAs is that overdose with this class of agents often results in serious morbidity and even death.

Therapeutic Considerations

Significant Warnings and Precautions
TCAs may lower the seizure threshold and should be used cautiously in patients with a history of or at risk of seizures. Due to TCAs' propensity to cause anticholinergic side effects, take precautions when prescribing for patients with urinary retention, constipation, narrow-angle glaucoma, or those with increased intraocular pressure. TCAs should be used cautiously in patients with cardiovascular disorders as TCAs may contribute to the development of arrhythmias, conduction defects, and postural hypotension. Of particular importance for patients with weight challenges and type 2 diabetes, TCAs often contribute to weight gain with some patients gaining in excess of 25% of their pre-antidepressant starting body weight.

As with all antidepressants, TCAs carry a black box warning regarding suicidal ideation and suicidality in children, adolescents, and young adults.

Special Populations
TCAs should be dosed cautiously and conservatively in patients with hepatic impairment. Specific guidelines for dosage adjustment in patients with renal impair-

ment are not available and most likely no dose adjustments are required. Older patients should be started on lower doses initially due to age-related decreases in hepatic function, concomitant disease states, and the need for multiple drug therapies to treat these accompanying disease states.

Most TCAs are pregnancy category C with amitriptyline, imipramine, and nortriptyline being category D. Caution is warranted in breastfeeding mothers as TCAs are excreted into breast milk. The American Academy of Pediatrics categorizes most TCAs as drugs whose effect on nursing infants are unknown and may be of concern.

Adverse Effects and Monitoring

Potential adverse effects are numerous, however sedation and peripheral and central anticholinergic side effects are most frequent. Fortunately, tolerance often develops to the aforementioned side effects and may be attenuated with using low initial dosages with gradual upward dose titration. Cardiovascular, CNS, and urinary side effects may develop and should be assessed with subsequent decisions made to decrease the dose or discontinue altogether.

Baseline and periodic WBC with differential and LFTs are recommended. Additionally, perform ECG assessment prior to initiation of therapy, particularly in older patients and those with pre-existing cardiac abnormalities, with periodic follow-up cardiac evaluation at appropriate intervals thereafter.

Drug Interactions

In general, TCAs are highly protein bound, with metabolism occurring in the liver (CYP2D6). Potential drug interactions are numerous with this class of agents. See **Table 19.2** or refer to the full prescribing information for the drug in for a complete listing of clinically relevant drug interactions.

Dosage and Administration

TCAs are often dosed orally once daily and should be started at low doses and gradually titrated. Dosing parameters vary depending on the specific agent used. Refer to information regarding individual agents for specific dosing and administration information, or see **Table 19.1**.

SUGGESTED READING

Anderson B, Funnell M. *The Art of Empowerment*. American Diabetes Association. Alexandria, VA.

Ciechanowski P, Katon WJ, Russo JE. Depression and diabetes: Impact of depressive symptoms on adherence, function and costs. *Arch Intern Med*. 2000;160:3278-3285.

Engum A, Mykletun A, Midthjell K, Holen A, Dahl AA. Depression and diabetes: a large population-based study of sociodemographic, lifestyle, and clinical factors associated with depression in type 1 and type 2 diabetes. *Diabetes Care*. 2005;28:1904-1909.

Goodnick PJ, Henry JH, Buki VMV. Treatment of depression in patients with diabetes mellitus. *J Clin Psychiatry*. 1995;56:128-136.

Katon W, Von Korff M, Ciechanowski P, Russo J, Lin E, Simon G, et al. Behavioral and clinical factors associated with depression among individuals with diabetes. *Diabetes Care.* 2004; 27: 914-920.

Kinder LS, Kamarchk TW, Baum A, Orchard TJ. Depressive symptomatology and coronary heart disease in type 1 diabetes mellitus: a study of possible mechanisms. *Health Psychology.* 2002;21:542-552.

Lustman PJ, Clouse RE, Alrakawi A, Rubin EH, Gelenberg AJ. Treatment of major depression in adults with diabetes: a primary care perspective. *Clin Diabetes.* 1997;May/June:122-126.

Lustman, PJ, Clouse RE, Nix BD, Freedland KE, Rubin EH, Ciechanowski PS, et al. Sertraline for prevention of depression recurrence in diabetes: a randomized, double-blind, placebo-controlled trial. *Arch Gen Psych.* 2006;63:521-529.

Lustman PJ, Griffith LS, Clouse RE, Freedland KE, Eisen SA, et al. Effects of nortriptyline on depression and glycemic control in diabetes: results of a double-blind, placebo-controlled trial. *Psychsom Med.* 1997;59:241-250.

Lustman PJ, Clouse RE, Sayuk GS, Williams MM, Nix BD. Factors influencing glycemic control in type 2 diabetes during acute- and maintenance-phase treatment of major depressive disorder with bupropion. *Diabetes Care.* 2007 Mar;30(3):459-66.

Lustman PJ, Clouse RE, Greedland KE. Management of major depression in adults with diabetes: implications of recent clinical trails. *Semin Clin Neuropsychiatry.* 1998;3:102-114.

Mann JJ. The medical management of depression. *N Engl J Med.* 2005;353:1819-1834.

Polonsky WH, Parkin CG. Depression in patients with diabetes: seven facts every healthcare provider should know. *Practical Diabetology.* 2001 (December):20-29.

Polonsky WH. Diabetes Burnout: What to do when you can't take it anymore. American Diabetes Association. Alexandria, VA.

Simon G, Katon W, Lin EHB, Rutter C, Manning WG, Ciechanowski P, et al. Cost-effectiveness of systematic depression treatment among people with diabetes mellitus. *Arch Gen Psychiatry.* 2007:64, 65-72.

Table 19.1. Prescribing Information for Antidepressants

GENERIC (BRAND)	FORM/ STRENGTH	DOSAGE	WARNINGS/PRECAUTIONS & CONTRAINDICATIONS	ADVERSE REACTIONS
AMINOKETONES				
Bupropion HBr (Aplenzin)	Tab, Extended-Release: 174mg, 348mg, 522mg	*Adults:* ≥18 yrs: Give in morning. Swallow whole. Initial: 174mg qd. Titrate: May increase to 348mg qd on Day 4 if tolerated. Max: 522mg/day given as single dose if no clinical improvement after several weeks. **Switching from Wellbutrin, Wellbutrin SR, or Wellbutrin XL:** Give equivalent dose. 522mg bupropion HBr = 450mg bupropion HCl; 348mg bupropion HBr = 300mg bupropion HCl; 174mg bupropion HBr = 150mg bupropion HCl. **Mild-Moderate Hepatic Cirrhosis/ Renal Impairment:** Reduce frequency and/or dose. **Severe Hepatic Cirrhosis:** Max: 174mg every other day.	**BB:** Antidepressants increased the risk of suicidal thinking and behavior (suicidality) in short-term studies in children, adolescents, and young adults with major depressive disorder (MDD) and other psychiatric disorders. Bupropion is not approved for use in pediatric patients. **W/P:** May worsen depression and/or emergence of suicidal ideation and behavior; monitor closely. May precipitate manic episodes in bipolar disorder. Dose-related risk of seizures; d/c and do not restart if seizure occurs. Extreme caution with history of seizure, cranial trauma, severe hepatic cirrhosis, concomitant medications that lower seizure threshold. Agitation, insomnia, psychosis, confusion, and other neuropsychiatric signs reported. Caution with hepatic impairment (including mild to moderate hepatic cirrhosis). Anorexia/ weight loss may occur. HTN reported; caution with recent history of MI or unstable heart disease. Anaphylactoid/ anaphylactic reactions reported; d/c if any occur. **Contra:** Seizure disorder, bulimia or anorexia nervosa, within 14 days of MAOIs, other forms of bupropion, abrupt discontinuation of alcohol or sedatives (including benzodiazepines). **P/N:** Category C, not for use in nursing.	Dry mouth, nausea, insomnia, dizziness, pharyngitis, abdominal pain, agitation, anxiety, tremor, palpitations, tremor, sweating, tinnitus, myalgia, anorexia, urinary frequency, rash.
Bupropion HCl (Wellbutrin, Wellbutrin SR)	Tab: 75mg, 100mg; Tab, Extended-Release: 100mg, 150mg, 200mg	*Adults:* ≥18 yrs: (Tab, Extended-Release) Initial: 150mg qd, may increase to 150mg bid after 3 days. Usual: 150mg bid. Max: 200mg bid. Separate doses by at least 8 hrs. **Severe Hepatic Cirrhosis:** 100mg/day or 150mg every other day. **Mild-Moderate Hepatic Cirrhosis/Renal Impairment:** Reduce frequency and/or dose. (Tab) Initial: 100mg bid, may increase to 100mg tid after 3 days. Usual: 100mg tid. Max: 450mg/day, given in divided doses of not more than 150mg each. **Severe Hepatic Cirrhosis:** Max: 75mg qd.	**BB:** Antidepressants increased the risk of suicidal thinking and behavior (suicidality) in short-term studies in children, adolescents, and young adults with Major Depressive Disorder (MDD) and other psychiatric disorders. Bupropion is not approved for use in pediatric patients. **W/P:** Dose-related risk of seizures. D/C and do not restart if seizure occurs. Extreme caution with history of seizure, cranial trauma, severe hepatic cirrhosis. Agitation, insomnia, psychosis, confusion and other neuropsychiatric signs reported. Caution with bipolar disorder, recent MI, unstable heart disease, renal impairment. Altered appetite/weight, allergic reactions, HTN reported. Monitor for clinical worsening and/or suicidality, especially at initiation of therapy or dose changes. **Contra:** Seizure disorder, bulimia or anorexia nervosa, within 14 days of MAOIs, other forms of bupropion, abrupt discontinuation of alcohol or sedatives. **P/N:** Category C, not for use in nursing.	Headache, dry mouth, nausea, insomnia, dizziness, pharyngitis, infection, abdominal pain, constipation, diarrhea, tinnitus, agitation, anxiety, rash, anorexia.
Bupropion HCl (Wellbutrin XL)	Tab, Extended-Release: 150mg, 300mg	*Adults:* ≥18 yrs: Give in AM. Swallow whole. **MDD:** Initial: 150mg qd. May increase to 300mg qd on Day 4. Usual: 300mg qd. Max: 450mg qd. **SAD:** Start in autumn; stop in early spring. Initial: 150mg qd. May increase to 300mg after 1 week. Usual/Max: 300mg qd. Taper dose for 2 weeks prior to discontinuation. **Mild-Moderate Hepatic Cirrhosis/Renal Impairment:** Reduce frequency and/or dose. **Severe Hepatic Cirrhosis:** Max: 150mg every other day.	**BB:** Antidepressants increased the risk of suicidal thinking and behavior (suicidality) in short-term studies in children, adolescents, and young adults with Major Depressive Disorder (MDD) and other psychiatric disorders. Bupropion is not approved for use in pediatric patients. **W/P:** Dose-related risk of seizures. D/C and do not restart if seizure occurs. Extreme caution with history of seizure, cranial trauma, severe hepatic cirrhosis. Agitation, insomnia, psychosis, confusion	Headache, dry mouth, nausea, insomnia, dizziness, pharyngitis, abdominal pain, agitation, diarrhea, palpitations, myalgia, anxiety, tinnitus, constipation, sweating, rash.

BB = black box warning; **W/P** = warnings/precautions; **Contra** = contraindications; **P/N** = pregnancy category rating and nursing considerations.

Table 19.1. Prescribing Information for Antidepressants

GENERIC (BRAND)	FORM/ STRENGTH	DOSAGE	WARNINGS/PRECAUTIONS & CONTRAINDICATIONS	ADVERSE REACTIONS
AMINOKETONES *(Cont.)*				
Bupropion HCl (Wellbutrin XL) *(Cont.)*			and other neuropsychiatric signs reported. Caution with bipolar disorder, recent MI, unstable heart disease, renal impairment. Altered appetite/weight, allergic reactions, HTN reported. Monitor for clinical worsening and/or suicidality, especially at initiation of therapy or dose changes. **Contra:** Seizure disorder, bulimia or anorexia nervosa, within 14 days of MAOIs, other forms of bupropion, abrupt discontinuation of alcohol or sedatives. **P/N:** Category C, not for use in nursing.	
MONOAMINE OXIDASE INHIBITORS				
Phenelzine sulfate (Nardil)	**Tab:** 15mg	***Adults:*** Initial: 15mg tid. Titrate: Increase to 60-90mg/day at a fairly rapid pace until maximum benefit. Maint: Reduce slowly over several weeks to 15mg qd or 15mg every other day.	**BB:** Antidepressants increased the risk of suicidal thinking and behavior (suicidality) in short-term studies in children, adolescents, and young adults with Major Depressive Disorder (MDD) and other psychiatric disorders. Phenelzine is not approved for use in pediatric patients. **W/P:** Hypertensive crisis, postural hypotension reported; monitor BP frequently. Caution with epilepsy, asthma, DM, or psychosis. D/C if palpitations or headache occur. Excessive stimulation in schizophrenics. D/C 10 days prior to elective surgery. Avoid abrupt withdrawal. **Contra:** Pheochromocytoma, CHF, history of liver disease, abnormal LFTs, severe renal impairment or renal disease, meperidine, MAOIs, dextromethorphan, CNS depressants, alcohol, certain narcotics, sympathomimetic drugs (eg, amphetamines, cocaine, methylphenidate, dopamine, epinephrine, norepinephrine), or related compounds (eg, methyldopa, L-dopa, L-tryptophan, L-tyrosine, phenylalanine), high tyramine-containing food (eg, cheese, pickled herring, beer, wine, yeast extract, salami, yogurt), excessive caffeine and chocolate, dextromethorphan, CNS depressants, buspirone, serotoninergic agents (eg, dexfenfluramine, fluoxetine, fluvoxamine, paroxetine, sertraline, venlafaxine), bupropion, guanethidine. **P/N:** Safety in pregnancy and nursing not known.	Dizziness, headache, drowsiness, sleep disturbances, constipation, dry mouth, GI disturbances, elevated serum transaminases, weight gain, edema, sexual disturbances.
Selegiline[†] (Emsam)	**Patch:** 6mg/24hrs, 9mg/24hrs, 12mg/24hrs [30ˢ]	***Adults:*** Apply to dry, intact skin on the upper torso, upper thigh, or outer surface of upper arm once every 24 hrs. Initial/Target Dose: 6mg/24hrs. Titrate: May increase in increments of 3mg/24hrs at intervals no less than 2 weeks. Max: 12mg/24hrs. **Elderly:** 6mg/24hrs. Increase dose cautiously and monitor closely.	**BB:** Antidepressants increased the risk of suicidal thinking and behavior (suicidality) in short-term studies in children, adolescents and young adults with Major Depressive Disorder and other psychiatric disorders. Selegiline transdermal system is not approved for use in pediatric patients. **W/P:** Hypertensive crisis may occur with ingestion of foods with a high concentration of tyramine. Postural hypotension may occur; consider dosage adjustment with orthostatic symptoms. Activation of mania/hypomania may occur; caution with history of mania. Caution with disorders or conditions that can produce altered metabolism or hemodynamic responses. Avoid elective surgery requiring general anesthesia.	Headache, diarrhea, dyspepsia, insomnia, dry mouth, pharyngitis, sinusitis, application site reaction, rash.

† Selective MAO inhibitor (type B).
BB = black box warning; **W/P** = warnings/precautions; **Contra** = contraindications; **P/N** = pregnancy category rating and nursing considerations.

Table 19.1. Prescribing Information for Antidepressants

GENERIC (BRAND)	FORM/ STRENGTH	DOSAGE	WARNINGS/PRECAUTIONS & CONTRAINDICATIONS	ADVERSE REACTIONS
Selegiline[†] (Emsam) *(Cont.)*			**Contra:** Pheochromocytoma. Concomitant SSRIs (eg, fluoxetine, sertraline, paroxetine), dual serotonin and norepinephrine reuptake inhibitors (eg, venlafaxine, duloxetine), TCAs (eg, imipramine, amitriptyline), bupropion, buspirone, meperidine, analgesic agents (eg, tramadol, methadone, and propoxyphene), dextromethorphan, St. John's wort, mirtazapine, cyclobenzaprine, carbamazepine, oxcarbazepine, sympathetic amines (including amphetamines), cold products and weight-reducing preparations that contain vasoconstrictors (eg, pseudoephedrine, phenylephrine, phenylpropanolamine, ephedrine), oral selegiline, other MAOIs (eg, isocarboxazid, phenelzine, tranylcypromine), general anesthesia agents, cocaine, or local anesthesia containing sympathomimetic vasoconstrictors. Dietary modifications required with 9mg/24hrs and 12mg/24hrs systems. **P/N:** Category C, caution in nursing.	
Tranylcypromine sulfate (Parnate)	**Tab:** 10mg	***Adults:*** Usual: 30mg/day in divided doses. Titrate: After 2 weeks, may increase by 10mg/day every 1-3 weeks depending on signs of improvement. Max: 60mg/day.	**BB:** Antidepressants increased the risk of suicidal thinking and behavior (suicidality) in short-term studies in children, adolescents, and young adults with Major Depressive Disorder and other psychiatric disorders. Tranylcypromine is not approved for use in pediatric patients. **W/P:** Use in patients who are resistant to other therapies. Hypotension reported. Drug dependency possible in doses excessive of the therapeutic range. May suppress anginal pain in myocardial ischemia. Caution with hyperthyroidism, renal dysfunction, diabetes, elderly. May aggravate depression symptoms. May lower seizure threshold. Inhibits MAO 10 days after discontinuation. D/C at least 10 days before elective surgery. D/C if palpitations or frequent headaches occur. **Contra:** Cardiovascular or cerebrovascular disorder, HTN, history of headache, pheochromocytoma. Concomitant MAOIs, dibenzazepine derivatives, sympathomimetics (including amphetamines), some CNS depressants (including narcotics and alcohol), antihypertensives, diuretics, antihistamines, sedatives, anesthetics, bupropion, buspirone, meperidine, SSRIs, dexfenfluramine, dextromethorphan, foods with high tyramine content (cheese) and excessive quantities of caffeine. Elective surgery requiring general anesthesia. History of liver disease or abnormal LFTs. Caution with anti-parkinsonism drugs. **P/N:** Safety in pregnancy and nursing not known.	Restlessness, insomnia, weakness, drowsiness, nausea, diarrhea, tachycardia, anorexia, edema, tinnitis, muscle spasm, overstimulation, dizziness, dry mouth, blood dyscrasias.
SEROTONIN/NOREPINEPHRINE REUPTAKE INHIBITORS (SNRIs)				
Desvenlafaxine (Pristiq)	**Tab, Extended-Release:** 50mg, 100mg	***Adults:*** ≥18 yrs: 50mg qd. **Renal Impairment (24-hr CrCl<30mL/min) or ESRD:** 50mg every other day. Supplemental doses should not be given to patients after dialysis. **Hepatic Impairment:** Max: 100mg/day. Upon	**BB:** Antidepressants increased the risk of suicidal thinking and behavior (suicidality) in short-term studies in children, adolescents, and young adults with Major Depressive Disorder (MDD) and other psychiatric disorders. Desvenlafaxine is	Headache, nausea, dry mouth, diarrhea, dizziness, insomnia, somnolence, hyperhidrosis, fatigue, constipation, vomiting,

[†] Selective MAO inhibitor (type B).
BB = black box warning; **W/P** = warnings/precautions; **Contra** = contraindications; **P/N** = pregnancy category rating and nursing considerations.

Table 19.1. Prescribing Information for Antidepressants

GENERIC (BRAND)	FORM/ STRENGTH	DOSAGE	WARNINGS/PRECAUTIONS & CONTRAINDICATIONS	ADVERSE REACTIONS
SEROTONIN/NOREPINEPHRINE REUPTAKE INHIBITORS (SNRIs) *(Cont.)*				
Desvenlafaxine (Pristiq) *(Cont.)*		discontinuation of therapy, gradual reduction in the dose (giving 50mg less frequently) rather than abrupt cessation is recommended. Do not divide, crush, chew or place in water.	not approved for use in pediatric patients. **W/P:** May experience worsening of depression and/or emergence of suicidal behavior. Serotonin syndrome reported; caution with concomitant serotonergic drugs. May cause sustained increases in BP; monitor BP regularly. May increase the risk of bleeding events. Monitor with increased IOP or if at risk of acute narrow-angle glaucoma. Activation of mania/hypomania reported. Caution with cardiovascular or cerebrovascular disease, recent MI, renal impairment, and patients with seizure disorder. Cholesterol and triglyceride elevation; consider monitoring. Discontinuation symptoms have occurred; taper dose and monitor symptoms. Hyponatremia may occur. Patients who present with progressive dyspnea, cough or chest discomfort should consider the possibility of interstitial lung disease and eosinophilic pneumonia. **Contra:** Concomitant MAOI therapy. **P/N:** Category C, not for use in nursing.	palpitations, anxiety, decreased appetite, specific male sexual disorders.
Duloxetine HCl (Cymbalta)	**Cap, Delayed-Release:** 20mg, 30mg, 60mg	***Adults: MDD:*** Initial: 40mg/day (given as 20mg bid) to 60mg/day (given qd or as 30mg bid). Re-evaluate periodically. **Diabetic Peripheral Neuropathic Pain:** 60mg/day given qd. May lower starting dose if tolerability a concern. **Renal Impairment:** Consider lower starting dose with gradual increase. **GAD:** Initial: 60mg qd or 30mg qd for 1 week to adjust before increasing to 60mg qd. Titrate: May increase by increments of 30mg qd if needed. Max: 120 mg qd. Do not chew or crush.	**BB:** Antidepressants increased the risk of suicidal thinking and behavior (suicidality) in short-term studies in children, adolescents, and young adults with major depressive disorder (MDD) and other psychiatric disorders. Not approved for use in pediatric patients. **W/P:** Monitor for clinical worsening and/or suicidality. May increase risk of serum transaminase elevations. May cause hepatotoxicity. Avoid with chronic liver disease. May increase BP; obtain baseline and monitor periodically. Orthostatic hypotension and syncope reported. Avoid abrupt cessation and with severe renal impairment/ESRD or hepatic insufficiency. Caution with conditions that may slow gastric emptying, history of mania or seizures. May increase risk of mydriasis; caution in patients with controlled narrow-angle glaucoma. Serotonin syndrome may occur; caution with concomitant use of serotonergic drugs. Hyponatremia reported. May affect urethral resistance. May increase risk of abnormal bleeding; caution with aspirin, NSAIDs, warfarin. Increases the risk of elevation of serum transaminase levels. **Contra:** Concomitant use of MAOIs, uncontrolled narrow-angle glaucoma. **P/N:** Category C, not for use in nursing.	Nausea, dry mouth, constipation, diarrhea, vomiting, decreased appetite, fatigue, dizziness, somnolence, increased sweating, blurred vision, insomnia, agitation, erectile dysfunction.
Nefazodone HCl*	**Tab:** 50mg, 100mg*, 150mg*, 200mg, 250mg *scored	***Adults:*** Initial: 100mg bid. Usual: 300-600mg/day. Titrate: May increase by 100-200mg/day at intervals of no less than 1 week. **Elderly/Debilitated:** Initial: 50mg bid.	**BB:** Antidepressants increased the risk of suicidal thinking and behavior (suicidality) in short-term studies in children, adolescents, and young adults with Major Depressive Disorder (MDD) and other psychiatric disorders. Nefazodone is not approved for use in pediatric patients. Life-threatening hepatic failure reported. Avoid with active liver disease or elevated serum transaminases. D/C and do not retreat if symptoms of hepatic disease develop or if ALT/AST ≥3x ULN. **W/P:**	Hepatic failure, somnolence, dry mouth, nausea, dizziness, insomnia, agitation, constipation, asthenia, lightheadedness, blurred vision, confusion, abnormal vision.

* Available only in generic form.
BB = black box warning; **W/P** = warnings/precautions; **Contra** = contraindications; **P/N** = pregnancy category rating and nursing considerations.

Table 19.1. Prescribing Information for Antidepressants

GENERIC (BRAND)	FORM/ STRENGTH	DOSAGE	WARNINGS/PRECAUTIONS & CONTRAINDICATIONS	ADVERSE REACTIONS
Nefazodone HCl* *(Cont.)*			May cause postural hypotension. Caution with cardiovascular or cerebrovascular disease that could be exacerbated by hypotension and conditions with predisposition to hypotension (eg, dehydration, hypotension). May activate mania/hypomania. Priapism reported. Caution with history of MI, unstable heart disease, seizures, liver cirrhosis. Avoid with active liver disease. **Contra:** Coadministration of terfenadine, astemizole, cisapride, pimozide, carbamazepine, triazolam. Liver injury from previous treatment. **P/N:** Category C, caution in nursing.	
Venlafaxine HCl (Effexor)	**Tab:** 25mg*, 37.5mg*, 50mg*, 75mg*, 100mg* *scored	**Adults:** ≥18 yrs: Initial: 75mg/day given bid-tid with food. Titrate: Increase by 75mg/day at no less than 4 day intervals. Max: 375mg/day. **Hepatic Impairment (moderate):** Reduce dose by 50%. **Renal Impairment (mild to moderate):** Reduce dose by 25%. **Hemodialysis:** Reduce dose by 50%. Withhold dose until after hemodialysis treatment completed. If drug used 6 weeks or longer, taper gradually (over 2 weeks or more) when discontinuing treatment.	**BB:** Antidepressants increased the risk of suicidal thinking and behavior (suicidality) in short-term studies in children, adolescents, and young adults with Major Depressive Disorder (MDD) and other psychiatric disorders. Venlafaxine is not approved for use in pediatric patients. **W/P:** May cause sustained increases in BP. Treatment-emergent anxiety, nervousness, insomnia, and anorexia reported. Caution with history of mania or seizures and conditions affecting hemodynamic responses. Monitor with increased IOP or if at risk of acute narrow angle glaucoma. Activation of mania/ hypomania reported. Risk of hyponatremia, SIADH, skin and mucous membrane bleeding. Caution with hyperthyroidism, heart failure, recent MI, renal or hepatic impairment. Serotonin syndrome may occur. Caution with concomitant serotonergic drugs. Patients who present with progressive dyspnea, cough or chest discomfort should consider the possibility of interstitial lung disease and eosinophilic pneumonia. **Contra:** Concomitant MAOIs. **P/N:** Category C, not for use in nursing.	Asthenia, sweating, nausea, constipation, anorexia, vomiting, insomnia, somnolence, dry mouth, dizziness, nervousness, anxiety, tremor, blurred vision, abnormal ejaculation/ orgasm, impotence in men.
Venlafaxine HCl (Effexor XR)	**Cap, Extended-Release:** 37.5mg, 75mg, 150mg	**Adults:** MDD/GAD/SAD: Initial: 75mg qd, or 37.5mg qd increase to 75mg qd after 4-7 days. Titrate: May increase by 75mg/day at no less than 4 day intervals. Max: 225mg/day. **PD:** Initial: 37.5mg qd for 7 days. Titrate: May increase 75mg/day, as needed at no less than 7 day intervals. Max: 225mg/day. **Moderate Hepatic Impairment:** Reduce initial dose by 50%. **Renal Impairment:** Reduce total daily dose by 25-50%. **Hemodialysis:** Reduce total daily dose by 50%. Withhold dose until after hemodialysis treatment completed. If drug used 6 weeks or longer, taper gradually (over 2 weeks or more) when discontinuing treatment. Periodically reassess need for maintenance therapy. Take with food in the am or pm, the same time each day. May sprinkle on spoonful of applesauce. Do not divide, crush, chew or place in water.	**BB:** Antidepressants increased the risk of suicidal thinking and behavior (suicidality) in short-term studies in children, adolescents, and young adults with Major Depressive Disorder (MDD) and other psychiatric disorders. Venlafaxine is not approved for use in pediatric patients. **W/P:** May cause sustained increases in BP; monitor BP regularly. Treatment-emergent nervousness, insomnia and anorexia reported. Caution with seizures, conditions affecting hemodynamic responses or metabolism, volume-depletion, the elderly. Risk of mydriasis; monitor those with raised IOP or risk of acute narrow angle glaucoma. Abnormal bleeding (eg, ecchymosis) and activation of mania/hypomania reported. Risk of hyponatremia, SIADH. Caution with recent MI, hyperthyroidism, heart failure, renal or hepatic impairment. Serotonin syndrome may occur; caution with concomitant use of serotonergic drugs. Patients who present with progressive dyspnea, cough or chest discomfort should consider the possibility of interstitial lung disease and eosinophilic	Asthenia, sweating, headache, nausea, constipation, anorexia, dry mouth, dizziness, insomnia, nervousness, somnolence, abnormal ejaculation, abnormal dreams.

* Available only in generic form.
BB = black box warning; **W/P** = warnings/precautions; **Contra** = contraindications; **P/N** = pregnancy category rating and nursing considerations.

Table 19.1. Prescribing Information for Antidepressants

GENERIC (BRAND)	FORM/ STRENGTH	DOSAGE	WARNINGS/PRECAUTIONS & CONTRAINDICATIONS	ADVERSE REACTIONS
SEROTONIN/NOREPINEPHRINE REUPTAKE INHIBITORS (SNRIs) *(Cont.)*				
Venlafaxine HCl (Effexor XR) *(Cont.)*			pneumonia. D/C if impaired balance occured. Cases of clinically significant hyponatremia in elderly patients. **Contra:** Concomitant MAOI therapy. **P/N:** Category C, not for use in nursing.	
SELECTIVE SEROTONIN REUPTAKE INHIBITORS (SSRIs)				
Citalopram HBr (Celexa)	**Sol:** 10mg/5mL [240mL]; **Tab:** 10mg, 20mg*, 40mg* *scored	***Adults:*** Initial: 20mg qd, in the am or pm. Titrate: Increase by 20mg at intervals of no less than 1 week. Max: 40mg/day (nonresponders may require 60mg/day). **Elderly/Hepatic Impairment:** 20mg/day; titrate to 40mg/day in nonresponders. suicidal thinking and behavior	**BB:** Antidepressants increased the risk of (suicidality) in short-term studies in children, adolescents, and young adults with Major Depressive Disorder (MDD) and other psychiatric disorders. Citalopram is not approved for use in pediatric patients. **W/P:** Activation of mania/hypomania, SIADH, hyponatremia reported. Close supervision with high risk suicide patients. Caution with history of mania or seizures, hepatic impairment, severe renal impairment, conditions that alter metabolism or hemodynamic responses. May impair judgment, thinking, or motor skills. **Contra:** Concomitant MAOI or pimozide therapy. **P/N:** Category C, not for use in nursing.	Nausea, dyspepsia, vomiting, diarrhea, dry mouth, somnolence, insomnia, increased sweating, ejaculation disorder, rhinitis, anxiety, anorexia, skeletal pain, agitation.
Escitalopram oxalate (Lexapro)	**Sol:** 5mg/5mL [240mL]; **Tab:** 5mg, 10mg*, 20mg* *scored	***Adults:*** Initial: 10mg qd, in am or pm. Titrate: May increase to 20mg after a minimum of 1 week. **Elderly/Hepatic Impairment:** 10mg qd. Re-evaluate periodically.	**BB:** Antidepressants increased the risk of suicidal thinking and behavior (suicidality) in short-term studies in children, adolescents, and young adults with Major Depressive Disorder (MDD) and other psychiatric disorders. Escitalopram is not approved for use in pediatric patients. **W/P:** Avoid abrupt withdrawal. Activation of mania/hypomania, hyponatremia reported. SIADH reported with citalopram. Caution with history of mania or seizures, hepatic impairment, severe renal impairment, conditions that alter metabolism or hemodynamic responses, suicidal tendencies. May impair mental/ physical abilities. Consider tapering dose during 3rd trimester of pregnancy. **Contra:** Concomitant MAOI or pimozide therapy. **P/N:** Category C, not for use in nursing.	Nausea, insomnia, ejaculation disorder, increased sweating, somnolence, fatigue, diarrhea.
Fluoxetine HCl (Prozac, Prozac Weekly)	**Cap:** 10mg, 20mg, 40mg; **Sol:** 20mg/5mL [120mL] **Cap, Extended- Release:** 90mg	***Adults:* MDD:** Daily Dosing: Initial: 20mg qam; increase dose if no improvement after several weeks. Doses >20mg/day, give qam or bid (am and noon). Max: 80mg/day. **(Cap, ER):** One 90mg cap every week starting 7 days after last daily dose of fluoxetine 20mg. **OCD:** Initial: 20mg qam; may increase dose if no significant improvement after several weeks. Maint: 20-60mg/day given qd-bid, am and noon. Max: 80mg/day. **Bulimia Nervosa:** 60mg qam. Max: 60mg/day. **Panic Disorder:** Initial: 10mg/day. May increase to 20mg/day after 1 week. May increase further after several weeks if no clinical improvement. Max: 60mg/day. **Hepatic Impairment/Elderly:** Use lower or less frequent dosage. ***Pediatrics:* MDD: ≥8 yrs: Higher Weight Peds:** Initial: 10 or 20mg/day. After 1 week at 10mg/day, may increase to 20mg/day. **Lower Weight Peds:** Initial: 10mg/day. Titrate: May increase to 20mg/day after several weeks if clinical improvement is not observed. **OCD: ≥7 yrs: Adolescents and Higher Weight Peds:** Initial: 10mg/day. Titrate: Increase to 20mg/day	**BB:** Antidepressants increased the risk of suicidal thinking and behavior (suicidality) in short-term studies of children, adolescents, and young adults with Major Depressive Disorder (MDD) and other psychiatric disorders. **W/P:** D/C if unexplained allergic reaction occurs. Monitor for symptoms of mania/ hypomania. Caution with diseases or conditions that could affect metabolism or hemodynamic responses, diabetes, history of seizures, suicidal tendencies. Altered platelet function, hyponatremia reported. Periodically monitor height and weight in pediatrics. Monitor for clinical worsening and/or suicidality, especially at initiation of therapy or dose changes. Avoid abrupt withdrawal. Monitor for discontinuation symptoms. Caution in third trimester of pregnancy due to risk of serious neonatal complications. May interfere with cognitive and motor performance. **Contra:** During or within 14 days of MAOI therapy. Thioridazine during or within 5 weeks of discontinuation. Concomitant use of pimozide. **P/N:** Category C, not for use	Nausea, diarrhea, insomnia, anxiety, nervousness, dizziness, somnolence, tremor, decreased libido, sweating, anorexia, asthenia, dry mouth, dyspepsia, headache.

BB = black box warning; **W/P** = warnings/precautions; **Contra** = contraindications; **P/N** = pregnancy category rating and nursing considerations.

Table 19.1. Prescribing Information for Antidepressants

GENERIC (BRAND)	FORM/ STRENGTH	DOSAGE	WARNINGS/PRECAUTIONS & CONTRAINDICATIONS	ADVERSE REACTIONS
Fluoxetine HCl (Prozac, Prozac Weekly) *(Cont.)*		after 2 weeks. Consider additional dose increases after several more weeks if clinical improvement is not observed. Usual: 20-60mg/day. **Lower Weight Peds:** Initial: 10mg/day. Titrate: Consider additional dose increases after several weeks if clinical improvement is not observed. Usual: 20-30mg/day. Max: 60mg/day.	in nursing.	
Paroxetine HCl (Paxil)	**Sus:** 10mg/5mL [250mL]; **Tab:** 10mg*, 20mg*, 30mg, 40mg *scored	*Adults:* Give qd, usually in the AM. **MDD:** Initial: 20mg/day. Max: 50mg/day. **OCD:** Initial: 20mg qd. Usual: 40mg qd. Max: 60mg/day. **Panic Disorder:** Initial: 10mg qd. Usual: 40mg/day. Max: 60mg/day. **GAD:** Initial: 20mg/day. Usual: 20-50mg/day. **SAD:** Initial/Usual: 20mg/day. Max: 60mg/day. **PTSD:** Initial: 20mg/day. Usual: 20-50mg/day. To titrate, may increase weekly by 10mg/day. **Elderly/Debilitated/Severe Renal/Hepatic Impairment:** Initial: 10mg qd. Max: 40mg/day.	**BB:** Antidepressants increased the risk of suicidal thinking and behavior (suicidality) in short-term studies in children, adolescents, and young adults with Major Depressive Disorder (MDD) and other psychiatric disorders. Paroxetine is not approved for use in pediatric patients. **W/P:** Caution with history of mania or seizures, conditions that affect metabolism or hemodynamic responses, narrow angle glaucoma. D/C if seizures occur. Altered platelet function, hyponatremia, mydriasis reported. Avoid abrupt withdrawal. Re-evaluate periodically. Monitor for clinical worsening and/or suicidality, especially at initiation of therapy or dose changes. **Contra:** Concomitant MAOIs, thioridazine, or pimozide. **P/N:** Category D, caution in nursing.	Somnolence, insomnia, nausea, asthenia, abnormal ejaculation, dry mouth, constipation, dizziness, diarrhea, decreased libido, sweating.
Paroxetine HCl (Paxil CR)	**Tab, Controlled-Release:** 12.5mg, 25mg, 37.5mg	*Adults:* Give qd, usually in the AM. Swallow whole. **MDD:** Initial: 25mg/day. Titrate: May increase weekly by 12.5mg/day. Max: 62.5mg/day. **Panic Disorder:** Initial: 12.5mg/day. May increase weekly by 12.5mg/day. Max: 75mg/day. **SAD:** Initial: 12.5mg/day. May increase weekly by 12.5mg/day. Max: 37.5mg/day. **PMDD:** Initial: 12.5mg/day continuous or limited to luteal phase of cycle. May increase weekly by 12.5mg/day. **Elderly/ Debilitated/Severe Renal/Hepatic Impairment:** Initial: 12.5mg/day. Max: 50mg/day.	**BB:** Antidepressants increased the risk of suicidal thinking and behavior (suicidality) in short-term studies in children, adolescents, and young adults with Major Depressive Disorder (MDD) and other psychiatric disorders. Paroxetine is not approved for use in pediatric patients. **W/P:** Caution with history of mania or seizures, conditions that affect metabolism or hemodynamic responses, narrow angle glaucoma. D/C if seizures occur. Hyponatremia, mydriasis reported. Avoid abrupt withdrawal. Re-evaluate periodically. Monitor for clinical worsening and/or suicidality, especially at initiation of therapy or dose changes. **Contra:** Concomitant MAOIs, thioridazine, or pimozide. **P/N:** Category C, caution in nursing.	Somnolence, insomnia, nausea, asthenia, abnormal ejaculation, dry mouth, constipation, dizziness, diarrhea, decreased libido, sweating.
Paroxetine mesylate (Pexeva)	**Tab:** 10mg, 20mg, 30mg, 40mg	*Adults:* **MDD:** Initial: 20mg/day. Max: 50mg/day. **OCD:** Initial: 20mg/day. Titrate: Increase by 10mg/day. Usual: 40mg/day. Max: 60mg/day. **Panic Disorder:** Initial: 10mg/day. Titrate: 10mg/day increments at intervals of at least 1 week. Max: 60mg/day. **GAD:** Initial: 20mg/day. Titrate: Increase by 10mg/day. Max: 50mg/day. **Elderly/ Debilitated/Severe Renal or Hepatic Impairment:** Initial: 10mg qd. Max: 40mg/day.	**BB:** Antidepressants increased the risk of suicidal thinking and behavior (suicidality) in short-term studies in children, adolescents, and young adults with Major Depressive Disorder (MDD) and other psychiatric disorders. Pexeva is not approved for use in pediatric patients. **W/P:** Caution with history of mania, seizures, history of suicidal thoughts or attempts (adolescents have an increased risk of suicidal thoughts and/or attempts), conditions that affect metabolism or hemodynamic responses, narrow angle glaucoma. Risk of serotonin syndrome with contomitant use of triptans, tramadol, and other serotonergic agents. D/C if seizures occur. Altered platelet function, hyponatremia, mydriasis reported. Avoid abrupt withdrawal. Re-evaluate periodically. Monitor for clinical worsening and/or suicidality, especially at initiation	Asthenia, sweating, nausea, decreased appetite, somnolence, dizziness, insomnia, tremor, nervousness, abnormal ejaculation, dry mouth, constipation, decreased libido, impotence, headache, tinnitus.

BB = black box warning; **W/P** = warnings/precautions; **Contra** = contraindications; **P/N** = pregnancy category rating and nursing considerations.

Table 19.1. Prescribing Information for Antidepressants

GENERIC (BRAND)	FORM/ STRENGTH	DOSAGE	WARNINGS/PRECAUTIONS & CONTRAINDICATIONS	ADVERSE REACTIONS
SELECTIVE SEROTONIN REUPTAKE INHIBITORS (SSRIs) *(Cont.)*				
Paroxetine mesylate (Pexeva) *(Cont.)*			of therapy or dose changes. **Contra:** Concomitant MAOIs, thioridazine, and pimozide. **P/N:** Category D, increased risk of cardiovascular malformations (ventrciular/ atrial septal defects) in newborns; avoid unless benefit outweighs risk.	
Sertraline HCl (Zoloft)	**Sol:** 20mg/mL [60mL]; **Tab:** 25mg*, 50mg*, 100mg* *scored	***Adults: MDD/OCD:*** 50mg qd. Titrate: Adjust dose at 1 week intervals. Max: 200mg/day. **Panic Disorder/PTSD/SAD:** Initial: 25mg qd. Titrate: Increase to 50mg qd after 1 week. Adjust dose at 1 week intervals. Max: 200mg/day. **PMDD:** Initial: 50mg qd continuous or limited to luteal phase of cycle. Titrate: Increase 50mg/cycle if needed up to 150mg/day for continuous or 100mg/day for luteal phase dosing. If 100mg/day is established for luteal phase dosing, a 50mg/day titration step for 3 days should take place at the beginning of each luteal phase dosing period. **Hepatic Impairment:** Use lower or less frequent doses. Dilute sol with 4oz water, ginger ale, lemon/lime soda, lemonade or orange juice. Take immediately after mixing. ***Pediatrics: OCD: Initial: 6-12 yrs:*** 25mg qd. **13-17 yrs:** 50mg qd. Titrate: Adjust dose at 1 week intervals. Max: 200mg/day. **Hepatic Impairment:** Use lower or less frequent doses. Dilute sol with 4oz water, ginger ale, lemon/lime soda, lemonade or orange juice. Take immediately after mixing.	**BB:** Antidepressants increased the risk of suicidal thinking and behavior (suicidality) in short-term studies in children, adolescents, and young adults with Major Depressive Disorder (MDD) and other psychiatric disorders. Sertraline HCl is not approved for use in pediatric patients except for patients with obsessive compulsive disorder (OCD). **W/P:** Activation of mania/hypomania reported. Monitor weight loss. Caution with conditions that could affect metabolism or hemodynamic responses, seizure disorder. Dose adjust with liver dysfunction. Altered platelet function and hyponatremia reported. Weak uricosuric effects reported. Caution with latex sensitivity; solution dropper dispenser contains rubber. Monitor for clinical worsening and/or suicidality, especially at initiation of therapy or dose changes. Avoid abrupt withdrawal. Monitor for discontinuation symptoms. **Contra:** Concomitant use with MAOIs or pimozide. Concomitant disulfiram with solution. **P/N:** Category C, caution in nursing.	Ejaculation failure, dry mouth, increased sweating, somnolence, tremor, anorexia, dizziness, headache, vomiting, diarrhea, dyspepsia, nausea, agitation, insomnia, nervousness, abnormal vision.
TETRACYCLIC ANTIDEPRESSANTS				
Mirtazapine (Remeron, Remeron SolTab)	**Tab:** 15mg*, 30mg*, 45mg; **Tab, Disintegrating:** 15mg, 30mg, 45mg *scored	***Adults:*** Initial: 15mg qhs. Titrate: May increase every 1-2 weeks. Max: 45mg/day. Disintegrating tabs disintegrate rapidly on tongue and can be swallowed with saliva; no water needed. Do not cut tabs in half.	**BB:** Antidepressants increased the risk of suicidal thinking and behavior (suicidality) in short-term studies in children, adolescents, and young adults with Major Depressive Disorder (MDD) and other psychiatric disorders. Mirtazapine is not approved for use in pediatric patients. **W/P:** Risk of agranulocytosis. D/C if sore throat, fever, or stomatitis, along with low WBC count, develop. May increase appetite, cholesterol, and triglycerides. Caution in history of seizures, mania/ hypomania, hepatic or renal impairment, altered metabolic or hemodynamic conditions, elderly. Somnolence, dizziness reported. Close supervision with high risk suicide patients. May impair judgment, thinking, or motor skills. **P/N:** Category C, caution in nursing.	Somnolence, appetite increase, weight gain, dizziness, dry mouth, constipation, asthenia, flu syndrome, abnormal dreams.
TRIAZOLOPYRIDINE ANTIDEPRESSANTS				
Trazodone HCl*	**Tab:** 50mg*, 100mg*, 150mg*, 300mg* *scored	***Adults:*** Initial: 150mg/day in divided doses pc. Titrate: May increase by 50mg/day every 3-4 days. Max: (Outpatient) 400mg/day, (Inpatient) 600mg/day.	**BB:** Antidepressants increased the risk of suicidal thinking and behavior (suicidality) in short-term studies in children and adolescents with Major Depressive Disorder (MDD) and other psychiatric disorders. Trazodone is not approved for use in pediatric patients. **W/P:** Avoid during initial recovery phase of MI. Caution in cardiac disease. D/C prior to elective surgery. **P/N:** Category C, caution in nursing.	Dry mouth, edema, constipation, blurred vision, fatigue, nervousness, drowsiness, dizziness, headache, insomnia, nausea, vomiting, musculoskeletal pain, hypotension, confusion, priapism.

* Brand not available, available only in generic form.
BB = black box warning; **W/P** = warnings/precautions; **Contra** = contraindications; **P/N** = pregnancy category rating and nursing considerations.

Table 19.1. Prescribing Information for Antidepressants

GENERIC (BRAND)	FORM/ STRENGTH	DOSAGE	WARNINGS/PRECAUTIONS & CONTRAINDICATIONS	ADVERSE REACTIONS
TRICYCLIC ANTIDEPRESSANTS				
Amitriptyline HCl*	**Inj:** 10mg/mL; **Tab:** 10mg, 25mg, 50mg, 75mg, 100mg, 150mg	**Adults: PO:** Initial: (Outpatient) 75mg/day in divided doses or 50-100mg qhs. (Inpatient) 100mg/day. Titrate: (Outpatient) Increase by 25-50mg qhs. (Inpatient) Increase to 200mg/day. Maint: 50-100mg qhs. Max: (Outpatient) 150mg/day. (Inpatient) 300mg/day. **IM:** Initial: 20-30mg qid. **Elderly:** 10mg tid or 20mg qhs.	**BB:** Antidepressants increased the risk of suicidal thinking and behavior (suicidality) in short-term studies in children, adolescents, and young adults with Major Depressive Disorder (MDD) and other psychiatric disorders. **W/P:** Caution with history of seizures, urinary retention, angle-closure glaucoma, increased IOP, hyperthyroidism, cardiovascular disorders, liver dysfunction. Increases symptoms with schizophrenia and manic-depression. D/C several weeks before elective surgery. May alter blood glucose levels. **Contra:** MAOI use or within 14 days, acute recovery period following MI. **P/N:** Category C, not for use in nursing.	MI, stroke, seizure, paralytic ileus, urinary retention, constipation, blurred vision, dry mouth, hyperpyrexia, rash, bone marrow depression, testicular swelling, gynecomastia (male), breast enlargement (female), alopecia, edema.
Amoxapine*	**Tab:** 25mg*, 50mg*, 100mg*, 150mg* *scored	**Adults:** Initial: 50mg bid-tid. Titrate: May increase to 100mg bid-tid by end of first week. Usual: 200-300mg/day. Max: Outpatients: 400mg/day; Inpatients: 600mg/day. **Elderly:** Initial: 25mg bid-tid. Titrate: May increase to 50mg bid-tid by end of first week. Max: 300mg/day. Doses ≤300mg/day may be given as single dose at bedtime.	**BB:** Antidepressants increased the risk of suicidal thinking and behavior (suicidality) in short-term studies in children, adolescents, and young adults with Major Depressive Disorder (MDD) and other psychiatric disorders. **W/P:** D/C if NMS, TD, rash and/or drug fever occur. Caution with history of urinary retention, angle-closure glaucoma, or increased IOP, suicidal tendencies. May induce sinus tachycardia, changes in conduction time, arrhythmias. MI, stroke reported. Extreme caution with history of seizure disorders. Activation of mania, increased psychosis reported. May impair mental/physical abilities. **Contra:** During or within 14 days of MAOIs; recent MI. **P/N:** Category C, caution in nursing.	Drowsiness, dry mouth, constipation, blurred vision.
Clomipramine HCl (Anafranil*)	**Cap:** 25mg, 50mg, 75mg	**Adults:** Initial: 25mg/day with meals. Titrate: Increase within 2 weeks to 100mg/day. Increase further over several weeks. Max: 250mg/day. Maint: May give total daily dose at bedtime. **Pediatrics: >10 yrs:** Initial: 25mg/day with meals. Titrate: Increase within 2 weeks to 3mg/kg or 100mg/day, whichever is smaller. Increase further over several weeks. Max: 3mg/kg/day or 200mg/day. Maint: May give total daily dose at bedtime.	**BB:** Antidepressants increased the risk of suicidal thinking and behavior (suicidality) in short-term studies in children, adolescents, and young adults with Major Depressive Disorder (MDD) and other psychiatric disorders. Clomipramine is not approved for use in pediatric patients except for patients with OCD. **W/P:** Pooled analyses of short-term placebo-controlled trials of antidepressant drugs showed that these drugs increase the risk of suicidal thinking and behavior (suicidality) in children, adolescents, and young adults (ages 18-24) with major depressive disorder (MDD) and other psychiatric disorders. Increased risks with electroconvulsive therapy. D/C prior to elective surgery. Avoid abrupt withdrawal. Caution with seizure disorder, conditions predisposing to seizures (eg, brain damage, alcoholism), urinary retention, narrow-angle glaucoma, adrenal medulla tumors, increased IOP, hyperthyroidism, cardiovascular disorders, liver dysfunction, significant renal dysfunction. Monitor hepatic enzymes with liver dysfunction. Weight changes, sexual dysfunction, blood dyscrasias, elevated liver enzymes reported. Hypomania/mania reported with affective disorder. Psychosis reported with schizophrenia. All patients	Dry mouth, constipation, nausea, dyspepsia, anorexia, weight gain, increased sweating, increased appetite, myoclonus, nervousness, libido change, dizziness, tremor, somnolence, impotence, visual changes.

* Brand name discontinued; generic version is still available.
BB = black box warning; **W/P** = warnings/precautions; **Contra** = contraindications; **P/N** = pregnancy category rating and nursing considerations.

Table 19.1. Prescribing Information for Antidepressants

GENERIC (BRAND)	FORM/ STRENGTH	DOSAGE	WARNINGS/PRECAUTIONS & CONTRAINDICATIONS	ADVERSE REACTIONS
TRICYCLIC ANTIDEPRESSANTS *(Cont.)*				
Clomipramine HCl* (Anafranil) *(Cont.)*			being treated with antidepressants for any indication should be monitored appropriately and observed closely for clinical worsening, suicidality, and unusual changes in behavior, especially during the initial few months of therapy or at times of dose changes. **Contra:** MAOI use within 14 days, acute recovery period following MI. **P/N:** Category C, not for use in nursing.	
Desipramine HCl (Norpramin)	**Tab:** 10mg, 25mg, 50mg, 75mg, 100mg, 150mg	***Adults:*** Usual: 100-200mg/day given qd or in divided doses. Max: 300mg/day. **Elderly/Adolescents:** Usual: 25-100mg/day given qd or in divided doses. Max: 150mg/day.	**BB:** Antidepressants increased the risk of suicidal thinking and behavior (suicidality) in short-term studies in children, adolescents, and young adults with Major Depressive Disorder (MDD) and other psychiatric disorders. Desipramine is not approved for use in pediatric patients. **W/P:** Hypomania with manic-depressive disease. D/C prior to elective surgery. Do not withdraw abruptly. Extreme caution with urinary retention, glaucoma, seizure disorders, cardiovascular disease, thyroid disease, alcohol abuse. May exacerbate psychosis; caution with schizophrenia. May impair mental or physical abilities. May alter blood glucose levels. **Contra:** MAOI use within 14 days, acute recovery period following MI. **P/N:** Safety in pregnancy and nursing not known.	Arrhythmias, hypotension, HTN, tachycardia, confusion, hallucination, dizziness, anxiety, numbness, tingling, ataxia, tremors, dry mouth, urinary retention, urticaria, photosensitivity, SIADH, altered libido.
Doxepin HCl (Sinequan)	**Cap:** 10mg, 25mg, 50mg, 75mg, 100mg, 150mg; **Sol, Concentrate:** 10mg/mL [120mL]	***Adults: Very Mild Illness:*** Usual: 25-50mg/day. **Mild to Moderate Severity:** Initial: 75mg/day. Usual: 75-150mg/day. **Severely Ill:** May increase up to 300mg/day. Dilute solution with 120mL of water, milk or juice. Give once daily or in divided doses. Divide dose if >150mg. **Elderly:** Use lower doses and monitor closely.	**BB:** Antidepressants increased the risk of suicidal thinking and behavior (suicidality) in short-term studies in children, adolescents, and young adults with Major Depressive Disorder (MDD) and other psychiatric disorders. Doxepin is not approved for use in pediatric patients. **W/P:** Monitor for suicidal tendencies and increased symptoms of psychosis. Avoid abrupt discontinuation. **Contra:** Glaucoma, urinary retention. **P/N:** Safety in pregnancy and nursing not known.	Drowsiness, dry mouth, blurred vision, constipation, urinary retention, hypotension, tachycardia, rash, edema, photosensitization, pruritus, eosinophilia, nausea, dizziness.
Imipramine HCl (Tofranil)	**Tab:** 10mg, 25mg, 50mg	***Adults:* Depression:** Initial: (Inpatient) 100mg/day in divided doses. Titrate: Increase to 200mg/day; up to 250-300mg/day after 2 weeks if needed. (Outpatient) 75mg/day. Titrate: Increase to 150mg/day. Maint: 50-150mg/day. Max: 200mg/day. **Elderly/Adolescents:** Initial: 30-40mg/day. Max: 100mg/day. ***Pediatrics:* Depression: Adolescents:** Initial: 30-40mg/day. Max: 100mg/day. **Enuresis: ≥6 yrs:** Initial: 25mg/day 1 hour before bedtime. Titrate: **6-12 yrs:** If inadequate response in 1 week, increase to 50mg before bedtime. **≥12 yrs:** Increase to 75mg before bedtime after 1 week if needed. Max: 2.5mg/kg/day.	**BB:** Antidepressants increased the risk of suicidal thinking and behavior (suicidality) in short-term studies in children, adolescents, and young adults with Major Depressive Disorder (MDD) and other psychiatric disorders. Imipramine HCl is not approved for use in pediatric patients except for patients with nocturnal enuresis. **W/P:** Caution with elderly, serious depression, cardiovascular disease, hyperthyroidism, urinary retention, narrow-angle glaucoma, increased IOP, seizure disorders, renal and hepatic impairment. May activate psychosis in schizophrenia; reduce dose. Limit electroshock therapy. May alter blood glucose levels. Photosensitivity reported. D/C prior to elective surgery, or with hypomanic or manic episodes. D/C with pathological neutrophil depression. **Contra:** Within 14 days of MAOI therapy, or during acute recovery period following MI. **P/N:** Safety in pregnancy not known; not for use in nursing.	Orthostatic hypotension, HTN, confusion, hallucinations, numbness, tremors, dry mouth, urticaria, nausea, vomiting, diarrhea, gynecomastia (male), breast enlargement (female), galactorrhea.

* Available only in generic form.
BB = black box warning; **W/P** = warnings/precautions; **Contra** = contraindications; **P/N** = pregnancy category rating and nursing considerations.

Table 19.1. Prescribing Information for Antidepressants

GENERIC (BRAND)	FORM/ STRENGTH	DOSAGE	WARNINGS/PRECAUTIONS & CONTRAINDICATIONS	ADVERSE REACTIONS
Imipramine pamoate (Tofranil-PM)	**Cap:** 75mg, 100mg, 125mg, 150mg	**Adults:** (Inpatient) Initial: 100-150mg/day. Titrate: May increase to 200mg/day. After 2 weeks may increase up to 250-300mg/day if needed. (Outpatient) Initial: 75mg/day. Titrate: May increase to 150mg/day. Max: 200mg/day. (Inpatient/Outpatient) Maint: Following remission, maintain at lowest possible dose. Usual: 75-150mg/day. **Elderly/ Adolescents:** Initiate with Tofranil 25-50mg/day. Switch to Tofranil-PM with doses ≥75mg. Max: 100mg/day. **Pediatrics: Adolescents:** Initiate with Tofranil 25-50mg/day. Switch to Tofranil-PM with doses ≥75mg. Max: 100mg/day.	**BB:** Antidepressants increased the risk of suicidal thinking and behavior (suicidality) in short-term studies in children, adolescents, and young adults with Major Depressive Disorder (MDD) and other psychiatric disorders. Imipramine pamoate is not approved for use in pediatric patients. **W/P:** Caution with elderly, serious depression, cardiovascular disease, hyperthyroidism, urinary retention, narrow-angle glaucoma, increased IOP, seizure disorders, renal and hepatic impairment. May activate psychosis in schizophrenia; reduce dose. Limit electroshock therapy. May alter blood glucose levels. Photosensitivity reported. D/C prior to elective surgery, or with hypomanic or manic episodes. D/C with pathological neutrophil depression. **Contra:** Within 14 days of MAOI therapy or during acute recovery period following MI. **P/N:** Safety in pregnancy not known; not for use in nursing.	Orthostatic hypotension, HTN, confusion, hallucinations, numbness, tremors, dry mouth, urticaria, nausea, vomiting, diarrhea, gynecomastia (male), breast enlargement (female), galactorrhea.
Nortriptyline HCl (Pamelor)	**Cap:** 10mg, 25mg, 50mg, 75mg; **Sol:** 10mg/5mL	**Adults:** 25mg tid-qid. Max: 150mg/day. Total daily dose may be given once a day. Monitor serum levels if dose >100mg/day. **Elderly/Adolescents:** 30-50mg/day in single or divided doses.	**BB:** Antidepressants increased the risk of suicidal thinking and behavior (suicidality) in short-term studies in children, adolescents, and young adults with Major Depressive Disorder (MDD) and other psychiatric disorders. Nortriptyline is not approved for use in pediatric patients. **W/P:** MI, arrhythmia, strokes have occurred. Caution with cardiovascular disease, glaucoma, history of urinary retention, hyperthyroidism. May lower seizure threshold, exacerbate psychosis or activate schizophrenia, cause symptoms of mania in bipolar disease, or alter glucose levels. D/C several days prior to elective surgery. **Contra:** MAOI use within 14 days, acute recovery period following MI. **P/N:** Safety during pregnancy and nursing not known.	Arrhythmias, hypotension, HTN, tachycardia, MI, heart block, stroke, confusion, hallucination, insomnia, tremors, ataxia, anxiety, dry mouth, blurred vision, skin rash, extrapyramidal symptoms, photosensitivity, SIADH, anorexia.
Protriptyline HCl (Vivactil)	**Tab:** 5mg, 10mg	**Adults:** Usual: 15-40mg/day taken tid-qid. Titrate: May increase to 60mg/day. Max: 60mg/day tid. **Elderly:** Initial: 5mg tid. Titrate: Increase gradually if needed. Monitor cardiovascular system with doses >20mg/day. **Pediatrics: Adolescents:** Initial: 5mg tid. Titrate: Increase gradually if needed.	**BB:** Antidepressants increased the risk of suicidal thinking and behavior (suicidality) in short-term studies in children, adolescents, and young adults with Major Depressive Disorder (MDD) and other psychiatric disorders. Protriptyline is not approved for use in pediatric patients. **W/P:** Caution with history of seizures, urinary retention, increased IOP, cardiovascular disorders, hyperthyroidism, elderly. May aggravate psychotic symptoms in schizophrenia, manic symptoms in manic-depressive psychosis, and anxiety/agitation in overactive/agitated patients. D/C several days before elective surgery. Both elevation and lowering of blood sugar levels reported. **Contra:** Within 14 days of MAOI therapy, cisapride, acute recovery period following MI. **P/N:** Safety in pregnancy and nursing not known.	Tachycardia, hypotension, confusion, anxiety, insomnia, nightmares, seizures, EPS, dizziness, headache, anticholinergic effects, rash, photosensitivity, blood dyscrasias, GI effects, impotence, decreased libido, flushing.
Trimipramine maleate (Surmontil)	**Cap:** 25mg, 50mg, 100mg	**Adults:** Outpatient: Initial: 75mg/day in divided doses. Titrate: Increase to 150mg/day. Maint: 50-150mg/day. Max: 200mg/day. **Hospitalized Patients:** Initial: 100mg/day in divided doses. Titrate:	**BB:** Antidepressants increased the risk of suicidal thinking and behavior (suicidality) in short-term studies in children, adolescents, and young adults with Major Depressive Disorder (MDD) and	Hypotension, HTN, arrhythmia, confusion, insomnia, incoordination, GI complaints, allergic reactions, gynecomastia,

BB = black box warning; **W/P** = warnings/precautions; **Contra** = contraindications; **P/N** = pregnancy category rating and nursing considerations.

Table 19.1. Prescribing Information for Antidepressants

GENERIC (BRAND)	FORM/ STRENGTH	DOSAGE	WARNINGS/PRECAUTIONS & CONTRAINDICATIONS	ADVERSE REACTIONS
TRICYCLIC ANTIDEPRESSANTS *(Cont.)*				
Trimipramine maleate (Surmontil) *(Cont.)*		Increase gradually to 200mg/day. If no improvement after 2-3 weeks, may increase up to 250-300mg/day. **Elderly:** Initial: 50mg/day. Titrate: Increase gradually to 100mg/day. Take hs for at least 3 months. ***Pediatrics: Adolescents:*** Initial: 50mg/day. Titrate: Increase gradually to 100mg/day. Take hs for at least 3 months.	other psychiatric disorders. Trimipramine is not approved for use in pediatric patients. **W/P:** Caution with cardiovascular disease, increased IOP, urinary retention, narrow-angle glaucoma, hyperthyroidism, seizure disorder, liver dysfunction. May impair ability to operate machinery. May alter glucose levels. May activate psychosis in schizophrenia. Manic or hypomanic episodes may occur. May increase hazards with electroshock therapy. **Contra:** Acute recovery period post-MI, within 14 days of MAOI therapy. **P/N:** Category C, safety in nursing not known.	blood dyscrasias, dry mouth, blurred vision, urinary retention.

BB = black box warning; **W/P** = warnings/precautions; **Contra** = contraindications; **P/N** = pregnancy category rating and nursing considerations.

Table 19.2. Drug Interactions for Antidepressants

AMINOKETONES

Bupropion HBr (Aplenzin)

Alcohol	May cause neuropsychiatric events or reduce alcohol tolerance.
Amantadine	May increase adverse reactions.
Cimetidine	May increase AUC and C_{max} of metabolites of bupropion.
CYP2B6 substrates or inhibitors (eg, orphenadrine, thiotepa, cyclophosphamide)	May inhibit metabolism of bupropion.
CYP2D6 substrates (eg, SSRIs, nortriptyline, imipramine, desipramine, fluoxetine, haloperidol, risperidone, thioridazine, metoprolol, propafenone, flecainide)	Caution with concomitant use; may potentiate effects of these agents.
Efavirenz	May inhibit hydroxylation of bupropion.
Fluvoxamine	May inhibit hydroxylation of bupropion.
Levodopa	May increase adverse reactions.
MAO inhibitors (eg, phenelzine)	May increase toxicity of bupropion.
Nelfinavir	May inhibit hydroxylation of bupropion.
Nicotine transdermal system	May cause hypertension.
Norfluoxetine	May inhibit hydroxylation of bupropion.
Paroxetine	May inhibit hydroxylation of bupropion.
Ritonavir	May inhibit hydroxylation of bupropion.
Seizure threshold-lowering drugs (eg, antipsychotics, antidepressants, theophylline, systemic steroids)	Caution with concomitant use; may increase risk of seizures.
Sertraline	May inhibit hydroxylation of bupropion.

Buproprion HCl (Wellbutrin, Wellbutrin XL, Wellbutrin SR)

Alcohol	Contraindicated in patients undergoing abrupt discontinuation of alcohol; may increase the risk of seizures in patients using excessive amounts of alcohol; ingestion of alcohol should be minimized or avoided.
Amantadine	Caution with concomitant use; buproprion doses should initially be low and gradually titrated.
Anoretics	Concomitant use may increase the risk of seizures.
Antiarrhythmics (type IC)	Caution with concomitant use; initiate at the lower end of the dose range of the concomitant medication.
Antidepressants	Extreme caution should be taken with concomitant use.

Table 19.2. Drug Interactions for Antidepressants

Antidiabetic drugs (insulin, oral hypoglycemic drugs)	Concomitant use may increase the risk of seizures.
Antipsychotics	Extreme caution should be taken with concomitant use.
Benzodiazepines	Contraindicated, in patients undergoing abrupt discontinuation of sedatives; may increase the risk of seizures in patients using excessive amounts of sedatives.
Beta-blockers	Caution with concomitant use; initiate at the lower end of the dose range of the concomitant medication.
Buproprion	Contraindicated, avoid use of other preparations containing buproprion.
Carbamazepine	Concomitant use may induce the metabolism of buproprion.
Cimetidine	Concomitant use may induce the metabolism of buproprion.
Cocaine (or stimulant addiction)	Concomitant use may increase the risk of seizures.
Cyclophosphamide	Caution with concomitant use.
CYP2B6 substrates or inhibitors	Caution with concomitant use.
CYP2D6-metabolized drugs	Caution with concomitant use; initiate at the lower end of the dose range of the concomitant medication.
Levodopa	Caution with concomitant use; buproprion doses should initially be low and gradually titrated.
MAO inhibitors	Contraindicated, avoid concomitant use; allow at least 14 days between discontinuation of an MAOI and initiation of buproprion.
Opioids	Concomitant use may increase the risk of seizures.
Orphenadrine	Caution with concomitant use.
Phenobarbital	Concomitant use may induce the metabolism of buproprion.
Phenytoin	Concomitant use may induce the metabolism of buproprion.
Sedatives (eg, benzodiazepines)	Contraindicated, in patients undergoing abrupt discontinuation of sedatives; may increase the risk of seizures in patients using excessive amounts of sedatives.
Seizure threshold lowering drugs	Extreme caution should be taken with concomitant use.
SSRIs	Caution with concomitant use; initiate at the lower end of the dose range of the concomitant medication.
Steroids (systemic)	Extreme caution should be taken with concomitant use.
Stimulants (OTC)	Concomitant use may increase the risk of seizures.
TCAs	Caution with concomitant use; initiate at the lower end of the dose range of the concomitant medication.
Theophylline	Extreme caution should be taken with concomitant use.
Thiopeta	Caution with concomitant use.
Transdermal nicotine	Concomitant use may cause hypertension; monitor blood pressure levels.

Table 19.2. Drug Interactions for Antidepressants

MONOAMINE OXIDASE INHIBITORS

Phenelzine sulfate (Nardil)

Alcohol	Avoid concomitant use.
Amphetamines	Concomitant use may lead to a hypertensive crisis.
Anesthesia (local, general, or spinal)	Avoid concomitant use.
Antihypertensives	Concomitant use may produce exaggerated hypotensive effects.
Barbiturates	Caution, barbiturates should be given at a reduced dose.
Beta-blockers	Concomitant use may produce exaggerated hypotensive effects.
Bupropion	Concomitant use is contraindicated; at least 14 days should elapse between discontinuation of phenelzine and initiation of bupropion.
Buspirone	Avoid concomitant use; at least 14 days should elapse between discontinuation of phenelzine and initiation of buspirone.
Caffeine	Contraindicated, avoid excessive amounts of caffeine.
CNS depressants	Avoid concomitant use.
Cocaine	Concomitant use may lead to a hypertensive crisis.
Dexfenfluramine	Concomitant use is contraindicated, serious reactions have been reported.
Dextromethorphan	Avoid concomitant use.
Dopamine	Concomitant use may lead to a hypertensive crisis.
Epinephrine	Concomitant use may lead to a hypertensive crisis.
Fluoxetine	Concomitant use is contraindicated, serious reactions have been reported; 14 days should elapse following discontinuation of a serotonin reuptake inhibitor and initiation of phenelzine; 5 wks should elapse between discontinuation of fluoxetine and initiation of phenelzine; 2 wks should also elapse if starting an SSRI (including fluoxetine) and discontinuing phenelzine.
Fluvoxamine	Concomitant use is contraindicated, serious reactions have been reported; 14 days should elapse following discontinuation of a serotonin reuptake inhibitor and initiation of phenelzine; 2 wks should also elapse if starting an SSRI (including fluoxetine) and discontinuing phenelzine.
Guanethidine	Concomitant use is contraindicated.
L-dopa	Concomitant use may lead to a hypertensive crisis.
L-tryptophan	Concomitant use may lead to a hypertensive crisis.
L-tyrosine	Concomitant use may lead to a hypertensive crisis.
MAO inhibitors	Concomitant use with another MAOI is contraindicated and may lead to a hypertensive crisis or convulsive seizures; allow 10 days after stopping phenelzine before starting another MAOI.
Meperidine	Contraindicated, avoid concomitant use; may produce excitation, seizures, delirium, hyperpyrexia, circulatory collapse, coma, and possible death.
Methyldopa	Concomitant use may lead to a hypertensive crisis.
Methylphenidate	Concomitant use may lead to a hypertensive crisis.
Narcotic analgesics	Avoid concomitant use with some narcotics.

Table 19.2. Drug Interactions for Antidepressants

Paroxetine	Concomitant use is contraindicated, serious reactions have been reported; 14 days should elapse following discontinuation of a serotonin reuptake inhibitor and initiation of phenelzine; 2 wks should also elapse if starting an SSRI (including fluoxetine) and discontinuing phenelzine.
Phenylalanine	Concomitant use may lead to a hypertensive crisis.
Rauwolfia alkaloids	Caution with concomitant use.
Serotonergic agents	Concomitant use is contraindicated, serious reactions have been reported; 14 days should elapse following discontinuation of a serotonin reuptake inhibitor and initiation of phenelzine; 5 wks should elapse between discontinuation of fluoxetine and initiation of phenelzine; 2 wks should also elapse if starting an SSRI (including fluoxetine) and discontinuing phenelzine.
Sertraline	Concomitant use is contraindicated, serious reactions have been reported; 14 days should elapse following discontinuation of a serotonin reuptake inhibitor and initiation of phenelzine; 2 wks should also elapse if starting an SSRI (including fluoxetine) and discontinuing phenelzine.
Sympathomimetic drugs (eg, amphetamines, cocaine, methylphenidate, dopamine, epinephrine, norephinephrine) or related compounds (eg, methyldopa, L-dopa, L-tryptophan, L-tyrosine, phenylalanine)	Concomitant use may lead to a hypertensive crisis.
Thiazide diuretics	Concomitant use may produce exaggerated hypotensive effects.
Tyramine-containing foods (eg, cheese, pickled herring, beer, wine, yeast extract, salami, yogurt)	Contraindicated, concomitant use may lead to a hypertensive crisis.
Venlafaxine	Concomitant use is contraindicated, serious reactions have been reported; 14 days should elapse following discontinuation of a serotonin reuptake inhibitor and initiation of phenelzine; 2 wks should also elapse if starting an SSRI (including fluoxetine) and discontinuing phenelzine.
Selegiline (Emsam)	
Alcohol	Avoid concomitant use.
Amitriptyline	Concomitant use is contraindicated.
Amphetamines	Concomitant use is contraindicated.
Analgesic agents (eg, tramadol, methadone, propoxyphene)	Concomitant use is contraindicated.
Anesthesia agents (general)	Contraindicated, patients should avoid undergoing elective surgery requiring general anesthesia.
Anesthesia agents (local)	Local anesthesia agents containing sympathomimemtic vasoconstrictors is contraindicated.
Bupropion	Concomitant use is contraindicated.

Table 19.2. Drug Interactions for Antidepressants

Buspirone	Concomitant use is contraindicated.
Carbamazepine	Concomitant use is contraindicated.
Cocaine	Concomitant use is contraindicated.
Cyclobenzaprine	Concomitant use is contraindicated.
Dextromethorphan	Concomitant use is contraindicated.
Duloxetine	Concomitant use is contraindicated.
Ephedrine	Concomitant use is contraindicated.
Fluoxetine	Concomitant use is contraindicated.
Imipramine	Concomitant use is contraindicated.
Isocarboxazid	Contraindicated, avoid concomitant use with other MAOIs.
MAO inhibitors (eg, isocarboxazid, phenelzine, tranylcypromine)	Contraindicated, avoid concomitant use with other MAOIs.
Meperidine	Concomitant use is contraindicated.
Methadone	Concomitant use is contraindicated.
Mirtazapine	Concomitant use is contraindicated.
Oxcarbazepine	Concomitant use is contraindicated.
Paroxetine	Concomitant use is contraindicated.
Phenelzine	Contraindicated, avoid concomitant use with other MAOIs.
Phenylephrine	Concomitant use is contraindicated.
Propoxyphene	Concomitant use is contraindicated.
Pseudoephedrine	Concomitant use is contraindicated.
Selegiline	Concomitant use with oral selegiline is contraindicated.
Sertraline	Comcomitant use is contraindicated.
SSRIs (eg, fluoxetine, sertraline, paroxetine)	Concomitant use is contraindicated.
SNRIs (eg, venlafaxine, duloxetine)	Concomitant use is contraindicated.
St. John's wort	Concomitant use is contraindicated.
Sympathetic amines (including amphetamines)	Concomitant use is contraindicated.
Tramadol	Concomitant use is contraindicated.
Tranylcypromine	Contraindicated, avoid concomitant use with other MAOIs.
Tricyclic antidepressants (eg, imipramine, amitriptyline)	Concomitant use is contraindicated.

Table 19.2. Drug Interactions for Antidepressants

Tyramine containing foods (eg, cheese, pickled herring, beer, wine, yeast extract, salami, yogurt)	Contraindicated in selegiline medication systems containing 9mg of selegline per 24 hrs or 12mg of selegline per 24 hrs.
Venlafaxine	Concomitant use is contraindicated.
Tranylcypromine sulfate (Parnate)	
Alcohol	Warning concomitant use of some CNS depressants is contraindicated.
Amphetamines	Concomitant use is contraindicated.
Anesthetics	Contraindicated, avoid concomitant use; patients should not undergo elective surgery with general anesthesia; local anesthesia containing sympathomimetic vasoconstrictors should also be avoided.
Antihistamines	Concomitant use is contraindicated.
Antihypertensive drugs	Concomitant use is contraindicated.
Anti-parkinsonism drugs	Caution with concomitant use.
Bupropion	Contraindicated, avoid concomitant use; at least 14 days should elapse between discontinuation of tranylcypromine and initiation of bupropion.
Buspirone	Contraindicated, avoid concomitant use; at least 10 days should elapse between discontinuation of tranylcypromine and initiation of buspirone.
Caffeine	Contraindicated, avoid excessive amounts of caffeine.
CNS depressants (eg, alcohol, narcotics)	Warning concomitant use of some CNS depressants is contraindicated.
Dexfenfluramine	Concomitant use is contraindicated.
Dextromethorphan	Concomitant use is contraindicated.
Dibenzapine derivatives	Concomitant use is contraindicated.
Disulfiram	Caution with concomitant use.
Diuretics	Concomitant use is contraindicated.
MAO inhibitors	Concomitant use with another MAOI is contraindicated; may lead to a hypertensive crisis or severe convulsive seizures; a week between initiating or discontinuing therapy with tranylcypromine should be allowed before using another MAOI.
Meperidine	Contraindicated, avoid concomitant use; may produce coma, severe hypertension or hypotension, severe respiratory depression convulsions, malignant hyperpyrexia, excitation, peripheral vascular collapse, and death.
Metrizamide	Avoid concomitant use; discontinue tranylcypromine 48 hrs before myelography, may resume therapy with tranylcypromine 24 hrs following the procedure.
Narcotic Analgesics	Warning concomitant use of some CNS depressants is contraindicated.
Phenothiazines	Concomitant use may produce additive hypotensive effects.
Sedatives	Concomitant use is contraindicated.
SSRIs	Concomitant use is contraindicated, serious reactions have been reported; 14 days should elapse following discontinuation of tranylcycpromine and initiation of an SSRI; 5 wks should elapse between discontinuation of fluoxetine and initiation of tranylcypromine; 2 wks should elapse after discontinuation of sertraline or paroxetine before initiation of tranylcypromine.

Table 19.2. Drug Interactions for Antidepressants

Sympathomimetic drugs (eg, amphetamines)	Concomitant use is contraindicated.
Tryptophan	Concomitant use may precipitate disorientation, memory impairment and other behavioral and neurological syndromes.
Tyramine containing foods (eg, cheese, pickled herring, beer, wine, yeast extract, salami, yogurt)	Contraindicated, concomitant use may lead to a hypertensive crisis.

SEROTONIN/NOREPINEPHRINE REUPTAKE INHIBITORS (SNRIs)

Desvenlafaxine (Pristiq)

Alcohol	Avoid concomitant use.
Anticoagulants	Increased risk of bleeding with concomitant use.
Aspirin	Increased risk of bleeding with concomitant use.
CNS-active drugs	Caution with concomitant use.
CYP2D6 inhibitors (potent)	Caution with concomitant use.
CYP3A4 inhibitors (potent)	Caution with concomitant use.
Desvenlafaxine	Avoid other products containing desvenlafaxine.
Lithium	Caution with concomitant use.
MAO inhibitors	Concomitant use is contraindicated; desvenlafaxine should not be used within 14 days following discontinuation of an MAOI; allow 7 days after stopping desvenlafaxine before starting an MAOI.
NSAIDs	Increased risk of bleeding with concomitant use.
Serotonergic drugs	Caution with concomitant use.
SNRIs	Caution with concomitant use.
SSRIs	Caution with concomitant use.
Tramadol	Caution with concomitant use.
Triptans	Caution with concomitant use.
Tryptophans	Caution with concomitant use.
Venlafaxine	Avoid products containing venlafaxine.
Warfarin	Increased risk of bleeding with concomitant use.

Duloxetine HCI (Cymbalta)

Alcohol	Avoid substantial alcohol use.
Antiarrhythmics (type IC)	Caution with concomitant use.
CNS-active drugs	Caution with concomitant use.
CYP1A2 inhibitors (eg, quinolone antibiotics)	Avoid concomitant use.
CYP2D6 inhibitors	Concomitant use may cause increases in levels of duloxetine.

Table 19.2. Drug Interactions for Antidepressants

CYP2D6-metabolized drugs (with a narrow therapeutic index; eg, TCAs, phenothiazines, type 1C antiarrhythmics)	Caution with concomitant use.
Drugs affecting gastric acidity	Caution, may interact.
Fluoxetine	Concomitant use may cause increases in levels of duloxetine.
Fluvoxamine	Avoid concomitant use.
MAO inhibitors	Concomitant use is contraindicated; do not use duloxetine within 14 days of discontinuing treatment with an MAOI; at least 5 days should be allowed after stopping duloxetine before starting an MAOI.
Paroxetine	Concomitant use may cause increases in levels of duloxetine.
Phenothiazines	Caution with concomitant use.
Protein-bound drugs	Concomitant use may increase free concentrations of the highly protein-bound drugs.
Quinidine	Concomitant use may cause increases in levels of duloxetine.
Serotonergic drugs (eg, triptans, tramadol, SNRIs)	Caution with concomitant use.
SNRIs	Caution with concomitant use.
TCAs	Caution with concomitant use.
Thioridazine	Avoid concomitant use.
Tramadol	Caution with concomitant use.
Triptans	Caution with concomitant use.
Nefazodone HCl*	
Alcohol	Avoid concomitant use.
Alprazolam	Increases plasma concentrations of alprazolam; if used concomitantly, dose of alprazolam should be reduced by 50%.
Astemizole	Concomitant use is contraindicated.
Buspirone	May increase buspirone levels; decrease buspirone dose to 2.5mg qd.
Carbamazepine	Concomitant use is contraindicated.
Cisapride	Concomitant use is contraindicated.
CNS-active drugs	Caution with concomitant use.
Cyclosporine	Concomitant use increases plasma levels of cyclosporine.
CYP3A4-metabolized drugs	Caution with concomitant use.
Digoxin	Caution with concomitant use; monitor digoxin plasma levels.
Fluoxetine	Institute a wash-out period and lower the doses of nefazodone if used after fluoxetine therapy.
General anesthetics	Nefazodone should be discontinued prior to elective surgery.

*Available only in generic form.

Table 19.2. Drug Interactions for Antidepressants

Haloperidol	Concomitant use may require dosage adjustment of haloperidol.
Lovastatin	Caution, reports of rhabdomyolysis reported.
MAO inhibitors	Warning, concomitant use with an MAOI is contraindicated; nefazodone should not be used within 14 days of discontinuing treatment with an MAOI.
Pimozide	Concomitant use is contraindicated.
Plasma protein-bound drugs	Caution with concomitant use.
Simvastatin	Caution, reports of rhabdomyolysis reported.
Tacrolimus	Concomitant use increases plasma levels of tacrolimus.
Terfenadine	Concomitant use is contraindicated.
Triazolam	Causes significant increases in plasma levels of triazolam; triazolam dose should be reduced by 75%; avoid concomitant use in the elderly.
Venlafaxine HCl (Effexor, Effexor XR)	
Alcohol	Avoid concomitant use.
Cimetidine	Caution with concomitant use in patients who are elderly, have hypertension, or hepatic dysfunction.
CNS-active drugs (eg, triptans, SSRIs, lithium)	Caution with concomitant use.
CYP2D6 inhibitors	Caution with concomitant use of drugs that are strong inhibitors of both CYP3A4 and CYP2D6.
CYP3A4 inhibitors	Caution with concomitant use of drugs that are strong inhibitors of both CYP3A4 and CYP2D6.
Desipramine	Concomitant use increases the plasma levels of desipramine.
Diuretics	Caution with concomitant use.
Haloperidol	Concomitant use decreases the clearance of haloperidol.
Indinavir	Concomitant use decreases the plasma levels of indinavir.
Lithium	Caution with concomitant use.
MAO inhibitors	Concomitant use is contraindicated; venlafaxine should not be used within 14 days of therapy with an MAOI; following discontinuation of venlafaxine, at least 7 days should elapse before starting therapy with an MAOI.
Risperidone	Concomitant use may increase plasma levels of risperidone.
SSRIs	Caution with concomitant use.
Serotonergic drugs (eg, tramadol, tryptophans, SSRIs)	Caution with concomitant use.
Tramadol	Caution with concomitant use.
Triptans	Caution with concomitant use.
Tryptophans	Caution with concomitant use.

SELECTIVE SEROTONIN REUPTAKE INHIBITORS (SSRIs)

Citalopram HBr (Celexa)	
Alcohol	Avoid concomitant use.
Aspirin	Caution, may increase the risk of bleeding.

Table 19.2. Drug Interactions for Antidepressants

Carbamazepine	Caution with concomitant use.
Cimetidine	Caution with concomitant use.
CNS drugs	Caution with concomitant use.
Lithium	Caution with concomitant use; monitor plasma lithium levels.
MAO inhibitors	Concomitant use is contraindicated; citalopram should not be used within 14 days following discontinuing treatment with an MAOI; at least 14 days should be allowed after stopping citalopram before starting an MAOI.
Metoprolol	Concomitant use may increase metoprolol levels which leads to decreased cardioselectivity.
NSAIDs	Caution, may increase the risk of bleeding.
Pimozide	Concomitant use is contraindicated.
CYP2C19 inhibitors (eg, omeprazole)	Concomitant use may decrease the clearance of citalopram.
CYP3A4 inhibitors	Concomitant use may decrease the clearance of citalopram.
Ketoconazole	Concomitant use may decrease the clearance of citalopram.
Itraconazole	Concomitant use may decrease the clearance of citalopram.
Fluconazole	Concomitant use may decrease the clearance of citalopram.
Erythromycin	Concomitant use may decrease the clearance of citalopram.
Sumatriptan	Caution, weakness, hyperreflexia, and incoordination have been reported with concomitant use.
TCAs	Caution with concomitant use.
Warfarin	Caution, may increase the risk of bleeding.
Escitalopram oxalate (Lexapro)	
Alcohol	Avoid concomitant use.
Anticoagulants	Increased risk of bleeding with concomitant use.
Aspirin	Increased risk of bleeding with concomitant use.
Carbamazepine	Caution with concomitant use.
Cimetidine	Caution with concomitant use.
Citalopram	Avoid concomitant use.
CNS drugs	Caution with concomitant use.
CYP2D6 metabolized drugs (eg, desipramine)	Caution with concomitant use.
Desipramine	Caution with concomitant use.
Linezolid	Warning, serotonin syndrome reported with concomitant use.
Lithium	Caution with concomitant use; monitor plasma lithium levels.
MAO inhibitors	Concomitant use is contraindicated; escitalopram should not be used within 14 days following discontinuation from an MAOI; at least 14 days should be allowed after stopping escitalopram before starting an MAOI.
NSAIDs	Increased risk of bleeding with concomitant use.

Table 19.2. Drug Interactions for Antidepressants

Pimozide	Concomitant use is contraindicated.
Sumatriptan	Caution, weakness, hyperreflexia, and incoordination have been reported with concomitant use.
Warfarin	Increased risk of bleeding with concomitant use.
Fluoxetine HCl (Prozac, Prozac Weekly)	
Alcohol	Avoid concomitant use.
Alprazolam	Concomitant use increases plasma levels of alprazolam.
Anticoagulants	Increased risk of bleeding with concomitant use.
Antidepressants	Concomitant use may potentiate effects of other antidepressants.
Antidiabetic drugs (insulin, oral hypoglycemic drugs)	Concomitant use may require dosage adjustments of antidiabetic drugs.
Antipsychotics (eg, haloperidol, clozapine)	Concomitant use may raise blood levels of antipsychotics.
Aspirin	Increased risk of bleeding with concomitant use.
Carbamazepine	Concomitant use may increase carbamazepine levels.
Clozapine	Concomitant use may raise blood levels of antipsychotics.
CNS drugs	Caution with concomitant use.
Coumadin	Concomitant use with other drugs that are highly bound to plasma proteins may cause a shift in concentrations of one of the drugs.
CYP2D6-metabolized drugs	Concomitant use may potentiate drugs metabolized by CYP2D6.
Digoxin	Concomitant use with other drugs that are highly bound to plasma proteins may cause a shift in concentrations of one of the drugs.
Haloperidol	Concomitant use may raise blood levels of antipsychotics.
Lithium	Concomitant use may increase or decrease lithium levels; monitor lithium levels.
MAO inhibitors	Concomitant use is contraindicated; fluoxetine should not be used within 14 days following discontinuation of an MAOI; at least 5 wks should be allowed after stopping fluoxetine before starting an MAOI.
NSAIDs	Increased risk of bleeding with concomitant use.
Phenytoin	Concomitant use may increase phenytoin levels.
Pimozide	Concomitant use is contraindicated.
Plasma protein-bound drugs (eg, coumadin, digoxin)	Concomitant use with other drugs that are highly bound to plasma proteins may cause a shift in concentrations of one of the drugs.
Thioridazine	Concomitant use is contraindicated; thioridazine should not be administered within 5 wks after fluoxetine has been discontinued.
Triptans	Caution, concomitant use may cause serotonin syndrome; monitor for signs of serotonin syndrome.
Tryptophan	Concomitant use may increase incidence of adverse effects (eg, agitation, restlessness, GI distress).
Warfarin	Increased risk of bleeding with concomitant use.

Table 19.2. Drug Interactions for Antidepressants

Paroxetine HCl (Paxil, Paxil CR)

Alcohol	Avoid concomitant use.
Antiarrhythmics (type IC)	Caution with concomitant use.
Anticoagulants	Increased risk of bleeding with concomitant use.
Antidepressants	Caution with concomitant use.
Aspirin	Increased risk of bleeding with concomitant use.
Atomoxetine	Concomitant use may increase levels of atomoxetine; dosage adjustment of atomoxetine may be necessary and initiation of atomoxetine should be done at a reduced dose.
Cimetidine	Caution with concomitant use, may increase plasma levels of paroxetine.
CYP2D6 inhibitors (eg, quinidine)	Caution with concomitant use.
CYP2D6-metabolized drugs (eg, antidepressants, phenothiazines, Type 1C antiarrhythmics)	Caution with concomitant use.
Digoxin	Caution with concomitant use.
Diuretics	Caution with concomitant use.
Fosamprenavir	Concomitant use may significantly decrease plasma levels of paroxetine.
Linezolid	Concomitant use is contraindicated.
Lithium	Caution with concomitant use; increased risk of serotonin syndrome.
MAO inhibitors	Concomitant use is contraindicated; paroxetine should not be used within 14 days of discontinuation from an MAOI; at least 2 wks should be allowed after stopping paroxetine before starting an MAOI.
NSAIDs	Caution with concomitant use; may increase the risk of bleeding.
Phenobarbital	Caution with concomitant use.
Phenothiazines	Caution with concomitant use.
Phenytoin	Caution with concomitant use.
Pimozide	Concomitant use is contraindicated; may increase plasma levels of pimozide.
Plasma protein-bound drugs	Concomitant use with other drugs that are highly bound to plasma proteins may cause a shift in concentrations of one of the drugs.
Procyclidine	Caution with concomitant use; dose of procyclidine should be reduced if anticholinergic effects occur.
Quinidine	Caution with concomitant use.
Risperidone	Concomitant use may increase levels of risperidone.
Ritonavir	Concomitant use may significantly decrease plasma levels of paroxetine.
Serotonergic drugs (eg, triptans, serotonin reuptake inhibitors, lithium, tramadol, St. John's wort)	Caution with concomitant use; increased risk of serotonin syndrome.
SSRIs	Caution with concomitant use; increased risk of serotonin syndrome.

Table 19.2. Drug Interactions for Antidepressants

St. John's wort	Caution with concomitant use; increased risk of serotonin syndrome.
Theophylline	Concomitant use may increase theophylline levels; monitor levels.
Thioridazine	Concomitant use is contraindicated.
Tramadol	Caution with concomitant use; increased risk of serotonin syndrome.
TCAs	Concomitant use may inhibit the metabolism of TCAs; may need to monitor plasma levels of TCAs.
Triptans	Caution, concomitant use may cause serotonin syndrome; monitor for signs of serotonin syndrome.
Tryptophan	Avoid concomitant use.
Warfarin	Increased risk of bleeding with concomitant use.
Paroxetine mesylate (Pexeva)	
Antiarrhythmics (type IC)	Caution with concomitant use.
Anticoagulants	Increased risk of bleeding with concomitant use.
Antidepressants	Caution with concomitant use.
Aspirin	Increased risk of bleeding with concomitant use.
Cimetidine	Caution with concomitant use, may increase plasma levels of paroxetine.
CYP2D6-metabolized drugs (eg, antidepressants, phenothiazines, type 1C antiarrhythmics)	Caution with concomitant use.
Digoxin	Caution with concomitant use.
Diuretics	Caution with concomitant use.
Fosamprenavir	Concomitant use may significantly decrease plasma levels of paroxetine.
Lithium	Caution with concomitant use.
MAO inhibitors	Concomitant use is contraindicated; paroxetine should not be used within 14 days of discontinuation from an MAOI; allow at least 2 wks after stopping paroxetine before starting an MAOI.
NSAIDs	Increased risk of bleeding with concomitant use.
Phenobarbital	Caution with concomitant use.
Phenothiazines	Caution with concomitant use.
Phenytoin	Caution with concomitant use.
Pimozide	Concomitant use is contraindicated; levels of pimozide may be increased.
Plasma protein-bound drugs	Concomitant use with other drugs that are highly bound to plasma proteins may cause a shift in concentrations of one of the drugs.
Procyclidine	Caution with concomitant use; dose of procyclidine should be reduced if anticholinergic effects occur.
Quinidine	Caution with concomitant use.
Ritonavir	Concomitant use may significantly decrease plasma levels of paroxetine.
SNRIs	Avoid concomitant use with other selective serotonin reuptake inhibitors.

Table 19.2. Drug Interactions for Antidepressants

SSRIs	Avoid concomitant use with other SSRIs.
Theophylline	Concomitant use may increase theophylline levels; monitor levels.
Thioridazine	Concomitant use is contraindicated.
TCAs	Concomitant use may inhibit the metabolism of TCAs; may need to monitor plasma levels of TCAs.
Triptans	Caution, concomitant use may cause serotonin syndrome; monitor for signs of serotonin syndrome.
Warfarin	Increased risk of bleeding with concomitant use.
Sertraline HCl (Zoloft)	
Alcohol	Avoid concomitant use.
Antiarrhythmics (type 1C)	Concomitant use may increase plasma levels of drugs metabolized by CYP2D6.
Aspirin	Increased risk of bleeding with concomitant use.
Cimetidine	Concomitant use may increase the levels of sertraline.
Cisapride	Concomitant use may induce the metabolism of cisapride.
CNS-active drugs (eg, diazepam)	Caution with concomitant use.
CYP2D6-metabolized drugs (eg, Type 1C antiarrhythmics)	Concomitant use may increase plasma levels of drugs metabolized by CYP2D6.
Diazepam	Caution with concomitant use.
Digitoxin	Concomitant use with other drugs that are highly bound to plasma proteins may cause a shift in concentrations of one of the drugs.
Disulfiram	Concomitant use with the oral concentrate form of sertraline is contraindicated.
Lithium	Caution with concomitant use; monitor lithium plasma levels.
MAO inhibitors	Concomitant use is contraindicated; sertraline should not be used within 14 days of discontinuation with an MAOI; allow at least 2 wks after stopping sertraline and starting an MAOI.
NSAIDs (nonselective)	Increased risk of bleeding with concomitant use.
Pimozide	Concomitant use is contraindicated.
Plasma protein-bound drugs (eg, warfarin, digitoxin)	Concomitant use with other drugs that are highly bound to plasma proteins may cause a shift in concentrations of one of the drugs.
Sumatriptan	Caution, weakness, hyperreflexia, and incoordination have been reported with concomitant use.
Tolbutamide	Concomitant use decreases clearance of tolbutamide.
TCAs	Concomitant use may inhibit the metabolism of TCAs; may need to monitor plasma levels of TCAs.
Warfarin	Concomitant use with other drugs that are highly bound to plasma proteins may cause a shift in concentrations of one of the drugs. Increased risk of bleeding with concomitant use; monitor PT.

Table 19.2. Drug Interactions for Antidepressants

TETRACYCLIC ANTIDEPRESSANTS
Mirtazapine (Remeron, Remeron SolTab)

Alcohol	Avoid concomitant use; increase in cognitive and motor skill impairment.
Diazepam	Avoid concomitant use; increases impairment of motor skills.
MAO inhibitors	Warning, avoid concomitant use; mirtazapine should not be used within 14 days using an MAOI.

TRIAZOLOPYRIDINE ANTIDEPRESSANTS
Trazodone HCl*

Alcohol	Concomitant use may enhance the response to alcohol.
Antihypertensive drugs	Caution, concomitant use may require a reduction in the dosing of the antihypertensive drug.
Barbiturates	Concomitant use may enhance the response to barbiturates.
Carbamazepine	Concomitant use may decrease plasma levels of trazodone.
CNS depressants	Concomitant use may enhance the response to CNS depressants.
CYP3A4 inhibitors	Concomitant use with potent CYP3A4 inhibitors may increase levels of trazodone.
Digoxin	Concomitant use increases serum digoxin levels.
Indinavir	Concomitant use with potent CYP3A4 inhibitors may increase levels of trazodone.
Itraconazole	Concomitant use with potent CYP3A4 inhibitors may increase levels of trazodone.
Ketoconazole	Concomitant use with potent CYP3A4 inhibitors may increase levels of trazodone.
MAO inhibitors	Caution with concomitant use.
Nefazodone	Concomitant use with potent CYP3A4 inhibitors may increase levels of trazodone.
Phenytoin	Concomitant use increases serum phenytoin levels.
Ritonavir	Concomitant use with potent CYP3A4 inhibitors may increase levels of trazodone.
Warfarin	Caution, concomitant use may affect prothrombin time.

TRICYCLIC ANTIDEPRESSANTS
Amitriptyline HCl*

Alcohol	Concomitant use potentiates the effects of alcohol.
Anticholinergic drugs	Monitor closely for increased anticholinergic effects; may cause paralytic ileus and hyperpyrexia.
Barbiturates	Concomitant use potentiates the effects of barbituates.
Cimetidine	Increases plasma levels of amtriptyline; dosage adjustments of amitriptyline or the other drug may be necessary.

*Available only in generic form.

Table 19.2. Drug Interactions for Antidepressants

Citalopram	Caution when switching to or from an SSRI; >5 wks may be needed before initiating treatment with amtriptyline following withdrawal from fluoxetine.
CNS depressants	Potentiates effects of CNS depressants.
CYP2D6 inhibitors (eg, quinidine, cimetidine, SSRIs)	Increases plasma levels of amtriptyline; dosage adjustments of amitriptyline or the other drug may be necessary.
CYP2D6 substrates (eg, phenothiazines, propafenone, flecainide)	Increases plasma levels of amtriptyline.
Disulfiram	Caution, delirium reported with concomitant use.
Escitalopram	Caution when switching to or from an SSRI; >5 wks may be needed before initiating treatment with amtriptyline following withdrawal from fluoxetine.
Ethchlorvynol	Caution, delirium reported with concomitant use.
Flecainide	Increases plasma levels of amtriptyline.
Fluoxetine	Caution when switching to or from an SSRI; >5 wks may be needed before initiating treatment with amtriptyline following withdrawal from fluoxetine.
Guanethidine	May block antihypertensive effects of guanethidine.
MAO inhibitors	Contraindicated, do not give concomitantly or within at least 2 wks of treatment with an MAOI.
Neuroleptics	Monitor patients closely who are receiving concomitant therapy; hyperpyrexia reported.
Paroxetine	Caution when switching to or from an SSRI; >5 wks may be needed before initiating treatment with amtriptyline following withdrawal from fluoxetine.
Phenothiazines	Increases plasma levels of amtriptyline.
Propafenone	Increases plasma levels of amtriptyline.
Quinidine	Increases plasma levels of amtriptyline; dosage adjustments of amitriptyline or the other drug may be necessary.
SSRIs (eg, fluoxetine, citalopram, escitalopram, sertraline, paroxetine)	Caution when switching to or from an SSRI; >5 wks may be needed before initiating treatment with amtriptyline following withdrawal from fluoxetine.
Sertraline	Caution when switching to or from an SSRI; >5 wks may be needed before initiating treatment with amtriptyline following withdrawal from fluoxetine.
Sympathomimetic drugs	Monitor closely if using concomitantly.
Thyroid drugs	Monitor closely if using concomitantly.
Amoxapine*	
Alcohol	Concomitant use may potentiate the response to alcohol.
Antidepressants	Concomitant use may increase levels of amoxapine.
Barbiturates	Concomitant use may potentiate the effects of barbiturates.
Cimetidine	Concomitant use may increase levels of amoxapine.

*Available only in generic form.

Table 19.2. Drug Interactions for Antidepressants

CNS depressants	Concomitant use may potentiate the effects of CNS depressants.
CYP2D6 metabolizers	Concomitant use with poor metabolizers of CYP2D6 may increase the levels of amoxapine.
Flecainide	Concomitant use may increase levels of amoxapine.
Fluoxetine	Caution when switching to or from an SSRI; at least 5 wks may be needed before starting therapy with amoxapine following discontinuation of fluoxetine.
MAO inhibitors	Concomitant use is contraindicated; a minimum of 14 days should pass before amoxapine replaces an MAOI.
Paroxetine	Caution when switching to or from an SSRI; at least 5 wks may be needed before starting therapy with amoxapine following discontinuation of fluoxetine.
Phenothiazines	Concomitant use may increase levels of amoxapine.
Propafenone	Concomitant use may increase levels of amoxapine.
Quinidine	Concomitant use may increase levels of amoxapine.
SSRIs (eg, fluoxetine, sertraline, paroxetine)	Caution when switching to or from an SSRI; at least 5 wks may be needed before starting therapy with amoxapine following discontinuation of fluoxetine.
Sertraline	Caution when switching to or from an SSRI; at least 5 wks may be needed before starting therapy with amoxapine following discontinuation of fluoxetine.
Clomipramine HCl (Anafranil*)	
Alcohol	Concomitant use may potentiate the effects of alcohol.
Anticholinergic drugs	Caution with concomitant use; monitor patient closely.
Barbiturates	Concomitant use may potentiate the effects of barbiturates.
Cimetidine	Concomitant use may increase plasma levels of clomipramine.
Clonidine	Caution, may block the effects of clonidine.
CNS depressants	Concomitant use may potentiate the effects of CNS depressants.
CNS-active drugs	Caution with concomitant use.
CYP2D6 enzyme substrates (eg, phenothiazines, propafenone, flecainide)	Concomitant use may increase plasma levels of clomipramine.
CYP2D6 inhibitors (eg, quinidine, cimetidine, SSRIs)	Concomitant use may increase plasma levels of clomipramine; dosage adjustments of clomipramine or the other drug may be necessary.
Digoxin	Concomitant use with other drugs that are highly bound to plasma proteins may cause a shift in concentrations of one of the drugs.
Flecainide	Concomitant use may increase plasma levels of clomipramine.
Fluoxetine	Caution when switching to or from an SSRI; at least 5 wks may be needed before starting therapy with clomipramine following discontinuation of fluoxetine.
Fluvoxamine	Caution when switching to or from an SSRI; at least 5 wks may be needed before starting therapy with clomipramine following discontinuation of fluoxetine.
Guanethidine	Caution, may block the effects of guanethidine.

* Brand name discontinued; generic version is still available.

Table 19.2. Drug Interactions for Antidepressants

Haloperidol	Concomitant use increases the plasma levels of clomipramine.
Hepatic enzyme inducers (eg, barbiturates, phenytoin)	Concomitant use may decrease plasma levels of clomipramine.
MAO inhibitors	Contraindicated; do not give concomitantly or within at least 2 wks of treatment with an MAOI.
Methylphenidate	Concomitant use may increase plasma levels of methylphenidate.
Neuroleptics	Warning, concomitant use may produce neuroleptic malignant syndrome.
Paroxetine	Caution when switching to or from an SSRI; at least 5 wks may be needed before starting therapy with clomipramine following discontinuation of fluoxetine.
Phenobarbital	Concomitant use increases plasma levels of phenobarbital.
Phenothiazines	Concomitant use may increase plasma levels of clomipramine.
Phenytoin	Concomitant use may decrease plasma levels of clomipramine.
Plasma protein-bound drugs (eg, warfarin, digoxin)	Concomitant use with other drugs that are highly bound to plasma proteins may cause a shift in concentrations of one of the drugs.
Propafenone	Concomitant use may increase plasma levels of clomipramine.
Quinidine	Concomitant use may increase plasma levels of clomipramine.
SSRIs (eg, fluoxetine, sertraline, paroxetine, fluvoxamine)	Caution when switching to or from an SSRI; at least 5 wks may be needed before starting therapy with clomipramine following discontinuation of fluoxetine.
Sertraline	Caution when switching to or from an SSRI; at least 5 wks may be needed before starting therapy with clomipramine following discontinuation of fluoxetine.
Sympathomimetic drugs	Caution with concomitant use; monitor patient closely.
Thyroid drugs	Caution with concomitant use; risk of cardiotoxicity.
Warfarin	Concomitant use with other drugs that are highly bound to plasma proteins may cause a shift in concentrations of one of the drugs.
Desipramine HCl (Norpramin)	
Alcohol	Concomitant use potentiates the effects of alcohol.
Anticholinergic drugs	Monitor closely for increased anticholinergic effects.
Antidepressants	Concomitant use increases plasma levels of desipramine.
Benzodiazepines (eg, diazepam, chlordiazepoxide)	Caution, additive sedative effects.
Chlordiazepoxide	Caution, additive sedative effects.
Cimetidine	Increases plasma levels of desipramine; dosage adjustment of desipramine or the other drug may be necessary.
Citalopram	Caution when switching to or from an SSRI.
CNS depressants (eg, sedatives/hypnotics, psychotropics)	Caution, additive sedative effects.

Table 19.2. Drug Interactions for Antidepressants

CYP2D6 inhibitors (eg, quinidine, cimetidine, SSRIs)	Increases plasma levels of desipramine; dosage adjustment of desipramine or the other drug may be necessary.
CYP2D6 substrates (eg, many other antidepressants, phenothiazines, propafenone, flecainide)	Concomitant use increases plasma levels of desipramine.
Diazepam	Caution, additive sedative effects.
Escitalopram	Caution when switching to or from an SSRI.
Flecainide	Concomitant use increases plasma levels of desipramine.
Fluoxetine	Caution when switching to or from an SSRI; at least 5 wks may be needed before initiating treatment with desipramine following withdrawal from fluoxetine.
Guanethidine	May block antihypertensive effects of guanethidine.
MAO inhibitors	Contraindicated; do not give concomitantly or within at least 2 wks of treatment with an MAOI.
Paroxetine	Caution when switching to or from an SSRI.
Phenothiazines	Concomitant use increases plasma levels of desipramine.
Propagenone	Concomitant use increases plasma levels of desipramine.
Psychotropics	Caution, additive sedative effects.
Quinidine	Increases plasma levels of desipramine; dosage adjustment of desipramine or the other drug may be necessary.
Sedatives/hypnotics	Caution, additive sedative effects.
SSRIs (eg, fluoxetine, citalopram, escitalopram, sertraline, paroxetine)	Caution when switching to or from an SSRI; at least 5 wks may be needed before initiating treatment with desipramine following withdrawal from fluoxetine.
Sertraline	Caution when switching to or from an SSRI.
Sympathomimetic drugs	Monitor closely if using concomitantly.
Thyroid drugs	Monitor closely; may cause cardiac arrhythmias.
Doxepin HCI (Sinequan)	
Alcohol	Warning, increased risk of doxepin overdose; potentiates effects of alcohol.
Anticholinergic drugs	Monitor closely for increased anticholinergic effects.
Antidepressants	Concomitant use increases plasma levels of doxepin.
Cimetidine	Concomitant use increases plasma levels of doxepin; dosage adjustment of doxepin or the other drug may be necessary.
Citalopram	Caution when switching to or from an SSRI.
CYP2D6 inhibitors (eg, cimetidine, quinidine, SSRIs)	Concomitant use increases plasma levels of doxepin; dosage adjustment of doxepin or the other drug may be necessary.

Table 19.2. Drug Interactions for Antidepressants

CYP2D6-metabolized drugs	Caution with concomitant use.
CYP2D6 substrates (eg, many other antidepressants, phenothiazines, propafenone, flecainide)	Concomitant use increases plasma levels of doxepin.
Escitalopram	Caution when switching to or from an SSRI.
Flecainide	Concomitant use increases plasma levels of doxepin.
Fluoxetine	Caution when switching to or from an SSRI; at least 5 wks may be needed before initiating treatment with doxepin following withdrawal from fluoxetine.
MAO inhibitors	Warning, do not give concomitantly or within at least 2 wks of treatment with an MAOI.
Paroxetine	Caution when switching to or from an SSRI.
Phenothiazines	Concomitant use increases plasma levels of doxepin.
Propafenone	Concomitant use increases plasma levels of doxepin.
Quinidine	Concomitant use increases plasma levels of doxepin; dosage adjustment of doxepin or the other drug may be necessary.
SSRIs (eg, fluoxetine, citalopram, escitalopram, sertraline, paroxetine)	Caution when switching to or from an SSRI; at least 5 wks may be needed before initiating treatment with doxepin following withdrawal from fluoxetine.
Sertraline	Caution when switching to or from an SSRI.
Tolazamide	Warning, hypoglycemia reported with concomitant use.
Imipramine HCl (Tofranil)	
Alcohol	Concomitant use potentiates the effects of alcohol.
Anticholinergic drugs	Monitor closely for increased anticholinergic effects; risk of paralytic ileus.
Antidepressants	Concomitant use increases plasma levels of imipramine.
Barbiturates	May decrease imipramine plasma levels.
Blood pressure lowering drugs	Caution with concomitant use.
Cimetidine	Increases imipramine plasma levels; dosage adjustment of imipramine or the other drug may be necessary.
Citalopram	Caution when switching to or from an SSRI.
Clonidine	Concomitant use may block the effects of clonidine.
CNS depressants	Potentiates effects of CNS depressants.
CYP2D6 inhibitors (eg, quinidine, cimetidine, SSRIs)	Increases imipramine plasma levels; dosage adjustment of imipramine or the other drug may be necessary.
CYP2D6 substrates (eg, phenothiazines, many other antidepressants, propafenone, flecainide)	Concomitant use increases plasma levels of imipramine.

Table 19.2. Drug Interactions for Antidepressants

Epinephrine	Caution, avoid concomitant use of any drugs containing sympathomimetic amines; may potentiate catecholamine effects.
Escitalopram	Caution when switching to or from an SSRI.
Flecainide	Concomitant use increases plasma levels of imipramine.
Fluoxetine	Caution when switching to or from an SSRI; at least 5 wks may be needed before initiating treatment with imipramine following withdrawal from fluoxetine.
Guanethidine	Concomitant use may block the effects of guanethidine.
Hepatic enzyme inducers (eg, barbiturates, phenytoin)	May decrease imipramine plasma levels.
MAO inhibitors	Contraindicated, do not give concomitantly or within at least 2 wks of treatment with an MAO inhibitor.
Methylphenidate	May increase imipramine plasma levels.
Norepinephrine	Caution, avoid concomitant use of any drugs containing sympathomimetic amines; may potentiate catecholamine effects.
Paroxetine	Caution when switching to or from an SSRI.
Phenothiazines	Concomitant use increases plasma levels of imipramine.
Phenytoin	May decrease imipramine plasma levels.
Propafenone	Concomitant use increases plasma levels of imipramine.
Quinidine	Increases imipramine plasma levels; dosage adjustment of imipramine or the other drug may be necessary.
SSRIs (eg, fluoxetine, citalopram, escitalopram, sertraline, paroxetine)	Caution when switching to or from an SSRI; at least 5 wks may be needed before initiating treatment with imipramine following withdrawal from fluoxetine.
Sertraline	Caution when switching to or from an SSRI.
Sympathomimetic amines (eg, epinephrine, norepinephrine)	Caution, avoid cocomitant use of any drugs containing sympathomimetic amines; may potentiate catecholamine effects.
Thyroid drugs	Monitor closely; risk of cardiovascular toxicity.
Imipramine pamoate (Tofranil-PM)	
Alcohol	Concomitant use may potentiate the CNS depressant effects of alcohol.
Anticholinergic drugs	Monitor closely for increased anticholinergic effects; risk of paralytic ileus.
Antidepressants	Concomitant use increases plasma levels of imipramine.
Barbiturates	May decrease imipramine plasma levels.
Blood pressure lowering drugs	Caution with concomitant use.
Cimetidine	Increases imipramine plasma levels; dosage adjustment of imipramine or the other drug may be necessary.
Clonidine	Concomitant use may block the effects of clonidine.
CNS depressants	Concomitant use may potentiate the effects of CNS depressants.

Table 19.2. Drug Interactions for Antidepressants

CYP2D6 inhibitors (eg, quinidine, cimetidine, SSRIs)	Increases imipramine plasma levels; dosage adjustment of imipramine or the other drug may be necessary.
CYP2D6 substrates (eg, phenothiazines, many other antidepressants, propafenone, flecainide)	Concomitant use increases plasma levels of imipramine.
Epinephrine	Caution, avoid concomitant use of any drugs containing sympathomimetic amines; may potentiate catecholamine effects.
Flecainide	Concomitant use increases plasma levels of imipramine.
Fluoxetine	Caution when switching to or from an SSRI; at least 5 wks may be needed before initiating treatment with imipramine following withdrawal from fluoxetine.
Guanethidine	Concomitant use may block the effects of guanethidine.
Hepatic enzyme inducers (eg, barbiturates, phenytoin)	May decrease imipramine plasma levels.
MAO inhibitors	Contraindicated, do not give concomitantly or within at least 2 wks of treatment with an MAO inhibitor.
Methylphenidate	May increase imipramine plasma levels.
Norepinephrine	Caution, avoid concomitant use of any drugs containing sympathomimetic amines; may potentiate catecholamine effects.
Paroxetine	Caution when switching to or from an SSRI.
Phenothiazines	Concomitant use increases plasma levels of imipramine.
Phenytoin	May decrease imipramine plasma levels.
Propafenone	Concomitant use increases plasma levels of imipramine.
Quinidine	Increases imipramine plasma levels; dosage adjustment of imipramine or the other drug may be necessary.
SSRIs (eg, fluoxetine, sertraline, paroxetine)	Caution when switching to or from an SSRI; at least 5 wks may be needed before initiating treatment with imipramine following withdrawal from fluoxetine.
Sertraline	Caution when switching to or from an SSRI.
Sympathomimetic amines (eg, epinephrine, norepinephrine)	Caution, avoid cocomitant use of any drugs containing sympathomimetic amines; may potentiate catecholamine effects.
Thyroid drugs	Caution with concomitant use, risk of cardiovascular toxicity.
Nortriptyline HCl (Pamelor)	
Alcohol	May potentiate effects of alcohol.
Anticholinergic drugs	Monitor closely if using concomitantly.
Antidepressants	Concomitant use increases the plasma levels of nortriptyline.
Chlorpropamide	Caution, may cause hypoglycemia.
Cimetidine	Increases plasma levels of nortriptyline.

Table 19.2. Drug Interactions for Antidepressants

Citalopram	Caution when switching to or from an SSRI.
CYP2D6 inhibitors (eg, quinidine)	Increases plasma levels of nortriptyline; dosage adjustment of nortriptyline or the other drug may be necessary.
CYP2D6 substrates (eg, phenothiazines, many other antidepressants, propafenone, flecainide)	Concomitant use increases the plasma levels of nortriptyline.
Escitalopram	Caution when switching to or from an SSRI.
Flecainide	Concomitant use increases the plasma levels of nortriptyline.
Fluoxetine	Caution when switching to or from an SSRI.
Guanethidine	May block the antihypertensive effects of guanethidine.
MAO inhibitors	Contraindicated, do not give concomitantly or within at least 2 wks of treatment with an MAOI.
Paroxetine	Caution when switching to or from an SSRI.
Phenothiazines	Concomitant use increases the plasma levels of nortriptyline.
Propafenone	Concomitant use increases the plasma levels of nortriptyline.
Quinidine	Increases plasma levels of nortriptyline; dosage adjustment of nortriptyline or the other drug may be necessary.
Reserpine	May produce a stimulating effect in depressed patients.
SSRIs	Caution when switching to or from an SSRI; at least 5 wks may be needed before initiating treatment with nortriptyline following withdrawal from fluoxetine.
Sertraline	Caution when switching to or from an SSRI.
Sympathomimetic drugs	Monitor closely if using concomitantly.
Thyroid drugs	Monitor closely; cardiac arrhythmias may develop.
Protriptyline HCl (Vivactil)	
Alcohol	Concomitant use may potentiate the response to alcohol.
Anticholinergic drugs	Monitor closely; risk of hyperpyrexia with concomitant use.
Antidepressants	Increases plasma levels of protriptyline; dosage adjustment of protriptyline or the other drug may be necessary.
Barbiturates	Concomitant use may potentiate the response to barbiturates.
Cimetidine	Concomitant use reduces hepatic metabolism and increases plasma levels of protriptyline.
Cisapride	Contraindicated; risk of adverse cardiac interactions with concomitant use.
CNS depressants	Concomitant use may potentiate the response to CNS depressants.
CYP2D6 enzyme inhibitors (eg, quinidine, many other antidepressants, phenothiazines, propafenone, flecainide, SSRIs)	Increases plasma levels of protriptyline; dosage adjustment of protriptyline or the other drug may be necessary.

Table 19.2. Drug Interactions for Antidepressants

Flecainide	Increases plasma levels of protriptyline; dosage adjustment of protriptyline or the other drug may be necessary.
Fluoxetine	Caution when switching to or from an SSRI; at least 5 wks may be needed before initiating treatment with protriptyline following withdrawal from fluoxetine.
Guanethidine	Concomitant use may block the antihypertensive effect of guanethidine.
MAO inhibitors	Contraindicated, do not give concomitantly or within at least 2 wks of treatment with an MAOI.
Neuroleptic drugs	Risk of hyperpyrexia with concomitant use.
Paroxetine	Caution when switching to or from an SSRI.
Phenothiazines	Increases plasma levels of protriptyline; dosage adjustment of protriptyline or the other drug may be necessary.
Propafenone	Increases plasma levels of protriptyline; dosage adjustment of protriptyline or the other drug may be necessary.
Quinidine	Increases plasma levels of protriptyline; dosage adjustment of protriptyline or the other drug may be necessary.
SSRIs (eg, fluoxetine, sertraline, paroxetine)	Caution when switching to or from an SSRI; at least 5 wks may be needed before initiating treatment with protriptyline following withdrawal from fluoxetine.
Sertraline	Caution when switching to or from an SSRI.
Tramadol	Concomitant use may increase the risk of seizures.
Trimipramine maleate (Surmontil)	
Alcohol	Concomitant use may potentiate the effects of alcohol.
Anticholinergic drugs	Caution with concomitant use; may potentiate anticholinergic effects.
Antidepressants	Concomitant use increases plasma levels of trimipramine.
Catecholamines	Caution with concomitant use, may potentiate effects of catecholamines.
Cimetidine	Concomitant use may inhibit elimination of trimipramine.
CYP2D6 inhibitors (eg, quinidine)	Concomitant use increases plasma levels of trimipramine; dosage adjustment of trimipramine or the other drug may be necessary.
CYP2D6 substrates (eg, many other antidepressants, phenothiazines, propafenone, fleccainide)	Concomitant use increases plasma levels of trimipramine.
Flecainide	Concomitant use increases plasma levels of trimipramine.
Fluoxetine	Caution when switching to or from an SSRI; at least 5 wks may be needed before initiating treatment with trimipramine following withdrawal from fluoxetine.
MAO inhibitors	Contraindicated; do not give concomitantly or within at least 2 wks of treatment with an MAOI.
Paroxetine	Caution when switching to or from an SSRI.
Phenothiazines	Concomitant use increases plasma levels of trimipramine.
Propafenone	Concomitant use increases plasma levels of trimipramine.

Table 19.2. Drug Interactions for Antidepressants

Quinidine	Concomitant use increases plasma levels of trimipramine; dosage adjustment of trimipramine or the other drug may be necessary.
SSRIs (eg, fluoxetine, sertraline, paroxetine)	Caution when switching to or from an SSRI; at least 5 wks may be needed before initiating treatment with trimipramine following withdrawal from fluoxetine.
Sertraline	Caution when switching to or from an SSRI.

Chapter 20

Hypoglycemia

Megan R. Undeberg, PharmD

INTRODUCTION

Hypoglycemia, as the name implies, is a state of low blood glucose. Hypoglycemia is likely the most confounding factor influencing tight glycemic control in the patient with diabetes. In the patient without diabetes, the body maintains glucose concentrations within a narrow range throughout the day: between 80-100 mg/dL in the fasting state, <135 mg/dL after ingestion of meals. However, the diabetic patient may discover that even with diligent monitoring and titration of insulin doses, or proper use of oral antidiabetic agents and other blood glucose-lowering interventions, blood glucose values may vary widely.

The human body has established an exquisitely sensitive system to detect falling blood glucose concentration in the body, and to then activate appropriate systems to resolve hypoglycemia. Of utmost importance is ensuring the brain has a constant supply of glucose to utilize for energy. Elsewhere in the body, glucose may be provided through the catabolism of fat and protein stores; this is not the case for the brain. As a result, through a blend of homeostatic mechanisms and a variety of hormones, including insulin, glucagon, epinephrine, cortisol, growth hormone, and others, the body mobilizes stored glucose for immediate use if and when necessary.

Glucose-sensitive neurons are located throughout the body, especially in the brain, which trigger an immediate series of neurohormonal interventions that are virtually undetected by the patient without diabetes. Increased sympathetic and parasympathetic activities occur that result in a quick inhibition of insulin secretion and an increased release of glucagon, epinephrine, cortisol, and growth hormone. These compensatory actions result in mobilization of stores of glucose from the liver for immediate use, a shunting of glucose for preferential use by the brain, and limitation of use of glucose by nonessential tissues. Insulin, glucagon, and epinephrine are central to the management of hypoglycemia; cortisol and growth hormone play a minor role, typically through their ability to slow the consumption of glucose by nonessential tissue.

These activities occur in a very systematic manner (see **Figure 1**). Around 80 mg/dL, the body will initiate the inhibition and suppression of endogenous insulin secretion from the pancreatic β-cells. If the blood glucose concentration continues to fall, at around 65 mg/dL, glucagon, epinephrine, cortisol, and growth hormone will be secreted in a further attempt to reverse hypoglycemia. With a continued decrease in blood glucose levels, physical and mental changes will be noted. Autonomic symptoms include such characteristics as tremors, shakiness, increased nervousness and anxiety, increased heart rate and palpitations, sweating, clamminess, extreme hunger, and

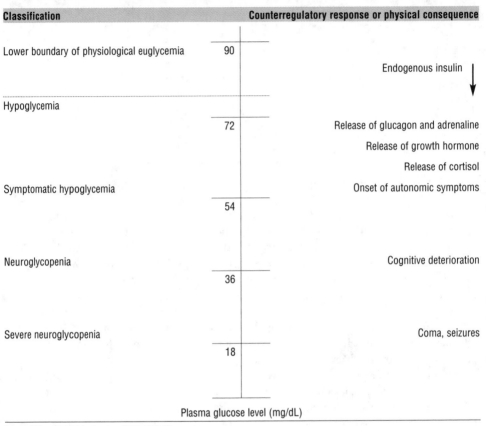

Figure 1. Glycemic Threshold Values for Counterregulatory Responses to and Physical Consequences of Insulin-Induced Hypoglycemia.

Classification		Counterregulatory response or physical consequence
Lower boundary of physiological euglycemia	90	Endogenous insulin
Hypoglycemia	72	Release of glucagon and adrenaline
		Release of growth hormone
		Release of cortisol
Symptomatic hypoglycemia	54	Onset of autonomic symptoms
Neuroglycopenia	36	Cognitive deterioration
Severe neuroglycopenia	18	Coma, seizures

Plasma glucose level (mg/dL)

Source: White, JR. *Diabetes Spectrum* 2007; 20:77-80.

sometimes pallor. Changes in mental status, including anger, irrational thinking and actions, confusion, tingling, numbness, drunken gait, blurred vision, headaches, as well as seizures and coma are typical of neuroglycopenic symptoms. Both autonomic and neuroglycopenic symptoms frequently are noticeable when the blood glucose concentration is nearing 50-60 mg/dL. If unregulated or untreated, hypoglycemia may lead to death (see **Table 20.1**).

In the patient with diabetes, particularly the type 1 patient, there is an association between the lack of endogenous insulin pro-duction and secretion that affects the body's ability to increase endogenous glucagon and epinephrine secretion when blood glucose levels are falling and hypoglycemia is developing. Compounding this situation is the fact that if insulin has been injected there is no mechanism by which to turn off or down-regulate the amount of insulin that is in the body, which is seen in patients without diabetes in the first compensatory attempts to balance hypoglycemia. As a result, hypoglycemia is a serious complication of treatment and management of diabetic patients.

Table 20.1. Autonomic and Neuroglypenic Symptoms Associated with Hypoglycemia

Autonomic	Neuroglypenic
Tremors	Anger
Shakiness	Irrational thinking and/or actions
Increased nervousness	Confusion
Anxiety	Tingling, often in hands or feet
Increased heart rate and palpitations	Numbness
Sweating	Changes in gait (ataxia)
Clammy hands, extremities	Blurred vision
Extreme hunger	Seizures
Pallor, paleness	Coma

The risk of hypoglycemia can be exacerbated by other factors. A diabetic status alone increases the risk of hypoglycemia, simply related to the progression of the disease state. Over time, with progressive loss of pancreatic β-cell function, and with a blunting of the sympathetic and parasympathetic nervous system responses after repeated hypoglycemic episodes, a patient with diabetes is less aware of early symptoms of hypoglycemia. Exercise, which increases the peripheral body tissue use of glucose, may result in a change in the affect of circulating insulin doses. Stress, acute illness, or surgery, which may result in rapidly changing blood glucose levels, may lead to varying degrees of hyper- or hypoglycemia. Additionally, medications may alter the response to blood glucose. For example, those with type 2 diabetes typically do not experience hypoglycemia from oral antidiabetic agents. One class in particular, however, stimulates the pancreas to increase the endogenous production of insulin. These medications, such as chlorpropamide, glipizide, glyburide, and others, belong to the sulfonylurea class of drugs. Patients must be educated about the risks of these medications, as well as how to manage the hypoglycemia that may accompany their use, whether taken as monotherapy or in combination with other classes, including biguanides or thiazolidinediones. Beta-blockers, a common class of medications used to treat a variety of conditions from hypertension to arrhythmias to post-MI management, may mask the autonomic response so the patient may not recognize he or she is experiencing hypoglycemia until the symptoms progress. Monoamine oxidase inhibitors (MAOIs), haloperidol, and some selective serotonin reuptake inhibitors (SSRIs) have also been associated with episodes of hypoglycemia.

INTERVENTIONS

Glucose Replacement

The main agents utilized in the treatment of hypoglycemia focus on the need to supply glucose to the body as quickly as possible to reverse the hypoglycemic state. One method is the direct replacement of glucose through oral or intravenous administration of a glucose product; the other is to mobilize stores of glucose from the liver through the parenteral administration of glucagon.

Fast-acting oral glucose products are easily available and simple to administer. Current products include chewable tablets, oral gels, liquid shots, and sprays. As long as a patient is conscious or demonstrates no difficulty in breathing or swallowing, oral glucose replacement therapy in the management of hypoglycemia is safe. Counsel patients on the amount of product that must be administered to raise blood glucose quickly. For example, it is advisable to ingest 15-24 g of a carbohydrate/glucose product to reverse hypoglycemia. This means that a patient will have to ingest 3-4 tablets of a commercially available glucose product or a minimum of 1 glucose gel tube.

Counsel patients with diabetes to carry with them at all times a source of fast-acting glucose. Patients also need to be educated that 1/2 cup (4 ounces) of regular fruit juice or 5-6 pieces of hard candy are acceptable substitutes to ingest to raise the blood glucose level when a person is experiencing early symptoms of hypoglycemia. Other alternatives include regular (not diet) soda, corn syrup, table sugar, honey, and commercial frosting in a tube that is typically used for cake decorating. The ultimate goal is to provide a hypoglycemic patient a quick source of a minimum of 15 g of glucose in an easily absorbable form.

Patients experiencing hypoglycemia should initially avoid ingesting high-fat or protein-based food or drinks. Both will impact and slow the absorption of glucose into the system, which counteracts what is attempting to be accomplished.

Following ingestion of a rapidly absorbed source of glucose, the patient with diabetes should check their blood glucose with their blood glucose meter in 15 to 20 minutes. At that point, if their blood glucose is still low (50-70 mg/dL), the patient should repeat the dosage of 15-24 g of digestible carbohydrate. If the blood glucose has risen to a normal range or is trending upward, the patient should follow the rapid glucose load with a balanced snack that includes a blend of carbohydrates, fat, and protein. Basic examples include a peanut butter and jelly sandwich, a meat sandwich, or crackers and cheese. After experiencing a hypoglycemic episode, the patient needs to continue with normal snacks and meals, and regular testing of their blood glucose for the remainder of the day. The patient should also contact their physician and discuss the episode to ascertain whether treatment adjustment is needed.

Alternatively, if a patient experiencing hypoglycemia is experiencing difficulty swallowing or has fallen unconscious, the risk of aspiration or choking is a concern with regard to consuming oral glucose products. The other option is the parenteral use of glucagon.

Glucagon

In the human body, glucagon is secreted by the α-2 cells located in the islets of Langerhans in the pancreas where it naturally mobilizes glucose stores in the liver. Glucagon in the liver triggers adenylate cyclase, which in turn catalyzes the conversion of AMP to cAMP. Activation of cAMP induces a sequential activation of enzymatic processes, which culminates in phosphorylase enzymes degrading stored glycogen to rapid-acting glucose. This process of glycogenolysis results in a near-immediate release of glucose to the bloodstream, resulting in a return to a euglycemic state in normally a few minutes. Glucagon for emergency replacement, typically for hypoglycemic patients, was formerly derived from animal sources, namely pork and beef. With advances in recombinant technology, glucagon is now produced entirely through this process, utilizing an *E. coli* vector. Glycogen supplied exogenously serves the same purpose and action as endogenous glycogen.

It is essential to recognize that those with potentially depleted stores of glycogen, including the elderly, the very thin, the cachetic, and chronic alcoholics, may have a reduced response or no response to glucagon. In these instances, it is imperative that the patient receives immediate medical attention to ensure methods are employed that raise the blood glucose level, including the intravenous administration of dextrose.

Glucagon in the treatment of hypoglycemia is administered parenterally via an intravenous, intramuscular, or subcutaneous injection in a dose of 1 mg to patients weighing more than 44 lbs (22 kg). Patients less than that weight, including pediatric patients, should be administered a 0.5 mg dose, or for the smallest pediatric patients, a weight-derived dosing of 20-30 mcg/kg per dose, not to exceed 1 mg per dose. Prior to administration, the lyophilized glucagon powder is reconstituted with sterile water, or equivalent diluent supplied by the manufacturer, to a concentration of 1 mg/mL. This reconstituted solution should be visually examined for clarity; there should not be any undissolved particles or foreign objects in the solution. If any anomalies are detected, discard the reconstituted product and do not inject into the patient. Discard unused solution and do not store for later use.

Glucagon is usually administered when the patient is unconscious. A clinical response and return to consciousness should occur within 15 minutes after an injection of glucagon. A second dose of glucagon may be administered if an insufficient clinical response is obtained. However, caution must be exercised, as the greatest concern is ensuring the brain is receiving an adequate supply of glucose. Immediate glucose replacement via an intravenous 50% dextrose solution may be preferred to ensure an adequate blood glucose concentration is achieved. This is also essential, particularly if there is a concern that the patient does not have adequate glycogen stores to be mobilized from the use of glucagon.

Once a conscious state is obtained, the patient should ingest carbohydrates, including examples as discussed above, with glucose replacement therapy. Patients should consume a fast-acting carbohydrate, followed by a long-acting carbohydrate that can be combined with some protein and small amounts of fat. All patients should receive some type of glucose replacement to replenish glycogen stores in the liver, as well as to prevent a recurrent episode of hypoglycemia. The selection of intravenous or oral routes will depend on the clinical situation.

Glucagon is relatively well tolerated. The major side effect associated with the use of glucagon is nausea and vomiting, which also may be compounded by the body's hypoglycemic response. Glucagon also has positive inotropic and chronotropic effects, thus patients with underlying cardiovascular disorders including arrhythmias and hypertension should be monitored closely following glucagon administration. Patients with a history of pheochromocytoma or insulinoma must also be carefully monitored for adverse side effects. There have been instances of generalized allergic reactions secondary to an injection of glucagon, including hives, itching, and difficulty breathing. For more prescribing information, see **Table 20.2**.

The use of glucagon in combination with anticoagulants such as warfarin and derivatives thereof has demonstrated an increased risk of bleeding. This is particularly noted in much larger doses of glucagon, usually 25 to 50 mg administered daily over several days. While it is important to recognize patients taking warfarin may be at an increased risk of bleeding, it is equally prudent to be cognizant of the comparative doses of glucagon at which the interactions appear to occur.

SUMMARY

Hypoglycemia is a commonly experienced condition that accompanies diabetes. With proper education and management techniques, hypoglycemia can be managed appropriately and efficiently. Therapeutic options include oral replacement utilizing fast-acting glucose products or mobilization of glucose stores in the liver through the injection of glucagon via an IM, IV, or SQ route.

SUGGESTED READING

Allen C, LeCaire T, Palta M, Daniels K, Meredith M, D'Alessio DJ. Risk factors for frequent and severe hypoglycemia in type 1 diabetes. *Diabetes Care*. 2001; 24(11):1878-81.

American Diabetes Association Workgroup on Hypoglycemia. Defining and reporting hypoglycemia in diabetes. *Diabetes Care*. 2005; 28(5):1245-49.

Cryer PE. Mechanisms of hypoglycemia-associated autonomic failure and its component syndromes in diabetes. *Diabetes*. 2005; 54:3592-3601.

Cryer PE, Davis SN, Shamoon H. Hypoglycemia in diabetes. *Diabetes Care*. 2003; 26:1902-12.

Fisher SJ, Bruning JC, Lannon S, Kahn CR. Insulin signaling in the central nervous system is critical for the normal sympathoadrenal response to hypoglycemia. *Diabetes*. 2005; 54:1447-51.

Pearson T. Glucagon as a treatment of severe hypoglycemia: Safe and efficacious but under-utilized. *The Diabetes Educator*. 2008; 34(1):128-34.

Rosetti P, Porcellati F, Bolli GB, Fanelli CG. Prevention of hypoglycemia while achieving good glycemic control in type 1 diabetes. *Diabetes Care*. 2008; 31:S113-S120.

Sigal RJ, Kenny GP, Wasserman DH, Castanesa-Sceppa C. Physical activity/exercise and type 2 diabetes. *Diabetes Care*. 2004; 27(10):2518-39.

White JR. The contribution of medications to hypoglycemia unawareness. *Diabetes Spectrum*. 2007; 20(2):77-80.

Zammitt NN, Frier BM. Hypoglycemia in type 2 diabetes: Pathophysiology, frequency, and effect of different treatment modalities. *Diabetes Care*. 2005; 28(12):2948-61.

Table 20.2. Prescribing Information for Glucagon

GENERIC NAME	FORM/ STRENGTH	DOSAGE	WARNINGS/PRECAUTIONS & CONTRAINDICATIONS	ADVERSE REACTIONS
Glucagon	Inj: 1mg	*Adults:* **Severe Hypoglycemia:** 1mg (1 U) SQ/IM/IV. May give another dose after 15 min if patient does not respond, but IV glucose would be a better alternative. Use immediately after reconstitution; discard unused portion. After patient responds, give supplemental carbohydrate. **Diagnostic Aid: Duodenum/Small Bowel:** 0.25-0.5mg (0.25-0.5 U) IV, or 1mg (1 U) IM, or 2mg (2 U) IV/IM before procedure. **Stomach:** 0.5mg (0.5 U) IV or 2mg (2 U) IM before procedure. **Colon:** 2mg (2 U) IM 10 min before procedure. *Pediatrics:* **Severe Hypoglycemia:** ≥20kg: 1mg (1 U) SQ/IM/IV. **<20kg:** 0.5mg (0.5 U) or 20-30mcg/kg. May give another dose after 15 min if patient does not respond, but IV glucose would be a better alternative. Use immediately after reconstitution; discard unused portion. After patient responds, give supplemental carbohydrate.	**W/P:** Caution with history suggestive of insulinoma and/or pheochromocytoma. Glucagon can cause pheochromocytoma tumor to release catecholamines, which may result in a sudden and marked increase in BP. Effective in treating hypoglycemia only if sufficient liver glycogen is present. Glucagon is not effective in states of starvation, adrenal insufficiency, or chronic hypoglycemia; use glucose to treat instead. **Contra:** Pheochromocytoma. **P/N:** Category B, caution in nursing.	Nausea, vomiting, allergic reactions, urticaria, respiratory distress, hypotension.

W/P = warnings/precautions; **Contra** = contraindications; **P/N** = pregnancy category rating and nursing considerations.

Defining and Reporting Hypoglycemia in Diabetes

American Diabetes Association

Iatrogenic hypoglycemia causes recurrent morbidity in most people with type 1 diabetes and in many with type 2 diabetes and is sometimes fatal. It also impairs defenses against subsequent hypoglycemia. Furthermore, the barrier of hypoglycemia precludes maintenance of euglycemia over a lifetime of diabetes; thus, full realization of the benefits of glycemic control is rarely achieved. Therefore, hypoglycemia is the critical limiting factor in the glycemic management of diabetes in both the short and long term (1).

Clinicians have recognized the problem of iatrogenic hypoglycemia since the first use of insulin in 1922 (2). The problem was underscored 70 years later by the finding that intensive glycemic therapy both decreased the frequency of long-term complications and increased the frequency of hypoglycemia in the Diabetes Control and Complications Trial (DCCT) (3,4). Despite steady improvements in the glycemic management of diabetes, and perhaps because of the impetus for glycemic control that resulted from the DCCT (3,4) and the U.K. Prospective Diabetes Study (5,6), recent population-based data indicate that hypoglycemia continues to be a major problem for people with both type 1 and type 2 diabetes (7–9).

The ultimate goal of the glycemic management of diabetes is a lifetime of euglycemia without hypoglycemia. That will undoubtedly require glucose-regulated insulin replacement or secretion (10). Pending that, the goal of new drugs, devices, or management strategies to be used for the glycemic management of diabetes is to both improve glycemic control and reduce the frequency and severity of hypoglycemia. How should new drugs, devices, or strategies be evaluated and reported from the perspective of hypoglycemia?

The American Diabetes Association assembled a Workgroup on Hypoglycemia in June of 2004 to discuss that issue and, in part, to advise the U.S. Food and Drug Administration as to how hypoglycemia should be used as an end point in studies of new treatments for diabetes. After reviewing the background of hypoglycemia in diabetes, the Workgroup discussed three questions: 1) How should hypoglycemia be defined? 2) How should hypoglycemia be reported? 3) What constitutes a meaningful reduction in hypoglycemia?

Address correspondence and reprint requests to Philip E. Cryer, MD, Washington University School of Medicine, Department of Endocrinology/Metabolism, CB 8127 WashU, 660 S. Euclid Ave., Saint Louis, MO 63110. E-mail: pcryer@wustl.edu
Abbreviations: DCCT, Diabetes Control and Complications Trial

HYPOGLYCEMIA IN DIABETES

The topic of hypoglycemia in diabetes has been reviewed in detail recently (1,11). The clinical syndrome is most convincingly documented by Whipple's triad (12): symptoms consistent with hypoglycemia, a low plasma glucose concentration, and relief of those symptoms when the plasma glucose concentration is raised. In people with diabetes, hypoglycemia has been classified as "asymptomatic" or "biochemical," which is particularly common, and "symptomatic" or "severe," which requires the assistance of another individual. Symptoms of hypoglycemia may be idiosyncratic, but individuals often learn to recognize their unique symptoms. Neurogenic (autonomic) symptoms include, but are not limited to, palpitations, tremor, hunger, and sweating. Neuroglycopenic symptoms often include behavioral changes, difficulty thinking, and/or frank confusion, but neuroglycopenic manifestations can include seizure, coma, and even death.

In people with diabetes, hypoglycemia is the result of the interplay of relative or absolute insulin excess and compromised physiological defenses against falling plasma glucose concentrations (1,11). Insulin excess from time to time is the result of the pharmacokinetic imperfections of all insulin preparations and insulin secretagogues used to treat diabetes in the context of an array of factors such as food intake, exercise, drug (including alcohol) interactions, altered sensitivity to insulin, and insulin clearance. Compromised physiological defenses against falling plasma glucose concentrations are the result of the pathophysiology of glucose counterregulation—the mechanisms that normally prevent or rapidly correct hypoglycemia—at least in type 1 and advanced type 2 diabetes. That pathophysiology includes impairment of all three key defenses against falling plasma glucose

levels in the endogenous insulin deficient state: 1) insulin levels do not decrease, 2) glucagon levels do not increase, and 3) the increase in epinephrine levels is typically attenuated (i.e., the glycemic threshold for epinephrine secretion is shifted to a lower plasma glucose concentration). In the setting of absent insulin and glucagon responses, the attenuated epinephrine response causes the syndrome of defective glucose counterregulation. The attenuated sympathoadrenal (sympathetic neural as well as adrenomedullary) response also causes the clinical syndrome of hypoglycemia unawareness, i.e., loss of the warning symptoms that previously allowed the patient to recognize developing hypoglycemia and take corrective action. While the absent insulin and glucagon responses are persistent defects, it is now recognized that the reduced sympathoadrenal response to a given level of hypoglycemia is a dynamic process typically induced by recent antecedent iatrogenic hypoglycemia (1,11). The concept of hypoglycemia-associated autonomic failure in type 1 diabetes (13) and advanced type 2 diabetes (14) posits that recent antecedent hypoglycemia causes both defective glucose counterregulation (by reducing the epinephrine response in the setting of absent insulin and glucagon responses) and hypoglycemia unawareness (by reducing the sympathoadrenal and the resulting symptomatic responses) and thus a vicious cycle of recurrent hypoglycemia (1,11). That concept has been extended recently to include exercise- and sleep-related hypoglycemia-associated autonomic failure (11). Thus, hypoglycemia unawareness is reversible in most affected patients, and the reduced epinephrine component of defective glucose counterregulation is variably improved, by as little as 2–3 weeks of scrupulous avoidance of iatrogenic hypoglycemia (15–19). Importantly, antecedent plasma glucose levels as high as

70 mg/dL (3.9 mmol/L) cause reduced sympathoadrenal responses to subsequent hypoglycemia (20).

Iatrogenic hypoglycemia often has a profound impact on the lives of people with diabetes (as well as on their physiological defenses against subsequent hypoglycemia). The experience of an episode can range from unrecognized to extremely uncomfortable and disrupting. As a group, people with diabetes fear hypoglycemia more than they fear the long-term complications of diabetes. The degree of cognitive-motor dysfunction, particularly slowing of cognitive and motor processing speed, during an episode depends on the magnitude of hypoglycemia. The psychological reactions can be quite frightening and can extend beyond the patient to include family, friends, and coworkers. If neuroglycopenia occurs while the individual is performing a critical task, such as driving, the individual and others are placed at risk of injury and death. The rational fear of hypoglycemia can lead to worsening of metabolic control as well as tension with, and a restriction of personal freedoms and responsibilities by, anxious and over-protective loved ones, colleagues, or employers.

Risk factors for hypoglycemia (1,11) include: 1) endogenous insulin deficiency, which also predicts a deficient glucagon response; 2) a history of hypoglycemia, hypoglycemia unawareness, or both; 3) aggressive glycemic therapy per se as evidenced by lower glycemic goals, lower HbA1c levels, or both; 4) recent moderate or intensive exercise; 5) sleep; and 6) renal failure. However, a history of severe hypoglycemia and lower HbA_{1c} levels have limited ability to predict additional episodes. These two parameters accounted for 9% of future episodes of severe hypoglycemia in the DCCT (4) and, when combined with a specific autonomic score, for 18% of future severe hypoglycemic episodes (21).

Mild hypoglycemic episodes frequently precede severe hypoglycemia (22). Indeed, >50% of hypoglycemia can be predicted based on risk analysis of self-monitored plasma glucose data over time (23). This reflects the fact, discussed earlier, that recent antecedent hypoglycemia, with prior plasma glucose concentrations as high as 70 mg/dL (3.9 mmol/L) (20), causes defective glucose counterregulation and hypoglycemia unawareness (1,11). Thus, episodes of hypoglycemia not only cause recurrent physical and psychological morbidity and risk of death in the short term but also preclude euglycemia in the long term. In addition, episodes lead to a vicious cycle of recurrent hypoglycemia.

QUESTIONS

A) How should hypoglycemia be defined?

The Workgroup first established a set of guiding principles regarding the ideal definition of hypoglycemia in individuals with diabetes. First, the optimal definition should be applicable to clinical decision-making by people with diabetes and their care providers as well as to studies of diabetes drugs, devices, or management strategies, although the standards for documenting and reporting hypoglycemia in studies need to be more stringent than those in the clinical setting. Second, the definition should be 1) free from reporting biases, 2) clinically important, 3) applicable to all persons with diabetes, 4) applicable to any time of day, 5) measurable by practical and widely available methods, and 6) reportable in a standardized fashion.

Given these parameters, the Workgroup's overarching definition of hypoglycemia includes all episodes of an abnormally low plasma glucose concentration that expose the individual to potential harm. With regard to the latter issue, it is not only the nadir glucose concentration and the duration of hypoglycemia that may be inherently dangerous; frequent hypoglycemic events interfere with daily living and, even if asymptomatic, lead to defective glucose counterregulation and hypoglycemia unawareness (1,11,13,14,20). Since these episodes increase the risk of subsequent hypoglycemia substantially, all hypoglycemic events can harm the individual with diabetes in the short or long term.

In addition to glucose counterregulatory systems that are triggered at an (arterialized venous) plasma glucose concentration of 65–70 mg/dL (3.6–3.9 mmol/L) in nondiabetic people (24–26), warning symptoms of hypoglycemia are critical to permit interventions that also restore the plasma glucose concentration toward normal. Thus, symptoms of a low plasma glucose, it can be argued, may be included in a definition of hypoglycemia. It is acknowledged that symptoms are idiosyncratic and nonspecific and may either not be recognized as such or be absent. Alternatively, it could be argued that hypoglycemia—literally low blood glucose—is by definition diagnosed by a low plasma glucose value. Thus, the question arises as to whether symptoms associated with hypoglycemia should ever replace a glucose value. Although it is appreciated that people with diabetes often know when they are hypoglycemic, there is also the very gray area that occurs when comorbid conditions or therapies produce symptoms similar to those that occur during hypoglycemia (e.g., palpitations, tremor, hunger, or sweating) or in patients with hypoglycemia unawareness. Clearly, it is important for patients to measure their glucose levels when they think they are hypoglycemic. The reality, however, is that a plasma glucose level is not always obtained.

Finally, the question arises as to how a glucose level used to define hypoglycemia should be measured. Although a precise laboratory-based plasma glucose measurement would be ideal, monitor-based estimates (or those with a validated glucose sensor) are the only practical method. Albeit a function of mean glycemia and therefore a useful index of overall glycemic control and generally inversely related to the frequency of hypoglycemia, the HbA_{1c} level is not an alternative to plasma glucose values. Given that they likely have periods of hyperglycemia, patients with near-normal HbA_{1c} levels likely have periods of hypoglycemia (e.g., during the night) whether they are detected or not.

The Workgroup definition describes a classification of hypoglycemic events based on the above considerations. A hypoglycemic episode could be:

1) Severe hypoglycemia

An event requiring assistance of another person to actively administer carbohydrate, glucagons, or other resuscitative actions. These episodes may be associated with sufficient neuroglycopenia to induce seizure or coma. Plasma glucose measurements may not be available during such an event, but neurological recovery attributable to the restoration of plasma glucose to normal is considered sufficient evidence that the event was induced by a low plasma glucose concentration.

2) Documented symptomatic hypoglycemia

An event during which typical symptoms of hypoglycemia are accompanied by a measured plasma glucose concentration 70 mg/dL (3.9 mmol/L).

3) Asymptomatic hypoglycemia

An event not accompanied by typical symptoms of hypoglycemia but with a measured plasma glucose concentration 70 mg/dL (3.9 mmol/L). Since the glycemic threshold for activation of glucagon and epinephrine secretion as glucose levels decline is normally 65–70 mg/dL (3.6–3.9 mmol/L) (24–26) and since antecedent plasma glucose concentrations of 70 mg/dL (3.9 mmol/L) reduce sympathoadrenal responses to subsequent hypoglycemia (1,11,20), this criterion sets the lower limit for the variation in plasma glucose in nondiabetic, nonpregnant individuals as the conservative lower limit for individuals with diabetes.

4) Probable symptomatic hypoglycemia

An event during which symptoms of hypoglycemia are not accompanied by a plasma glucose determination (but that was presumably caused by a plasma glucose concentration 70 mg/dL [3.9 mmol/L]). Since many people with diabetes choose to treat symptoms with oral carbohydrate without a test of plasma glucose, it is important to recognize these events as "probable" hypoglycemia. Such self-reported episodes that are not confirmed by a contemporaneous low plasma glucose determination may not be suitable outcome measures for clinical studies that are aimed at evaluating therapy, but they should be reported.

5) Relative hypoglycemia

An event during which the person with diabetes reports any of the typical symptoms of hypoglycemia, and interprets those as indicative of hypoglycemia, but with a measured plasma glucose concentration >70 mg/dL (3.9 mmol/L). This category reflects the fact that patients with chronically poor glycemic control can experience symptoms of hypoglycemia at plasma glucose levels >70 mg/dL (3.9 mmol/L) as plasma glucose concentrations decline toward that level (27,28). Though causing distress and interfering with the patient's sense of well-being, and potentially limiting the

achievement of optimal glycemic control, such episodes probably pose no direct harm and therefore may not be a suitable outcome measure for clinical studies that are aimed at evaluating therapy, but they should be reported.

B) How should hypoglycemia be reported?

At a minimum, hypoglycemic events should be reported in each of the first three categories: severe hypoglycemia, documented symptomatic hypoglycemia, and asymptomatic hypoglycemia. Thus, since severe hypoglycemia is infrequent, the vast majority of reported episodes will require a corresponding plasma glucose concentration <70 mg/dL (3.9 mmol/L), with (documented symptomatic hypoglycemia) or without (asymptomatic hypoglycemia) symptoms. Such relatively stringent criteria are appropriate for studies of new drugs, devices, or management strategies. Nonetheless, their use alone will underestimate the frequency of symptomatic episodes attributed to hypoglycemia. Therefore, it would be useful to also report episodes of probable symptomatic and relative hypoglycemia, even though these are not used as statistical outcome variables.

Currently there is no standardized convention for reporting the frequency of hypoglycemia in clinical studies. The Workgroup recommends that both the proportion (percentage) of patients affected and the event rates (e.g., episodes per patient-year or 100 patient-years) for each of the categories of hypoglycemic events be reported. These provide complementary information.

At least in type 1 diabetes, hypoglycemia occurs most frequently during sleep (3,4). Episodes of nocturnal hypoglycemia range from asymptomatic to severe and are potentially fatal if untreated. In addition, even asymptomatic nocturnal hypoglycemia impairs defenses against subsequent hypoglycemia (29,30), i.e., it causes defective glucose counterregulation and hypoglycemia unawareness (1,11). Therefore, it is appropriate to separate hypoglycemic events into nocturnal and daytime episodes.

Finally, if patients at high risk for hypoglycemia are excluded from clinical studies, that exclusion should be made clear. Similarly, it should be made clear if patients at low risk are excluded. Obviously, the exclusion/inclusion criteria can affect the frequency of hypoglycemic events.

C) What constitutes a meaningful reduction in hypoglycemia?

Clearly, clinical approaches that reduce the severity of hypoglycemia, as well as those that reduce the frequency of hypoglycemia, would be worthwhile. The Workgroup concluded that any significant reduction in severe hypoglycemia (that requiring the assistance of another individual), even by as little as 10–20%, would be advantageous. It was the consensus of the Workgroup that a significant reduction in the frequency of documented hypoglycemia (plasma glucose <70 mg/dL [3.9 mmol/L]), with or without symptoms, of 30% by a new drug, device, or management strategy would represent a clinically important improvement over existing therapies. That could be a 30% reduction in the proportion of patients affected by hypoglycemia, the hypoglycemia event rates, or both. (Again, both the proportion of patients affected and the event rates should be reported.) The reduction in hypoglycemia could be over any clinically relevant period of time; if limited to a segment of the day, e.g., during the night, it should not be offset by an increase in the frequency of hypoglycemia in the remainder of the day. Finally, a clinically important reduction in hypoglycemia should not be accompanied by an increase in mean glycemia (e.g., HbA_{1c}). Indeed, as

mentioned earlier, the goal is to reduce both hypoglycemia and glycemia.

Rates of hypoglycemia can vary within a given clinical study. The frequency of hypoglycemia could increase sharply early in a study with intensification of treatment only to decrease to a lower steady state when a plateau of stable glycemic control is achieved. This initial phase of increased hypoglycemia can be variable and depends on factors such as the pharmacokinetics and pharmacodynamics of a new drug; the investigator and patient learning curve with a new drug, device, or strategy; and the rapidity of intensification of glycemic control. On the other hand, since the frequency of hypoglycemia is linked to glycemic control, a study that improves glucose levels slowly may produce a pattern of increasing rates of hypoglycemia over months. A third scenario is an experimental design that tests a chronic intervention over years.

Therefore, the experimental question is a key factor driving the assessment of the frequency of hypoglycemia. The sample size is, of course, another key variable. Thus, the metrics that should be considered in designing a study aimed at determining the frequency of hypoglycemia include: 1) the time required to achieve the glycemic target, 2) the duration of stable glycemic control, 3) the target level of glycemic control, and 4) the number of participants.

APPENDIX

Members of the ADA Workgroup on Hypoglycemia
Belinda P. Childs, ARNP, MN, CDE; Nathaniel G. Clark, MD, MS, RD; Daniel J. Cox, PhD; Philip E. Cryer, MD (chair); Stephen N. Davis, MD, Monica M. DiNardo, MSN, CRNP, CDE; Richard Kahn, PhD; Boris Kovatchev, PhD; and Harry Shamoon, MD.

ACKNOWLEDGMENTS

The meeting of this workgroup and the resulting report were made possible by unrestricted educational grants from Abbott Diabetes Care, Amylin Pharmaceuticals, Eli Lilly and Company, LifeScan, Medtronic Diabetes, and Novo Nordisk Pharmaceuticals. The authors acknowledge the review and comments on the manuscript by Scott Jacober, DO, CDE; David L. Horwitz, MD, PhD; Alan O. Marcus, MD; and Fannie E. Smith, MD, PhD.

REFERENCES

1. Cryer PE, Davis SN, Shamoon H: Hypoglycemia in diabetes. *Diabetes Care* 26:1902–1912, 2003[Abstract/Free Full Text]
2. Fletcher AA, Campbell WR: The blood sugar following insulin administration and the symptom complex: hypoglycemia. *J Metab Res* 2:637–649, 1922
3. The Diabetes Control and Complications Trial Research Group: The effect of intensive treatment of diabetes on the development and progression of long-term complications in insulin-dependent diabetes mellitus. *N Engl J Med* 329:977–986, 1993
4. The Diabetes Control and Complications Trial Research Group: Hypoglycemia in the Diabetes Control and Complications Trial. *Diabetes* 46:271–286, 1997
5. Intensive blood-glucose control with sulphonylureas or insulin compared with conventional treatment and risk of complications in patients with type 2 diabetes (UKPDS 33): UK Prospective Diabetes Study (UKPDS) Group. *Lancet* 352:837–853, 1998
6. Effect of intensive blood-glucose control with metformin on complications in overweight patients with type 2 diabetes: the United Kingdom Prospective Diabetes Study Group. *Lancet* 352: 854–865, 1998
7. Bulsara MK, Holman CDJ, Davis EA, Jones TW: The impact of a decade of changing treatment on rates of severe hypoglycemia in a population-based cohort of children with type 1 diabetes. *Diabetes Care* 27:2293–2298, 2004
8. Holstein A, Plaschke A, Egberts E-H: Clinical characterization of severe hypoglycemia: a prospective population-based study. *Exp Clin Endocrinol Diabetes* 111:364–369, 2003
9. Leese GP, Wang J, Broomhall J, Kelly P, Marsden A, Morrison W, Frier BM, Morris AD, DARTS/MEMO Collaboration: Frequency of severe hypoglycemia requiring emergency treatment in type 1 and type 2 diabetes: a population-based study of health service resource use. *Diabetes Care* 26:1176–1180, 2003
10. Ryan EA, Shandro T, Green K, Paty BW, Senior PA, Bigam D, Shapiro AMJ, Vantyghem M-C: Assessment of the severity of hypoglycemia and glycemic lability in type 1 diabetic subjects undergoing islet transplantation. *Diabetes* 53:955–962, 2004
11. Cryer PE: Diverse causes of hypoglycemia-associated autonomic failure in diabetes. *N Engl J Med* 350:2272–2279, 2004
12. Whipple AO: The surgical therapy of hyperinsulinism. *J Int Chir* 3:237–276, 1938
13. Dagogo-Jack SE, Craft S, Cryer PE: Hypoglycemia-associated autonomic failure in insulin-dependent diabetes mellitus. *J Clin Invest* 91:819–828, 1993
14. Segel SA, Paramore DS, Cryer PE: Hypoglycemia-associated autonomic failure in advanced type 2 diabetes. *Diabetes* 51:724–733, 2002
15. Fanelli CG, Epifano L, Rambotti AM, Pampanelli S, Di Vincenzo A, Modarelli F, Lepore M, Annibale B, Ciofetta M, Bottini P, Porcellati F, Scionti L, Santeusanio F, Brunetti P, Bolli GB: Meticulous prevention of hypoglycemia normalizes the glycemic thresholds and magnitude of most of neuroendocrine responses to, symptoms of, and cognitive function during hypoglycemia in intensively treated patients with short-term IDDM. *Diabetes* 42:1683–1689, 1993
16. Cranston I, Lomas J, Maran A, Macdonald I, Amiel SA: Restoration of hypoglycaemia awareness in patients with long-duration insulin-dependent diabetes. *Lancet* 344:283–287, 1994
17. Fanelli C, Pampanelli S, Epifano L, Rambotti AM, Di Vincenzo A, Modarelli F, Ciofetta M, Lepore M, Annibale B, Torlone E, Perriello G, De Feo P, Santeusanio F, Brunetti P, Bolli GB: Long-term recovery from unawareness, deficient counterregulation and lack of cognitive dysfunction during hypoglycaemia, following institution of rational, intensive insulin therapy in IDDM. *Diabetologia* 37:1265–1276, 1994
18. Dagogo-Jack S, Rattarasarn C, Cryer PE: Reversal of hypoglycemia unawareness, but not defective glucose counterregulation in IDDM. *Diabetes* 43:1426–1434, 1994
19. Liu D, McManus RM, Ryan EA: Improved counter-regulatory hormonal and symptomatic responses to hypoglycemia in patients with insulin-dependent diabetes mellitus after 3 months of less strict glycemic control. *Clin Invest Med* 19:71–82, 1996
20. Davis SN, Shavers C, Mosqueda-Garcia, Costa F: Effects of differing antecedent hypoglycemia on subsequent counterregulation in normal humans. *Diabetes* 46:1328–1335, 1997
21. Gold AE, Frier BM, MacLeod KM, Deary IJ: A structural equation model for predictors of severe hypoglycaemia in patients with insulin-dependent diabetes mellitus. *Diabet Med* 14:309–315, 1997
22. Kovatchev BP, Cox DJ, Farhy LS, Straume M, Gonder-Frederick LA, Clarke WL: Episodes of severe hypoglycemia in type 1 diabetes are preceded, and followed, within 48 hours by measurable disturbances in blood glucose. *J Clin Endocrinol Metab* 85:4287–4292, 2000
23. Kovatchev BP, Cox DJ, Kumar A, Gonder-Frederick L, Clarke WL: Algorithmic evaluation of metabolic control and risk of severe hypoglycemia in type 1 and type 2 diabetes using self-monitoring blood glucose data. *Diabetes Technol Ther* 5:817–828, 2003
24. Schwartz NS, Clutter WE, Shah SD, Cryer PE: Glycemic thresholds for activation of glucose counterregulatory systems are higher than the threshold for symptoms. *J Clin Invest* 79:777–781, 1987
25. Mitrakou A, Ryan C, Veneman T, Mokan M, Jenssen T, Kiss I, Durrant J, Cryer P, Gerich J: Hierarchy of glycemic thresholds for counterregulatory hormone secretion, symptoms, and cerebral dysfunction. *Am J Physiol Endocrinol Metab* 260:E67–E74, 1991
26. Fanelli C, Pampanelli S, Epifano L, Rambotti AM, Ciofetta M, Modarelli F, Di Vincenzo A, Annibale B, Lepore M, Lalli C, Sindaco P, Brunetti P, Bolli G: Relative roles of insulin and hypoglycaemia on induction of neuroendocrine responses to, symptoms of, and deterioration of cognitive function in hypoglycaemia in male and female humans. *Diabetologia* 37:797–807, 1994
27. Boyle PJ, Schwartz NS, Shah SD, Clutter WE, Cryer PE: Plasma glucose concentrations at the onset of hypoglycemic symptoms in patients with poorly controlled diabetes and in nondiabetics. *N Engl J Med* 318:1487–1492, 1988
28. Amiel SA, Sherwin RS, Simonson DC, Tamborlane WV: Effect of intensive insulin therapy on glycemic thresholds for counterregulatory hormone release. *Diabetes* 37:901–907, 1988
29. Veneman T, Mitrakou A, Mokan M, Cryer P, Gerich J: Induction of hypoglycemia unawareness by asymptomatic nocturnal hypoglycemia. *Diabetes* 42:1233–1237, 1993
30. Fanelli CG, Paramore DS, Hershey T, Terkamp C, Ovalle F, Craft S, Cryer PE: Impact of nocturnal hypoglycemia on hypoglycemic cognitive dysfunction in type 1 diabetes. *Diabetes* 47:1920–1927, 1998

Section IV
Future Medications

Chapter 21

New Products in Development for Patients with Diabetes

Danial E. Baker, PharmD, FASHP, FASCP
Terri L. Levien, PharmD

INTRODUCTION

A number of new drugs for the treatment of diabetes and its complications are under development. Information on these agents was obtained by a review of the medical literature, abstracts from recent endocrinology and diabetes meetings, Wolters Kluwer Health's Adis R&D Insight database, the Pharmaceutical Research and Manufacturers of America database, and press releases from numerous information services.

The new products furthest along in development are described in some detail, if they have not been discussed in a previous chapter, and those in phase I through preregistration are summarized in **Table 21.1**.

The references for each entry can be found at the end of this chapter, under the entry's name.

DIABETES

Alogliptin

Alogliptin is an oral dipeptidyl peptidase-4 (DPP-4) antagonist for the treatment of type 2 diabetes as an adjunct to diet and exercise to improve glycemic control. It may be indicated for use as monotherapy or as combination therapy with metformin, sulfonylureas, thiazolidinediones, or insulin when a single agent does not provide adequate control. Its new drug application (NDA) has been submitted to the U.S. Food and Drug Administration.

DPP-4 inhibitors are thought to work by slowing the inactivation of incretin hormone GLP-1 (glucagon-like peptide 1) and glucose-dependent insulinotropic peptide (GIP). These agents are released by the gastrointestinal tract in response to food and are involved with the stimulation of glucose-dependent insulin secretion.

The first marketed DPP-4 inhibitor was sitagliptin. Alogliptin belongs to a different chemical class than the other DPP-4 inhibitors. Alogliptin is a dioxo-dihydropyrimidine compound, while sitagliptin is a triazole-pyrazine compound and vildagliptin and saxagliptin are pyrrolidine-carbonitrile compounds.

Very little information has been published on the clinical efficacy and safety of alogliptin. The information on the common adverse reactions reported in the clinical trials with alogliptin is very limited, but has included reports of hypoglycemia with an incidence similar to the placebo control group.

Balaglitazone

Balaglitazone belongs to the class of agents known as thiazolidinediones. It works as an insulin sensitizer and peroxisome proliferator-activated receptor gamma agonist. Phase III clinical trials are ongoing to determine its efficacy and safety in the treatment patients with type 2 diabetes.

Dapagliflozin

Dapagliflozin is a selective sodium glucose cotransporter 2 inhibitor in the early portion of phase III development for use as a monotherapy agent or in combination with other oral hypoglycemic agents. It is hoped that this agent will improve plasma glucose levels and decrease body weight in patients with type 2 diabetes. The drug was well tolerated in pharmacokinetic studies, with the most common adverse reactions being constipation, nausea, and diarrhea.

Exenatide LAR

This is a long-acting release formulation of exenatide that is in Phase III development. It is intended for once-weekly subcutaneous administration for the treatment of type 2 diabetes. This agent was discussed in more detail in Chapter 11.

Liraglutide

Liraglutide is a human analog of the glucagon-like peptide-1 (GLP-1). As a GLP-1 analog, it induces its activity through a glucose-dependent stimulation of insulin secretion, inhibition of glucagon secretion, slowing of gastric emptying, and reduction in appetite. Liraglutide is administered by subcutaneous injection in the upper arm, abdomen, or thigh. It has a half-life of 11 to 15 hours allowing for once-daily administration.

Liraglutide is under evaluation for use in the treatment of patients with type 2 diabetes as an adjunct to diet and exercise, either as monotherapy or in combination with commonly used diabetes medications, including sulfonylureas and metformin. In clinical trials, liraglutide has been associated with a reduction in HbA_{1c} and fasting plasma glucose with either weight loss or no change in body weight. Significant reductions in HbA_{1c} have been observed at doses of 0.1 mg to 2 mg administered subcutaneously once daily.

A randomized, double-dummy study has compared the addition of liraglutide to glimepiride therapy with glimepiride monotherapy or the addition of rosiglitazone to glimepiride in 1041 patients with type 2 diabetes and baseline HbA_{1c} of 8.4%. Patients received liraglutide 0.6 mg/day, 1.2 mg/day, or 1.8 mg/day in combination with glimepiride, placebo plus glimepiride 2 to 4 mg per day, or rosiglitazone 4 mg daily plus glimepiride for 26 weeks. HbA_{1c} was reduced 1.08% with liraglutide 1.2 mg and by 1.13% with liraglutide 1.8 mg, compared with a reduction of 0.44% with the addition of rosiglitazone and an increase of 0.23% with glimepiride monotherapy ($P<0.0001$). HbA_{1c} <6.5% was achieved in 22% treated with liraglutide 1.2 mg plus glimepiride and 21% treated with liraglutide 1.8 mg plus glimepiride, compared with 4% treated with glimepiride monotherapy, and 10% treated with rosiglitazone plus glimepiride ($P<0.0003$).

Liraglutide has also been evaluated in combination with metformin therapy in a randomized, double-blind study enrolling 1091 patients with type 2 diabetes and baseline HbA_{1c} of 8.4%. Patients received liraglutide 0.6 mg, 1.2 mg, or 1.8 mg once daily added to metformin 1 g twice daily, placebo plus metformin, or glimepiride 4 mg once daily added to metformin for 26 weeks. HbA_{1c} was reduced 0.7% with liraglutide 0.6 mg, and 1% with liraglutide 1.2 mg and 1.8 mg plus metformin, compared with an increase of 0.1% with metformin monotherapy, and a reduction of 1% with glimepiride plus metformin ($P<0.05$ vs. liraglutide plus metformin vs placebo plus metformin).

HbA$_{1c}$ <6.5% was achieved in 11.3% of patients treated with liraglutide 0.6 mg plus metformin, 19.8% treated with liraglutide 1.2 mg plus metformin, 24.6% treated with liraglutide 1.8 mg plus metformin, compared with 4.2% treated with placebo plus metformin, and 22.2% treated with glimepiride plus metformin. Weight loss was greater in all three liraglutide plus metformin groups than in the glimepiride plus metformin group.

Liraglutide has also been compared with insulin glargine as add-on to therapy with metformin and glimepiride in a study enrolling 581 patients with type 2 diabetes and a baseline HbA$_{1c}$ of 8.2%. Patients received liraglutide 1.8 mg once daily, liraglutide placebo, or insulin glargine in addition to metformin 1 g twice daily and glimepiride 2-4 mg once daily for 26 weeks. HbA$_{1c}$ was reduced 1.33% with the addition of liraglutide, 0.24% with the addition of placebo, and 1.09% with the addition of insulin glargine (P<0.05 for liraglutide vs placebo and insulin glargine). HbA$_{1c}$ <6.5% was achieved in 37.1% treated with liraglutide compared with 10.9% in the placebo group, and 23.6% in the insulin glargine group. A weight loss of 1.81 kg was observed in the liraglutide group, compared with a loss of 0.42 kg in the placebo group and a weight gain of 1.62 kg in the insulin glargine group.

Additional ongoing studies are assessing liraglutide in combination with rosiglitazone plus metformin; comparing liraglutide with glimepiride and glyburide as monotherapy; comparing liraglutide and glimepiride added to metformin; and comparing liraglutide and exenatide in patients on metformin, a sulfonylurea, or metformin and a sulfonylurea.

Adverse effects associated with liraglutide therapy have included headache, dizziness, nausea, and vomiting.

Saxagliptin

Saxagliptin is an oral DPP-4 antagonist in phase III development for the treatment of type 2 diabetes as an adjunct to diet and exercise to improve glycemic control. Saxagliptin belongs to a different chemical class than alogliptin and sitagliptin. However, it is in the same chemical class as vildagliptin. It may be indicated for use as monotherapy or as combination therapy with metformin, a sulfonylurea, or a thiazolidinedione when a single agent does not provide adequate control.

Very little information has been published on the clinical efficacy and safety of saxagliptin. Saxagliptin is capable of decreasing the average HbA$_{1c}$ level in patients alone or in combination with metformin. Treatment with saxagliptin alone has been weight neutral. Common adverse reactions reported in the clinical trials with saxagliptin include nasopharyngitis, headache, diarrhea, upper respiratory infections, influenza and urinary tract infection, and hypoglycemia.

Succinobucol

Succinobucol is an oral antioxidant, lipid peroxidation inhibitor, and vascular cell adhesion molecule antagonist that is in phase III development for the treatment of atherosclerosis and type 2 diabetes. It is a monosuccinate ester of probucol, a previously approved lipid-lowering agent.

The first of these studies failed to achieve its primary endpoint in the treatment of patients with acute coronary syndrome. The double-blind, placebo-controlled multicenter trial was designed to evaluate the efficacy of succinobucol in the treatment of acute coronary syndrome. Patients were randomized to succinobucol 300 mg/day or placebo. The primary endpoint for the study was the composite of cardiovascular death, resuscitated cardiac arrest, myocardial infarction, stroke, unstable angina, or coronary revascularization. The secondary endpoints were primary composite endpoint with all-cause death, primary composite endpoint without coronary revascularization; and primary composite endpoint without coronary revascularization or unstable angina. After 24 months of treatment, the primary endpoint of the study was the same in both the succinobucol and placebo groups (17.2% vs 17.3%, respectively; $P= 0.99$). However, the secondary endpoint of cardiovascular death, cardiac arrest, myocardial infarction, or stroke was lower in patients randomized to succinobucol (6.7% vs 8.2%, $P= 0.028$)

The interim report from the AGI-1067 study included results from 806 patients who had completed three months of treatment. The HbA$_{1c}$ were decreased from baseline and better than those achieved with placebo. The primary endpoint for the study is the change in HbA$_{1c}$ at the end of six months of therapy.

Tagatose

Tagatose is a naturally occurring, sweet-tasting, low-calorie monosaccharide hexoketose found in dairy products. It was originally developed as a sugar substitute for calorie and weight control. It was granted "Generally Recognized as Safe" status for use as a sweetener in foods and beverages by the U.S. Food and Drug Administration in 2001.

The product under development by Spherix for the treatment of diabetes is being produced from whey. Oral administration of this product decreases the postprandial glucose peaks seen in patients with type 2 diabetes when it is administrated prior to a meal. The current clinical trial to demonstrate the efficacy of tagatose in the treatment of type 2 diabetes is scheduled for completion in 2009.

Vildagliptin

Vildagliptin is an oral DPP 4 antagonist for the treatment of type 2 diabetes as an adjunct to diet and exercise to improve glycemic control. It may be indicated for use as monotherapy or as combination therapy with metformin, a sulfonylurea, a thiazolidinedione, or insulin when a single agent does not provide adequate control.

Vildagliptin received an approvable letter from the FDA in 2007 for the treatment of diabetes and has been approved for use in Europe. However, the FDA approvable-letter requested additional data on the safety and efficacy of vildagliptin in renally impaired patients.

Vildagliptin alone or in combination with metformin, a thiazolidinedione, or insulin is capable of decreasing fasting plasma glucose levels and improving HbA$_{1c}$ levels in patients with type 2 diabetes.

The efficacy of vildagliptin in drug-naïve patients with type 2 diabetes and "mild" hyperglycemia was evaluated in multicenter, double-blind, randomized, placebo-controlled, parallel-group study that enrolled 306 patients. The baseline HbA$_{1c}$ for this population ranged from 6.2% to 7.5% and averaged 6.7% in the vildagliptin group and 6.8% in the placebo group. Patients were randomized to treatment with vildagliptin 50 mg or placebo once daily for 52 weeks. The change in the HbA$_{1c}$ level was -0.2% in the vildagliptin group and 0.1% in the placebo group; the difference between groups was 0.3%. Fasting plasma glucose and postprandial plasma glucose all improved with vildagliptin compared with placebo. The patients' mean body weight decreased by 0.5 kg with vildagliptin therapy and increased by 0.2 kg with placebo therapy. Both drug therapies were well tolerated.

Patients who were inadequately controlled with a sulfonylurea were treated with either vildagliptin or placebo in another multicenter, randomized, double-blind, placebo-controlled study. All 515 type 2 diabetes patients enrolled in this trial received glimepiride 4 mg once daily plus their assigned study medication for 24 weeks. The vildagliptin was administered either as 50 mg once daily or 50 mg twice daily. Both vildagliptin doses were better than placebo in improving the patients' HbA_{1c} level. The between-group difference (vildagliptin – placebo) for HbA_{1c} was -0.6% with vildagliptin 50 mg once daily and -0.7% with vildagliptin 50 mg twice daily ($P<0.001$ vs placebo).

The efficacy of vildagliptin was compared with acarbose in drug-naïve patients with type 2 diabetes in a multicenter, randomized, double-blind, parallel-arm study. Patients were given either vildagliptin 50 mg twice daily (n=441) or acarbose (n=220) given in three equally divided doses (up to 300 mg daily) for 24 weeks. The average baseline HbA_{1c} level in both groups was 8.6%. At the end of 24 weeks, the adjusted mean change from baseline was -1.4% in the vildagliptin group and -1.3% in the acarbose group. The decrease in plasma glucose was -1.2 mmol/L with vildagliptin and -1.5 mmol/L with acarbose. The body weight of the vildagliptin group remained unchanged (-0.4 +/- 0.1 kg) and decreased by 1.7 +/- 0.2 kg in the acarbose group.

Adverse reactions reported in the clinical trials have included cough, nasopharyngitis, headache, hypoglycemia, dizziness, dyspepsia, nausea, constipation, and diarrhea. It had no impact on the patient's weight in the majority of studies.

DIABETIC FOOT ULCER

Pexiganan

Pexiganan is being developed as a topical cream for the treatment of diabetic foot ulcers. It is a 22 amino acid-containing peptide that has activity against both gram-negative and gram-positive bacteria, including methicillin-resistant *Staphylococcus aureus* (MRSA).

Its mechanism of action is disruption of the integrity of the bacteria's cell membrane. Pexiganan is believed to have a low potential for induction of resistance and no cross-resistance with existing antimicrobial agents.

Results from phase III comparative trials with oral ofloxacin found no significant difference between the bacteriological eradication rate with both treatments in patients with mildly infected diabetic foot ulcers; the combined overall bacteriological eradication rate from the two clinical trials was 66% with pexiganan 1% cream and 82% with the oral ofloxacin. The topical pexiganan 1% cream was applied to the infected site and the ofloxacin 400 mg was taken orally twice daily for 14 to 28 days.

No significant adverse reactions have been reported with topical pexiganan. The incidence of adverse reactions with the pexiganan therapy was lower than the incidence reported with the ofloxacin therapy in the comparative clinical trial. Adverse reactions reported in these clinical trials have included insomnia, diarrhea, headache, pain, nausea, rash, vesiculobullous rash, cellulitis, and osteomyelitis.

DIABETIC MACULAR EDEMA AND DIABETIC RETINOPATHY

Pegaptanib

Pegaptanib is approved for the treatment of patients with neovascular (wet) age-related macular degeneration. It is also under development (phase III) for the treatment of diabetic macular edema and diabetic retinopathy.

Pegaptanib is a selective vascular endothelial growth factor (VEGF) antagonist. This polyethylene glycol-conjugated oligonucleotide binds to the major soluble human VEG isoform $VEGF_{165}$ with high specificity and selectivity, and inhibits $VEGF_{165}$ binding to all three of its receptors (VEGF-R1, VEGF-R2, Npn-1).

Changes in VEGF concentrations are thought to contribute to the progression of the neovascular form of age-related macular degeneration. The binding of pegaptanib to

VEGF prevents the interaction of VEGF with its receptors on the surface of endothelial cells, reducing endothelial cell proliferation, vascular leakage, and new blood vessel formation. Similar effects are thought to occur in patients with diabetic macular edema.

Pegaptanib was assessed in two pivotal phase II/III randomized, double-blind, placebo-controlled, dose-finding studies, enrolling 1,190 patients with neovascular age-related macular degeneration. One study enrolled patients from 58 sites in the United States and Canada, and the other enrolled patients from 59 sites in Europe, Israel, Australia, and South America. Both studies enrolled patients ≥50 years (mean age 77 years) with active subfoveal choroidal neovascularization secondary to exudative neovascular age-related macular degeneration. Best-corrected visual acuity was between 20/40 and 20/320 in the study eye and at least 20/800 in the fellow eye. Patients with all angiographic subtypes of lesions were enrolled, and lesions with a total size up to 12 optic-disk area (including blood, scar or atrophy, and neovascularization) were permitted. Patients were randomized to receive sham injections (298 patients) or pegaptanib 0.3 mg (295 patients), 1 mg (301 patients), or 3 mg (296 patients) as an intravitreal injection every 6 weeks for 54 weeks. All pegaptanib injection volumes were 100 microliters. Patients receiving sham injections underwent the same ocular antisepsis procedure and received injected subconjunctival anesthetic, but rather than the intravitreal injection these patients had an identical syringe (without needle) pressed against the eye wall to mimic the active doses. The efficacy analysis included 1,186 patients; 92% of enrolled patients completed the full study and a mean 8.5 treatments out of a possible 9 were received across all treatment arms. The primary endpoint was the percent of patients losing less than 15 letters of visual acuity by week 54 on the Early Treatment of Diabetic Retinopathy Study (ETDRS) chart.

In the combined population, the percentage of patients achieving the primary endpoint was more favorable for each pegaptanib dosage group compared with placebo ($P< 0.05$). A loss of fewer than 15 letters was observed at 54 weeks in 206 of 294 (70%) treated with pegaptanib 0.3 mg ($P<0.001$), 213 of 300 (71%) treated with pegaptanib 1 mg ($P<0.001$), and 193 of 296 (65%) treated with pegaptanib 3 mg ($P=0.03$), compared with 164 of 295 (55%) assigned sham injections. In one study, less than 15 letters of visual acuity were lost by 73.2% of patients treated with the 0.3 mg dose of pegaptanib and 75.3% of patients treated with the 1 mg dose. In the other study, less than 15 letters of visual acuity were lost by 67.4% of patients treated with the 0.3 mg dose. At the 0.3 mg dose of pegaptanib, less than 3 lines of vision were lost by 70% of the pegaptanib-treated patients compared with 55% of the placebo-treated patients ($P<0.05$). In addition, more patients at this dose compared with the placebo group gained 15 letters of visual acuity (6% vs. 2%, $P<0.05$) and maintained or gained vision (33% vs. 23%, $P<0.05$). Pegaptanib demonstrated similar effects at each dose and in all subtypes of neovascular age-related macular degeneration. Severe vision loss (loss of 30 letters or more or six lines on the study eye chart) occurred in 22% of sham injection recipients compared with 10% of patients treated with pegaptanib 0.3 mg ($P<0.001$), 8% treated with pegaptanib 1 mg ($P<0.001$), and 14% treated with pegaptanib 3 mg ($P=0.01$).

At one year, approximately 1,050 patients were re-randomized for a total study duration of 102 weeks. Patients treated initially with pegaptanib were re-randomized to either stop therapy or continue with the same pegaptanib regimen. Patients initially in the placebo group were re-randomized to stop therapy, continue sham injections, or receive pegaptanib at one of the three doses. Patients continuing therapy in Year 2 received a mean of 16 treatments out of a possible 17 overall. Pegaptanib was less effective during the second year. Loss of less than 15 letters from baseline to week 102 occurred in 38 of 67 (57%) treated with pegaptanib 0.3 mg compared with 30 of 54 (56%) treated with sham injections in one study, and 40 of 66 (61%) treated with pegaptanib 0.3 mg compared with 18 of 53 (34%) treated with sham injections in the other study.

Pegaptanib has also been assessed in a randomized, double-blind, phase II study enrolling 172 patients with diabetic macular edema involving the center of the macula and best correct visual acuity between 20/50 and 20/320 in the study eye. Patients received intravitreous pegaptanib 0.3 mg, 1 mg, or 3 mg, or sham injection at study entry, Week 6, and Week 12. At final assessment at Week 36, median visual acuity was better in the pegaptanib-treated eyes compared with the sham-treated eyes. A gain of at least 10 letters in visual acuity (approximately two lines) was observed in 34% of patients treated with the 0.3-mg dose compared with 10% in the sham treatment group ($P=0.003$). Photocoagulation was deemed necessary in 25% of patients in the 0.3 mg group compared with 48% in the sham treatment group ($P=0.04$).

The most common adverse effects associated with pegaptanib therapy have included anterior chamber inflammation, blurred vision, cataracts, conjunctival hemorrhage, corneal edema, eye discharge, eye irritation, eye pain, hypertension, increased intraocular pressure, ocular discomfort, punctate keratitis, reduced visual acuity, visual disturbance, vitreous floaters, and vitreous opacities in patients with neovascular (wet) age-related macular degeneration.

Ranibizumab

Ranibizumab is also approved for the treatment of patients with neovascular (wet) age-related macular degeneration. It is also under development (phase III) for the treatment of diabetic macular edema and retinal vascular occlusion.

Ranibizumab is the antigen-binding fragment of an antivascular endothelial growth factor (VEGF) antibody. This antibody is capable of binding to the receptor binding site of active forms of VEGF-A, including the biologically active VEGF110. VEGF-A has been shown to cause neovascularization and leakage in animal models of ocular angiogenesis. Like pegaptanib, these changes are thought to contribute to the progression of the neovascular form of age-related macular degeneration. The binding of ranibizumab to VEGF-A prevents the interaction of VEGF-A with its receptors (VEGFR1 and VEGFR2) on the surface of endothelial cells, reducing endothelial cell proliferation, vascular leakage, and new blood vessel formation. Similar effects are thought to occur in patients with diabetic macular edema.

Ranibizumab has been assessed in a six-month open-label study enrolling 64 patients with primary or recurrent predominantly or minimally classic subfoveal choroidal neovascularization due to age-related macular degeneration. In the first part of the study, patients were randomized to monthly intravitreal ranibizumab for three months (four injections of 0.3 mg [25 patients] or one injection of 0.3 mg followed by three injections of 0.5 mg [28 patients]) or usual care (11 patients). Randomization was stratified based on investigator's screening assessment of those with predominantly classic lesions (50% or more classic choroidal neovascularization) and no prior photodynamic therapy; minimally classic (<50% classic choroidal neovascularization) and no prior photodynamic therapy; and previously treated with photodynamic therapy.

In the second part of the study, subjects could continue their regimen for three additional months or crossover to the alternative treatment. Sixty-two patients completed the six-month study. Twenty of 25 (80%) randomized to ranibizumab 0.3 mg and 22 of 28 (79%) randomized to 0.5 mg ranibizumab in the first part of the study continued on that treatment in the second part; nine of 11 (82%) randomized to usual care crossed over to ranibizumab in the second part. After four ranibizumab injections (day 98), mean visual acuity had increased 9.4±13.3 and 9.1±17.2 letters in the 0.3 and 0.5 mg groups, respectively, but had decreased 5.1±9.6 letters with usual care. At day 98, two of 53 ranibizumab-treated patients (3.8%) had lost 15 or more letters from baseline compared with two of 11 usual-care patients (18.2%). The percentage of patients with reduction in visual acuity to 20/200 or worse was 45.5% in the usual-care group (95% CI 16.7%-76.6%), compared with 24% in the 0.3-mg group (95% CI 9.4%-45.1%) and 10.7% in the 0.5 mg group (95% CI 2.3%-28.2%). In the second part (Day 210), visual acuity had increased from baseline 12.8±14.7 and 15±14.2 letters in subjects continuing on ranibizumab 0.3 and 0.5 mg, respectively. Visual acuity improved by 15 letters or more from baseline in 26% (Day 98) and 45% (Day 210) of patients initially randomized to and continuing on ranibizumab therapy. No patient in the usual-care group had a 15-letter or greater improvement in visual acuity at Day 98. Angiographic results revealed growth of choroidal neovascularization by at least 0.3 disc diameters from baseline in two of 25 patients (8%) in the 0.3-mg group and eight of 27 patients (29.6%) in the 0.5-mg group, compared with four of 10 patients (40%) in the usual-care group (P=0.0428 for 0.3 mg vs usual care).

The MARINA study is a long-term study assessing ranibizumab in 716 patients with minimally classic (264 eyes) or occult (451 eyes) choroidal neovascularization. Patients received ranibizumab 0.3 mg, ranibizumab 0.5 mg, or sham injection monthly for two years. At one year, 95% of subjects receiving ranibizumab 0.5 mg lost <15 letters of visual acuity compared with 62% of sham-treated patients (P<0.0001; estimated difference 32%, 95% CI 26%-39%). At two years, 90% of ranibizumab 0.5-mg treated patients lost <15 letters of visual acuity compared with 53% of sham-treated patients (P<0.01; estimated difference 37%, 95% CI 29%-44%). A gain of 15 letters or more of visual acuity was achieved in 4% of sham-treated patients compared with 33% of ranibizumab 0.5-mg treated patients at two years (P<0.01; estimated difference 29%, 95% CI 23%-35%). The mean change in visual acuity at two years was a loss of 14.9 letters in the sham group compared with a gain of 5.5 letters in the ranibizumab 0.5-mg group (P<0.01; estimated difference 21.1 letters; 95% CI 18.1-24.1).

The most common adverse effects associated with ranibizumab therapy have included iris and uveal tract inflammation, iridocyclitis, iritis, conjunctival hemorrhage, eye pain, injection-site reactions (erythema, hemorrhage), increased intraocular pressure, and reduced visual acuity in patients with neovascular (wet) age-related macular degeneration.

Ruboxistaurin

Ruboxistaurin is an oral protein kinase C β-selective inhibitor in phase III clinical development for the treatment of diabetic macular edema and in preregistration for the treatment of diabetic retinopathy. Increased protein kinase C β activity induces retinal vascular permeability and neovascularization. Inhibition of this enzyme reduces diabetes-induced retinal vascular permeability and ischemia-induced retinal neovascularization in animal models.

The safety and efficacy of ruboxistaurin in the treatment of patients with diabetic macular edema were evaluated using a multicenter, double-masked, randomized, placebo-controlled study. The study enrolled 686 patients with diabetic macular edema. Patients were randomly assigned to oral treatment with placebo or ruboxistaurin (4, 16, or 32 mg/day) for 30 months. The primary outcome was progression to sight-threatening diabetic macular edema or application of focal/grid photocoagulation for diabetic macular edema. At the end of 30 months, the delay in progression to the primary outcome was not significant (ruboxistaurin 32 mg vs placebo, $P=0.14$ [unadjusted]; 95% CI 0.53-1.0; $P=0.06$). However, application of focal/grid photocoagulation prior to progression to sight-threatening diabetic macular edema varied by site, and a secondary analysis of progression to sight-threatening diabetic macular edema alone showed a reduction in progression with ruboxistaurin 32 mg compared with placebo ($P=0.054$ [unadjusted]; 95% CI 0.47-0.93; $P=0.02$).

A pilot study of 123 patients with type 2 diabetes and persistent albuminuria (despite therapy with renin-angiotensin system inhibitors) treated with ruboxistaurin 32 mg/day for one year had a favorable impact on their nephropathy. At the end of the year, there was no difference in between-group differences in the albumin-to-creatinine ratio and the estimated glomerular filtration rate, but the study was not powered for this type of analysis. There was a trend for reduction in the albumin-to-creatinine ratio and appeared to be a benefit in stabilizing the estimated glomerular filtration rate. Another group of patients (n=1157) being treated for diabetic eye disease were also included in an evaluation of the impact of ruboxistaurin on kidney function. The median follow-up period was 33 to 39 months. During this time, both the placebo-treated patients and the ruboxistaurin-treated patients did not differ in the rate of doubling of serum creatinine, development of advanced chronic kidney disease, and death. The frequency of doubling of serum creatinine was 6%, progression to advanced chronic kidney disease was 4.1%, and death was 4.1% in the

combined placebo and ruboxistaurin groups. Based on these results, prospective trials in patients with diabetic nephropathy will need to be conducted to determine the efficacy and safety of ruboxistaurin in this patient population.

The adverse reactions associated with ruboxistaurin therapy have included cough, headache, hypertension, atrioventricular block, asthma, dysuria, and nasopharyngitis.

DIABETIC NEPHROPATHIES

Aliskiren

Aliskiren is approved for the treatment of hypertension, alone or in combination with other antihypertensive agents. It is still undergoing development for the prevention of diabetic nephropathy.

Aliskiren is an orally active, direct renin inhibitor that decreases plasma renin activity and inhibits the conversion of angiotensinogen to angiotensin I. The results of the efficacy clinical trials for aliskiren in the prevention of diabetic nephropathy are not available at this time.

The common adverse reactions reported with aliskiren therapy in the treatment of hypertension have included diarrhea, rash, headache, nasopharyngitis, dizziness, fatigue, upper respiratory tract infection, back pain, and cough.

Valsartan

Valsartan is approved for the treatment of hypertension (alone or in combination with other antihypertensive agents), treatment of heart failure (NYHA class II-IV), and post-myocardial infarction to reduce cardiovascular mortality. It is still undergoing development for the prevention of diabetic nephropathy.

Valsartan is an orally active, angiotensin receptor blocker. Valsartan is able to block the vasoconstrictive and aldosterone-secreting effects of angiotensin II by selectively blocking the binding of angiotensin II to the AT_1 receptor. It is thought to decrease the risk of diabetic nephropathy, similar to the improvements seen with angiotensin converting enzyme inhibitors.

The common adverse reactions reported with valsartan therapy in the treatment of hypertension have included fatigue, abdominal pain, dry cough, orthostatic effects, and dizziness.

DIABETIC NEUROPATHIES

Dextromethorphan/quinidine
The combination of dextromethorphan and quinidine is being evaluated for the oral treatment of various pain conditions, including diabetic neuropathy. Dextromethorphan is a dextrorotatory analogue of levorphanol and is a noncompetitive N-methyl-D-aspartate (NMDA) receptor antagonist. Dextromethorphan also appears to be an agonist of the omega-1 receptor that produces a suppression of the release of excitatory neurotransmitters and effect on the N-type calcium channels. The quinidine component of the drug regimen is used to take advantage of a drug-drug interaction. Quinidine decreases the metabolism of the dextromethorphan and its metabolite (dextrorphan) by inhibition of the cytochrome P450 2D6 isozyme. Administration of low-dose quinidine results in a boost in the plasma levels of the dextromethorphan and dextrorphan; a situation similar to the use of ritonavir in HIV-drug regimens.

In an open-label study with 33 adults with painful diabetic peripheral neuropathy, the combination of dextromethorphan and quinidine sulfate was able to decrease the patients' pain and discomfort after 29 days of therapy. The starting dose of drug was one capsule containing dextromethorphan 30 mg and quinidine sulfate 30 mg per day. The dose could be titrated at weekly intervals to a maximum dose of 4 capsules per day. Additional ongoing studies are assessing a combination with a lower quinidine dose to minimize the risk of adverse cardiovascular effects.

The most commonly reported adverse reactions in the clinical trials with the combination of dextromethorphan and quinidine were nausea, dizziness, and headache.

Lacosamide
Lacosamide, the R-enantiomer of 2-acetamido-N-benzyl-3-methoxypropionamide, is an oral anticonvulsant and analgesic agent from the acetamide class that is being evaluated for the treatment of diabetic neuropathies, migraine, fibromyalgia, and as an adjunctive therapy in partial onset seizures. It is listed as being in the preregistration phase for the treatment of diabetic neuropathies and epilepsy.

Lacosamide works by modulating the sodium channel by selective enhancement of sodium channel slow inactivation without affecting its fast inactivation and/or modulation of collapsing-response protein (CRMP)-2. The exact mechanism of action for its anticonvulsant and analgesic activity is unknown.

A pooled analysis of the phase II (SP614) and phase III (SP742, SP743, SP768) clinical trials for the treatment of diabetic neuropathic pain is available but unpublished. All the clinical trials were placebo-controlled and demonstrated that the lacosamide 400 mg therapy was better than placebo in producing a meaningful reduction in pain in three of the four studies. A meta-analysis of the four studies found the mean reduction in pain score (primary outcome) was -2.14 for the lacosamide group and -1.57 for the control group. General reduction in pain (secondary outcome) was achieved in all four studies.

The most commonly reported adverse reactions associated with lacosamide therapy have included dizziness, nausea, diarrhea, blurred vision, headache, tremor, nasopharyngitis, and vertigo.

Mexiletine

Oral mexiletine has been available for years for the treatment of arrhythmias. It has also been used as an alternative form of therapy for the treatment of diabetic neuropathy.

The analgesic activity of mexiletine may be related to membrane stabilization as a result of the antagonism of the Na+-channel. Several of the published clinical trials have shown a trend for some benefit in the treatment of pain, paresthesia, and global assessment, but the majority did not reach statistical significance. The patients that might benefit the most from mexiletine therapy are those with burning or stabbing pain.

Mexiletine needs to be used with caution in patients with underlying cardiac abnormalities (ie, arrhythmias, angina, chest pain) because of the risk of worsening some arrhythmias or exacerbating some cardiovascular conditions. The most common adverse reactions associated with the use of mexiletine include nausea, vomiting, dyspepsia, dysphagia, lightheadedness, dizziness, tremor, and ataxia.

Tapentadol

Tapentadol is an oral analgesic agent in phase III clinical development that works by inhibiting norepinephrine reuptake and as an agonist at the mu-opioid receptor. The drug is being developed for the treatment of postoperative and chronic pain, including diabetic neuropathy.

A clinical trial using an extended release formulation is ongoing to assess the efficacy of tapentadol in the treatment of patients with moderate to severe pain from diabetic peripheral neuropathy in a 12-week study. The extended-release formulation will be given twice daily with the total daily dose ranging from 100 mg to 250 mg per day.

The most commonly reported adverse reactions associated with tapentadol therapy have included nausea, vomiting, constipation, somnolence, and dizziness.

Topiramate

Topiramate is an oral antiepileptic drug approved for the treatment of epilepsy and migraine headaches and in phase III development for the treatment of diabetic neuropathy and obesity. Its exact mechanism of action in these various conditions is unknown, but is thought to be related to its ability to block voltage-dependent sodium channels; augment the activity of the neurotransmitter gamma-aminobutyrate at some subtypes of the GABA-A receptor; antagonize the AMPA/kainate subtype of the glutamate receptor; and inhibit the carbonic anhydrase enzyme, particularly isozymes II and IV.

Like mexiletine, some of the placebo-controlled clinical trials have shown no statistical benefit from the topiramate therapy for the treatment of the patient's diabetic neuropathy, however, in a subsequent clinical trial, other investigators were able to show a benefit with the topiramate therapy. The primary endpoint in these studies was the change in pain intensity at baseline and at follow-up visits using the 100-mm pain visual analog scale. The reason for the difference in these results may be because the negative studies had a much higher response to the placebo therapy than did the positive study. In addition, the patients enrolled in the positive study had a higher baseline pain score than those enrolled in the negative studies. Based on this information, it appears that topiramate therapy may have a role in the treatment of patients with more severe diabetic neuropathy.

The positive study was a 12-week, multicenter, randomized, double-blind placebo-controlled clinical trial that enrolled 323 patients with painful diabetic neuropathy with a pain visual analog score of at least 40 mm (on a 0 to 100 scale with 0 representing no pain and 100 representing the worst possible pain). Patients were randomized to treatment with placebo or topiramate and the dose of the study medication was titrated based on their clinical response. The starting dose of the topiramate was 25 mg at bedtime and titrated up to 400 mg/day or the maximum tolerated dose over 8 weeks. At the end of Week 12, the topiramate therapy reduced the pain visual score from 68 mm to 46.2 mm, while the placebo decreased the score from 69.1 mm to 54 mm ($P=0.038$). A clinical response, defined as a >30% reduction in the pain visual score, was achieved by 49.5% with topiramate and 33.9% with placebo ($P=0.004$). A 50% reduction in the visual pain scale was achieved by 35.6% with topiramate and 21.1% with placebo ($P=0.005$). The topiramate therapy was also associated with a reduction in worst pain intensity and improvement in sleep disruption.

The other focus for topiramate is the treatment of obese patients with type 2 diabetes. These clinical trials are designed to determine if the weight loss observed with topiramate in the treatment of patients with epilepsy will occur in patients with diabetes and produce an improvement in glycemic control. The published studies have shown a decrease in body weight and fat and an improvement in HbA_{1c}.

One-hundred and eleven (111) obese patients with type 2 diabetes were enrolled in a randomized, placebo-controlled study. The inclusion criteria included a body mass index >27 kg/m^2 and an HbA_{1c} between 6.5% and 11%. All patients had to be treated with diet and exercise alone or in combination with metformin. The starting dose of the controlled-release study medication was 25 mg. The dose could be titrated up to 175 mg/day during the seven-week titration phase and maintained during the nine-week maintenance phase. At the end of the 16-week study period, the placebo group had lost 2.5 kg (2.3%) of body weight and the topiramate group had lost 6 kg (5.8%; $P<0.001$). The proportion of patients who lost ≥10% of their baseline weight at Week 16 was 19% in the placebo group and 50% in the topiramate group ($P<0.001$). Waist circumference was reduced by 2.3 cm in the placebo group and 4.2 cm in the topiramate group. HBA_{1c} improved from 7.4% in the placebo group to 7.1%, and from 7.6% to 6.7% in the topiramate group ($P<0.001$).

The most common adverse reactions associated with topiramate therapy include paresthesia, somnolence, fatigue, nervousness, anorexia, weight loss, dizziness, difficulty with memory, concentration or attention, confusion, and depression.

Table 21.1. Agents Under Development for the Treatment of Diabetes and Its Complications

Generic Name	Manufacturer	Phase of Development	Indication	Mechanism of Action
ABT 279	Abbott Laboratories	I	Diabetes	CD26 antigen antagonist
ABT 894	NeuroSearch/ Abbott Laboratories	II	Diabetic neuropathies	Nicotinic receptor modulator
ADL 5859	Adolor Corporation	II	Diabetic neuropathies	Opioid delta receptor agonist
Aflibercept	Regeneron Pharmaceuticals	I	Diabetic macular edema	Placental growth factor inhibitor; vascular endothelial growth factor A antagonist
AGN 203818	Allergan/ACADIA Pharmaceuticals	II	Diabetic neuropathies	Alpha adrenergic receptor agonists
AI 401 – oral insulin	AutoImmune	III	Diabetes, type 1 (prevention)	Ornithine decarboxylase stimulant; phosphokinase stimulant tyrosine aminotransferase stimulant
AKP 020	University of British Columbia	II	Diabetes, type 2	Insulin sensitizer
AKP 111	Akesis Pharmaceuticals	I	Diabetes, type 2	Glucose uptake stimulant, insulin sensitizer
Albiglutide	Human Genome Sciences	II	Diabetes, type 2	Glucagon-like peptide-1 agonist
Aleglitazar	Roche	II	Diabetes, type 2	Peroxisome proliferator-activated receptor alpha agonist; peroxisome proliferator-activated receptor gamma agonist
Aliskiren	Novartis	III*	Diabetic nephropathies	Renin inhibitor
Alogliptin	Takeda	Preregistration	Diabetes, type 2	CD26 antigen antagonist
AMG 221	Biovitrum	I	Diabetes, type 2	11-beta hydroxysteroid dehydrogenase inhibitor
AMG 222	Alantos Pharmaceuticals/ Amgen	II	Diabetes, type 2	CD26 antigen antagonist
AMG 477	Amgen	I	Diabetes, type 2	Glucagon receptor antagonist

Table 21.1.   Agents Under Development for the Treatment of Diabetes and Its Complications

ATG 002	CoMentis	I	Diabetic foot ulcer	Angiogenesis-inducing agent; nicotinic receptor agonist
AVE 0010	Zealand Pharma	II	Diabetes, type 2	Glucagon-like peptide-1 receptor agonist
Balaglitazone	Dr. Reddy's Laboratories	III	Diabetes, type 2	Insulin sensitizer; peroxisome proliferator-activated receptor gamma agonist
Bevasiranib	Opko Health	II	Diabetic macular edema	RNA interference; vascular endothelial growth factor antagonist
BHT 3021	Bayhill Therapeutics	I	Diabetes, type 1	Immunosuppressant
BI 1356 BS	Boehringer Ingelheim	II/III	Diabetes, type 2	CD26 antigen antagonists
Bicifadine	Wyeth	II	Diabetic neuropathies	Norepinephrine reuptake inhibitor; serotonin reuptake inhibitor
Bromocriptine	VeroScience LLC	III*	Diabetes, type 2	Dopamine D2 receptor agonist
Canakinumab	Novartis	II/III	Diabetes, type 2	Interleukin 1-β antagonist
Capsaicin topical	NeurogesX	II*	Diabetic neuropathies	Nociceptin receptor antagonist; TRPV cation channel agonist
CE 326597	Pfizer	II	Diabetes, type 2	Unknown
Cetilistat	Alizyme	II	Diabetes, type 2	Lipase inhibitor
Clonidine topical gel	Arcion Therapeutics	II*	Diabetic neuropathies	Alpha 2 adrenergic receptor agonist
Dapagliflozin	Bristol-Myers Squibb	III	Diabetes, type 2	Sodium glucose co-transporter type 2 inhibitor
Dapagliflozin/ metformin	Bristol-Myers Squibb	III	Diabetes, type 2	Sodium glucose co-transporter type 2 inhibitor; insulin sensitizer
Dexamethasone ophthalmic	Allergan	III*	Diabetic macular edema	Glucocorticoid receptor agonist

Table 21.1. Agents Under Development for the Treatment of Diabetes and Its Complications

Dextromethorphan/ quinidine	Center for Neurologic Study	III*	Diabetic neuropathies	Cytochrome P450 inhibitor; NMDA receptor antagonist; sigma-1 receptor agonist
Diabetic retinal therapeutic	VitreoRetinal Technologies	III	Diabetic retinopathy	Unknown
DIO 902	Cortendo	II	Diabetes, type 2	Lanosterol 14 alpha-demethylase inhibitor; Steroid 11-beta-hydroxylase inhibitor
Exenatide LAR	Alkermes	III*	Diabetes	Glucagon-like peptide-1 agonist
FG 3019	FibroGen	I	Diabetic nephropathies	Connective tissue growth factor inhibitor
Fibroblast growth factor 1	CardioVascular Bio Therapeutics	I	Diabetic foot ulcer	Fibroblast growth factor agonist
Fluocinolone acetonide ophthalmic	pSivida Inc	III*	Diabetic macular edema	Arachidonic acid antagonist; glucocorticoid receptor agonist
Gabapentin enacarbil	XenoPort	II*	Diabetic neuropathies	GABA receptor agonist
Gabapentin extended-release	Depomed	II*	Diabetic neuropathies	GABA receptor agonist
GAM 501	Tissue Repair Company	II	Diabetic foot ulcer	Gene transference; platelet derived growth factor; BB agonist
Gentamicin implant	Innocoll	II*	Diabetic foot ulcer	Protein 30s ribosomal subunit inhibitor
GLY 230	Exocell	I	Diabetic complications	Unknown
GSK 189075	Kissei Pharmaceutical	II	Diabetes, type 2	Sodium glucose co-transporter type 2 inhibitor
GSK 376501	GlaxoSmithKline	I	Diabetes, type 2	Peroxisome proliferator-activated receptor gamma agonist
GSK 625019	GlaxoSmithKline	I	Diabetes, type 2; Metabolic syndrome	Peroxisome proliferator-activated receptor agonist
HE 3286	Hollis-Eden Pharmaceuticals	I/II	Diabetes, type 2	Insulin sensitizer NF-kappa B inhibitor

Table 21.1.	Agents Under Development for the Treatment of Diabetes and Its Complications			
ICO 007	Isis Pharmaceuticals	I	Diabetic macular edema	Paf kinase inhibitor; RNA antagonist
INCB 13739	Incyte Corporation	II	Diabetes, type 2	11-beta-hydroxysteroid dehydrogenase inhibitor
INCB 19602	Incyte Corporation	I	Diabetes, type 2	HM74 protein agonist
INCB 20817	Incyte Corporation	I	Diabetes, type 2	Hydroxysteroid dehydrogenase inhibitor
INCB 3284	Incyte Corporation	II	Insulin resistance	CCR2 antagonist Chemokine receptor antagonist
Insulin glargine	sanofi-aventis	Preregistration*	Diabetic retinopathy	Insulin analog
Insulin inhalation	Baxter Healthcare	I	Diabetes	Insulin
Insulin inhalation	Coremed	I	Diabetes	Insulin
Insulin inhalation	QDose / MicroDose Technologies	I	Diabetes	Insulin
Insulin inhalation	MannKind Corporation	III	Diabetes	Insulin
Insulin oral	Coremed	I	Diabetes	Insulin
Insulin oral	Generex Biotechnology Corporation	III	Diabetes	Insulin - buccal
INT 131	Amgen	II	Diabetes, type 2	Peroxisome proliferator-activated receptor gamma agonist; Peroxisome proliferator-activated receptor modulator
INV 064	InVasc Therapeutics	II	Diabetes, type 2	Unknown
KRP 104	ActivX Biosciences Kyorin Pharmaceutical	I	Diabetes, type 2	CD26 antigen antagonist
Lacosamide	University of Houston	Preregistration	Diabetic neuropathies	CRMP2 protein regulator; sodium channel antagonist
Larazotide	University of Maryland	I	Diabetes, type 1	Membrane permeability inhibitor; zonulin antagonist
Liraglutide	Novo Nordisk	Preregistration	Diabetes, type 2	Glucagon receptor antagonist; glucagon-like peptide-1 agonist
MCC 257	Mitsubishi Pharma Corporation	II	Diabetic neuropathies	Unknown

Table 21.1.	Agents Under Development for the Treatment of Diabetes and Its Complications			
Mecamylamine ophthalmic	CoMentis	II*	Diabetic macular edema	Nicotinic receptor antagonist
Mexiletine	Boehringer Ingelheim	III*	Diabetic neuropathies	Neuromuscular blocking agent Sodium channel antagonist
Mitemcinal	Chugai Pharmaceuticals	II	Diabetic gastroparesis	Motilin agonist
MB 07803	Metabasis Therapeutics	II	Diabetes, type 2	Fructose bisphosphatase inhibitor; gluconeogenesis inhibitor
MBX 2982	Metabolex	I	Diabetes, type 2	GPR 119 protein agonist
Mitiglinide/ metformin	Kissei Pharmaceutical	III	Diabetes, type 2	Insulin sensitizer; potassium channel antagonist
MK 0893	Merck	II	Diabetes	Unknown
MK 0941	Merck	I	Diabetes	Unknown
MK 2662	Merck	I	Diabetes	Unknown
MK 8245	Merck	I	Diabetes	Unknown
MP 513	Mitsubishi Pharma	I	Diabetes, type 2	CD26 antigen antagonist
Netoglitazone	Mitsubishi Pharma	I	Diabetes, type 2	Insulin sensitizer; peroxisome proliferator-activated receptor agonist
NN 1250	Novo Nordisk	I	Diabetes, type 1 & 2	Ornithine decarboxylase stimulant; phosphokinase stimulant; protein tyrosine kinase stimulant
Nova 63035	Novagali Pharma	I	Diabetic macular edema	Steroid receptor agonist
Otelixizumab	Tolerx	II	Diabetes, type 1	CD3 antagonist; immunosuppressant
Pegaptanib	Gilead Sciences / OSI Pharmaceuticals	III*	Diabetic macular edema Diabetic retinopathy	Angiogenesis inhibitor; vascular endothelial growth factor antagonist
Pexiganan	MacroChem Corporation	III	Diabetic foot ulcer	Membrane permeability enhancer
PF 4603629	Pfizer	I	Diabetes	Unknown

Table 21.1. Agents Under Development for the Treatment of Diabetes and Its Complications

PHX 1149	Phenomix Corporation	II	Diabetes, type 2	CD26 antigen antagonist
PPM 201	Wyeth	I	Diabetes, type 2	Unknown
PPM 202	Wyeth	I	Diabetes, type 2	Unknown
PPM 204	Plexxikon / Wyeth	I	Diabetes, type 2	Peroxisome proliferator-activated receptor alpha agonist; peroxisome proliferator-activated receptor delta agonist; peroxisome proliferator-activated receptor gamma agonist
PS 433540	Bristol-Myers Squibb	I	Diabetic nephropathies	Angiotensin II receptor agonist: endothelin A receptor antagonist
Pyridoxamine	BioStratum	II	Diabetic nephropathies	Advanced glycation end product inhibitor
Ranibizumab	Genentech	III*	Diabetic macular edema	Vascular endothelial growth factor antagonist
Reboxetine	Pfizer	II	Diabetic neuropathies	Alpha 2 adrenergic receptor antagonist; norepinephrine reuptake inhibitor
Ruboxistaurin	Eli Lilly / Alcon	III Preregistration	Diabetic macular edema Diabetic retinopathy	Protein kinase C inhibitor
Saxagliptin	Bristol-Myers Squibb/ AstraZeneca	III	Diabetes, type 2	CD26 antigen antagonist
Saxagliptin / metformin	Bristol-Myers Squibb/ AstraZeneca	III	Diabetes, type 2	CD26 antigen antagonist; insulin sensitizer
SB 509	Sangamo BioSciences	II	Diabetic neuropathies	Gene transcription activated; vascular endothelial growth factor A agonist
SB 756050	GlaxoSmithKline	I	Diabetes, type 2	Unknown
Sergliflozin	Kissei Pharmaceutical GlaxoSmithKline	II	Obesity	Sodium glucose co-transporter type 2 inhibitor

Table 21.1. Agents Under Development for the Treatment of Diabetes and Its Complications

Sirolimus ophthalmic	MacuSight	I*	Diabetic macular edema	B cell inhibitor; immunosuppressant MTOR inhibitor; T cell inhibitor
Sodelgitazar	GlaxoSmithKline	II	Diabetes, type 2; Metabolic syndrome	Peroxisome proliferator-activated receptor agonist
Sonedenoson	New York University	II	Diabetic foot ulcer	Adenosine A2 receptor agonist
SSR 180575	sanofi-aventis	II	Diabetic neuropathies	Benzodiazepine receptor agonist
Succinobucol	AtheroGenics	III	Diabetes, type 2	Antioxidant; lipid peroxidation inhibitor; vascular cell adhesion molecule antagonist
Superoxide solution	Oculus Innovative Sciences	II	Diabetic foot ulcer	Membrane integrity antagonist
SYR 472	Takeda	II	Diabetes, type 2	CD26 antigen antagonist
TA 6666	Mitsubishi Tanabe	II	Diabetes, type 2	CD26 antigen antagonist
TA 7284	Mitsubishi Tanabe	I	Diabetes, type 2	Sodium glucose co-transporter type 2 inhibitor
Tagatose – Spherix	Spherix	III	Diabetes, type 2	Chelating agent
TAK 428	Takeda	II	Diabetic neuropathies	Nerve growth factor agonist
TAK 583	Takeda	II	Diabetic neuropathies	Unknown
Talactoferrin alfa	Agennix	II	Diabetic foot ulcer	Immunostimulant
Tapentadol	Grunenthal/Ortho-McNeil	III	Diabetic neuropathies	Norepinephrine reuptake inhibitor opioid mu receptor agonist
Teplizumab	MacroGenics/ Eli Lilly	II/III	Diabetes, type 1	CD3 antagonist
Topiramate	Johnson & Johnson	III*	Diabetic neuropathies	GABA receptor agonist; glutamate agonist; glutamate antagonist; sodium channel antagonist
Triamcinolone acetonide ophthalmic	SurModics	I*	Diabetic macular edema	Glucocorticosteroid receptor agonist

Table 21.1.	**Agents Under Development for the Treatment of Diabetes and Its Complications**			
TZP 101	Tranzyme	II	Gastroparesis	Ghrelin agonist ; growth hormone secretagogue receptor agonist
Valsartan	Novartis	III*	Diabetic nephropathies	Angiotensin II receptor antagonist
Vildagliptin	Novartis	Preregistration	Diabetes, type 2	CD26 antigen antagonist
Vildagliptin/ metformin	Novartis	Preregistration	Diabetes, type 2	CD26 antigen antagonist; Insulin sensitizer

*Active ingredient FDA-approved for another indication or in another dosage form.

References

New Medicines in Development Database: Diabetes [online database]. Pharmaceutical Research and Manufacturers of America. Available at http://www.phrma.org/. Accessed 14 May 2008.
Adis R&D Insight. Wolters Kluwer Health. Yardley, PA, 2008.

REFERENCES

Alogliptin

A study to evaluate SYR-322 plus pioglitazone HCl (Actos®), SYR-322 alone, or pioglitazone HCl alone for the treatment of type 2 diabetes. ClinicalTrials.gov (*http://clinicaltrials.gov*). Accessed 27 May 2008.

Covington P, Christopher R, Davenport M, Fleck P, Mekki QA, Wann ER, et al. Pharmacokinetic, pharmacodynamic, and tolerability profiles of the dipeptidyl peptidase-4 inhibitor alogliptin: A randomized, double-blind, placebo-controlled, multiple-dose study in adult patients with type 2 diabetes. *Clin Ther.* 2008;30(3):499-512.

Deacon CF. Alogliptin, a potent and selective dipeptidyl peptidase-IV inhibitor for the treatment of type 2 diabetes. *Curr Opin Investig Drugs.* 2008;9(4):402-13.

Long-term, open-label extension study to investigate the long-term safety in subjects with type 2 diabetes. ClinicalTrials.gov (*http://clinicaltrials.gov*) Accessed 27 May 2008.

Miller SA, Onge ELS, Taylor JR. DPP-IV inhibitors: A review of sitagliptin, vildagliptin, alogliptin, and saxagliptin. *Formulary* 2008;43(4):122-34.

Placebo-controlled study of the combination of SYR-322 and pioglitazone HCl in the treatment of type 2 diabetes. ClinicalTrials.gov (*http://clinicaltrials.gov*) Accessed 27 May 2008.

Study of SYR-322 combined with a sulfonylurea in the treatment of type 2 diabetes. ClinicalTrials.gov (*http://clinicaltrials.gov*) Accessed 27 May 2008.

Study of SYR-322 combined with pioglitazone in the treatment of type 2 diabetes. ClinicalTrials.gov (*http://clinicaltrials.gov*) Accessed 27 May 2008.

Study of SYR-322 in the treatment of type 2 diabetes. ClinicalTrials.gov (*http://clinicaltrials.gov*) Accessed 27 May 2008.

The effect of SYR-322 alone and in combination with pioglitazone on post-meal blood lipid levels in patients with type 2 diabetes. ClinicalTrials.gov (*http://clinicaltrials.gov*) Accessed 27 May 2008.

Thomas L, Eckhardt M, Langkopf E, Tadayyon M, Himmelsbach F, Mark M. (R)-8-(3-amino-piperidin-1-yl)-7-but-2-ynyl-3-methyl-1-(4-methyl-quinazolin-2-ylmethyl)-3,7-dihydro-purine-2,6-dione (BI 1356), a novel xanthine-based dipeptidyl peptidase-4 inhibitor, has a superior potency and longer duration of action compared with other dipeptidyl peptidase-4 inhibitors. *J Pharmacol Exp Ther.* 2008 Apr;325(1):175-82.

Balaglitazone
Efficacy and safety of treatment with balaglitazone in type 2 diabetes patients on stable insulin therapy (BALLET). ClinicalTrials.gov (*http://clinicaltrials.gov*) Accessed 2 June 2008.

Dapagliflozin
A phase III Study of BMS-512148 (dapagliflozin) in patients with type 2 diabetes who are not well controlled with diet and exercise. ClinicalTrials.gov (*http://clinicaltrials.gov*) Accessed 2 June 2008.

A Phase III Study of BMS-512148 (dapagliflozin) in patients with type 2 diabetes who are not well controlled on metformin alone. ClinicalTrials.gov (*http://clinicaltrials.gov*) Accessed 2 June 2008.

A pilot study of BMS-512148 in subjects with type 2 diabetes. ClinicalTrials.gov (*http://clinicaltrials.gov*) Accessed 2 June 2008.

Add-on to thiazolidinedione (TZD) failures. ClinicalTrials.gov (*http://clinicaltrials.gov*) Accessed 2 June 2008.

An efficacy and safety study of BMS-512148 in combination with metformin extended release tablets. ClinicalTrials.gov (*http://clinicaltrials.gov*) Accessed 2 June 2008.

Efficacy and safety of dapagliflozin in combination with glimepiride (a sulphonylurea) in type 2 diabetes patients. ClinicalTrials.gov (*http://clinicaltrials.gov*) Accessed 2 June 2008.

Efficacy and safety of dapagliflozin in combination with metformin in type 2 diabetes patients. ClinicalTrials.gov (*http://clinicaltrials.gov*) Accessed 2 June 2008.

Efficacy and safety of dapagliflozin, added to therapy of patients with type 2 diabetes with inadequate glycemic control on insulin. ClinicalTrials.gov (*http://clinicaltrials.gov*) Accessed 2 June 2008.

Feng Y, Zhang L, Komoroshki B, Pfister M. Population pharmacokinetic analysis of dapagliflozin in healthy and subjects with type 2 diabetes mellitus. [abstract] *Clin Pharmacol Ther.* 2008;83:S93.

Glycemic efficacy and renal safety study of dapagliflozin in subjects wwith type 2 diabetes mellitus and moderate renal impairment. ClinicalTrials.gov (*http://clinicaltrials.gov*) Accessed 2 June 2008.

Han S, Hagan DL, Taylor JR, Xin L, Meng W, Biller SA, et al. Dapagliflozin, a selective SGLT2 inhibitor, improves glucose homeostasis in normal and diabetic rats. *Diabetes.* 2008;57(6):1723-9.

Meng W, Ellsworth BA, Nirschi AA, McCann PJ, Patel M, Girotra RN, et al. Discovery of dapagliflozin: A potent, selective renal sodium-dependent glucose cotransporter 2 (SGLT2) inhibitor for the treatment of type 2 diabetes. *J Med Chem.* 2008;51(5):1145–49.

Exenatide LAR

A study to compare the glycemic effects, safety, and tolerability of exenatide once weekly to those of sitagliptin and a thiazolidinedione in subjects wwith type 2 diabetes treated with metformin (DURATION - 2). ClinicalTrials.gov (*http://clinicaltrials.gov*) Accessed 27 May 2008.

Effects of exenatide long-acting release on glucose control and safety in subjects with type 2 diabetes mellitus (DURATION - 1). ClinicalTrials.gov (*http://clinicaltrials.gov*) Accessed 27 May 2008.

Study examining exenatide long-acting release in subjects wwith type 2 diabetes. ClinicalTrials.gov (*http://clinicaltrials.gov*) Accessed 27 May 2008.

Liraglutide

Effect of liraglutide in combination with sulfonylurea (SU) on blood glucose control in subjects with type 2 diabetes. ClinicalTrials.gov (*http://clinicaltrials.gov*) Accessed June 2, 2008.

Effect of liraglutide on blood glucose control in subjects with type 2 diabetes (LEAD-4). ClinicalTrials.gov (*http://clinicaltrials.gov*) Accessed June 2, 2008.

Effect of liraglutide or exenatide added to an ongoing treatment on blood glucose control in subjects with type 2 diabetes (LEAD 6). ClinicalTrials.gov (*http://clinicaltrials.gov*) Accessed June 2, 2008.

Effect of liraglutide or glimepiride added to metformin on blood glucose control in subjects with type 2 diabetes. ClinicalTrials.gov *(http://clinicaltrials.gov)* Accessed June 2, 2008.

Elbrond B, Jakobsen G, Larsen S, Agerso H, Jensen EB, Rolan P, et al. Pharmacokinetics, pharmacodynamics, safety, and tolerability of a single-dose of NN2211, a long-acting glucagon-like peptide 1 derivative, in healthy male subjects. *Diabetes Care.* 2002;25:1398-1404.

Kapitza C, Flint A, Spitzer H, Hindsberger C, Zdravkovic M. The effect of three different injection sites on the pharmacokinetics of the once-daily human GLP-1 analogue liraglutide [abstract]. ADA 2008. Abstract 2146-PO.

Madsbad S, Schmitz O, Ranstam J, Jakobsen G, Matthews DR, NN2211-1310 International Study Group. Improved glycemic control with no weight increase in patients with type 2 diabetes after once-daily treatment with the long-acting glucagon-like peptide 1 analog liraglutide (NN2211). *Diabetes Care.* 2004;27:1335-1342.

Marre M, Shaw J, Brandle M, Debakar WMW, Kamaruddin NA, Strand J, et al. Liraglutide, a once-daily human GLP-1 analog, added to a sulfonylurea (SU) offers significantly better glycemic control and favorable weight change compared with rosiglitazone and SU combination therapy in subjects with type 2 diabetes [abstract]. ADA 2008. Abstract 13-OR.

Nauck MA, Frid A, Hermansen K, Shah NS, Tankova T, Mitha IH, et al. Liraglutide, a once-daily human GLP-1 analog, in type 2 diabetes provides similar glycemic control with reduced body weight compared with glimepiride when added to metformin [abstract]. ADA 2008. Abstract 504-P.

Nauck MA, Hompesch M, Filipczak R, Le TDT, Zdravkovic M, Gumprecht J. Five weeks of treatment with the GLP-1 analogue liraglutide improves glycemic control and lower body weight in subjects with type 2 diabetes. Exp Clin Endocrinol Diabetes 2006;114:417-23.

Russell-Jones D, Vaag A, Schmitz O, Sethi BK, Lalic N, Antic SS, et al. Significantly better glycemic control and weight reduced with liraglutide, a once-daily human GLP-1 analog, compared with insulin glargine: all as add-on to metformin and a sulfonylurea in type 2 diabetes [abstact]. ADA 2008. Abstract 536-P.

Seino Y, Rasmussen MF, Zdravkovic M, Kaku K. Dose-dependent improvement in glycemia with once-daily liraglutide without hypoglycemia or weight gain: a double-blind, randomized, controlled trial in Japanese patients with type 2 diabetes. *Diabetes Res Clin.* Pract 2008; epub ahead of print; doi:10.1016/j.diabres.2008.03.018.

To evaluate the effect of liraglutide versus glimepiride (Amaryl®) on haemoglobin A1C (LEAD 3). ClinicalTrials.gov *(http://clinicaltrials.gov)* Accessed June 2, 2008.

Vilsboll T, Zdravkovic M, Le-Thi T, Krarup T, Schmitz O, Courreges J-P, et al. Liraglutide, a long-acting human glucagon-like peptide-1 analog, given as monotherapy significantly improves glycemic control and lowers body weight without risk of hypoglycemia in patients with type 2 diabetes. *Diabetes Care.* 2007;30:1608-10.

Saxagliptin

18-Week add-on to metformin comparison of saxagliptin and sitagliptin. ClinicalTrials.gov (*http://clinicaltrials.gov*) Accessed 27 May 2008.

52-Week add-on to metformin ccomparison of saxagliptin and sulphonylurea. ClinicalTrials.gov (*http://clinicaltrials.gov*) Accessed 27 May 2008.

A Phase III Study of BMS-477118 in combination with metformin in subjects with type 2 diabetes who are not controlled with diet and exercise. ClinicalTrials.gov (*http://clinicaltrials.gov*) Accessed 27 May 2008.

A study assessing saxagliptin treatment in subjects with type 2 diabetes who are not controlled with diet and exercise. ClinicalTrials.gov (*http://clinicaltrials.gov*) Accessed 27 May 2008.

A study assessing saxagliptin treatment in type 2 diabetic subjects who are not controlled with TZD therapy alone. ClinicalTrials.gov (*http://clinicaltrials.gov*) Accessed 27 May 2008.

A study of saxagliptin in subjects with type 2 diabetes who have inadequate blood sugar control with sulfonylureas. ClinicalTrials.gov (*http://clinicaltrials.gov*) Accessed 27 May 2008.

Evaluate efficacy and safety of saxagliptin in combination with metformin in adult patients with type 2 diabetes. ClinicalTrials.gov (*http://clinicaltrials.gov*) Accessed 27 May 2008.

Miller SA, Onge ELS, Taylor JR. DPP-IV inhibitors: A review of sitagliptin, vildagliptin, alogliptin, and saxagliptin. *Formulary.* 2008;43(4):122-34.

Rosenstock J, Sankoh S, List JF. Glucose-lowering activity of the dipeptidyl peptidase-4 inhibitor saxagliptin in drug-naive patients with type 2 diabetes. *Diabetes Obes Metab.* 2008;10(5):376-86.

Safety and efficacy study of subjects that are taking saxagliptin added onto metformin XR compared to subjects taking metformin XR alone. ClinicalTrials.gov (*http://clinicaltrials.gov*) Accessed 27 May 2008.

Saxagliptin treatment in subjects with type 2 diabetes who are not controlled with diet and exercise. ClinicalTrials.gov (*http://clinicaltrials.gov*) Accessed 27 May 2008.

Study assessing saxagliptin treatment in type 2 diabetic subjects who are not ccontrolled with metformin alone. ClinicalTrials.gov (*http://clinicaltrials.gov*) Accessed 27 May 2008.

Study of BMS-477118 as monotherapy with titration in subjects with type 2 diabetes who are not controlled with diet and exercise. ClinicalTrials.gov (*http://clinicaltrials.gov*) Accessed 27 May 2008.

Thomas L, Eckhardt M, Langkopf E, Tadayyon M, Himmelsbach F, Mark M. (R)-8-(3-amino-piperidin-1-yl)-7-but-2-ynyl-3-methyl-1-(4-methyl-quinazolin-2-ylmethyl)-3,7-dihydro-purine-2,6-dione (BI 1356), a novel xanthine-based dipeptidyl peptidase 4 inhibitor, has a superior potency and longer duration of action compared with other dipeptidyl peptidase-4 inhibitors. *J Pharmacol Exp Ther*. 2008;325(1):175-82.

Treatment effect of saxagliptin compared with placebo in patients with Type 2 diabetes and renal impairment. ClinicalTrials.gov (*http://clinicaltrials.gov*) Accessed 27 May 2008.

Succinobucol
Tardif, JC, McMurray JJV, Klug E, Small R, Schumi J, Choi J, et al. Effects of succinobucol (AGI-1067) after an acute coronary syndrome: a randomised, double-blind, placebo-controlled trial. *Lancet*. 2008;371(9626):1761-68.

ANDES-AGI-1067 as a novel antidiabetic agent evaluation study. ClinicalTrials.gov (*http://clinicaltrials.gov*) Accessed 2 June 2008.

ARISE – Aggressive Reduction of Inflammation Stops Events. ClinicalTrials.gov (*http://clinicaltrials.gov*) Accessed 2 June 2008.

Tagatose
A clinical study to evaluate the effect of naturlose (Tagatose). ClinicalTrials.gov (*http://clinicaltrials.gov*) Accessed 2 June 2008.

Donner TW, Wilber JF, Ostrowski D. D-tagatose, a novel hexose: acute effects on carbohydrate tolerance in subjects with and without type 2 diabetes. *Diabetes Obes Metab*. 1999;1(5):285-91.

Levin GV. Tagatose, the new GRAS sweetener and health product. *J Med Food*. 2002;5(1):23-36.

Lu Y, Levin GV, Donner TW. Tagatose, a new antidiabetic and obesity control drug. *Diabetes Obes Metab*. 2008;10(2):109-34.

Moore MC. Drug evaluation: Tagatose in the treatment of type 2 diabetes and obesity. *Curr Opin Invest Drugs*. 2006;7(10):934-35.

Vildagliptin
A clinical study to assess the effect of vildagliptin on beta cell function in drug naive patients with type 2 diabetes. ClinicalTrials.gov (*http://clinicaltrials.gov*) Accessed 27 May 2008.

Assessment of the skin-concentration of vildagliptin 50 mg every 12 hours for 10 days in healthy subjects and patients with type 2 diabetes. ClinicalTrials.gov *(http://clinicaltrials.gov)* Accessed 27 May 2008.

Bolli G, Dotta F, Rochotte E, Cohen SE. Efficacy and tolerability of vildagliptin vs pioglitazone when added to metformin: a 24-week, randomized, double-blind study. *Diabetes Obes Metab*. 2008 Jan;10(1):82-90. Epub 2007 Nov 22.

Effect of LAF237 on glucagon secretion in patients with type 2 diabetes and in healthy subjects. ClinicalTrials.gov *(http://clinicaltrials.gov)* Accessed 27 May 2008.

Garber AJ, Foley JE, Banerji MA, Ebeling P, Gudbjörnsdottir S, Camisasca RP, Couturier A, Baron MA. Effects of vildagliptin on glucose control in patients with type 2 diabetes inadequately controlled with a sulphonylurea. *Diabetes Obes Metab*. 2008 Feb 18. [Epub ahead of print]

Kleppinger EL, Helms K. The role of vildagliptin in the management of type 2 diabetes mellitus. *Ann Pharmacother*. 2007 May;41(5):824-32

Miller SA, Onge ELS, Taylor JR. DPP-IV inhibitors: A review of sitagliptin, vildagliptin, alogliptin, and saxagliptin. *Formulary* 2008;43(4):122-34.

Pan C, Yang W, Barona JP, Wang Y, Niggli M, Mohideen P, Wang Y, Foley JE. Comparison of vildagliptin and acarbose monotherapy in patients with Type 2 diabetes: a 24-week, double-blind, randomized trial. *Diabet Med*. 2008 Apr;25(4):435-41.

Panina G. The DPP-4 inhibitor vildagliptin: robust glycaemic control in type 2 diabetes and beyond. *Diabetes Obes Metab*. 2007 Sep;9 (S1):32-9.

Pharmacokinetic study of vildagliptin in patients with renal impairment. ClinicalTrials.gov *(http://clinicaltrials.gov)* Accessed 27 May 2008.

Rosenstock J, Fitchet M. Vildagliptin: clinical trials programme in monotherapy and combination therapy for type 2 diabetes. Int *J Clin Pract Suppl*. 2008 Mar;(159):15-23.

Safety and tolerability of vildagliptin versus placebo in patients with type 2 diabetes and moderate or severe renal insufficiency. ClinicalTrials.gov *(http://clinicaltrials.gov)* Accessed 27 May 2008.

Safety and tolerability of vildagliptin versus sitagliptin in patients with type 2 diabetes and severe renal insufficiency. ClinicalTrials.gov *(http://clinicaltrials.gov)* Accessed 27 May 2008.

Scherbaum WA, Schweizer A, Mari A, Nilsson PM, Lalanne G, Jauffret S, Foley JE. Efficacy and tolerability of vildagliptin in drug-naïve patients with type 2 diabetes and mild hyperglycaemia. *Diabetes Obes Metab*. 2008 Feb 1. [Epub ahead of print]

Pexiganan

Ge Y, MacDonald D, Henry MM, Hait HI, Nelson KA, Lipsky BA, et al. In vitro susceptibility to pexiganan of bacteria isolated from infected diabetic foot ulcers. *Diagn Microbiol Infect Dis.* 1999;35(1);45-53.

Lamb HM, Wiseman LR. Pexiganan acetate. *Drugs.* 1998;56(6):1047-52.

MSI-78 Topical cream vs oral ofloxacin in the treatment of infected diabetic ulcers. ClinicalTrials.gov (*http://clinicaltrials.gov*) Accessed 16 May 2008.

Nelson EA, O'Meara S, Golder S, Dalton J, Craig D, Iglesias C. Systematic review of antimicrobial treatments for diabetic foot ulcers. *Diabetic Medicine.* 2006;23(4):348-59.

Pegaptanib

Eyetech Pharmaceuticals, Inc. Prescribing information for Macugen® (pegaptanib sodium injection). March 2006.

A multi-center trial to evaluate the safety and efficacy of pegaptanib sodium (Macugen®) injected into the eye every 6 weeks for up to 2 years for macular swelling associated with diabetes. ClinicalTrials.gov (*http://clinicaltrials.gov*) Accessed 16 May 2008.

Adamis AP, Altaweel M, Bressler NM, Cunningham ET, Davis MD, Goldbaum M, et al. Changes in retinal neovascularization after pegaptanib (Macugen) therapy in diabetic individuals. *Ophthalmology.* 2006;113(1):23-8.

Andreoli CM, Miller JW. Anti-vascular endothelial growth factor therapy for ocular neovascular disease. *Curr Opin Ophthalmol.* 2007;18(6):502-8.

Barouch FC, Miller JW. Anti-vascular endothelial growth factor strategies for the treatment of choroidal neovascularization from age-related macular degeneration. *Int Ophthalmol Clin.* 2004;44(3):23-32.

Colquitt JL, Jones J, Tan SC, Takeda A, Clegg AJ, Price A. Ranibizumab and pegaptanib for the treatment of age-related macular degeneration: a systematic review and economic evaluation. *Health Technol Assess.* 2008;12(16):1-222.

D'Amico DJ, Bird AC. VEGF inhibition study in ocular neovascularization-1 (VISION-1): safety evaluation from the pivotal Macugen™ (pegaptanib sodium) clinical trials [abstract]. *Invest Ophthalmol Vis Sci.* 2004;45:abstract 2363.

Effect of Macugen (pegaptanib) on surgical outcomes and VEGF levels in diabetic patients with PDR (diabetic retinopathy or CSDME (macular edema) (PEGAP001). ClinicalTrials.gov (*http://clinicaltrials.gov*) Accessed 16 May 2008.

Eyetech Study Group. Anti-vascular endothelial growth factor therapy for subfoveal choroidal neovascularization secondary to age-related macular degeneration: phase II study results. *Ophthalmology.* 2003;110:979-986.

Food and Drug Administration. Division of Anti-inflammatory, Analgesic and Ophthalmic Drug Products Advisory Committee meeting briefing package for Macugen (pegaptanib sodium injection) for the treatment of neovascular age-related macular degeneration. August 27, 2004. Available at: *www.fda.gov.* Accessed August 30, 2004.

Gragoudas ES, Adamis AP, Cunningham ET, Feinsod M, Guyer DR. Pegaptanib for neovascular age-related macular degeneration. *N Engl J Med.* 2004;351:2805-16.

Gragoudas ES. VEGF inhibition study in ocular neovascularization-1 (VISION-1): efficacy results from phase II/III Macugen™ (pegaptanib sodium) clinical trials [abstract]. *Invest Ophthalmol Vis Sci.* 2004;45:abstract 2364.

Klettner AK, Roider J. Comparison of bevacizumab, ranibizumab and pegaptanib in vitro: efficiency and possible additional pathways. *Investig Ophthalmol Vis Sci.* 2008; DOI:10.1167/iovs.08-2055.

Macugen Diabetic Retinopathy Study Group. A phase II randomized double-masked trial of pegaptanib, an anti-vascular endothelial growth factor aptamer, for diabetic macular edema. *Ophthalmology.* 2005;112:1747-57.

Ng E, Krilleke D, De Erkenez A, et al. VEGF RNA aptamer binding specificity and inhibition of ligand binding to VEGF receptors in vitro. [abstract]. *Invest Ophthalmol Vis Sci.* 2004; 45:abstract 1794/B605.

Pegaptanib sodium (Macugen) compared to sham injection in patients with diabetic macular edema (DME) involving the center of the macula. ClinicalTrials.gov *(http://clinicaltrials.gov)* Accessed 16 May 2008.

Pegaptanib sodium compared to sham injection in patients with DME involving the center of the macula. ClinicalTrials.gov *(http://clinicaltrials.gov)* Accessed 16 May 2008.

Tremolada G, Lattanzio R, Mazzolari G, Zerbini G. The therapeutic potential of VEGF inhibition in diabetic microvascular complications. *Am J Cardiovasc Drugs.* 2007;7(6):393-8.

Ranibizumab

Lucentis (ranibizumab injection) [package insert]. South San Francisco, CA: Genentech, Inc.; June 2006.

A randomized study comparing ranibizumab to sham in patients with macular edema secondary to CRVO. ClinicalTrials.gov *(http://clinicaltrials.gov)* Accessed 16 May 2008.

An extension study to evaluate the safety and tolerability of ranibizumab in subjects with choroidal neovascularization secondary to AMD. ClinicalTrials.gov *(http://clinicaltrials.gov)* Accessed 16 May 2008.

Antoszyk AN, Tuomi L, Chung CY, Singh A, FOCUS Study Group. Ranibizumab combined with verteporfin photodynamic therapy in neovascular age-related macular degeneration (FOCUS): year 2 results. *Am J Ophathalmol.* 2008;145(5):862-74.

Colquitt JL, Jones J, Tan SC, Takeda A, Clegg AJ, Price A. Ranibizumab and pegaptanib for the treatment of age-related macular degeneration: a systematic review and economic evaluation. *Health Technol Assess.* 2008;12(16):1-222.

Efficacy study of Lucentis in the treatment of diabetic macular edema. ClinicalTrials.gov *(http://clinicaltrials.gov)* Accessed 16 May 2008.

Efficacy/Safety of verteporfin photodynamic therapy and ranibizumab compared with ranibizumab in patients with subfoveal choroidal neovascularization. ClinicalTrials.gov *(http://clinicaltrials.gov)* Accessed 16 May 2008.

Gohel PS, Mandava N, Olson JL, Durairaj VD. Age-related macular degeneration: An update on treatment. *Am J Med.* 2008;121(4):279-81.

Klettner AK, Roider J. Comparison of bevacizumab, ranibizumab and pegaptanib in vitro: efficiency and possible additional pathways. *Investig Ophthalmol Vis Sci.* 2008; DOI:10.1167/iovs.08-2055.

Laser-ranibizumab-triamcinolone for diabetic macular edema (LRT for DME). ClinicalTrials.gov *(http://clinicaltrials.gov)* Accessed16 May 2008.

Lucentis for central retinal vein occlusion (CRVO)
Lucentis Utilizing Visudyne (LUV Trial) combination therapy in the treatment of age-related macular degeneration. ClinicalTrials.gov *(http://clinicaltrials.gov)* Accessed 16 May 2008.

Nguyen QD, Tatlipinar S, Shah SM, Haller JA, Quinlan E, Sung J, et al. Vascular endothelial growth factor is a critical stimulus for diabetic macular edema. *Am J Ophthalmol.* 2006;142(6):961-9.

Ranibizumab to treat type 2 idiopathic macular telangiectasia (RAMA-Trial). ClinicalTrials.gov *(http://clinicaltrials.gov)* Accessed 16 May 2008.

Reduced fluence PDT with visudyne in combination with Lucentis for age-related macular degeneration. ClinicalTrials.gov *(http://clinicaltrials.gov)* Accessed 16 May 2008.

Regillo CD, Brown DM, Abraham P, Yue H, Ianchuley T, Schneider S, Shams N. Randomized, double-masked, sham-controlled trial of ranibizumab for neovascular age-related macular degeneration: PIER Study year 1. *Am J Ophthalmol.* 2008;145(2):239-48.

Safety and tolerability of ranibizumab in patients with subfoveal choroidal neovascularization secondary to age-related macular degeneration. ClinicalTrials.gov *(http://clinicaltrials.gov)* Accessed 16 May 2008.

Study comparing ranibizumab monotherapy with ccombined verteporfin therapy in subfoveal CNV. ClinicalTrials.gov *(http://clinicaltrials.gov)* Accessed 16 May 2008.

SUSTAIN - study of ranibizumab in patients with subfoveal choroidal neovascularization secondary to age-related macular degeneration. ClinicalTrials.gov *(http://clinicaltrials.gov)* Accessed 16 May 2008.

The effects of bevacizumab and ranibizumab on ocular pulse amplitude in neovascular age-related macular degeneration (AMD). ClinicalTrials.gov *(http://clinicaltrials.gov)* Accessed 16 May 2008.

Triple Therapy - PDT Plus IVD and intravitreal ranibizumab versus Lucentis monotherapy to treat age-related macular degeneration (PDEX)

Ruboxistaurin

Effect of ruboxistaurin on clinically significant macular edema. ClinicalTrials.gov *(http://clinicaltrials.gov)* Accessed 16 May 2008.

Fraser-Bell S, Kaines A, Hykin PG. Update on treatments for diabetic macular edema. *Curr Opin Ophthalmol.* 2008;19(3):185-9.

Gilbert RE, Kim SA, Tuttle KR, Bakris GL, Toto RD, McGill JB, et al. Effect of ruboxistaurin on urinary transforming growth factor-β in patients with diabetic nephropathy and type 2 diabetes. *Diabetes Care.* 2007;30(4):995-6.

PKC-DMES Study Group. Effect of ruboxistaurin in patients with diabetic macular edema: thirty-month results of the randomized PKC-DMES clinical trial. *Arch Ophthalmol.* 2007;125(3):318-24.

Protein Kinase C (PKC) inhibitor-diabetic retinopathy Phase III study. ClinicalTrials.gov *(http://clinicaltrials.gov)* Accessed 16 May 2008.

Ruboxistaurin: LY 333531. *Drugs R D.* 2007;8(3):193-9.

Tuttle KR, Bakris GL, Toto RD, McGill JB, Hu K, Anderson PW. The effect of ruboxistaurin on nephropathy in type 2 diabetes. *Diabetes Care.* 2005;28(11):2686-90.

Tuttle KR, McGill JB, Haney DJ, Lin TE, Anderson PW, PKC-DRS, PKC-DMES, and PKC-DRS 2 Study Groups. Kidney outcomes in long-term studies of ruboxistaurin for diabetic eye disease. *Clin J Am Soc Nephrol.* 2007;2(4):631-6.

Aliskiren

Feldman DL, Jin L, Xuan H, Contrepas A, Zhou Y, Webb RL, et al. Effects of aliskiren on blood pressure, albuminuria, and (pro)renin receptor expression in diabetic TG(mREN-2)27 rats. *Hypertension*. 2008 (Epub ahead of print: 19 May 2008).

Kelly DJ, Zhang Y, Moe G, Naik G, Gilbert RE. Aliskiren, a novel renin inhibitor, is renoprotective in a model of advanced diabetic nephropathy in rats. *Diabetologia*. 2007;50(11):2398-2404.

Persson F, Rossing P, Schjoedt KJ, Juhl T, Tarnow L, Stehouwer CD, et al. Time course of the antiproteinuric and antihypertensive effects of direct renin inhibition in type 2 diabetes. *Kidney Int*. 2008; Epub ahead of print: doi:10.1038/ki.2008.68.

Uresin Y, Taylor AA, Kilo C, Tschope D, Santonastaso M, Ibram G, et al. Efficacy and safety of the direct renin inhibitor aliskiren and ramipril alone or in combination in patients with diabetes and hypertension. *J Renin Angiotensin Aldosterone Syst*. 2007;8(4):190-8.

Zhao C, Vaidyanathan S, Yeh CM, Maboudian M, Dieterich HA. Aliskiren exhibits similar pharmacokinetics in healthy volunteers and patients with type 2 diabetes mellitus. *Clin Pharmacokinet*. 2006;45(11):1125-34.

Valsartan

A study in patients with diabetes mellitus type 2 of the effect on albuminuria of 24-week treatment with valsartan, benazepril, and valsartan+benazepril. ClinicalTrials.gov (*http://clinicaltrials.gov*) Accessed 21 May 2008.

Effect of valsartan on proteinuria in patients with hypertension and diabetes mellitus. ClinicalTrials.gov (*http://clinicaltrials.gov*) Accessed 21 May 2008.

Long-term study of nateglinide+valsartan to prevent or delay type 2 diabetes mellitus and cardiovascular complications (Navigator). ClinicalTrials.gov (*http://clinicaltrials.gov*) Accessed 21 May 2008.

To assess the effects of valsartan on albuminuria/proteinuria in hypertensive patients with type 2 diabetes mellitus. ClinicalTrials.gov (*http://clinicaltrials.gov*) Accessed 21 May 2008.

To evaluate safety & efficacy of the combination of aliskiren, valsartan & hydrochlorothiazide in diabetic hypertensive nonresponder patients. ClinicalTrials.gov (*http://clinicaltrials.gov*) Accessed 21 May 2008.

SMOOTH - blood pressure control in diabetic/obese patients. ClinicalTrials.gov (*http://clinical-trials.gov*) Accessed 21 May 2008.

Valsartan/hydrochlorothiazide combination vs amlodipine in patients with hypertension, diabetes, and albuminuria. ClinicalTrials.gov (*http://clinicaltrials.gov*) Accessed 21 May 2008.

1-Year trial telmisartan 80 mg versus valsartan 160 mg in hypertensive type 2 diabetic patients with overt nephropathy. ClinicalTrials.gov *(http://clinicaltrials.gov)*   Accessed 21 May 2008.

Comparison of morning and evening dosing of valsartan and lisinopril in patients with diabetes. ClinicalTrials.gov *(http://clinicaltrials.gov)* Accessed 21 May 2008.

Antiproteinuric effect of valsartan and lisinopril. ClinicalTrials.gov *(http://clinicaltrials.gov)* Accessed 21 May 2008.

A 16-week study to evaluate the effect on insulin. ClinicalTrials.gov *(http://clinicaltrials.gov)* Accessed 21 May 2008.

Sensitivity of valsartan (320 mg) and hydrochlorothiazide (25 mg) combined and alone, in patients with metabolic syndrome. ClinicalTrials.gov *(http://clinicaltrials.gov)* Accessed 21 May 2008.

A randomized, double-blind, placebo-controlled, forced-titration, phase IV study comparing telmisartan 80 mg + hydrochlorothiazide 25 mg [Micardis HCT] versus valsartan 160 mg + hydrochlorothiazide 25 mg [Diovan HCT] taken orally for eight weeks in patients with stage 1 and stage 2 hypertension. ClinicalTrials.gov *(http://clinicaltrials.gov)* Accessed 21 May 2008.

Dextromethorphan and Quinidine
Safety and efficacy of dextromethorphan and quinidine in the treatment of the pain of diabetic neuropathy. ClinicalTrials.gov *(http://clinicaltrials.gov)* Accessed 21 May 2008.

Thisted RA, Klaff L, Schwartz SL, Wymer JP, Culligan NW, Gerard G, et al. Dextromethorphan and quinidine in adult patients with uncontrolled painful diabetic peripheral neuropathy: A 29-day, multicenter, open-Label, dose-escalation study. *Clin Ther.* 2006;28(10):1607-18.

Werling LL, Lauterbach EC, Calef U. Dextromethorphan as a potential neuroprotective agent with unique mechanisms of action. *Neurologist.* 2007;13(5):272-93.

Lacosamide
A follow-on trial to assess the long term safety and efficacy of SPM 927 in painful distal diabetic neuropathy. ClinicalTrials.gov *(http://clinicaltrials.gov)* Accessed 16 May 2008.

A trial to assess the efficacy and safety of 400mg/day lacosamide in subjects with painful diabetic neuropathy. ClinicalTrials.gov *(http://clinicaltrials.gov)* Accessed 16 May 2008.

A trial to assess the efficacy and safety of SPM 927 (Lacosamide) in Subjects with painful distal diabetic neuropathy. ClinicalTrials.gov *(http://clinicaltrials.gov)* Accessed 16 May 2008.

A trial to assess the long-term safety and efficacy of lacosamide in subjects with painful diabetic neuropathy. ClinicalTrials.gov *(http://clinicaltrials.gov)* Accessed 16 May 2008.

Beyreuther B, Callizot N, Stohr T. Antinociceptive efficacy of lacosamide in a rat model for painful diabetic neuropathy. *Eur J Pharmacol.* 2006;539(1-2):64-70.

Beyreuther B, Freitag J, Heers C, Krebsfanger N, Scharfenecker U, Stohr T. Lacosamide: A review of preclinical properties. *CNS Drug Rev.* 2007;13(1):21-42.

Chong MS, Hester J. Diabetic painful neuropathy: current and future treatment options. *Drugs.* 2007;67(4):569-85.

Ghailbani A, Bongardt S, Ommerville K. Evaluation of lacosamide in diabetic neuropathic pain trials. [abstract] 60th Annual Meeting of the American Academy of Neurology: 12 April 2008 (*www.aan.com*).

Open-label, follow-on trial to assess the long-term safety and efficacy of lacosamide in subjects with painful distal diabetic neuropathy. ClinicalTrials.gov (*http://clinicaltrials.gov*) Accessed 16 May 2008.

Rauck RL, Shaibani A, Biton V, Simpson J, Koch B. Lacosamide in painful diabetic peripheral neuropathy - A phase 2 double-blind placebo-controlled study. *Clin J Pain.* 2007;23(2):150-8.

Trial to assess the efficacy and safety of SPM 927 (200, 400, and 600mg/day) in subjects with painful distal diabetic neuropathy. ClinicalTrials.gov (*http://clinicaltrials.gov*) Accessed 16 May 2008.

Mexiletine

Duby JJ, Campbell RK, Setter SM, White JR, Rasmussen KA. Diabetic neuropathy: An intensive review. *Am J Health Syst Pharm.* 2004;61:160-76.

Jarvis B, Coukell AJ. Mexiletine: A review of its therapeutic use in painful diabetic neuropathy. *Drugs.* 1998;58(4):691-707.

Oskarasson P, Ljunggren JG, Lins PE, The Mexiletine Study Group. Efficacy and safety of mexiletine in the treatment of painful diabetic neuropathy. *Diabetes Care.* 1997;20(10):1594-97.

Phase III randomized, double-blind, placebo-controlled study of mexiletine for painful diabetic neuropathy. ClinicalTrials.gov (*http://clinicaltrials.gov*) Accessed 31 May 2008.

Tapentadol

A safety and efficacy study for tapentadol (CG5503) extended release for patients with painful diabetic peripheral neuropathy. ClinicalTrials.gov (*http://clinicaltrials.gov*) Accessed 16 May 2008.

Rauschkolb-Loeffler C, Okamoto A, Steup A, Lange C. Efficacy and tolerability of tapentadol for relief of moderate-to-severe chronic pain due to osteoarthritis of the knee. [abstract] Ann Rheumatic Dis. 2007;66(suppl 2):507.

Tzschentke TM, Christoph T, Kogel B, Schiene K, Hennies HH, Englberger W, et al. (-)-(1R,2R)-3-(3-dimethylamino-1-ethyl-2-methyl-propyl)-phenol hydrochloride (tapentadol HCl): a novel mu-opioid receptor agonist/norepinephrine reuptake inhibitor with broad-spectrum analgesic properties. *J Pharmacol Exp Ther.* 2007;323(1):265-76.

Topiramate
A study of safety and efficacy of topiramate in male patients with abdominal obesity condition: obesity. ClinicalTrials.gov (*http://clinicaltrials.gov*) Accessed 31 May 2008.

A study of the efficacy and safety of topiramate in the treatment of obese, type 2 diabetic patients treated with metformin. ClinicalTrials.gov (*http://clinicaltrials.gov*) Accessed 31 May 2008.

A study of the safety and effectiveness of topiramate on insulin sensitivity in overweight or obese patients with type 2 diabetes. ClinicalTrials.gov (*http://clinicaltrials.gov*) Accessed 31 May 2008.

A study of the safety and efficacy of topiramate in the treatment of obese, type 2 diabetes patients on a controlled diet. ClinicalTrials.gov (*http://clinicaltrials.gov*) Accessed 31 May 2008.

A study on efficacy and safety of topiramate in maintaining weight loss in obese patients following an intensive, non-pharmacologic weight loss program. ClinicalTrials.gov (*http://clinicaltrials.gov*) Accessed 31 May 2008.

A study on efficacy and safety of topiramate in the treatment of patients with obesity. ClinicalTrials.gov (*http://clinicaltrials.gov*) Accessed 31 May 2008.

A study on efficacy and safety of topiramate OROS® controlled-release in obese, type 2 diabetic subjects managed with diet or metformin. ClinicalTrials.gov (*http://clinicaltrials.gov*) Accessed 31 May 2008.

A study to evaluate the effect of topiramate on clinical and electrophysiological parameters in subjects with diabetic peripheral polyneuropathy. ClinicalTrials.gov (*http://clinicaltrials.gov*) Accessed 31 May 2008.

A study using DNA samples from patients who participated in previous topiramate obesity and type 2 diabetes studies. ClinicalTrials.gov (*http://clinicaltrials.gov*) Accessed 31 May 2008.

A VI-0521 Study to Evaluate the Long-Term Safety and Efficacy in Type 2 Diabetic Adults Condition: Diabetes. ClinicalTrials.gov (*http://clinicaltrials.gov*) Accessed 31 May 2008.

Carroll DG, Kline KM, Malnar KF. Role of topiramate for the treatment of painful diabetic peripheral neuropathy. *Pharmacotherapy.* 2004;24(9):1186-93.

Chang MS, Hester J. Diabetic painful neuropathy: Current and future treatment options. *Drugs.* 2007;67(4):569-85.

Donofrio PD, Raskin P, Rosenthal NR, Hewitt DJ, Jordan DM, Xiang J, et al. Safety and effectiveness of topiramate for the management of painful diabetic peripheral neuropathy in an open-label extension study. *Clin Ther*. 2005;27(9):1420-31.

Eliasson B, Gudbjornsdottir S, Cederholm, J, Liang Y, Vercruysse F, Smith U. Weight loss and metabolic effects of topiramate in overweight and obese type 2 diabetic patients: Randomized double-blind placebo-controlled trial. *Int J Obesity*. 2007;31:1140-47.

Raskin P, Donofrio PD, Rosenthal NR, Hewitt DJ, Jordan DM, Xiang J, et al. Topiramate vs placebo in painful diabetic neuropathy: Analgesic and metabolic effects. *Neurology*. 2004;63:865-73.

Rosenstock J, Hollander P, Gadde KM, Sun X, Strauss R, Leung A, et al. A randomized, double-blind, placebo-controlled, multicenter study to assess the efficacy and safety of topiramate controlled release in the treatment of obese type 2 diabetic patients. *Diabetes Care*. 2007;30:1480-86.

Study of VI-0521 compared to placebo in treatment of diabetes and obesity in adults with obesity-related co-morbid conditions. ClinicalTrials.gov (*http://clinicaltrials.gov*) Accessed 31 May 2008.

The Topiramate Diabetic Neuropathic Pain Study Group, Thienel U, Neto W, Schwabe SK, Vijapurkar U. Topiramate in painful diabetic polyneuropathy: Findings from three double-blind placebo-controlled trials. *Acta Neurol Scand*. 2004;110:221-31.

Appendix
Sugar-Free Products

Sugar-Free Products

Listed below, by therapeutic category, is a selection of drug products that contain no sugar. When recommending these products to diabetic patients, keep in mind that many may contain sorbitol, alcohol, or other sources of carbohydrates. This list should not be considered all-inclusive. Generics and alternate brands of some products may be available. Check product labeling for a current listing of inactive ingredients.

PRODUCT	MANUFACTURER
ANALGESICS	
Addaprin Tablet	Dover
Aminofen Tablet	Dover
Aminofen Max Tablet	Dover
Aspirtab Tablet	Dover
Back Pain-Off Tablet	Medique
Backprin Tablet	Hart Health and Safety
Buffasal Tablet	Dover
Dyspel Tablet	Dover
I-Prin Tablet	Medique
Medi-Seltzer Effervescent Tablet	Medique
Methadose Solution	Mallinckrodt
Ms.-Aid Tablet	Medique
Silapap Children's Elixir	Silarx
ANTACIDS/ANTIFLATULENTS	
Alcalak Chewable Tablet	Medique
Dimacid Chewable Tablet	Otis Clapp & Son
Diotame Chewable Tablet	Medique
Diotame Suspension	Medique
Mylanta Gelcaplet	Johnson & Johnson/Merck
Mylanta Tablets	Johnson & Johnson/Merck
Neutralin Tablet	Dover
Pepto-Bismol Tablets	Procter & Gamble
Tums E-X Chewable Tablet	GlaxoSmithKline Consumer
ANTI-ASTHMATIC/RESPIRATORY AGENTS	
Jay-Phyl Syrup	Pharmakon

PRODUCT	MANUFACTURER
ANTIDIARRHEALS	
Diarrest Tablet	Dover
Imogen Liquid	Pharm Generic
BLOOD MODIFIERS/IRON PREPARATIONS	
I.L.X. B-12 Elixir	Kenwood
Nephro-Fer Tablet	R & D
CORTICOSTEROID	
Pediapred Solution	Celltech
COUGH/COLD/ALLERGY PREPARATIONS	
Accuhist Drops	Pediamed
Accuhist PDX Drops Solution	Pediamed
Alacol DM Syrup	Ballay
Alacol Solution	Ballay
Amerifed DM Liquid	Ambi
Amerifed Liquid	Ambi
Amerituss AD Solution	Ambi
Anaplex DM Syrup	ECR
Anaplex DMX Syrup	ECR
Anaplex HD Syrup	ECR
Andehist DM NR Syrup	Cypress
Andehist NR Syrup	Cypress
Aquatab C Tablets	Deston
Aridex Solution	Gentex
Baltussin Solution	Ballay
Benadryl-D Allergy & Sinus Children's Solution	Johnson & Johnson
Bromhist-DM Solution	Cypress
Bromhist Pediatric Solution	Cypress
Bromphenex DM Solution	Breckenridge

PRODUCT	MANUFACTURER	PRODUCT	MANUFACTURER
Bromphenex HD Solution	Breckenridge	Despec-SF Liquid	International Ethical
Bromplex DM Solution	Prasco	Diabetic Tussin Allergy Relief Liquid	Health Care Products
Bromplex HD Solution	Prasco	Diabetic Tussin Allergy Relief Tablet	Health Care Products
Bromtuss DM Solution	Breckenridge		
Broncotron Liquid	Seyer Pharmatec	Diabetic Tussin Cold & Flu Gelcaplet	Health Care Products
Broncotron-D Suspension	Seyer Pharmatec	Diabetic Tussin DM Liquid	Health Care Products
B-Tuss Liquid	Blansett		
Carbaphen 12 Ped Suspension	Gil	Diabetic Tussin EX Liquid	Health Care Products
Carbaphen 12 Suspension	Gil		
Carbatuss-12 Suspension	GM	Diabetic Tussin Solution	Health Care Products
Carbatuss-CL Solution	GM	Diphen Capsule	Medique
Carbetaplex Solution	Breckenridge	Donatussin Solution	Laser
Carbofed DM Liquid	Hi-Tech	Double-Tussin DM Liquid	Reese
Carbofed DM Syrup	Hi-Tech	Drocon-CS Solution	Cypress
Carbofed DM Drops	Hi-Tech	Duratuss DM Solution	Victory
Cardec DM Syrup	Qualitest	Dynatuss HC Solution	Breckenridge
Cardec Solution	Qualitest	Dytan-CS Tablet	Hawthorn
Cetafen Cough & Cold Tablets	Hart Health and Safety	Dytan-HC Suspension	Hawthorn
Cetafen Cold Tablet	Hart Health and Safety	Emagrin Forte Tablet	Otis Clapp & Son
Cheratussin DAC Liquid	Qualitest	Emagrin Tablets	Otis Clapp & Son
Chlordex GP Syrup	Cypress	Endacof DM Solution	Larken Laboratories
Codal-DM Syrup	Cypress	Endacof HC Solution	LarkenLaboratories
Codiclear DH Solution	Victory	Endacof XP Solution	Larken Laboratories
ColdCough HC Syrup	Breckenridge	Endacof-PD Solution	Larken Laboratories
ColdCough HCM Solution	Breckenridge	Endal HD Plus Liquid	Pediamed
ColdCough PD Solution	Breckenridge	Ganidin NR Liquid	Cypress
ColdCough Solution	Breckenridge	Gani-Tuss NR Liquid	Cypress
ColdCough XP Solution	Breckenridge	Gani-Tuss-DM NR Liquid	Cypress
Coldonyl Tablet	Dover	Genebronco-D Liquid	Pharm Generic
Colidrops Pediatric Liquid	A.G. Marin	Genecof-HC Liquid	Pharm Generic
Cordron-D NR Solution	Cypress	Genecof-XP Liquid	Pharm Generic
Cordron-DM Solution	Cypress	Genedel Syrup	Pharm Generic
Cordron-DM NR Solution	Cypress	Genedotuss-DM Liquid	Pharm Generic
Cordron-HC Solution	Cypress	Genelan Liquid	Pharm Generic
Cordron-HC NR Solution	Cypress	Genetuss-2 Liquid	Pharm Generic
Cordron NR Solution	Cypress	Genexpect DM Liquid	Pharm Generic
Corfen DM Solution	Cypress	Genexpect-PE Liquid	Pharm Generic
Coughtuss Solution	Breckenridge	Genexpect-SF Liquid	Pharm Generic
Crantex HC Syrup	Breckenridge	Gilphex TR Tablet	Gil
Crantex Syrup	Breckenridge	Giltuss Liquid	Gil
Dacex-DM Solution	Cypress	Giltuss Ped-C Solution	Gil
Dallergy Solution	Laser	Giltuss Pediatric Liquid	Gil
De-Chlor DM Solution	Cypress	Giltuss TR Tablet	Gil
De-Chlor DR Solution	Cypress	Guiadex DM Solution	Breckenridge
De-Chlor HD Solution	Cypress	Guiaplex HC Solution	Breckenridge
Despec Liquid	International Ethical	Halotussin AC Liquid	Axiom
		Halotussin DAC Solution	Axiom

PRODUCT	MANUFACTURER
Histinex HC Syrup	Ethex
Histinex PV Syrup	Ethex
Hydro-Tussin CBX Solution	Ethex
Hydro-Tussin DHC Solution	Ethex
Hydro-Tussin DM Elixir	Ethex
Hydro-Tussin HC Syrup	Ethex
Hydro-Tussin HD Liquid	Ethex
Hydro-Tussin Exp Solution	Ethex
Hydro-Tussin XP Syrup	Ethex
Jaycof Expectorant Syrup	Pharmakon
Jaycof-HC Liquid	Pharmakon
Jaycof-XP Liquid	Pharmakon
Liquicough DM Solution	Breckenridge
Liquicough HC Solution	Breckenridge
Lodrane Liquid	ECR
Lodrane D Suspension	ECR
Lodrane XR Suspension	ECR
Lohist-LQ Solution	Larken
Lohist-PD Solution	Larken
Lortuss DM Solution	Proethic Laboratories
Marcof Expectorant Syrup	Marnel
Maxi-Tuss HCG Solution	MCR American.
Maxi-Tuss HCX Solution	MCR American
M-Clear Solution	McNeil, R.A.
M-Clear Jr Solution	McNeil, R.A.
Metanx Tablet	Pamlab
Mintuss NX Solution	Breckenridge
Nalex DH Liquid	Blansett
Nalex-A Liquid	Blansett
Nasop Suspension	Hawthorn
Neo DM Drops	Laser
Neo DM Suspension	Laser
Neotuss-D Liquid	A.G. Marin
Neotuss S/F Liquid	A.G. Marin
Niferex Elixir	Ther-Rx
Norel DM Liquid	U.S. Pharmaceutical
Nycoff Tablet	Dover
Organidin NR Liquid	MedPointe
Organidin NR Tablet	MedPointe
Pancof EXP Syrup	Pamlab
Pancof HC Solution	Pamlab
Pancof XP Solution	Pamlab
Panmist DM Syrup	Pamlab
Pediatex HC Solution	Zyber
Phanasin Syrup	Pharmakon
Phanasin Diabetic Choice Syrup	Pharmakon

PRODUCT	MANUFACTURER
Phanatuss Syrup	Pharmakon
Phanatuss DM Diabetic Choice Syrup	Pharmakon
Phanatuss-HC Diabetic Choice Solution	Pharmakon
Phena-HC Solution	GM
Phenabid Tablets	Gil
Phenabid DM Tablet	Gil
Phena-S 12 Suspension	GM
Phena-S Liquid	GM
Phendacof HC Syrup	Larken
Phendacof Plus Solution	Larken
Poly Hist DM Solution	Poly
Poly Hist HC Solution	Poly
Poly Hist PD Solution	Poly
Poly-Tussin Solution	Poly
Poly-Tussin DM Syrup	Poly
Poly-Tussin HD Syrup	Poly
Poly-Tussin XP Solution	Poly
Pro-Clear Solution	Pro-Pharma
Pro-Red Solution	Pro-Pharma
Prolex DM Liquid	Blansett
Quintex Syrup	Qualitest
Relacon-HC Solution	Cypress
Rescon-DM Liquid	Capellon
Rindal HD Liquid	Breckenridge
Rindal HD Plus Solution	Breckenridge
Rondec Solution	Alliant
Rondec DM Solution	Alliant
Ru-Tuss DM Solution	Carwin
Safetussin Liquid	Kramer
Scot-Tussin Diabetes CF Liquid	Scot-Tussin
Scot-Tussin DM Cough Chasers Lozenge	Scot-Tussin
Scot-Tussin DM Solution	Scot-Tussin
Scot-Tussin Expectorant Solution	Scot-Tussin
Scot-Tussin Senior Solution	Scot-Tussin
Siladryl Allergy Solution	Silarx
Sildec Syrup	Silarx
Sildec-DM Syrup	Silarx
Sildec PE-DM Solution	Silarx
Sildec-PE Solution	Silarx
Silexin Syrup	Otis Clapp & Son
Silexin Tablet	Otis Clapp & Son
Sil-Tex Liquid	Silarx

PRODUCT	MANUFACTURER
Siltussin DAS Liquid	Silarx
Siltussin DM DAS Cough Formula Syrup	Silarx
Siltussin SA Syrup	Silarx
Statuss Green Liquid	Magna
Sudafed Children's Cold & Cough Solution	Pfizer
Sudafed Children's Solution	Pfizer
Sudanyl Tablet	Dover
Sudatuss-SF Liquid	Pharm Generic Developers
Supress DX Pediatric Drops	Kramer-Novis
Suttar-SF Syrup	Gil
Tanacof XR Suspension	Larken
Triant-HC Solution	Hawthorn
Tricodene Syrup	Pfeiffer
Trituss Solution	Everett
Tri-Vent DM Solution	Ethex
Tri-Vent DPC Syrup	Ethex
Tusdec-DM Solution	Cypress
Tusnel Solution	Llorens
Tussafed Syrup	Everett
Tussafed-EX Pediatric Drops	Everett
Tussafed-HC Syrup	Everett
Tussafed-HCG Solution	Everett
Tussall Solution	Everett
Tussi-Organidin DM NR Solution	Victory
Tussi-Organidin DM-S NR Solution	Victory
Tussi-Organidin NR Solution	Victory
Tussi-Organidin-S NR Solution	Victory
Tussplex DM Solution	Breckenridge
Tussi-Pres Liquid	Kramer-Novis
Vazol Solution	Wraser
Vi-Q-Tuss Syrup	Qualitest
Welltuss EXP Solution	Prasco
Z-Cof HC Solution	Zyber
Z-Cof HCX Solution	Zyber
Z-Tuss DM Syrup	Magna
Ztuss Expectorant Solution	Magna

FLUORIDE PREPARATIONS

PRODUCT	MANUFACTURER
Fluor-A-Day Tablet	Pharmascience
Fluor-A-Day Liquid	Pharmascience
Flura-Loz Tablet	Kirkman
Lozi-Flur Lozenge	Dreir
Sensodyne w/Fluoride Gel	GlaxoSmithKline Consumer

PRODUCT	MANUFACTURER
Sensodyne w/Fluoride Tartar Control Toothpaste	GlaxoSmithKline Consumer
Sensodyne w/Fluoride Toothpaste	GlaxoSmithKline Consumer

LAXATIVES

PRODUCT	MANUFACTURER
Benefiber Powder	Novartis
Citrucel Powder	GlaxoSmithKline Consumer
Colace Solution	Purdue Products
Fiber Choice Tablets	CNS
Fiber Ease Liquid	Plainview
Fibro-XL Capsule	Key
Genfiber Powder	Teva
Konsyl Easy Mix Formula Powder	Konsyl
Konsyl-Orange Powder	Konsyl
Konsyl Powder	Konsyl
Metamucil Smooth Texture Powder	Procter & Gamble
Reguloid Powder	Rugby
Senokot Wheat Bran	Purdue Products

MISCELLANEOUS

PRODUCT	MANUFACTURER
Acidoll Capsule	Key
Alka-Gest Tablet	Key
Bicitra Solution	Ortho-McNeil
Cafergot Tablets	Sandoz
Colidrops Pediatric Drops	A.G. Marin
Cytra-2 Solution	Cypress
Cytra-K Solution	Cypress
Cytra-K Crystals	Cypress
Mason Natural Drinkin' Buddy Tablets	Mason
Melatin Tablet	Mason Vitamins
Namenda Solution	Forest
Neutra-Phos Powder	Ortho-McNeil
Neutra-Phos-K Powder	Ortho-McNeil
Polycitra-K Solution	Ortho-McNeil
Polycitra-LC Solution	Ortho-McNeil
Prosed-DS Tablets	Esprit
Questran Light Powder	Par
Soltamox Solution	Cytogen

MOUTH/THROAT PREPARATIONS

PRODUCT	MANUFACTURER
Cepacol Dual Relief Sore Throat Spray	Combe
Cepacol Maximum Strength Spray	Combe
Cepacol Sore Throat + Coating Relief Lozenge	Combe
Cepacol Sore Throat Lozenges	Combe

PRODUCT	MANUFACTURER
Cheracol Sore Throat Spray	Lee
Chloraseptic Spray	Prestige
Cylex Lozenges	Pharmakon
Diabetic Tussin Cough Drops	Health Care Products
Diabetic Tussin Cough Lozenges	Health Care Products
Fisherman's Friend Lozenges	Mentholatum
Fresh N Free Liquid	Geritrex
Larynex Lozenges	Dover
Listerine Pocketpaks Film	Pfizer Consumer
Luden's Lozenges	Johnson & Johnson
Medikoff Drops	Medique
N'ice Lozenges	Heritage/Insight
Oragesic Solution	Parnell
Orajel Dry Mouth Moisturizing Gel	Del
Orajel Dry Mouth Moisturizing Spray	Del
Orasept Mouthwash/ Gargle Liquid	Pharmakon
Sepasoothe Lozenges	Medique
Thorets Maximum Strength Lozenges	Otis Clapp & Son
Throto–Ceptic Spray	S.S.S.
Triaminic Sore Throat Spray	Novartis

VITAMINS/MINERALS/SUPPLEMENTS

PRODUCT	MANUFACTURER
Action-Tabs Made For Men	Action Labs
Adaptosode For Stress Liquid	HVS
Adaptosode R+R For Acute Stress Liquid	HVS
Alamag Tablet	Medique
Alcalak Tablet	Medique
Apetigen Elixir	Kramer-Novis
Apptrim Capsule	Physician Therapeutics
Apptrim-D Capsule	Physician Therapeutics
Bevitamel Tablet	Westlake
Biosode Liquid	HVS
Biotect Plus Caplet	Gil
Bugs Bunny Complete Tablets	Bayer
C & M Caps-375 Capsule	Key
Cal-Cee Tablet	Key
Calcet Plus Tablet	Mission Pharmacal
Calcimin-300 Tablet	Key
Cal-Mint Chewable Tablet	Freeda Vitamins
Cerefolin Tablet	Pamlab
Choice DM Liquid	Bristol-Myers Squibb
Chromacaps Tablet	Key

PRODUCT	MANUFACTURER
Delta D3 Tablet	Freeda Vitamins
Detoxosode Liquids	HVS
Dexfol Tablet	Rising
DHEA Capsule	ADH Health Products
Diatx ZN Tablet	Pamlab
Diet System 6 Gum	Applied Nutrition
Dimacid Tablet	Otis Clapp & Son
Diucaps Capsule	Legere
Dl-Phen-500 Capsule	Key
Electrotab Tablet	Hart Health And Safety
Ensure Nutra Shake Pudding	Ross Products
Enterex Diabetic Liquid	Victus
Essential Nutrients Plus Silica Tablet	Action Labs
Evening Primrose Oil Capsule	National Vitamin
Evolve Softgel	Bionutrics Health Products
Ex-L Tablet	Key
Extress Tablet	Key
Eyetamins Tablet	Rexall Consumer
Fem-Cal Citrate Tablets	Freeda Vitamins
Fem-Cal Tablet	Freeda Vitamins
Fem-Cal Plus Tablet	Freeda Vitamins
Ferrocite F Tablet	Breckenridge
Ferrocite Plus Tablets	Breckenridge
Folacin-800 Tablet	Key
Folbee Plus Tablet	Breckenridge
Folbee Tablets	Breckenridge
Foleve Plus Tablets	Cura
Foleve Tablets	Cura
Folplex 2.2 Tablet	Breckenridge
Foltx Tablet	Pamlab
Gabadone Capsule	Physician Therapeutics
Gram-O-Leci Tablet	Freeda Vitamins
Herbal Slim Complex Capsule	ADH Health Products
Hypertensa Capsules	Physician Therapeutics
Lynae Calcium/Vitamin C Chewable Tablet	Boscogen
Lynae Chondroitin/ Glucosamine Capsule	Boscogen
Lynae Ginse-Cool Chewable Tablet	Boscogen
Mag-Caps Capsule	Rising
Mag-Ox 400 Tablet	Blaine
Mag-SR Tablet	Cypress
Magimin Tablet	Key Company
Maginex Tablets	Logan

PRODUCT	MANUFACTURER	PRODUCT	MANUFACTURER
Magnacaps Capsule	Key Company	Ribo-100 T.D. Capsule	Key
Mag-SR Plus Calcium Tablets	Cypress	Samolinic Softgel	Key
		Sea Omega 30 Softgel	Rugby
Mangimin Tablet	Key Company	Sea Omega 50 Softgel	Rugby
Medi-Lyte Tablet	Medique	Sentra AM Capsule	Physician Therapeutics
Metanx Tablet	Pamlab	Sentra PM Capsule	Physician Therapeutics
Multi-Delyn w/Iron Liquid	Silarx	Soy Care for Menopause Capsule	Inverness Medical
Natelle C Tablet	Pharmelle		
Natelle Tablets	Pharmelle	Span C Tablet	Freeda Vitamins
Nephro-Fer Tablet	Watson	Strovite Forte Syrup	Everett
Neutra-Phos Powder	Ortho-Mcneil	Sunnie Tablet	Green Turtle Bay Vitamin
Neutra-Phos-K Powder	Ortho-Mcneil		
New Life Hair Tablet	Rexall Consumer	Sunvite Tablet	Rexall Naturalist
Niferex Elixir	Ther-Rx	Super Dec B100 Tablet	Freeda Vitamins
Nutrisure OTC Tablet	Westlake	Super Quints-50 Tablet	Freeda Vitamins
Nutrivit Solution	Llorens	Supervite Liquid	Seyer Pharmatec
Ob Complete Tablets	Vertical	Suplevit Liquid	Gil
O-Cal Fa Tablet	Pharmics	Theramine Capsule	Physician Therapeutics
Os-Cal 500+D Tablets	Glaxosmithkline	Triamin Tablet	Key
Plenamins Plus Tablet	Rexall Consumer	Triamino Tablet	Freeda Vitamins
Powervites Tablet	Green Turtle Bay Vitamin	Ultramino Powder	Freeda Vitamins
		Uro-Mag Capsule	Blaine
Prostaplex Herbal Complex Capsule	ADH Health Products	Vitafol Tablets	Everett
		Vitamin C/Rose Hips Tablet	ADH Health Products
Prostatonin Capsule	Pharmaton Natural Health	Vitrum Jr Chewable Tablet	Mason Vitamins
Protect Plus Liquid	Gil		
Protect Plus NR Softgel	Gil	Xtramins Tablet	Key
Pulmona Capsule	Physician Therapeutics	Yohimbe Power Max 1500 For Women Tablet	Action Labs
Quintabs-M Tablet	Freeda Vitamins		
Replace Capsule	Key	Yohimbized 1000 Capsule	Action Labs
Replace w/o Iron Capsule	Key	Ze-Plus Softgel	Everett
Resource Arginaid Powder	Novartis Nutrition		

Index

In addition to chapter topics, this index lists drugs by therapeutic class (shown in bold and italic) as well as brands, generics, and common drug groups (shown in bold). Entries that appear in prescribing or drug interaction tables are marked with "t" following the page number.